Oxford Textbook of

Psychiatry of Intellectual Disability

OXFORD TEXTBOOKS IN PSYCHIATRY

Oxford Textbook of Psychiatry of Intellectual Disability
Edited by Sabyasachi Bhaumik and Regi Alexander

Oxford Textbook of Inpatient Psychiatry
Edited by Alvaro Barrera, Caroline Attard, and Rob Chaplin

Oxford Textbook of Attention Deficit Hyperactivity Disorder
Edited by Tobias Banaschewski, David Coghill, and Alessandro Zuddas

Oxford Textbook of Correctional Psychiatry
Edited by Robert Trestman, Kenneth Appelbaum, and Jeffrey Metzner

Oxford Textbook of Old Age Psychiatry
Edited by Tom Dening and Alan Thomas

Oxford Textbook of Community Mental Health
Edited by Graham Thornicroft, George Szmukler, Kim T. Mueser, and Robert E. Drake

Oxford Textbook of Suicidology and Suicide Prevention
Edited by Danuta Wasserman and Camilla Wasserman

Oxford Textbook of Women and Mental Health
Edited by Dora Kohen

Oxford Textbook of

Psychiatry of Intellectual Disability

EDITED BY

Sabyasachi Bhaumik

Leicestershire Partnership NHS Trust and University of Leicester, UK

Regi Alexander

Hertfordshire Partnership University NHS Foundation Trust and University of Leicester, UK

OXFORD
UNIVERSITY PRESS

OXFORD
UNIVERSITY PRESS

Great Clarendon Street, Oxford, OX2 6DP,
United Kingdom

Oxford University Press is a department of the University of Oxford.
It furthers the University's objective of excellence in research, scholarship,
and education by publishing worldwide. Oxford is a registered trade mark of
Oxford University Press in the UK and in certain other countries

First Edition published in 2020

Published in the United States of America by Oxford University Press
198 Madison Avenue, New York, NY 10016, United States of America

British Library Cataloguing in Publication Data
Data available

Library of Congress Control Number: 2019947978

ISBN 978–0–19–879458–5

Dedication

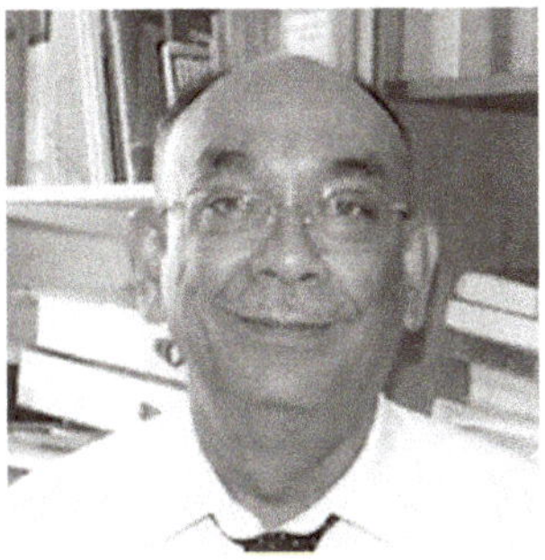

Professor Sabyasachi Bhaumik (1952–2019)

For 27 years as an NHS consultant, Sab Bhaumik lived a particular routine on Saturdays. He would turn up in his office at Leicester Frith Hospital to carry out the still pending bits of his academic work which invariably included teaching. Turning up to benefit from his generosity, would be a large number of students—from psychiatrists preparing for the Royal College's membership exams to registrars getting ready for consultant interviews and consultants seeking guidance on assorted issues—clinical and otherwise. I often teased him that these Saturday gatherings were his *durbar* and the response from this large-hearted man was always a loud guffaw, as he continued with his long sustained routine. As a close friend remarked, Sab Bhaumik died the way he lived—on a Saturday afternoon in the grounds of Leicester Frith—albeit this time the cardiac ICU of Glenfield Hospital, surrounded by a large number of people he had taught over the years, an extended family that owed so much to this professor who always cared, who always had time.

Sab graduated in medicine from RG Kar Medical College in Calcutta in 1978 and then went on to work in the West Bengal Health Service in a place called Khatra. This rural outpost was as much a contrast as possible from the teeming metropolis that was Calcutta. What was lacking there in equipment, medication, and infra structure, Sab made up with his commitment, compassion, and honesty. These were traits that particularly endeared him to his patients who often travelled from miles around to see him. When he left after 3 years there were at least 200 people around the bus, waiting to see him off. Sab went on to join an MD programme in Pharmacology at the Benares Hindu University and it was with the medical students there that he honed the teaching skills that would go on to make him an inspirational communicator.

Coming to the United Kingdom in 1985, Sab Bhaumik chose Psychiatry, a medical specialty where he truly found his calling. Starting with the psychiatry rotation in North Wales in a hospital where his only son now works, he went on to complete a Diploma in Psychiatry from the University of London and then the MRCPsych. In February 1992, he joined Leicester Frith Hospital as a Consultant in the Psychiatry of Learning Disability. Over the next 27 years, he would remain with what is now Leicestershire Partnership NHS Trust, working in a variety of roles—lead clinician, clinical director, medical director, and then after his retirement in 2013, a consultant psychiatrist and senior medical advisor to the board.

His influence in shaping policy went beyond the local. Within the Royal College of Psychiatrists, he was elected first as Chair of its Trent division and later as the Chair of the Faculty of Psychiatry of Intellectual Disability. He was credited with pioneering the tiered approach to mental healthcare provision and developing accessible information on medication for people with intellectual disability. An author of over 100 peer-reviewed publications and book chapters, Sab edited two editions of the internationally acclaimed Frith guidelines for psychotropic medication use, was a member of the NICE guidelines panel on mental health problems in people with learning disability, and edited with me, the *Oxford Textbook of Psychiatry of Intellectual Disability*, due to be published in January 2020. His work with diaspora organizations within the RCPsych, the struggle to gain equity of treatment outcomes for patients from BAME communities, and the campaign to target differential attainment among trainees from ethnically diverse backgrounds were some of his passionate causes.

The honours were many too. In 2005, he was the winner of the Hospital Doctor Award for Psychiatry Team of the Year, in 2006 he was awarded the OBE for services to medicine, and in 2015, the Royal College of Psychiatrists gave him its highest honour, the Honorary Fellowship. Through all this, Sab remained his usual self deprecating self, never taking himself too seriously. Through all this, his greatest attribute was that he remained a true fighter for his patients—a marginalized group of people with developmental disabilities and mental health difficulties who often had neither equity of access to healthcare nor equity of treatment outcomes. In his struggle to secure this equity, he was willing, sometimes at considerable personal cost, to speak out against what Susan Sontag called the 'anti-intellectual pieties and facile compassion, all so triumphant in contemporary medicine', that effectively disadvantaged patients from marginalized groups.

Sab Bhaumik died on 9 November 2019 at the age of 66, following a massive myocardial infarction. He is survived by his wife Susmita and son Sugato. Susmita, for long his anchor and arguably the only person who could possibly tell him no, found in the depths of her unexpected loss, the words that describe him best—'He had that magnetic quality to attract people—his honesty, sincerity, compassion, and ability to rise above petty jealousies made him one of a kind. Like a comet he blazed into our lives touching everyone with love, laughter, and hope—the world darkening as he left'.

Regi Alexander

Foreword

The diagnosis and treatment of mental disorders in people with intellectual and developmental disorders is a particularly challenging area of psychiatric practice. The presence of a neurodevelopmental disorder can have a profound effect on the subsequent development of psychopathology. The interface between physical conditions, psychiatric problems and environmental factors, while relevant for all of psychiatry, has a particular resonance in this population. Until fairly recently the evidence base in this field has been limited but it is now expanding rapidly as a result of high-quality research. In the last five years in the United Kingdom, the National Institute for Health and Care Excellence (NICE) has published three treatment guidelines in this area, learning disability and challenging behaviour, learning disability and mental health and learning disability service models. It is particularly pleasing that a significant part of the research literature in this area has come from practising clinicians and academics working closely with patients and family members. This textbook is edited by two highly regarded practising clinicians who have a long track record in this field. Professor Sabyasachi Bhaumik and Dr Regi Alexander are very experienced consultant psychiatrists and they have done a remarkable job in bringing together an array of opinion leaders to write on their respective areas of expertise. The 73 authors of the book's 28 chapters are drawn from over 21 universities and 20 service providers from across the world- they include psychiatrists, neurologists, general practitioners, psychologists, pharmacists, neuro-scientists, epidemiologists, social workers, nurses and above all patients and family members. The chapters cover a wide range of topics, from clinical assessment and bedside diagnosis to measuring outcomes using rating scales, from the full range of psychiatric conditions to epilepsy and physical health issues and from psychological or pharmacological treatments to the most recent developments in the relationship between neurodevelopmental disorders and schizophrenia. The *Oxford Textbook of the Psychiatry of Intellectual Disability* is an essential read for everyone practicing in this field who wishes to provide up to date evidenced-based care for their patients.

Professor Wendy Burn
President, Royal College of Psychiatrists
June 2019

Preface

Since intellectual disability is not a mental illness, many often question why psychiatrists are involved in the field at all. It is a question that has an additional resonance because of the dark shadow of institutionalization. There was a time when people could be committed to institutions, not merely because they were mentally ill, but also because they were developmentally delayed. This meant that the old asylums had psychiatrists who treated those with a mental illness along with others called the 'mental handicap specialists' who were responsible for all aspects of healthcare for those with that condition. This is no longer the case. Today, in much of the Western world and beyond, the vast majority of people with an intellectual disability live meaningful lives in the community. It is clear however, that they are as likely and in some cases more likely than the general population to develop mental health problems. When people with an intellectual disability develop mental health problems, there can be crucial differences in their clinical presentations, the process of diagnosis, and response to treatment, both in the short and long term. Psychiatrists who specialize in the care of people with an intellectual disability today focus on these aspects.

Structured training in the Psychiatry of Intellectual Disability is unique to the United Kingdom and focuses on the nuances of how developmental disorders affect the clinical presentation of psychopathology, how the same clinical presentation may occur due to physical health reasons rather than psychopathology, and how people presenting with apparent behavioural problems are not necessarily an amalgam of various disorders, but unique individuals shaped by biopsychosocial factors. This training has created a critical mass of professionals who deliver high quality care for a marginalized patient group and enable them to have the equity of outcome that they deserve. While this book is targeted to some extent at psychiatric trainees, we believe it offers a useful introduction and overview for those in allied professions, families, carers, and all those involved in any way with organizing or delivering care and treatment for people with intellectual disability and mental health problems. Throughout, we aim to address the issues that are of relevance to those on the frontline and hence most chapters offer examples of clinical issues that come up in day-to-day practice. There are also a number of single response multiple choice questions that will serve as an aid to learning.

Sabyasachi Bhaumik†
Regi Alexander

Contents

Abbreviations

AAMD	American Association on Mental Retardation
ABA	applied behaviour(al) analysis
ABAS	adaptive behaviour assessment system
ABC	aberrant behaviour checklist
ABS	adaptive behaviour scales
ADHD	attention deficit hyperactivity disorder
ADI-R	autism diagnostic interview—revised
ADOS-2	autism diagnostic observation schedule 2
AS	Angelman syndrome
ASD	autism/autistic spectrum disorder
BAS	British ability scale
BMI	body mass index
BPAD	bipolar affective disorder
BT	behaviour therapy
BVPS	British picture vocabulary scales
CAARS	Conners' Adult ADHD Rating Scales
CAMHS	Child and Adolescent Mental Health Services
CBI	challenging behaviour interview
CBT	cognitive behaviour(al) therapy
CdLS	Cornelia De Lange syndrome
CIPOLD	confidential inquiry into the deaths of people with a learning disability
CMA	chromosomal micro-array
CNVs	copy number variants(variations)
COMT	catechol-O-methyltransferase
CP	cerebral palsy
CT	computed tomography
DASH	diagnostic assessment for the severely handicapped
DBT	dialectical behaviour therapy
DC-LD	diagnostic criteria for psychiatric disorders for use with adults with learning disabilities/mental retardation
DID	intellectual or developmental disability
DISCO	diagnostic interview for social and communication disorders
DM-ID	diagnostic manual: intellectual disability (ID)
DoLS	deprivation of liberty safeguards
DS	Down syndrome
DSM	Diagnostic and Statistical Manual of Mental Disorders
DTI	diffusion tensor imaging
ECT	electroconvulsive therapy
EEG	electroencephalography
eMC	electronic medicines compendium
ESSENCE	early symptomatic syndromes eliciting neurodevelopmental clinical examination
EUPD	emotionally unstable personality disorder
FFM	five factor model
FISH	fluorescent *in situ* hybridization
FMRP	fragile X mental retardation protein
FSIQ	full-scale IQ
GAD	generalized anxiety disorder
GAI	general abilities index
GP	general practitioner(s)
GSD-LD	Glasgow depression scale for people with a learning disability
hCG	human chorionic gonadotropin
HoNOS-LD	Health of the Nation Outcome Scales-LD
IASSID	International Association for the Scientific Study of ID
IBI	intensive behaviour intervention
ICD	International Classification of Diseases
ID	intellectual disability
IDD	intellectual and developmental disabilities or intellectual development disorder
IMCA	independent mental capacity advocate
IPDE	international personality disorder examination
IQ	intelligence quotient
K-Bit	Kauffman brief intelligence test
KCH	Kwai Chung Hospital
LPFS	level of personality functioning scale
MAOIs	monoamine oxidase inhibitors
MAS	motivation assessment scale
MCA	Mental Capacity Act 2005
MEDS	Matson evaluation of drug side-effects
Mini PAS-ADD	mini psychiatric assessment schedule for adults with a developmental disability
MMR	mumps, measles, rubella
MOAS	modified overt aggression scale
MRI	magnetic resonance imaging
NCAP	Northgate, Cambridge, and Abertay Pathways
NDDs	neuro developmental disorders
NEAD	non-epileptic attack disorder
NEWS	national early warning score
NGOs	non-governmental organizations
NICE	National Institute of Health and Care Excellence
OCD	obsessive compulsive disorder
OMIM	online Mendelian inheritance in man
PANDAS	paediatric autoimmune neuropsychiatric disorders associated with streptococcal infections
PASADD	psychopathology assessment schedule—adults with developmental disabilities

PBCL	problem behaviour check list
PBS	positive behavioural support
PD	personality disorder
PDA	pathological demand avoidance
PIMRA	psychopathology instrument for the mentally retarded
PKU	phenylketonuria
PNES	psychogenic non-epileptic seizures
PTSD	post traumatic stress disorder
PULD	psychiatric unit for learning disabilities
PWID	people with intellectual disabilities
PWS	Prader-Willi syndrome
QABF	questions about behavioural function scale
RCT	randomized controlled trials
SAP	standardized assessment of personality
SNVs	single nucleotide variants
SSCT	suitability for short-term cognitive therapy scale
SSD	schizophrenia spectrum disorders (SSD)
SSRIs	selective serotonin reuptake inhibitors
SUD	substance use disorder
SUDEP	sudden unexpected death in epilepsy
TEACCH	Treatment and Education of Autistic and related Communication Handicapped Children
TSC	tuberous sclerosis complex
TSI	test for severe impairment
UDHR	Universal Declaration of Human Rights
UK	United Kingdom
Vineland	Vineland Adaptive Behaviour Scales
VNS	vagus nerve stimulation
WAIS	Weschler Adult Intelligence Scale
WISC	Weschler Intelligence Scale for Children
WS	Williams-Beuren syndrome
XLID	X-linked disorders that cause ID
YMRS	Young Mania Rating Scale

Contributors

Regi Alexander Hertfordshire Partnership University NHS Foundation Trust and University of Leicester, UK

Bijil Arackal Sussex Partnership NHS Trust, UK

Mary Barrett Leicestershire Partnership NHS Trust, UK

Salah Basheer National Institute of Mental Health and Neurosciences, Bangalore, India

Tom Berney Newcastle University, UK

Sabyasachi Bhaumik[†] University of Leicester, UK

Sugato Bhaumik Medical University of Silesia, Poland

Asit Biswas Leicestershire Partnership NHS Trust, UK

David Branford Independent Consultant Pharmacist, UK

Traolach S. Brugha University of Leicester, UK

Tobias Buxton Sussex Partnership NHS Trust, UK

Umesh Chauhan General Practitioner and University of Central Lancashire, UK

Verity Chester Hertfordshire Partnership University NHS Foundation Trust, RADIANT and University of East Anglia, UK

Sally-Ann Cooper OBE University of Glasgow, Scotland Glasgow, United Kingdom

Sherva Cooray Central and North West London NHS Foundation Trust (retired), UK

Ken Courtenay Consultant Psychiatrist in Intellectual Disabilities, Barnet, Enfield and Haringey Mental Health NHS Trust, UK

Dasari Michael Humber Teaching NHS Foundation Trust, UK

John Devapriam Executive Medical Director, Worcestershire Health & Care NHS Trust and National Clinical Advisor, Care Quality Commission, UK

Divya Devulapally Leicestershire Partnership NHS Trust, UK

Karen Dodd Surrey and Borders Partnership NHS Foundation Trust, UK

Satheesh Kumar Gangadharan Leicestershire Partnership NHS Trust, UK

Shweta Gangavati Leicestershire Partnership NHS Trust, UK

Satheesh C. Girimaji National Institute of Mental Health and Neurosciences, Bangalore, India

Jackie Grace Priory Hospitals, St Johns House, Norfolk, UK

Rohit Gumber Leicestershire Partnership NHS Trust, Leicester, UK

Ignatius Gunaratna Hertfordshire Partnership University NHS Foundation Trust, St Johns House, Norfolk, UK

Jeremy Hall Cardiff University, Wales, UK

Marisa Hanney King's College London, London, UK

Angela Hassiotis King's College London, London, UK

Avinash Hiremath Leicestershire Partnership NHS Trust, Leicester

Matthew Hoghton General Practitioner and University of Bristol, UK

Anthony Holland University of Cambridge, UK

Laura Humphries Westminster Learning Disability Partnership, London, UK

Neil James University of East Anglia, UK

Sujeet Jaydeokar Cheshire and Wirral Partnership NHS Foundation Trust and Centre for Autism, Neurodevelopmental Disorders and Intellectual Disability (CANDDID), Chester, UK

Ian Jones Cardiff University, Wales, UK

Chaya Kapugama Leicestershire Partnership NHS Trust, UK

Tawakalitu Kehinde Hertfordshire Partnership University NHS Foundation Trust, UK

Kimberley Kendall MRC Centre for Neuropsychiatric Genetics and Genomics, Cardiff University, Wales, UK

Reza Kiani Leicestershire Partnership NHS Trust, Leicester and University of Leicester, UK

Peter E. Langdon Tizard Centre, University of Kent and Hertfordshire Partnership University NHS Foundation Trust, UK

William R. Lindsay[†] University of Abertay, Scotland, Bangor University, Wales, and Deakin University, Melbourne, Australia

Mark Lovell Tees, Esk, and Wear Valley NHS Foundation NHS Trust, UK

Yona Lunsky Centre for Addiction and Mental Health CAMH, University of Toronto, Canada

Caryl Marshall South London and Maudsley NHS Foundation Trust, UK

Jane McCarthy Waikato District Health Board, New Zealand and Kings College London, UK

Peter McGill Tizard Centre, University of Kent, UK

Glynis H. Murphy Tizard Centre, University of Kent, UK

Natalie Orr Leicestershire Partnership NHS Trust, Leicester

Sir Michael Owen Cardiff University, Wales, UK

Georgina Parkes Hertfordshire Partnership University NHS Foundation Trust, UK

Dheeraj Rai University of Bristol, UK

Ameeta Retzer University of Birmingham, UK

Ian Rogers Parent and Expert by Experience, UK

Ashok Roy Coventry and Warwickshire Partnership NHS Trust, UK

Meera Roy Leicestershire Partnership NHS Trust, UK

Rohit Shankar Cornwall Partnership NHS Foundation Trust

Andre Strydom Kings College London, London, UK

John L. Taylor Worcestershire Health and Care NHS Trust, UK

Priyanka Tharian East London Foundation NHS Trust, UK

Reena Tharian Community Pharmacist, Norfolk to Reena Tharian, Clinical Pharmacist, Norfolk & Suffolk NHS Foundation Trust, Norfolk, UK

Rupert Thurston University of Bristol, UK

Jennifer Torr Monash University, Melbourne, Australia

Samuel Tromans University of Leicester, and Leicestershire Partnership NHS Trust, UK

Freya Tyrer University of Leicester, UK

Peter Tyrer Imperial College, London, UK

Stephen Tyrer Institute of Neuroscience, Newcastle University, Newcastle, UK

Nwamaka Uchendu South London and Maudsley NHS Foundation Trust, UK

Atiq Umar Leicestershire Partnership NHS Trust, UK

Matthew Walker University College London Hospitals, UK

Suzanne Wilson Clinical Psychologist (independent practice), London, UK

Kiriakos Xenitidis South London and Maudsley NHS Foundation Trust, UK

Shazia Zahid South London and Maudsley NHS Foundation Trust, UK

[†] It is with great regret that we report the death of Sabyasachi Bhaumik and William R. Lindsay during the production of this textbook.

1

Definitions, Classification, and Epidemiology of Intellectual Disability

Sally-Ann Cooper

Introduction

This book provides a comprehensive overview of mental disorders experienced by people with intellectual disability (ID), and important related considerations. A starting point is to consider what is meant by ID, the terminology that is used in different countries; how ID is defined and classified; and to describe the epidemiology of ID, as far as it has been determined, including the factors that impact on prevalence of ID, and its variation by geography and over time. This chapter will address these initial points.

Terminology

Within the UK, the terms ID, intellectual disabilities, learning disability, learning disabilities, learning difficulty, and learning difficulties tend to be used interchangeably with the same meaning, depending upon the environment. Developmental delay or global developmental delay is also sometimes used for young children before a definitive diagnosis is made. In the USA, the terms ID, intellectual disabilities, or intellectual developmental disorder have equivalent meaning, but the terms learning disability, learning disabilities, or specific learning disorder do not, as these three terms refer to conditions such as dyslexia and dyscalculia, which are referred to as specific learning disability in the UK, and explicitly excluded from the UK use of the term 'learning disability'. In the USA, the term developmental disability refers to a wider grouping of disorders; those that can impair learning/functional ability, so as well as ID, it includes other mental or physical impairments or combination of impairments, for example, severe epilepsies, cerebral palsy, sensory impairments, and autism. Elsewhere globally, the terms intellectual disability/ies and mental retardation are widely used. The current draft of the International Classification of Diseases for Mortality and Morbidity Statistics, eleventh revision (1) (September 2019) uses the term disorders of intellectual development.

Clearly, the multiple terminology in use can cause unnecessary confusion, but reflects that language evolves and terminology must be acceptable to persons with ID and their families, and this may differ in different areas and over time. It does mean that practitioners and academics need to be careful when reading and interpreting reports and evidence, with regards to whom the population under consideration is, particularly when the terms learning disability or developmental disorder are used. In the past, terms such as mental handicap were acceptable (and mental retardation in the USA), but as language evolved, these terms and numerous previous other terms that were used came to be considered as derogatory and offensive, and hence became obsolete.

Definitions and classification of intellectual disability

Most definitions of ID apply an arbitrary cut-off of intellectual level and/or functional ability. This arbitrary approach is not uncommon for a wide range of conditions, but it is important to be aware that it is arbitrary cut-off of a continuum, and not necessarily related to biological aetiology. For example, genetic studies indicate that intelligence is highly heritable and can itself be conceptualized as a spectrum of syndromes (2). Many specific genetic syndromes can cause ID, but typically they shift the mean population IQ lower, with other family factors also influencing an individual's resultant IQ; an example is Prader-Willi syndrome, which is typically associated with mild ID, but also with low average intelligence. With regard to intelligence quotient (IQ), it is predominantly normally distributed, so the cut-off point is arbitrary, and indeed has changed over time in some classifications; the American Association of Intellectual and Developmental Disorders used an IQ cut-off of less than one standard deviation below the population mean (IQ<85) (3), until this was lowered in 1973 to two or more standard deviations below the population mean (IQ<70) (4), and revised in 1983 to IQ<70–75, recognizing test error (5). In view of the normal distribution of IQ in the population, such changes have substantial impact on the proportion of the population who fall under the cut-off.

ID is a social construct rather than purely a statistical one, reflecting developmental changes across the life-course, and the societal interaction of the individual. For a child with an IQ of 69, her/his *intellectual impairment* is likely to be disabling—an *intellectual disability*—and she/he would benefit from additional support at school. As she/he gradually learns and acquires skills, the intellectual impairment may not be disabling in adulthood, as she/he succeeds in living independently, in employment, relationships, and basic educational skills. Hence she/he no longer has an ID, despite the continuing intellectual impairment meaning she/he will always take longer to learn new skills. The person may no longer view themselves as having ID, will not be viewed by others as having ID, and so would not put demand upon services designed for people with ID (which is one important reason why we need to know the number of people with ID in a locality, to inform service planning). Clearly, this depends not just on the level of a person's IQ, but also on other health and personality factors (e.g. whether the person additionally has autism).

The standard classifications used all define ID socially, rather than purely statistically.

1. The ICD-10 Classification of Mental and Behavioural Disorders, Clinical Descriptions, and Diagnostic Guidelines (ICD-10) requires (i) a reduced level of intelligence (an IQ level of <70 is provided as a guide), (ii) impairment of skills (diminished ability to adapt to the daily demands of the normal social environment, based on global assessments of ability and not a specific impairment or skill), and (iii) onset during the developmental period (6). It further classifies it into mild, moderate, severe, and profound levels based on IQ and adaptive functioning (6).
2. The Diagnostic and Statistical Manual of Mental Disorders, fifth edition (DSM-5) requires (i) intellectual deficits (such as reasoning, problem solving, planning, abstract thinking, judgement, academic learning, and learning from experience; two standard deviations or more below the population mean, including a margin for measurement error, i.e. 70+/−5), (ii) adaptive functioning deficits in conceptual, social, and practical domains (resulting in failure to meet developmental and socio-cultural standards for personal independence and social responsibility, such as communication, social participation, and independent living, across multiple environments), and (iii) onset during the developmental period (7). It further classifies into mild, moderate, severe, and profound ID based on adaptive functioning rather than IQ (7).
3. The American Association of Intellectual and Developmental Disabilities requires significant limitations in (i) intellectual functioning (general mental capacity, such as learning, reasoning, problem solving; with an IQ test score of around 70 or as high as 75 indicating a limitation in intellectual functioning), (ii) adaptive behaviour, which covers many everyday social and practical skills (the collection of conceptual, social, and practical skills that are learned and performed by people in their everyday lives), along with (iii) originating before the age of 18 years (8).

Whilst we use the terms 'intelligence' and 'functional ability', these are not unitary attributes, as they comprise of many domains, and a person's intellectual ability and adaptive behaviours are not usually uniform across all domains. Consequently, referring to ID in the singular is technically inaccurate, but, as discussed in the terminology section of this chapter, both the terms intellectual disability and intellectual disabilities are used interchangeably, internationally.

There are of course many different causes of ID. Where these are known, when classifying using the International Statistical Classification of Diseases and Health Related Problems, 10th revision (9), one should record both the condition that is the cause of ID, in addition to recording that the individual *has* ID. The current draft of the eleventh revision of this classificatory manual also adopts this same approach (1). More detailed consideration of the causes of ID is provided in Chapter 2 of this book.

Prevalence of intellectual disability

ID is not rare. A meta-analysis of 52 studies reported the prevalence of ID to be 10.37/1,000 population (10). Prevalence varied according to age (highest rates in childhood/youth), income group of the country (higher rates from low-income countries), and study design. In high-income countries, rates for all ages combined were 9.2/1,000, with the highest rates for child/young person-only populations at 18.3/1,000, and lowest rates in adult-only populations at 4.9/1,000. Twenty-five of the studies included in the meta-analysis did not provide their age range, a further two did not report their observation period, and some studies were outliers in their findings. An earlier review of studies between 1960 and 1987 is of lesser relevance to today's population, given cohort effects, that almost all were studies in childhood/youth, and some provided very limited methodological information (11).

The majority of studies in the meta-analysis were of administrative samples such as people known to local authorities. These are the people who are making demands upon services, so the information is useful, but it may omit some people with ID, and include others using services who do not have ID.

Since the meta-analysis, three large studies have been reported from the UK. A study of people with a record of ID in their general practitioner medical records reported a rate of 5.4/1,000 patients aged 18 years and over from an English database of 451 practices (12). In high-income countries like England, people are likely to have been assessed once their developmental delay was reported by parents or schools, so a record is likely to exist in the general practitioner medical records. A rate of 4.9/1,000 aged 16 years and over (self/proxy report) was reported from analysis of Scotland's Census, 2011 (13), and 23/1,000 school-aged children/young persons (teacher report) was reported from Scotland's Pupil Census, 2015 (14). These two studies have the attraction of being large scale, and include whole country samples. Interestingly, the findings from the meta-analysis for high-income countries, the general practitioner medical records, Scotland's Census, 2011, and Scotland's Pupil Census, 2015 show reasonably similar prevalence rates at comparable ages, despite the different approaches.

Factors influencing prevalence of intellectual disability, and reported prevalence rates in individual studies

It is essential that careful considerations are given in interpreting the literature on prevalence of ID, both of individual studies and meta-analysis, for the following reasons.

As noted in the diagnostic criteria in the standard classification systems, measurement of IQ can incur test error, hence the +/−5 IQ points in the criteria. However, for a simple normal distribution of IQ, with a mean IQ of 100, and a standard deviation of 15, if no other factors were relevant, the proportion of the population between IQ of 70–75 (2.5%) is greater than the proportion with IQ<70 (2.3%), so the effect of test error can be substantial. There are several other factors that can influence test scores, alongside cultural appropriateness of the assessment tool, such as the person's concentration on the day, which might always be impaired, or may be temporarily impaired (e.g. because of a cold, day-to-day worry about something, or a mental disorder such as depression or schizophrenia). IQ results therefore need to be interpreted, rather than being considered an absolute measure.

It is also very apparent that the extent to which people with mild intellectual impairments are included in a study to determine the prevalence of ID will greatly influence the reported rate, as mild intellectual impairments are considerably more common than moderate-profound intellectual impairments, by a ratio of about 6:1. This accounts for much of the variation between study findings. Study findings will also vary according to whether IQ is measured (statistical approach), adaptive behaviour is measured, or both are measured (social approach, in keeping with the diagnostic criteria in most classificatory systems), particularly in adult populations. Where the population is drawn from is also relevant (i.e. whether or not it is population-based or biased). Hence the study methodology is crucial to interpreting its results.

Additionally, whilst the IQ cut-off is set at two or more standard deviations from the mean, the deviation from the normal distribution is greatest at the most extreme ends of the IQ spectrum. There is also the Flynn effect where measured IQ can produce overly high scores due to out-of-date test norms.

Cohort effects that need to be carefully considered when interpreting the literature are also present. The prevalence of ID is highly likely to vary geographically, and over time.

Geographic factors include the provision and quality of maternal, perinatal, neonatal, and infant health care; maternal nutrition; outbreaks such as the zika virus epidemic in South America in 2015–16 causing microcephaly; maternal exposure to other infections; provision of immunization; provision and societal views on termination of pregnancies and antenatal screening; regions of endemic iodine deficiency; regions with high rates of consanguinity and autosomal and sex-linked recessive conditions, such as the lipid disorder Tay-Sachs disease in Ashkenazi Jews, French Canadians, and the Cajun in Louisiana, although the condition is not common (about 1 in 3,500 births in these populations); neonatal screening for phenylketonuria and hypothyroidism; access to cardiac surgery for infants with Down syndrome. The prevalence of mild ID is influenced by many cultural and societal factors that determine whether a mild intellectual impairment is likely to result in a functional disability (e.g. rural communities versus highly technology-based communities), hence also contributing to geographic differences.

Temporal factors include many of these same issues. Prevalence of ID has been reduced over time in high-income countries due to immunization; improved antenatal, perinatal, and neonatal health care; identification and treatment of metabolic and endocrine causes of ID such as phenylketonuria and hypothyroidism; better childhood education. Other factors increase prevalence of ID over time: maternal smoking and particularly alcohol use; changes in termination rates of children with Down syndrome (currently falling (15), but could possibly increase again with introduction of first trimester diagnosis); access to cardiac surgery for infants and children with Down syndrome; increased survival of very low birthweight infants; improved lifestyles of people with ID, and their access to health care.

There is a clear advantage to being given the label of ID if it attracts additional resources, such as additional educational support for children provided in high-income countries. Hence there may be some flexibility around the cut-off, to benefit children with abilities in the 'borderline' range (low average intelligence just above the ID cut-off). Conversely, as these children progress through youth to adulthood, they are likely to have acquired basic educational skills and no longer identify as having ID.

Identified prevalence of ID increases in early childhood. Some individuals with ID are identified at birth or antenatally (e.g. with Down syndrome), others are identified as parents seek input when they recognize their child's development appears to be delayed compared with older siblings or children of friends or other family members. Some children with mild ID are not diagnosed until they attend school, where teachers note their impaired scholastic achievements and speed of learning compared to the rest of the class. Hence prevalence in infancy and childhood increases until about ages 5–7 years, with a further small increase on entering secondary school.

People with ID experience premature death, hence the proportion of the population with ID progressively falls within older age groups. The lifespan of people with Down syndrome has progressively increased over the last 50 years, with access to treatment for congenital heart disorders and improved surgical techniques and post-operative care accounting for much of this (16), although their lifespan remains 30 years shorter than for other people. Whilst the lifespan of people with ID has also shown some increase in recent decades, a recent systematic review of 27 studies has reported that it stubbornly remains 20 years lower than for the general population—there has been no narrowing of the inequality gap (17). More severe ID and/or additional co-morbidities were associated with the shortest life expectancy (hence in older age groups, the ratio of mild to moderate-profound ID is higher than in younger age groups). Standardized mortality rates showed a greater inequality for women than for men, for reasons that are unknown (17). The main causes of death amongst people with ID differed from the general population, with respiratory disease the most common, then circulatory diseases (with greater congenital and lesser ischaemic disease compared with the general population). Cancer was less common compared with the general population, and cancer profile differed from the general population (17).

Population prevalence of ID can also be affected at the local level by migration and clustering (e.g. congregate care facilities and colonies), which can be influenced by economic factors and local policy.

Some of the factors that account for a significant proportion of ID may well be amenable to change. For example, extreme prematurity has been shown to account for 17 per cent of ID; together, gestational age and birthweight centile have been reported to account for 26.6 per cent of ID (18). Month of conception (January–March conception compared with summer conception) has been reported to account for 15 per cent of ID, postulated to be related to Vitamin D deficiency or infections at the critical first trimester stage of development (19). Foetal alcohol syndrome is highly likely to be under-diagnosed, and has the potential to be influenced by policy such as alcohol pricing, and societal factors.

Prevalence could be increased if there was some closure of the life-span gap between people with ID and the general population. A confidential inquiry reviewed 247 deaths of people with ID, finding that avoidable deaths from causes that could have been amenable to good quality health care occurred in 37 per cent compared with only 13 per cent of the general population (20). Further large-scale study (16,666 people with ID; 656 deaths, compared with age-, gender-, and practice-matched controls, n = 113,562; 1,358 deaths) also found high rates of deaths amenable to good quality health care at 37.0 per cent, compared with 22.5 per cent in the general population (21), with the standard definition of amenable deaths used in the study excluding some types of deaths that could be considered to be amenable to health care, and which occurred more commonly in people with ID (21). These important studies highlight avenues for potential change and improvements in health care which in turn may impact on the prevalence of ID in high-income countries.

Key points on the epidemiology of intellectual disability

Despite the complexities in estimating epidemiological findings on ID, and the variations that exist geographically, temporally, and in administrative systems, the following are reasonably consistent reported findings:

1. In high-income countries, about 5/1,000 adults have ID, falling to about 2/1,000 over the age of 65 years.
2. Prevalence is higher in children and young people than in adults.
3. The majority of children with ID are identified by the ages of 5–7 years (i.e. identified on entry to the education system if not before).
4. Prevalence is higher in boys/men than girls/women; across the whole of Scotland, 58 per cent of people with ID are male (13).
5. Prevalence is higher in low-income countries than in high- and middle-income countries for multiple reasons including lifestyles and health care; although in areas that are less driven by technology, having mild intellectual impairments may be less disabling.
6. The great majority of people with intellectual impairments have mild intellectual impairments (6 mild impairment:1 moderate-profound impairment), and the majority of people with intellectual impairments in whom this is disabling have mild rather than severe ID.

REFERENCES

1. World Health Organisation. *International Classification of Diseases for Mortality and Morbidity Statistics, eleventh revision.* http://www.who.int/classifications/icd/revision/en/ [Accessed 8.5.17].
2. Davies G, Tenesa A, Payton A, et al. Genome-wide association studies establish that human intelligence is highly heritable and polygenic. *Molecular Psychiatry*, 2011;16:996–1005.
3. Herber R. *A Manual on Terminology and Classification on Mental Retardation (revised edition).* Washington DC: American Association on Mental Deficiency; 1961.
4. Grossman HJ. *A Manual on Terminology and Classification in Mental retardation (revised edition).* Washington, DC: American Association on Mental Deficiency; 1973.
5. Grossman HJ. *Classification in Mental Retardation (revised edition).* Washington, DC: American Association on Mental Deficiency; 1983.
6. World Health Organisation. *The ICD-10 Classification of Mental and Behavioural Disorders. Clinical Descriptions and Diagnostic Guidelines.* Geneva: World Health Organisation; 1992.
7. American Psychiatric Association. *The Diagnostic and Statistical Manual of Mental Disorders, fifth edition.* Arlington, VA: American Psychiatric Association; 2013.
8. American Association on Intellectual and Developmental Disabilities. *Intellectual Disability. Definition, Classification, and System of Supports. The 11th Edition of the ASIDD Definition Manual.* Washington, DC: American Association on Intellectual and Developmental Disabilities; 2010.
9. World Health Organisation. *The International Statistical Classification of Diseases and Health Related Problems, 10th revision.* Geneva: World Health Organisation; 1990.
10. Maulik PK, Mascarenhas MN, Mathers CD, Dua T, Saxena S. Prevalence of intellectual disability: A meta-analysis of population-based studies. *Research in Developmental Disabilities*, 2011;32:419–436.
11. Roeleveld N, Zielhuis GA, Gabreels F. The prevalence of mental retardation: A critical review of recent literature. *Developmental Medicine and Child Neurology*, 1997;39:125–132.
12. Carey IM, Shah SM, Hosking FJ, et al. Health characteristics and consultation patterns of people with intellectual disability: A cross-sectional database study in English general practice. *British Journal of General Practice*, 2016;66(645):e264–e270.
13. Hughes-McCormack LA, Rydzewska E, Henderson A, Rintoul, J, Macintyre C, Cooper S-A. Prevalence and general health status of people with intellectual disabilities in Scotland— A total population study. *Journal of Epidemiology and Community Health*, (2017);72:78–85.
14. Scottish Learning Disabilities Observatory. https://www.sldo.ac.uk/projects/children-young-people/pupil-census/ [Accessed 8.5.17].
15. Jacobs M, Cooper S-A, McGowan R, Nelson S, Pell J. Pregnancy outcome following prenatal diagnosis of chromosomal anomaly: a record linkage study of 26,261 pregnancies. *PLOS ONE*, 2016;11(12):e0166909.
16. Hijii T, Fukushige J, Igarashi H, et al. Life expectancy and social adaptation in individuals with Down syndrome with and without surgery for congenital heart disease. *Clinical Pediatrics*, 1997;37:327–332.
17. O'Leary L, Hughes-McCormack L, Cooper S-A. Life expectancy and causes of death of people with intellectual disabilities: A systematic review. *Journal of Applied Research in Intellectual Disabilities, Journal of Applied Research in Intellectual Disabilities*, 2017;31:325–342.
18. Mackay DF, Smith GCS, Dobbie R, Cooper S-A, Pell JP. Obstetrics factors and different causes of special educational need: Retrospective cohort study of 407,503 schoolchildren. *British Journal of Obstetrics and Gynaecology*, 2013;120:297–308.
19. Mackay DF, Smith GCS, Cooper S-A, et al. Month of conception and developmental disorders: A record-linkage study of 801,603 children. *American Journal of Epidemiology*, 2016;184:485–493.

20. Heslop P, Blair PS, Fleming P, Hoghton, M, Marriott, A, Russ, L. The confidential inquiry into premature deaths of people with intellectual disabilities in the UK: A population-based study. *The Lancet*, 2014;383(9920):889–895.

21. Hosking FJ, Carey IM, Shah SM, et al. Mortality among adults with intellectual disability in england: Comparisons with the general population. *American Journal of Public Health*, 2016;106(8):1483–1490.

2

Clinical Assessment Including Bedside Diagnosis

Sabyasachi Bhaumik†, Samuel Tromans, Rohit Gumber, and Shweta Gangavati

Introduction

Intellectual disability (ID) is a heterogeneous condition and includes people with wide-ranging abilities (i.e. from those with reasonable verbal skills to those who can only communicate through eye movements, facial expressions, or other simple gestures such as nodding or finger pointing). At the one end of the spectrum, it is possible to have a good verbal interaction especially with those with mild ID. However, at the other end, you may encounter people with ID with no verbal communication and very limited non-verbal expressions. Hence, interviewing someone with ID requires adaptations in line with the person's communication needs.

Many aspects of psychiatric assessment in People with Intellectual Disabilities (PWID) bear similarity to that of the general population. However, there are also considerable differences involving the areas of information gathering, psychiatric interviewing, mental state examination, and the importance of observational skills, especially for non-verbal patients. There is a considerable emphasis on physical examination, as the interface between the physical and mental states often overlap, having great influence of one another. In addition, there are also differences in interviewing techniques involving adults, children, and the older population. One of the key central issues is of how to take a psychiatric history that is meaningful for a non-verbal patient and interpreting one's findings in a systematic way. The symptomatology of psychiatric disorders are varied, but very often these symptoms present in an atypical fashion in those with ID.

A shift from the normative function of that person may indicate underlying mental health problems, physical health problems, environmental issues, or communication difficulties. To illustrate, we provide an example of a patient who presents with the symptoms of early morning wakening; however, on closer questioning and further enquiries you may find out that the person concerned has always been an early riser and tends to get up at around 4:30am. This symptomatology therefore does not fit into part of the symptom cluster for a depressive illness, but rather is a normative function for that person. When you complete your assessment and agree for a plan of interventions, your therapeutic goals should be to return to the baseline function of that person, otherwise there will be disappointments for the high expectations that you may have given to both carers and the person with ID in relation to the outcome of your interventions. So please go through the following sections carefully, bearing in mind that they highlight the key differences between the general interviewing process and the interviewing process for PWID.

This chapter will highlight some of these issues and hopefully help trainees feel more prepared to carry out effective psychiatric assessments in PWID.

Psychiatric interviewing

The main goals of a psychiatric interview in a PWID are to:

- Build rapport with the patient
- Arrive at a diagnosis if possible
- Understand the causation through contextual information

Fundamental to interviewing a PWID, and indeed psychiatric interviews more generally, is establishing a good level of rapport with the patient. A useful tip is to learn about the patient's likes and dislikes prior to the meeting; this can help inform how you can arrange the meeting in a way that is conducive to providing a supportive atmosphere that will cause them minimal distress. For example, many PWID find clinical environments intimidating or even frightening, and thus a natural setting such as the patient's own home, may be preferable. Sometimes PWID may require time to relax or settle into a meeting, and starting by discussing a topic of their interest may help in this regard, rather than immediately delving into the psychiatric interviewing process. The presence of a carer who knows the patient well is also a useful technique for putting the patient at ease.

Whilst arriving at a diagnosis is a central tenet of the psychiatric interview in a PWID, you may often only be able to arrive at a probable working diagnosis initially, with a clear diagnosis often emerging through the process of time and further information gathering. Diagnoses may have physical and psychiatric aspects

† It is with great regret that we report the death of Sabyasachi Bhaumik during the production of this textbook.

to them, and it is important to appreciate the marked effect that common physical health conditions (such as chronic pain) can have on behaviour and mental state. Also, it is essential to be mindful of the possibility of underlying psychological, physical, or sexual abuse, as this is more common in the ID population, and can lead to challenging behaviours that maintain a cycle of abuse (1). In situations where it is impossible to rule out other potential diagnoses, you might be best placed to begin the process of a therapeutic trial based on your priorities. For instance, if you strongly suspect a bipolar disorder but cannot be sure the patient is not suffering with paranoid psychosis, you might use a therapeutic trial. Commencing multiple therapies at the same time, especially medications, is not recommended as you will not know what agent has had the positive effect for the patient.

Contextual information is important, particularly from family carers, who will usually have known the patient for many years and likely be able to provide a wealth of relevant clinical information. In speaking to foster or professional carers, request to speak to those whom have known the patient for longer than six months, in order to improve one's chances of obtaining a meaningful history. Please also be mindful about the influence of the environment in which the patient lives, along with attitudes of care staff. Thus, it is important to make the patient the centre of any assessment approach. Additionally, observing the patient directly can be helpful in situations where you receive conflicting reports from carers.

Stages of the assessment process

Preparation and collection of information

Please ensure that you have gathered and gone through all the pertinent information from the relevant sources prior to the assessment. Occasionally, there may be a need to correspond further with the referrer prior to the assessment, especially if the information provided is perceived to be incomplete. Any further information gap might be filled up during the assessment process itself.

Of course, the assessment itself provides the main opportunity to obtain information relevant to the patient's current mental state and functioning, as well as filling in any informational gaps identified in the preparatory stage. Therefore, please be mindful that information collection during the process should not lead to ignoring the patient's wishes and missing the opportunity to establish rapport. Purely information collection alone is insufficient and one must make every effort to ensure that the assessment experience is a positive and valuable interaction for the patient as well. Thus, endeavouring to put the patient at ease, establishing rapport, and ascertaining the patient's wishes are all vital in any successful consultation. You may wish to consider inviting other healthcare professionals to the assessment, which might enable you to obtain their views and establish a multidisciplinary care plan.

An initial psychiatric assessment for a PWID typically takes between 60 to 90 minutes, though the time required may be more in patients with particularly complex needs. Follow-up clinic assessments for patients already known to services are often around 30 minutes duration, though again one needs to be flexible and individualize their approach according to the specific patient involved.

Using the information

Needless to say, simply collection of the relevant information is insufficient; it needs to be considered and formulated to develop an appropriate management plan, making the assessment a worthwhile endeavour for the patient and that their needs are suitably addressed.

Recording and communicating the information

The information collected from the assessment process needs to be accurately recorded in the patients clinical notes, to provide a reference point for other health professionals in working with the patient in the future. Additionally, these details need to be communicated to the professional who made the original referral to ID services, as well as any other appropriately involved parties.

Capacity to consent

Capacity assessment is essential to decisions made across all medical care, but additional challenges in PWID, pertaining to their ID as well as other factors such as communication impairments, make them an even more prominent part of day-to-day practice. It is imperative that every attempt to communicate the information in as simple terms as possible, via the patients preferred mode of communication.

In making treatment decisions for patients who lack the capacity to consent, ensure that all relevant parties have been consulted with regard to making a best interests decision, including closest relatives, professional carers and members of the multidisciplinary team. Additionally, be mindful that capacity is both decision and time-specific. For example, following antipsychotic treatment for an acute psychotic episode, a patient may have regained capacity to make her decision regarding whether to take this medication upon restoration of their baseline mental state.

It is worth recognizing that, as ID psychiatrists, we have specialist expertise in assessing capacity relative to many of our peers, and that we can support other professionals in making such judgements for PWID.

Sharing information with families and caregivers is an important part of working collaboratively with PWID. However, where the patient has capacity to make the decision about this, informed consent should be obtained. In instances where the patient lacks consent, a best interests decision should be made by the multidisciplinary team managing the patient's care on whether sharing such information is best for the patient. In most such instances, information sharing will likely have a positive effect on the patient's care, as well as empowering families and caregivers; however, in exceptional circumstances such as instances of suspected abuse, information may be withheld in the patient's best interests.

Communication skills

As discussed in the introduction, communication skills vary widely within the ID population, and one must modify their interview approach accordingly. Some patients may be able to communicate verbally on a level not too dissimilar to those in the non-ID population. However, it is important not to assume that relatively good communication skills necessarily indicate comprehension, and to check the patient's level of understanding throughout the assessment process, particularly with regard to any therapeutic decision-making.

It is important to appreciate that you may be seeing the patient at a time where there are concerns pertaining to their mental state and/or functioning, and as such, their communication skills may be similarly affected. Information from carers as well as previous clinical assessments are central to determining if this is the case. A speech and language therapist may have developed a communication passport for the patient following a detailed assessment, which can contain vital information of how best to approach your assessment.

Patients have different preferred means of communication, and predominantly verbally-based interaction with the patient may be inappropriate in some instances. It is worth considering why the patient prefers to communicate in a particular way, as the underlying basis for such inclinations may lie in an undiagnosed sensory deficit. Some patients respond well to a picture-based approach to communication, particularly with regard to explaining multi-step processes (e.g. visiting the doctor).

History

Developmental history

ID is a developmental disorder, and one of the key distinctions between taking a history from a PWID relative to someone without ID is the level of depth explored with regard to their development. Thus it is essential to have a good working understanding of the major developmental milestones (see Table 2.1). Often patients with suspected or known ID will have had previous assessments conducted during the developmental phase (0–18 years of age), and, where this information is available, the findings and conclusions can be invaluable in determining possible aetiology, characterizing their behavioural phenotype and understanding how their functioning has changed in the intervening period. Certain genetic syndromes associated with ID have characteristic behavioural phenotypes and associated ID severities (see Table 2.3), and thus gaining a thorough understanding of development can support one's clinical suspicions and prompt collaborative assessment with a clinical geneticist specializing in genetic causes of ID.

It is conceivable that a patient may now demonstrate measured intelligence and adaptive functioning consistent with ID, but that this was not always the case for them. Indeed, the definition of ID requires an onset before the age of 18 years (i.e. the developmental period), otherwise their impairments would instead be considered as an adult onset insult to brain. Conversely, if someone has acquired brain injury during the developmental period, he or she will come under the umbrella of ID.

Understanding adaptive functioning

Initially, information on adaptive functioning can be obtained from both patient and carer, as well as other informants. Assessing particular aspects of functioning (e.g. reading and writing) can sometimes be assessed directly as part of the assessment process, though it should be borne in mind that if the patient's mental state is not currently at its baseline level, their functioning will likely be similarly disrupted (see Table 2.2).

It can be invaluable to take a history of a 'typical day' for the patient, from first thing in the morning to last thing at night, where each daily task is discussed in detail with regard to the level of independence and/or degree of support the patient requires. In instances where the patients functioning has changed (e.g. due to psychiatric illness), the discrepancies between current and previous functioning can be ascertained and later used as a means of establishing their subsequent progress post-intervention.

Diagnostic criteria for ID include requirements for both intellectual and adaptive impairments. At present IQ tests are rarely carried out; where it is available, it is important to understand it clearly. However, there is a potential for fluctuation in IQ scores at different phases of life. In the absence of an available IQ score, you may wish to use certain measures of assessment of adaptive functioning, such as ABAS and Vineland adaptive behaviour scale, both of which will give a clear idea as to the patient's approximate mental age. In assessing intelligence, clinicians may choose between standardized measures of IQ, some of which measure overall intellectual ability by measuring two core domains—verbal and non-verbal reasoning skills, while others include additional domains such as information-processing. The most commonly used IQ tests, the Weschler Intelligence Scale for Children, fourth edition (WISC-IV) and the Weschler Adult Intelligence Scale, fourth edition (WAIS-IV), offer both a full-scale IQ (FSIQ) and general abilities index (GAI). The four index scores representing major components of intelligence are verbal comprehension index, perceptual reasoning index, working memory index, and processing speed index. Evidence suggests that the use of full scale IQ in ID diagnostic decision-making, which includes working memory and processing speed, is a more appropriate measure as these impairments are vital components in the efficiency of overall intellectual functioning (2,3). A number of measures for the assessment of adaptive functioning are currently available, the two most commonly used in the United Kingdom are the Adaptive Behaviour Assessment System, second edition (ABAS-II) (4) and the Vineland Adaptive Behaviour Scales, second edition (Vineland-3) (5).

The task of determining whether the individual has impaired social functioning (adaptive behaviour) an IQ less than 70, is not as straightforward as the definition implies. There are a number of problems associated with the tools used. The reliability of IQ tests has been called into question; it is well-known that IQ scores are only accurate to within about five points; however this may be considerably less accurate when applied to people with low IQ. There is also evidence to suggest that there is a lower retest reliability for individuals with low IQ. Even amongst the two most commonly used intelligence scales, there is evidence of significant lack of consistency in the low IQ ranges. Evidence suggests that the Weschler Intelligence Scale for Children, fourth edition (WISC-IV) may give IQ scores of approximately 12 points lower than the Weschler Adult Intelligence Scale, third edition (WAIS-III) (6, 7). The reliability of adaptive behaviour scales has also been called into question. The reliability of self-report measures are especially salient when respondents could have a potential stake in the outcome of the assessment. This may also hold true for third-party respondents where there may be a potential secondary gain. For the test results to be considered valid it is important that the individual gives full effort to the assessment process, and lack of motivation to do so or deliberately underperforming during formal assessment will clearly impact on results. Clinicians should consider and formally assess, where indicated, the person's efforts throughout the assessment. Conversely, in some circumstances it has also been suggested that individuals have a tendency to overestimate the competence and adaptive skills in an effort to appear more capable than they may actually be. The only instrument available that permits self-report is the ABAS-II, however the authors clearly state that they do not recommend relying on self-report for the purposes of ruling in or out a diagnosis of

Table 2.1 Summary of developmental milestones during the first 4 years of life

Average age	Milestone	Red flags
6 weeks	• Smiles • Follows eyes past midline	
4–6 months	• Sits with support • Rolls • Reaches out and grasps objects • Starts babbling	At 6 months if: • No smile • No grasp • Not rolling • Poor head control
6–9 months	• Crawls • Sits without support • Pulls to stand • Transfers objects between hands • Gives toy on request • Turns head to name • Responds to 'bye-bye' • Gestures with babbling • First tooth	At 9 months if: • No response to words • Lack of eye contact or facial expression • No gestures • No passing of toys from hand to hand • Not sitting without support or crawling
7–12 months	• Develops pincer grasp • Plays 'peek-a-boo' • Walks with a hand held • Waves goodbye	At 12 months if: • Unable to pick up small items • Not crawling/ bottom shuffling • Not standing when holding onto furniture • No babbled phrases
12–15 months	• Single words • Listens to stories • Drinks from cup • Builds 2-brick tower	
18 months	• Speaks 6 words • Able to walk up steps • Names pictures • Walks independently • Scribbles • Builds 3-brick tower • To-and-fro scribble	• Uninterested in playing with others • No clear words • Not walking without support • Not able to hold crayon • Unable to stack 2 blocks
2 years	• Kicks/ throws a ball • Runs • Jumps • 2-word sentences • Understands two-word commands (e.g. 'feed teddy') • Builds 6-brick tower • Turns pages • Uses a spoon • Helps with dressing • Circular scribble	At 2 years if: • Has <50 words • Difficulty handling small objects • Unable to climb stairs • No interest in feeding or dressing
3 years	• Stands on one leg momentarily • Asks 'what' and 'who' questions • Uses pronouns (e.g. 'I', 'me') • Understands three-word commands • Eats with fork and spoon • Participates in imaginative play • Draws circle	
4 years	• Hops • Can dress and undress (except for shoe laces) • Asks 'why', 'when' and 'how' questions • Can count up to 20 • Draws person with head, body, and legs	

If there is regression, or loss of a previously developed skill, this should be considered a red flag requiring immediate investigation. Other red flags at any age include poor interaction with others, differences in strength between right and left sides of body, abnormal tones and strong parental concern.

Adapted from *Oxford Handbook of Clinical Specialities*, 9th edition, Judith Collier, Murray Longmore, Keith Amarakone, p.219, 2013. Source data from *Training in Paediatrics*, Mark Gardiner, Sarah Eisen, Catherine Murphy (eds), 2009. By permission of Oxford University Press.

Table 2.2 Adaptive Functioning Across Levels of Intellectual Disability

	MILD IQ (69–50)	MODERATE IQ (49–35)	SEVERE/PROFOUND IQ (34–0)
Mental Age Equivalence	9yrs–<12yrs	6yrs–<9yrs	3yrs–<6yrs
Proportion	85% of the group	10% of the group	3%–4% of the group
Language Acquisition	Some delay Most achieve the ability to use speech for everyday purposes, hold conversations and engage in clinical interview. Executive speech problems may persist. and interfere with development of independence.	Slow in developing comprehension and use of language. Eventual achievement is limited but variable: from just enough language to communicate basic needs to being able to have simple conversations. May learn to use manual signs to compensate.	Acquire little or no communicative speech in early childhood years but may develop some speech during school-age period.
Expressive Language	Most achieve the ability to use speech for everyday purposes, hold conversations and engage in clinical interview. Executive speech problems may persist and interfere with development of independence.	From just enough language to communicate basic needs to simple conversations with limited vocabulary. May learn to use manual signs to compensate.	Limited to a few words only or absent speech May indicate choice through nodding or pointing.
Comprehension	Reasonable	Limited to simple instructions.	Very limited understanding if any
Non-verbal communication	Good	Limited	Rudimentary
Self-care & Continence	Most achieve full independence in washing, eating, dressing as well as bladder and bowel control.	Can attend to personal care with moderate assistance from carers. Mainly continent.	Achieve elementary skills only. Full support of carers needed. Mainly incontinent.
Independent Living	Full independence in practical and domestic skills possible. May be able to cook simple meals; participate in household chores; operate common household appliances (television, telephone, microwave, washing machine, etc.). May travel independently; do everyday shopping and use money. Regression in skills is common under unusual social or economic stress	Will need supervised living arrangements. Limited mastery of domestic tasks; will require support and assistance. Unlikely to shop or use public transport without support.	Full 24-hour supervision required.
Academic Skills	More likely to have left school without any qualifications; achievements up to approximately the sixth-grade level. May learn to read, write, and do simple maths but can have problems.	More likely to have attended a special school; achievements unlikely beyond the second-grade level. May develop some reading, writing and math skills.	Familiarity with the alphabet and simple counting. Simple sight reading of some words. May learn to copy/write. Simple visuospatial skills.
Adult Work	Capable of work demanding of practical rather than academic skills.	Simple practical work with supervision.	Most not capable of this.
Motor Skills	Normal mobility. Generally without problems with motor dexterity.	Delayed but usually fully mobile.	Frequent musculoskeletal abnormalities. Often severe restriction.
Social & Emotional Development	Some immaturity is present which can make demands of marriage, child-rearing, or fitting in with cultural traditions and expectations difficult.	Interaction may be as usual but difficulties in understanding social conventions may interfere with peer relationships	Maybe very limited. Autism common.
Associated Deficits	Organic aetiology identifiable in only a minority. Minimal sensorimotor impairment. Other deficits as in normal population.	Organic aetiology identifiable in a greater proportion. More frequent sensorimotor impairments with Increase in CNS disorders like epilepsy.	Organic aetiology frequently identifiable. Increased CNS disorders such as epilepsy and sensorimotor deficits including visual and hearing. Impairments.
Autism & other Pervasive Developmental Disorders	Present in varying proportions.	Present in a substantial minority and can impact clinical picture and type of management needed.	Increased prevalence affecting presentation and management.

Table 2.3 Overview of genetic disorders associated with ID

Genetic syndrome	Underlying genetic pathology	Degree of ID	Morphological features	Behavioural phenotype	Physical associations	Psychiatric associations
Angelman syndrome	Lack of maternal contribution to a portion of chromosome 15	Severe	Microcephaly, strabismus, coarse facial features, hypopigmentation of skin and eyes	Hand flapping, frequent laughter, happy demeanour, excitability, attraction towards water	Seizure disorder, ataxia, scoliosis	Speech impairment, sleeping difficulties
Cornelia de Lange syndrome	Can be due to mutations in different genes (e.g. NIBPL, SMC1A, SMC3, HDAC8, RAD21)	Moderate to severe	Microcephaly, unibrow (synophrys), small and upturned nose, low-set ears, large philtrum	Aggression, self-injurious behaviour	Congenital heart disease, cleft palate, hearing impairment, gastro-oesophageal reflux	Autism spectrum disorder or ASD-like traits
Cri du chat syndrome	Deletion of a section of the short arm of chromosome 5	Moderate to severe	Microcephaly, hypertelorism, low-set ears, round face, acrochordons (skin tags) in front of eyes	Cat-like cry, hyperactivity, aggression, repetitive movements	Congenital heart disease, feeding difficulties	Speech impairment
Di George (velocardiofacial) syndrome	Deletion of the 22q11.2 region of chromosome 22	Borderline to mild	Hypertelorism, cleft palate	Speech and language deficits, inattention	Congenital heart disease, hypoparathyroidism, hearing impairment, recurrent infections, rheumatoid arthritis, renal abnormalities, feeding difficulties	Schizophrenia, early-onset Parkinson's disease, anxiety, depression, bipolar disorder
Down syndrome	Trisomy of chromosome 21	Mild to moderate	Brachycephaly, large tongue, epicanthal folds persisting beyond infancy, Brushfield spots, single palmar crease, small neck	Inattention, cheerful, sociable, reduced rates of maladaptive behaviours compared to peers with ID (23)	Congenital heart disease, hypothyroidism, gastro-oesophageal reflux, coeliac disease, leukaemia	Early-onset Alzheimer's-type dementia, obsessive-compulsive symptoms, autistic spectrum disorder
Fragile X syndrome	Trinucleotide (CGG) repeat mutation in FMR1 gene on X chromosome	Mild to moderate	Long face, large ears, prominent jaw and forehead, joint hyperextensibility, macroorchidism in males (post-puberty)	Shyness, poor eye contact, inattention, impulsivity, hyperactivity	Seizure disorder, infertility (female patients), strabismus	Autistic spectrum disorder, social anxiety, ADHD, OCD
Klinefelter syndrome	An additional X chromosome (47, XXY). Please note that other variants can exist (such as 48, XXXY and 49, XXXXY)	Normal intellectual functioning to mild	Tall stature, gynaecomastia, microorchidism	Inattention,	Infertility, gynaecomastia, osteoporosis, thromboembolism	Dyslexia
Lesch-Nyhan syndrome	Hypoxanthine-guanine phyosphoribosyltransferase (HPRT) mutation on X chromosome	Moderate	Coarse facial features, short thumbs and great toes	Self-mutilation, involuntary muscle movements, hypotonia	Gout, renal and bladder calculi	Severe self-injury
Neurofibromatosis type 1	Mutations in the neurofibromin 1 (NF-1) gene	Normal intellectual functioning to mild	Café au lait spots, neurofibromas, macrocephaly	No characteristic behavioural phenotype	Increased cancer risk, scoliosis, hypertension, optic gliomas, epilepsy	ADHD, social anxiety, depression (24)
Phenylketonuria	Mutations in the gene for phenylalanine hydroxylase, which converts phenylalanine to tyrosine	Mild to severe	Often normal appearance, may have lighter skin than other family members	Motor dysfunction, impaired executive function, challenging behaviour	Epilepsy, eczema, mouse-like odour	Autism spectrum disorder, ADHD, Parkinson's disease (25)
Prader-Willi syndrome	Lack of paternal contribution to a portion of chromosome 15	Mild-moderate	Narrow forehead, almond-shaped eyes, triangular (downturned) mouth, short stature, light skin and hair	Hyperphagia, skin picking, aggression, stubbornness	Obesity, hypogonadism, infertility, scoliosis, type 2 diabetes	Compulsive behaviour, sleep disturbances
Rett syndrome	Mutation in MECP2 gene on X chromosome	Severe	Often normal appearance, may have microcephaly	Repetitive stereotypic hand movements (e.g. hand wringing),	Encephalopathy, seizures, scoliosis, cardiac abnormalities	Autistic-like features, sleep disturbances

Table 2.3 Continued

Genetic syndrome	Underlying genetic pathology	Degree of ID	Morphological features	Behavioural phenotype	Physical associations	Psychiatric associations
Smith-Magenis syndrome	Deletion of p11.2 region of chromosome 17	Moderate	Square face, deep-set eyes, full cheeks, large jaw	Self-hugging, aggression, hyperactivity, inattention, impulsivity, self-injury	Dental abnormalities, scoliosis, visual and hearing impairment	Self-injury, sleep disturbances
Turners syndrome	Absence or partial absence of one X chromosome (45, X)	Normal intellectual functioning to mild	Webbed neck, broad chest, widely-spaced nipples, low-set ears, lymphoedema of peripheries	No characteristic behavioural phenotype	Infertility, congenital heart disease, osteoporosis, hypothyroidism	ADHD (26)
Williams syndrome	Deletion of q11.23 region of chromosome 7	Mild to moderate	Broad forehead, short nose, full cheeks, wide mouth	Lack of social inhibition, hyperactivity, affectionate demeanour	Supravalvular aortic stenosis, strabismus, gastrointestinal and renal problems	ADHD, anxiety, phobias

ID. Obtaining input from individuals themselves will be critical to the assessment process but it is recommended that a person's adaptive behaviour should be assessed through involvement of multiple third-party respondents and multiple sources of information including background information such as schooling and development including evidence for deficits reported (8).

Many factors may impact on the assessment, and consequently result in false positive or false negative results. These may include underlying mental health problems, use of pharmacological agents or illicit substances etc. Individuals suffering from active symptoms of mental illness will neither be able to engage fully in the process nor be functioning at optimal level. There is also evidence that many pharmacological agents, including prescription and illicit substances can influence neuropsychological functioning, especially sedating psychotropic medication. It is generally accepted that medication will have greatest effect in the first few weeks of prescription and for two weeks after withdrawal, and this should be taken into account. Motor impairments such as seen in those with cerebral palsy may lead to significant impairments in adaptive functioning which may be accounted for by motor impairment rather than ID. Another confounding factor might be motor impairments such as cerebral palsy and presence or absence of any neurodevelopmental disorders. The impact of neuro development disorders and adaptive functioning has also been studied; there are significant differences in the pattern of deficits in those with neuro development disorders such as autism. Adaptive behaviour in people with autism shows disproportionate deficits in socialization and communication domains compared to comparison groups, and this pattern of adaptive behaviour, without impairments in other areas may result in false positive results if clinicians do not consider this. Adaptive functioning is generally lower in children with autism, relative to IQ matched comparison groups, and this discrepancy between intelligence and adaptive behaviour found in autism should be taken into consideration during the assessment of intellectual disability. It is well known that slowed processing speed and working memory deficits are a common characteristic of variety of neurodevelopmental disorders such as attention deficit hyperactivity disorder (ADHD), and this may in turn impact on the overall intellectual functioning and adaptive functioning of the individual (2).

Intellectual functioning and adaptive behaviour are not highly correlated (7), and clinicians should take into account that people with IQ below 70 may function adequately and that there are many people with IQs above 70 with additional neurodevelopmental disorders such as autism, who have significant functional impairments (9). Understanding an individual's distribution of adaptive behaviour scores is a key task in order to recognize individual needs of patients, and should be used to inform decisions about care.

Working with different groups of patients

Patients may present to an assessment in a range of different ways, and one needs to endeavour to nevertheless make the assessment process valuable and meaningful for them. In all of the examples outlined below, it is essential to explore the reasons why the patient may be presenting as they are, as through better understanding of this, we can work on addressing such issues with a more informed approach. Carer involvement can be instrumental in this regard, as they may not only understand the basis for the patient's presentation, but also of successful techniques previously used to understand and remedy such situations.

Significant agitation

In patients presenting with significant agitation, distraction techniques such as engaging the patient in a discussion about their favourite subject, can be helpful in reducing their distress and fostering a supportive atmosphere. You need to be mindful of not encroaching on their personal space, and respecting the fact that an assessment can in itself be a stressful experience for patients, adding to their agitation (indeed, in some cases, the assessment may be the underlying source of the patient's agitation).

Hyperactivity

Though not overtly agitated, some patients may present as hyperactive, often manifesting in ways such as pacing around the room or fidgeting while seated. Your approach would be similar to that for an extremely agitated patient, as well as discussing with carers.

Aggression

As with any patient, it is crucial to consider any risks prior to the assessment, and in patients who have historical risks, have strategies in place to minimize their impact. Again, respecting the patient's personal space can be an effective strategy, as well as reducing the degree of direct eye contact with the patient, so as not to appear confrontational. For home visits, ensure that you are accompanied by a colleague, as well as informing your workplace base beforehand of where you are going and how you can be contacted. The room within which you are conducting the assessment should be carefully determined, with clear potential exit pathways identified. It is imperative to avoid a situation where the patient is situated between yourself and the exit pathways for the room. If the assessment is conducted in a clinical environment, panic alarms are often available—it is important to check that the alarm is functioning correctly prior to the assessment commencing.

Autistic spectrum disorder

Despite conventional wisdom, there is no one approach for interviewing patients with Autistic Spectrum Disorder (ASD). As Lorna Wing described, some patients may be 'passive' or 'aloof', and any attempted physical contact, such as shaking their hand for example, might actually be detrimental to rapport. Other ASD patients may be 'active and odd', and can conversely be overly familiar and invade your own personal space (10). Additionally, patients with ASD may be hypersensitive to sensory stimuli, so it is key to avoid the room being too brightly lit or having extraneous sounds present (indeed, some patients will be markedly distressed by something as seemingly innocuous as the ticking of a wall clock). Though starting an assessment by discussing a topic of the patient's interest is a generally useful approach in fostering rapport, this is particularly the case for those with ASD, who often have intensely observed special interests. An additional consideration would be to assess the patient at their own home, as ASD patients are likely to be distressed by an unfamiliar environment.

Sensory impairment

Please refer to Chapter 24 on Sensory Impairment for further information pertaining to working with patients with ID and sensory impairments. When patients have sensory impairments, adaptations should be made to the assessment approach so that the means of communication with the patient is that which they are most comfortable and proficient with. Liaise with any carers beforehand regarding how they communicate with the patient, as well as ascertaining the severity of any sensory impairment and whether any other sensory modalities are concomitantly affected. The involvement of a speech and language therapist from an early stage can help greatly, both in facilitating communication during the assessment as well as potentially working with the patient in the longer term. This may include developing a communication passport to further inform others how best to communicate with the patient. Finally, it is also important to appreciate that sensory impairments are often missed in PWID (particularly severe ID), and can be misconstrued by others; for example, someone with hearing impairment may be seen as not wanting to listen or having poor attention (11). Undiagnosed sensory impairment can have a major impact on the patient's ability to compensate for their ID and further reduce their potential; if such impairments are suspected, promptly refer the patient for further specialist sensory assessment to determine the presence and extent of any impairment. Ophthalmology and audiology services have modified assessment procedures for PWID, but the presence of a carer and a community intellectual disability nurse can also help support the patient as well as offering further relevant information to the assessor.

Profound and multiple disabilities

For patients with profound and/or multiple disabilities, liaising with well-established carers is again of utmost importance, as they will be best positioned to advise on how the patient communicates. This may be in the form of subtle or seemingly non-specific gestures that might otherwise go by unnoticed by even the more keen-eyed clinician. Despite the best possible efforts, you will likely be more dependent on carer testimony in this group of patients, though the importance of being informed and utilizing your observational skills cannot be overstated.

Mental state examination

Introduction

Obtaining a good history from the patient as well as from the carers and carrying out a good mental state examination is vital to the process of diagnostic formulation of mental health problems in any PWID. This process can however pose certain challenges in PWID. This could be attributable to communication issues, sensory impairments, the environment in which the assessment is carried out, and the presence of other comorbidities such as ASD.

Equal importance must be levied on the setting in which the mental state examination is carried out. It is often found that when the person is assessed in their own natural environment such as their family homes, residential home or the day centre, they tend to be more relaxed compared to having to attend a hospital setting to see the psychiatrist. This is more so for people with ASD, who often find new settings anxiety-provoking.

Just as in the general adult population, every effort needs to be made to see the PWID separately. If communication issues are identified, enlisting the help of a speech and language therapist can assist in improving the quality of the mental state examination and the psychiatric interview. As highlighted before, the use of special communication apps, picture exchange cards, Makaton, British Sign Language, and often simple use of pictures can assist with the interview process.

Components of Mental State Examination (MSE)

Appearance and behaviour

Clothing, gait, rapport, use of aids such as hearing aids, walking aids, or helmet for epilepsy need to be commented upon. Special comments need to be made regarding any dysmorphic features associated with genetic disorders. Any abnormal movements and stereotypes should also be noted. In people with ASD, eye contact and general behaviour should be commented upon. Some patients, particularly those with severe ID may be wheelchair-bound. Some may also bring objects which are of value to them in their lives, such as a favourite toy, pieces of jewellery etc. People with ASD may be very particular about their personal belongings, or wear the same piece of clothing repeatedly irrespective of the weather.

Speech

Make sure to comment on the rate, tone, volume, and fluency in patients who are verbal. It is important to note for echolalia and the tone, especially in people with ASD. It is again useful to have an understanding of the patient's normal speech patterns, to identify any differences in the quality of the speech. For example, a patient with ASD may have a history of always speaking in whisper, and this could easily be mistaken for low volume secondary to depression. For people with other speech problems such as dysarthria or dysphasia, having carers who can understand and help with understanding the speech can also lead to vital clues in the mental state examination. Sometimes the clinician may not be able to comprehend the patient's speech and it is acceptable to acknowledge that and clarify what the patient is trying to say with the help of carers.

Mood

People with mild to moderate ID can often express their mood states. Nevertheless, some patients may struggle, and as such, using simple pictures of facial expressions (e.g. smiley face, sad face) can be of value. Across the ranges of ID, it is vital to obtain corroborative history from carers regarding the shift from the normative state, engagement in activities, interaction with family, carers, and any other behavioural changes. An example of this could be refusal to attend the day centre. Changes in biological functions such as sleep and appetite can be discerned through history and/or observation.

Affect

As in the general adult population, observe for range, congruency, and fluctuation in affect.

It may be difficult to accurately describe affect in people who have facial dysmorphic features due to an underlying genetic condition. For example, people with Angelman syndrome can always present as appearing happy, and this therefore will influence the description of affect. People with cerebral palsy can have a poor facial muscle tone and this again can make description of affect unreliable.

Thought

Every aspect of thought, such as content and form needs to be commented upon in the mental state examination in people who are verbal. It may sometimes be difficult to tease out the difference between overvalued ideas and delusions, and having a good background history of the patient can prove valuable in making this distinction. In addition, delusions usually lead to clear actions, which may not be observed with overvalued ideas. It is difficult to substantiate a diagnosis of schizophrenia in a patient with moderate/severe/profound ID, as some of the critical first rank symptoms cannot be elicited. In people with mild to moderate degrees of ID, delusions of reference, persecution, and grandeur can be identified; however, it may be difficult to identify delusions of guilt. Other thought abnormalities, such as flight of ideas can be identified in people with reasonably good verbal skills. People with ID can present with magical thinking and the level of their cognitive abilities need to be taken into consideration prior to establishing it to be pathological.

It is absolutely crucial to check explicitly for thoughts of self-harm or harm to others. Obsessive-compulsive thoughts can occur in ASD and obsessive-compulsive disorder.

However, the key difference is that the obsessions in obsessive-compulsive disorder have an egodystonic nature, in contrast to the egosyntonic quality in ASD, where the affected individual often gains pleasure from routines being followed in a certain manner.

Perception

Depending on verbal ability, hallucinatory experiences such as auditory hallucinations can be identified. Patients can describe 'hearing voices', however it may be difficult to identify whether they are in the second or third person. It is crucial that the patient understands the questions that are being asked to explore this symptomatology reliably. Clinicians need to refrain from asking leading questions as patients with ID are suggestible. Other hallucinatory experiences, such as in the visual, tactile, olfactory, and gustatory modalities need to be specifically enquired about. In residential homes or inpatient settings when there is a patient who has a history of hearing voices, other patients can often mimic this response and can themselves complain of hearing voices. It is important to bear in mind that people with ASD and ID often tend to talk to themselves and this can be misinterpreted as 'hearing voices'. Establishing the chronology of these behaviours often help to distinguish between psychosis and other aetiologies, including normative behaviour for that person.

Insight

It is important to identify the patient's awareness of their mental health problems and acceptance of the need for the treatment. This may be difficult in people with moderate to severe degrees of ID. Additionally, many patients with ID are recipients of passive care and hence may accept medications without questioning, but this does not constitute informed consent. Many ID psychiatry services have information leaflets available that are designed for different developmental levels, and can help to enhance insight.

Cognition

Keeping in mind the developmental age of the person, other cognitive functions such as attention, concentration and memory can be assessed. It is important for the clinician to have a clear idea about the approximate developmental age of the patient and presence or absence of other comorbidities. Assessing for memory problems is considered separately under dementia in Chapter 9.

Diagnostic formulation

In the clinical practice of ID psychiatry, arriving at a diagnosis involves primarily obtaining history from the patient (depending on their verbal ability), obtaining corroborative history from carers and family, and observation of the patient.

For non-verbal patients, often the use of simple pictorial aids can help in assessing mental state. For example, for assessing mood, drawing happy or sad smiley faces, and asking the patient to point out how they feel may be helpful. Observing the patient may clarify any issues related to behaviours, including those deemed to be challenging. Certain examples of descriptions of behaviours by family or carers are 'challenging behaviour', 'he is trying to be difficult', and 'he is having a tantrum and being naughty'. These descriptions may not only be misleading and pejorative but also could result in misdiagnosis.

As psychiatrists, we need to be aware that carers' own emotional states and perceptions around ID might contribute to wrong inferences in relation to behavioural problems. In case of conflicting reports, attempts need to be made to obtain information from staff who have known the patient for a long period of time and this can help in establishing accuracy of facts. Therefore, every attempt should be made by the clinicians to observe the patients prior to finalizing a diagnosis. Corroborative history from family and carers is absolutely crucial. As part of the history taking, having a good understanding of the patient's premorbid personality, 'what constitutes being normal' for the person, and any shift from this state will help in identifying any new behaviours or exaggeration of pre-existing behaviours. However, the experience of the staff, duration of familiarity with the patient, staff's own perceptions, and attitudes towards the patient, as well as expectations from healthcare services all play a major role in the clinician's understanding of the underlying mental health problem.

The importance and relevance of the environment in which the patient operates is also equally important in the diagnostic formulation. Other factors, such as sensory impairments, presence of physical health problems, abuse, bereavement, life events, substance misuse, side effects of medication, and environmental issues are relevant factors that will impact on the presentation of a mental illness and clinicians will have to consider the above prior to making a diagnosis.

Atypical presentations

Atypical presentations in people with ID are usually multifactorial and may be influenced by concurrent administration of medication for other conditions (e.g. anti-epileptic medications such as Levitiracetam may change the mental state of previously well patients), presence of co-morbidities (e.g. ASD), and influence of environment etc.

Observational features of mental health problems in non-verbal individuals

Depression

Patients can appear unkempt with poor hygiene. If there has been an impact on food and fluid intake, there could be signs of dehydration, such as dry mucous membranes. Some individuals take a keen interest in their appearance, and patients who are known to like jewellery and dressing well may simply lose interest in their self-appearance. Eye contact can be poor and tearfulness and psychomotor retardation may also be observed. Anhedonia can be observed through the patient's refusal or disinterest in the activities that they used to enjoy such as the day centre, going to the cinema etc. Patients can be observed to engage in self-harming behaviours, such as scratching themselves with sharp objects, head banging etc.

If the depression is associated with psychotic symptoms, hallucinatory experiences or delusions are observed in behaviours such as talking to themselves (unless it is habitual), or appearing to shout out. Staring at empty spaces and appearing frightened could be an indicator of visual hallucinations. Other obvious biological markers such as loss of weight, loss of appetite, and poor sleep pattern (early morning waking) are distinctly observable.

Anxiety

Anxiety can be reflected in the patient's appearance, where they may look tense, have increased respiratory rate, be clinging onto staff members/family, appear distressed, be tearful, as well as demonstrating psychomotor agitation, tremors, or sweating. Gastrointestinal symptoms such as nausea, vomiting, and diarrhoea can be an further indicators of anxiety.

Other signs include avoidance of certain places or people, marked distress at being in certain environments or around certain people, and comorbid features of depressive illness. Specific phobias present predominantly with avoidance and increase in anxiety at the specific trigger.

Some self-harming behaviours and self-mutilating behaviours can also be a manifestations of anxiety. In severe cases, physical aggression can be a marker of underlying anxiety. Simple procedures such as checking blood pressure and pulse can be a useful guide to the patient's current level of anxiety.

Psychosis

Psychosis can be identified by their appearance, which can be dishevelled, with an associated decline in their personal hygiene. They can appear fearful and can be seen talking when there is nobody around, which could be a reflection of auditory hallucinations (though further enquiry is often required to confirm this as new behaviour, rather than long-standing self-talking seen in ASD, for example). Delusions, such as delusions of persecution, can be identified by changing behaviours such as social isolation, refusal of participation in regular activities, appearing to be scared etc. It can be very difficult to identify thought alienation phenomena in a non-verbal individual.

Mania/hypomania

This can manifest as increased psychomotor restlessness, with irritability, poor concentration and insomnia. There may also be evidence of disinhibited behaviours as well as verbal or physical aggression. In many clinical situations, an elated mood state itself may not be readily apparent, but irritability, restlessness, and agitation can be more obvious.

Physical examination

Why is it important?

Physical examination in PWID is of paramount importance for numerous reasons. Firstly, the interface between physical and mental health problems is well established, and physical assessment provides an opportunity to ascertain whether the patient has an underlying physical sign that could contribute towards their current mental state. For example, tenderness in the suprapubic region of the abdomen could suggest an underlying urinary tract infection, and increased neuromuscular tone could be a manifestation of extrapyramidal side effects secondary to antipsychotic use.

Additionally, it is well established that PWID have an increased physical health burden relative to the non-ID population, as well as a significantly reduced life expectancy (12, 13). There are likely numerous contributory factors to this. Physical health problems, especially for those who lack verbal communication may be expressed through behaviours, and hence it is important to have a thorough assessment of the patient's physical health.

General approach

When conducting a physical examination, it is useful to have the patient's carer present, as they can be an invaluable source of support for them. Furthermore, if the carer is willing, it can sometimes help to 'act out' parts of the examination on the carer, to help educate the patient as to what is involved, as well as providing reassurance. As always, obtain consent from the patient before proceeding, including checking their level of understanding of what would be involved in your assessment. Where a patient is refusing physical examination but demonstrates a lack of capacity to do so, a best interest decision on the approach to take is warranted. If you and your colleagues feel that the patient is unlikely to be acutely unwell or have a life-threatening condition, it may be appropriate not to examine the patient to avoid causing undue distress and potentially lasting damage to the doctor-patient relationship.

If you identify any physical injury during your assessment, this could potentially indicate self-injurious behaviour or abuse. Try to establish how any injuries occurred and how these injuries are explained by patient and carers. In the event that you suspect possible abuse, document your findings clearly in the patient's clinical notes as well as urgently contacting the safeguarding team. If you do not feel the patient is safe then you may need to urgently look at alternative accommodation for them while the matter is investigated.

Assessment of dementia

There are multiple additional challenges to establishing a diagnosis of dementia in a PWID. Firstly, many PWID may have a history of significant variability in their cognition and functioning over time, and it can be difficult to determine whether their current presentation represents a progressive decline. Also, the patient may not always be able to provide a detailed account of their experiences due to deficits with regard to their communication skills, including sensory impairment (14).

In screening for dementia, it is important to recognize that PWID represents a heterogeneous group with significant variability in terms of baseline intelligence and adaptive functioning. For patients with mild ID, using tools designed for the non-ID population, such as the Mini-Mental State Examination (MMSE), may be of some value, particularly if there is a record of previous findings (15). However, for many PWID, such tools would be of limited use, as their cognition is significantly impaired at baseline relative to that of their non-ID peers. Instead, use tools that have been specifically designed for use with patients with ID, such as the Dementia Screening Questionnaire for Individuals with Intellectual Disabilities (DSQIID) or the Dementia Questionnaire for Persons with Learning Difficulties (DLD, previously the DMR) (16,17). Additionally, consider in detail the patient's current level of functioning, and in what ways (if any) it has deteriorated relative to their baseline; the Vineland Adaptive Behavioural Scale can be useful in this regard. Also enquire regarding recent life events and for signs of other forms of mental or physical illness, as there are a multitude of possible diagnostic explanations for a cognitive and/or functional decline.

A basic blood screen for possible reversible causes of dementia, including a full blood count, urea and electrolytes, liver function testing, lipid profile, thyroid function testing, B12, and folate is important. Additionally, one may wish to consider neuroimaging, though be mindful that many PWID find such an investigation distressing and require desensitization work beforehand. Additionally, in the case of patients with Down syndrome, many will have abnormal neuroimaging findings irrespective of dementia. Indeed, neuroimaging may be most useful as a means of ruling out other possible pathologies, such as space-occupying lesions or infarction (18).

Risk assessment

When conducting risk assessments with PWID the standard format of assessment should be followed as per NICE guidelines (19). This should be completed following a detailed assessment including a background history of risks, as well as a thorough assessment of the current risk related behaviours, including description of the behaviour, as well as its frequency, intensity, antecedents, and consequences. Mental health conditions impacting on, or resulting in the risk-related behaviour should be assessed. Previous and current records should be reviewed and informant-based information should be taken into account. This can lead to a more comprehensive risk assessment/formulation and management plan. Risk formulation should consider the factors above and can be summarized in a risk statement which highlights; 1) nature and magnitude of likely event, 2) probability of likely event, 3) precipitants of likely event, 4) imminence of risk, and 5) means/access to items related to risks. This should be developed with the individual, family members, carers, and carer workers, as appropriate, and with multidisciplinary input if appropriate. Certain risks are inherent to PWID and are influenced by their understanding and adaptability. Risk related to using kitchen utensils, understanding difference in temperatures and being aware of safety whilst handling sharp objects should be considered, along with risks related to road safety, poor personal hygiene, and vulnerability. These risks increase with increasing degree of ID.

Risk to self

Self-injurious behaviour is common, especially amongst those with severe ID and/or ASD. Numerous causes can be considered; often sensory needs and environmental triggers can be identified, and a risk management plan can be devised to minimize soft tissue damage and distress caused to individuals. In more able individuals, the risk of self-harm and suicide should be assessed, and factors such as personality and mental health problems may impact in this risk.

Risk to others

Background information indicating a risk to others is a key predictor of future aggression. A detailed assessment of challenging behaviour including antecedents, behaviours, and consequences should be carried out. Assessment of other risk factors for harm to others should include personal history of violence, lack of a meaningful occupation, substance misuse, active symptoms of mental health problems such as psychosis, low tolerance to frustration, difficulty understanding others' feelings and emotions, and plans to harm others. The risk posed to others should be understood in terms of potential triggers, intensity, and frequency, as well as to whom the risk is directed towards. Offending history or risk of serious harm to others could be assessed using structured tools, but this should not replace detailed clinical assessment and opinion. Careful consideration should be given to certain risks that may be infrequent but are of such high intensity that they have a significant impact on the patient and others (e.g. intense desire to swallow boiling water due to a lack of awareness of the consequences).

Risk of self-neglect and vulnerability

These risks are almost universal to individuals with ID. By definition, if one is functioning at a level of ID they have impairments in their ability to manage day-to-day life tasks and, if unsupported would be at risk of self-neglect. In addition, factors such as mental illness, dementia and ASD should be included in this area and these disorders may significantly increase the risks due to cognitive, social, and communication impairments. Exploitation and abuse of individuals with ID is not uncommon. Local safeguarding protocols should be followed in order to protect vulnerable individuals, which ensures good communication between services and within services to minimize risks.

Risk related to physical health

Risks to physical health to individuals with ID should be integral to the assessment. Increased risk of side effects, swallowing problems, risk of falls and deteriorating mobility, risk to skin integrity, and epilepsy-related risks should be considered, amongst others. Epilepsy risk assessments are essential as part of a preventative strategy for Sudden Unexpected Death in Epilepsy (SUDEP). Risks related to bathing, falls, and prolonged seizures should be disused, as well as supervision during both the day and overnight.

Risk management plan

A risk management plan should set out the potential factors that increase risk, as well as factors that mitigate risks, incorporating early warning signs and proactive, active, and reactive approaches, using a positive behaviour support model, if appropriate. Risk prevention such as engaging trust and working to ensure responsive support should be clearly articulated to both carers and family. Social, environmental, and pharmacological interventions for risks management including crisis and contingency plans, should be clearly documented. The care plan should be shared and good inter-agency communication is an essential aspect of risk management by the multidisciplinary team. Positive risk taking should be considered to support empowerment of individuals with ID and ensure that inappropriate restrictions are not put upon them. A protective framework should be constructed with clear boundaries as well as established and trusting working relationships before commencing positive risk taking plans.

Comorbidities in people with intellectual disabilities

Introduction

PWID are at greater risk for the development of both physical and psychiatric comorbidities relative to the non-ID population (20). This is due to interaction of a multitude of factors, including:

- *Biological factors*, including genetic predispositions associated with certain syndromes, such as cardiac anomalies, hypothyroidism, depression, and early onset dementia observed in persons with Down syndrome.
- *Psychological factors*, including reduced frustration tolerance and poor problem-solving skills, as well as maladaptive coping strategies for managing difficult life situations. They may also be the victims of stigmatization and various forms of abuse, the effects of which should never be underestimated.
- *Social and environmental influences*, as individuals with ID often have smaller social networks on which they can seek support, as well as reduced freedoms and opportunities in life, in part due to the limitations that their disabilities place on their independence.

Syndrome-specific comorbidity

Introduction

While for many persons the cause of their ID is unknown, some are associated with genetic syndromes. However, it is important to bear in mind that there are also non-syndromic genetic causes of ID (i.e. where no other symptoms or comorbid features are evident) (21).

Of the well-recognized genetic syndromes, the most common are Down syndrome and fragile X syndrome, though there are many other well-recognized causes. Summary details of specific genetic syndromes associated with ID are summarized in Table 2.3, though more general aspects of genetic disorders will now be discussed in further detail.

Dysmorphic features

As psychiatrists, it is important to be able to recognize the major dysmorphic presentations of genetic syndromes associated with ID. If you suspect a genetic syndrome, referral for assessment and further investigative testing by clinical geneticists is important, as this leads to a greater collective understanding of both their condition as well as the potential for current or future physical and psychiatric comorbidity, providing opportunities for early intervention.

Behavioural phenotypes

Flint (1996) described a behavioural phenotype as 'a behaviour, including cognitive processes and social interaction style that is consistently associated with, and specific to, a syndrome which has a chromosomal or a genetic aetiology (22)'. Nevertheless, it is important to recognize that a high degree of within-syndrome variation exists, and as such, a behavioural phenotype should be considered as a behaviour that is more prevalent in individuals with a specific genetic condition, rather than universal to all individuals with said condition. An example of a behavioural phenotype is ASD.

Physical and psychiatric associations

Genetic disorders associated with ID generally also have implications for the individual's physical and psychiatric health. This can manifest in a wide variety of ways, from schizophrenia observed in Di George syndrome, to obesity and hyperphagia in Prader-Willi syndrome, to Alzheimer's-type dementia in Down syndrome. For these reasons, patients with such disorders frequently require coordinated input from a range of professionals across multiple medical specialities.

Non-syndromic comorbidity

In assessing someone with ID, it is always important to consider the possibility of diagnostic overshadowing, whereby physical or psychiatric phenomena have been attributed to a patient's ID or mental illness, when in fact there is actually an unidentified comorbid condition.

Psychiatric comorbidity

The once-held notion that psychopathology did not occur in PWID has since been discredited, and it is now recognized that prevalence rates in this group exceed that of the general population (27). Furthermore, Bhaumik et al. found that use of psychiatric services increases with increasing severity of ID (28).

Neurodevelopmental conditions

Attention deficit hyperactivity disorder (ADHD) and autistic spectrum disorder (ASD) are the two most common psychiatric disorders in persons with ID (29). Identifying these disorders at an early age is important, as this can inform approaches on how best to understand their needs, as well as structure both their caregiving and education. ASD and ADHD are discussed in further detail in Chapters 7 and 8 respectively.

Affective disorders

Affective disorders are significantly more prevalent in persons with ID relative to the non-ID population, and are likely underdiagnosed, particularly in severe ID, where the usefulness of applying standardized diagnostic criteria is reduced, and clinicians often make judgements based on 'behavioural equivalents' (30). Affective disorders are discussed in further detail in Chapters 11 and 12.

Anxiety disorders

Anxiety disorders are frequently encountered in persons with ID, particularly following significant life events (31). Any psychological treatment approaches should be adjusted to the individual patient's level of understanding and intellectual function.

Psychotic disorders

Psychosis is more prevalent in persons with ID compared to the general population (12), though the true extent of this is difficult to establish as clinicians generally find it challenging to confidently diagnose schizophrenia in patients with moderate to profound levels of ID. Psychotic disorders are discussed further in Chapter 10.

Dementia

Dementia is an important comorbidity in patients with an ID, who can often develop symptoms at a younger age and declined more rapidly. Please refer to Chapter 9, which details dementia in persons with ID in greater detail.

Delirium

Delirium describes an acute change in cognitive functioning, associated with change in level of arousal, disturbance of the sleep-wake cycle, perceptual disturbances, and a fluctuating course. Delirium can be mistaken for dementia, and indeed these conditions can co-exist, but delirium classically has more of an acute onset, as well as a disturbance of conscious level and attentional deficits (which are generally only seen in the latter stages of dementia). PWID are particularly susceptible to developing delirium and are also at risk of this not being identified. The extent of changing their presentation from their baseline state may be less marked than for a person without ID. Additionally, delirium can present in both hyperactive (associated with an increase in arousal level and agitation) and hypoactive (associated with quietness and withdrawal) forms, and it is important to be aware of both possible manifestations.

Delirium has a multitude of possible causes, including infections, electrolyte imbalance, hypoxia, dehydration, medication side-effects, and constipation among others. In terms of management, it is essential to establish the root cause or causes of the delirium and treat these accordingly, as well as providing reassurance and reorientation to the patient during this time.

Neurological comorbidity

Along with psychiatric illness, neurological comorbidity is among the most common forms of comorbidity seen in persons with ID (32). This can manifest in a variety of ways, including motor and sensory impairments, as well as conditions such as epilepsy and cerebral palsy.

Many individuals with ID suffer from motor impairments and this is more noticeable in patients with severe/profound ID. Difficulties with ambulation are frequently observed and, if left unaddressed, can markedly limit the independence of a person with ID and be significantly detrimental to their overall quality of life. Physical exercise-based approaches focused on maintaining physical strength and balance are essential to optimizing the patient's functioning, as well as mobility aids where indicated. Additionally, fall prevention programmes and aids to minimize the impact in the event of falls occurring need to be considered.

Both visual and hearing impairment are more prevalent in PWID relative to their non-ID peers. It is essential to identify any visual or hearing deficits as early as possible in order to provide appropriate correction to minimize any additional impact of this on their development (33). PWID may not spontaneously report any deficits themselves, so referral for screening is often recommended; screening approaches can be modified according to the person's level of ID. The frequency of screening may need to be increased as persons with ID become older, as a means of identifying any progressive deterioration. In terms of hearing impairment, earwax (cerumen) build-up is a frequently-observed contributory factor that is readily treatable. Input from a Speech and Language Therapist can also provide further support with regards to speech production and comprehension problems.

Pain

PWID may struggle to articulate their pain experience to carers or medical professionals, and it is important to consider pain as a possible explanation for behavioural disturbance. Frequently observed causes of pain include dental pathology, musculoskeletal injury, and gastro-oesophageal reflux disease. Sensitivity to pain may vary amongst PWID, especially with those with ASD, where both hypo- and hypersensitivity is seen.

Epilepsy

Epilepsy is very common, with a lifetime prevalence of 30 per cent in PWID. Additionally, some individuals have Non-Epileptic

Attack Disorder (NEAD), with or without co-morbid epilepsy. Similarly, some behaviours during epileptic phenomena may be perceived to be challenging and misinterpreted as a behavioural problem. A careful joint assessment with a neurologist and appropriate investigations (e.g. electroencephalography, video-telemetry) may clarify the situation. SUDEP is more common in patients with ID relative to the non-ID epilepsy population (14). The risk of SUDEP can be minimized through optimization of seizure control as well as being aware of the risks associated with nocturnal seizures. Epilepsy in discussed in greater detail in Chapter 22.

Cerebral palsy

Cerebral palsy (CP) is often seen in individuals with ID but is not invariably associated with ID. Many individuals with CP have reasonable intellectual functioning but have significant functional impairment due to their underlying condition. A careful assessment of the person's cognitive abilities should distinguish between the two groups.

Other physical comorbidities

There is a greater prevalence of substandard oral health among persons with ID relative to the general population for many reasons, including a lack of motivation towards self-care, inadequate prompting from caregivers and barriers in regards to receiving appropriate dental care from professionals (34). It is important to bear in mind that pain due to poor dental care may be manifested through behaviours.

Other physical comorbidities commonly experienced by people with ID include constipation, which may have an impact on the person's behaviour and functioning. Similarly, many individuals with ID may suffer from obesity due to relative lack of physical exercise and poor dietary habits, or use of psychotropic medications. In addition, common physical health problems encountered include respiratory tract infections and cardiovascular disease, which may often lead to increased morbidity and mortality. Menstruation and associated pain can have a marked impact on the mental state of females with ID, and should be particularly considered when behavioural disturbance follows a cyclical pattern. People with ID have a greater prevalence of low Bone Mineral Density (BMD), potentially leading to fractures, the consequences of which can have devastating effects on mobility and long-term quality of life. However, another common cause of reduced BMD is due to long-term use of anti-epileptic drugs.

Key points

- There are numerous genetic disorders associated with ID that have different profiles of dysmorphic features and behaviours, as well as physical and psychiatric comorbidities.
- PWID are at increased risk of both psychiatric and physical comorbidity, and it is important to be vigilant in identifying any comorbid conditions rather than attributing them to their ID and/or previously recognized psychiatric illness.

Case study 1

Adam is a 21-year-old male. He communicates verbally and has basic reading and writing skills. He has difficulties with more complex communications such as business letters. He attended clinic with his mother and carer, with whom he spends 14 hours of one-to-one time per week. This time is used accessing community. He also attends a voluntary job in a local café. During the assessment a clear personal history and developmental history is obtainable from his mother, and his current functioning indicates that he is independent in some areas of adaptive functioning including self-care and domestic skills. There are deficits in academic skills, some evidence of communication deficits, especially in receptive communication, and he also needs support in areas such as community access and self-direction. He was referred because of complaints of high anxiety. As well as a detailed history of adaptive functioning, the assessment includes assessment of mental health, which reveals some features of anxiety specifically around social situations and routine changes. On mental state examination, he appears to have a long face, large ears and eye contact is poor. It is noted that he has some hand flapping behaviours. Based on collateral information, detailed assessment of personal and background history, and current mental state examination, you are confident that he presents with features consistent with mild ID and fragile X syndrome, with social anxiety appearing to have significant impact on his current functioning and quality of life. Referral is made to the local geneticist, further reviews are booked for assessment for autism spectrum disorder and treatment of social anxiety are commenced.

Case study 2

Sarah is a 30-year-old female who has been referred to the ID service due to high levels of agitation and aggressive behaviour. She attends with her carer, who has been supporting for approximately two months. She has basic communication skills but is repetitive, and two-way conversation is impaired. Her carer reports that her mental health has deteriorated, as she is now exhibiting self-injurious behaviour and aggression towards others. Unfortunately, there is no collateral information regarding background history or developmental history, and information about past psychiatric history including medication and non-pharmacological treatments is not available. Based on the history from her carer, Sarah needs support in most areas of adaptive skills, including self-care, continence, and independent living. She ordinarily communicates her distress through her behaviour, and has history of self-injurious behaviour which she appears to be exhibiting more often recently. She accesses the community regularly but frequently refuses to leave the car. On mental state examination, Sarah does not appear aggressive but repetitive speech is noted, as well as repetitive hand movements, including pressing her nails onto the skin. The carer is requesting medication for behaviour, however the clinician decided that more information is first required from collateral sources. Following contact with Sarah's father it is established that Sarah has always displayed repetitive behaviours, including self-injurious behaviour, which is normally response to demands not being met or environmental changes. She has always responded well to the use of items that vibrate, which helps her calm quickly. She has previously used pictures to communicate, which is not being used at present. Following collateral history, it is concluded that she presents with severe ID, and challenging behaviour related to environmental factors, including a change of her care staff. Communication skills need to be optimized, and so she is referred to the speech-language therapist. She is also referred to occupational therapy for sensory assessment. She is followed up for assessment of both ASD and challenging behaviour. The risk assessment indicates risk to self, others, and vulnerability. An appropriate risk management plan is developed, and the information gathered is shared amongst both the multidisciplinary and carer teams.

MULTIPLE CHOICE QUESTIONS

Questions

Please select the single most appropriate answer.

1. Assessment of Dementia in PWID does not usually involve?

A. Current level of functioning
B. MMSE
C. Neuroimaging
D. Thyroid Function Tests
E. Change in functioning

2. Risk formulation in PWID does not usually include?

A. Probability of likely event
B. Nature and magnitude of likely events
C. Precipitants of likely event
D. Imminence of risk
E. Use of restraint to manage behaviour

3. What is most common inherited cause of ID?

A. Down Syndome
B. Angelmans Syndrome
C. Williams Syndrome
D. Fragile X Syndrome
E. Tuberous Sclerosis

4. What is a behavioural phenotype?

A. A behaviour that is consistently associated with, and specific to, a syndrome which has a chromosomal or a genetic aetiology
B. A behaviour that is consistently associated with, and specific to, a specific gene
C. A genotype that consistently associated with, and specific to, a syndrome which has a chromosomal or a genetic aetiology

5. In which circumstance would concern be highlighted about a child's development?

A. Vocabulary of <50 words at age 2 years
B. Lack of eye contact or facial expression at 4 months
C. Unable to stack 2 blocks at 9 months
D. Unable to climb stairs at 18 months
E. Not walking without support at 12 months

Answers

1. B. MMSE has limited value in PWID, as their cognition is significantly impaired at baseline relative to that of their non-ID peers
2. E. The risk formulation is part of the risk assessment, use of restraint is part of a risk management plan
3. D. Fragile X Syndrome is the most common inherited cause, Down Syndrome is the most common genetic cause, but is not usually inherited
4. A. As described by Flint (1996)
5. A. Developmental milestones will vary from child to child but all normally developing children would be expected to have a vocabulary of >50 words at aged 2 years

REFERENCES

1. Sobsey D, Doe T. Patterns of sexual abuse and assault. *Sex Disab.*, 1991;9(3):243–259.
2. Koriakin TA, Mccurdy MD, Papazoglou A, Pritchard AE, Zabel TA, Mahone EM, et al. Classification of intellectual disability using the Wechsler Intelligence Scale for children: Full scale IQ or general abilities index? *Developmental Medicine and Child Neurology*, 2013;55(9):840–845.
3. Wechsler D. Wechsler *Adult Intelligence Scale*—Fourth Edition (WAIS-IV). San Antonio, TX: NCS Pearson, 2008;22:498.
4. Harrison P, Oakland T. *Adaptive Behavior Assessment System*—(ABAS-II). San Antonio, TX: The Psychological Corporation 2003.
5. Sparrow SS, Cicchetti DV, Saulnier CA. Vineland-3: Vineland adaptive behavior scales: *PsychCorp*: 2016.
6. Whitaker S. Intellectual disability: a concept in need of revision? *The British Journal of Development Disabilities*, 2008;54(106):3–9.
7. Gordon S, Duff S, Davidson T, Whitaker S. Comparison of the WAIS-III and WISC-IV in 16-Year-Old Special Education Students. *Journal of Applied Research in Intellectual Disabilities*, 2010;23(2):197–200.
8. Tassé MJ, Schalock RL, Balboni G, Bersani H Jr, Borthwick-Duffy SA, Spreat S, et al. The construct of adaptive behavior: Its conceptualization, measurement, and use in the field of intellectual disability. *American Journal on Intellectual and Developmental Disabilities*, 2012;117(4):291–303.
9. Carter AS, Volkmar FR, Sparrow SS, Wang J, Lord C, Dawson G, et al. The Vineland Adaptive Behavior Scales: Supplementary norms for individuals with autism. *J Autism Dev Disord.*, 1998;28(4):287–302.
10. Wing L, Gould J. Severe impairments of social interaction and associated abnormalities in children: Epidemiology and classification. *J Autism Dev Disord.*, 1979;9(1):11–29.
11. Carvill S. Sensory impairments, intellectual disability and psychiatry. *Journal of Intellectual Disability Research*, 2001;45(6):467–483.
12. Cooper SA, Smiley E, Morrison J, Williamson A, Allan L. Mental ill-health in adults with intellectual disabilities: Prevalence and associated factors. *Br J Psychiatry*, 2007 Jan;190:27–35.
13. Heslop P, Blair PS, Fleming P, Hoghton M, Marriott A, Russ L. The confidential inquiry into premature deaths of people with intellectual disabilities in the UK: A population-based study. *The Lancet*, 2014;383(9920):889–895.

14. Bhaumik S, Gangadharan S, Branford D, Barrett M. The Frith Prescribing Guidelines for People with Intellectual Disability. Wiley-Blackwell; 2015.
15. Folstein MF, Folstein SE, McHugh PR. 'Mini-mental state': A practical method for grading the cognitive state of patients for the clinician. *J Psychiatr Res*, 1975;12(3):189–198.
16. Evenhuis H. Further evaluation of the dementia questionnaire for persons with mental retardation (DMR). *Journal of Intellectual Disability Research*, 1996;40(4):369–373.
17. Deb S, Hare M, Prior L, Bhaumik S. Dementia screening questionnaire for individuals with intellectual disabilities. *Br J Psychiatry*, 2007 May;190:440–444.
18. Stanton LR, Coetzee RH. Down's syndrome and dementia. *Advances in Psychiatric Treatment*, 2004;10(1):50–58.
19. National Institute for Health and Care Excellence. Mental Health Problems in People with Learning Disabilities: Prevention. *Assessment and Management*, (NG 54). 2016.
20. Emerson E. Prevalence of psychiatric disorders in children and adolescents with and without intellectual disability. *Journal of Intellectual Disability Research*, 2003;47(1):51–58.
21. Kaufman L, Ayub M, Vincent JB. The genetic basis of non-syndromic intellectual disability: a review. *Journal of Neurodevelopmental Disorders*, 2010;2(4):182.
22. Flint J. Behavioral phenotypes: Conceptual and methodological issues. *Am J Med Genet.*, 1998;81(3):235–240.
23. Collacott RA, Cooper SA, Branford D, McGrother C. Behaviour phenotype for Down's syndrome. *Br J Psychiatry*, 1998 Jan;172:85–89.
24. Johnson NS, Saal HM, Lovell AM, Schorry EK. Social and emotional problems in children with neurofibromatosis type 1: Evidence and proposed interventions. *J Pediatr.*, 1999;134(6):767–772.
25. Blau N, van Spronsen FJ, Levy HL. Phenylketonuria. *The Lancet*, 2010;376(9750):1417–1427.
26. Russell HF, Wallis D, Mazzocco MM, Moshang T, Zackai E, Zinn AR, et al. Increased prevalence of ADHD in Turner syndrome with no evidence of imprinting effects. *J Pediatr Psychol.*, 2006 Oct;31(9):945–955.
27. Matson JL, Belva BC, Hattier MA, Matson ML. Scaling methods to measure psychopathology in persons with intellectual disabilities. *Res Dev Disabil.*, 2012;33(2):549–562.
28. Bhaumik S, Tyrer F, McGrother C, Ganghadaran S. Psychiatric service use and psychiatric disorders in adults with intellectual disability. *Journal of Intellectual Disability Research*, 2008;52(11):986–995.
29. Strømme P, Diseth TH. Prevalence of psychiatric diagnoses in children with mental retardation: Data from a population-based study. *Developmental Medicine and Child Neurology*, 2000;42(04):266–270.
30. Hurley AD. Mood disorders in intellectual disability. *Curr Opin Psychiatry*, 2006 Sep;19(5):465–469.
31. Reid K, Smiley E, Cooper S. Prevalence and associations of anxiety disorders in adults with intellectual disabilities. *Journal of Intellectual Disability Research*, 2011;55(2):172–181.
32. Arvio M, Sillanpää M. Prevalence, aetiology and comorbidity of severe and profound intellectual disability in Finland. *Journal of Intellectual Disability Research*, 2003;47(2):108–112.
33. Wilkinson JE, Culpepper L, Cerreto M. Screening tests for adults with intellectual disabilities. *J Am Board Fam Med.*, 2007 Jul–Aug;20(4):399–407.
34. Feldberg I, Merrick J. Intellectual disability and dental services: Experience from Israel. *Front Public Health*, 2014 Sep 30;2:133.

3

Intellectual Disability—Concepts, Aetiology, and Genetics

Satish C. Girimaji, Salah Basheer, Asit Biswas, and Satheesh Kumar Gangadharan

Intellectual Disability (ID)—Concepts

Background

Intelligence is a trait which is highly evolved in humans and sets them apart from other members of the animal kingdom. One of the earliest formulations of intelligence was by Wechsler, who defined it as 'The aggregate or global capacity of the individual to act purposefully, to think rationally, and to deal effectively with his environment' (1). We extensively use our intellectual abilities to learn, understand, imagine, remember, think, adapt, and modify our environments and differ from each other in these abilities. The terms cognition and intelligence, though used interchangeably, are different concepts. Cognition is a neuropsychological construct and indicates mental processes for acquiring knowledge such as attention, perception, reasoning, imagining, and abstract thinking, whereas intelligence is a much broader concept and includes behaviours and performances that are directed by cognitions.

Though the construct of intelligence is extensively used in clinical and scientific contexts, there have been major controversies about how to define intelligence. Definitions proposed by theorists such as Spearman, Cattell, Gardner, and others have their commonalities and differences. One major point of contention is to consider intelligence as unitary construct or as a conglomeration of numerous abilities. Modern theorists propose a small number of inter-related but independent abilities, such as the triarchic model of intelligence of Sternberg, which has three components—analytic, synthetic/creative, and practical (2). Cattell described fluid and crystallized forms of intelligence (3). Fluid intelligence refers to innate capability for reasoning, problem solving, and pattern recognition and crystallized intelligence is the learnt abilities or knowledge gained through life experiences and education. Large scale factor analysis of intelligence tests (e.g. WISC-IV) has identified 4 factors—verbal comprehension, perceptual reasoning, working memory, and processing speed (4).

IQ tests as a measure of intelligence have a long history and have been associated with numerous controversies. The main objection to IQ has been that they are not reliable and valid measures of intelligence—they do not reflect the true intellectual capacity of the individual in the given socio-cultural setting and often underestimate it. Though IQ scores continue to play a significant role in the definition and classification of ID, its importance has been diminishing over time.

The three different constructs of ID

Given the fact that intelligence plays such a crucial role in our lives, it is not surprising that a diminished intellectual capability puts significant limitations on the person's functioning. ID is perhaps the most disabling of all disabilities, with major consequences for the individual themselves, their families and the society. There are several ways of conceptualizing ID that are described briefly below:

1. Statistical or psychometric model: Intelligence as measured by IQ tests is normally distributed in the community, or follows a bell-shaped Gaussian distribution. ID can be viewed as extreme variation in the lower end of this Gaussian distribution, generally considered to be less than two standard deviations below the mean. However, this model does not explain the fact that this distribution in reality is skewed to the left with a hump in the lowest ranges, implying that there are more people with intelligence in the lower ranges.
2. Biomedical model: This perspective considers ID as a neurodevelopmental disorder (NDD), a disorder secondary to an impediment in the maturation and development of the brain. Anything that significantly interferes with the smooth, orderly, orchestrated process of brain maturation and development is likely to cause impairments in development of intelligence and thereby leads to ID. The limitation of this model is that in a proportion of cases, especially those with milder forms of ID, a biomedical basis cannot be identified.
3. Socio-cultural model: This is a disability perspective that states that people with lesser intelligence are lacking in their adaptive behaviours and face disadvantages in their societies and therefore have higher support needs. As per this model, it is not enough for someone to have lesser intelligence to be labelled as having ID; he or she must also have concurrent deficits in adaptive behaviours. These adaptive behaviours are now widely

accepted to have three components—conceptual, practical and social (5). However, this model cannot account for the fact that there are hundreds of medical diseases that are highly associated with ID.

Current approaches

The current classificatory systems acknowledge all the above three constructs to provide a descriptive definition of ID.

The Diagnostic and Statistical Manual-5 (DSM-5) defines ID or Intellectual Developmental Disorder (IDD) as a disorder with onset during developmental period that includes intellectual and adaptive functioning deficits in conceptual, practical and social domains. It further characterizes deficits in intellectual functioning as deficits in reasoning, problem solving, planning, abstract thinking, judgement, academic learning and learning from experience that can be ascertained either clinically or through individualized, standardized tests of intelligence. Similarly, deficits in adaptive functioning deficits are conceptualized as failure to meet the developmental and socio-cultural standards for personal independence and social responsibility. These adaptive deficits are thought to limit functioning in one or more activities of daily life (6). DSM-5 allows for coding the aetiology as a specifier and has also included a diagnosis of 'global developmental delay' in children below five years who have significant delays in two or more areas of development.

The ICD-11 draft version names the condition as 'disorders of intellectual development' and defines it as a 'group of etiologically diverse conditions originating during the developmental period characterized by significantly below-average intellectual functioning and adaptive behaviour that are approximately two or more standard deviations below the mean (approximately less than the 2.3rd percentile), based on appropriately normed, individually administered standardized tests. Where appropriately normed and standardized tests are not available, diagnosis of disorders of intellectual development requires greater reliance on clinical judgement based on appropriate assessment of comparable behavioural indicators' (7).

It is clear from these two definitions that ID is a clinical concept which calls for clinical judgement and does not rely on just IQ tests alone.

Aetiology

Starting from a single cell as zygote, the human embryo rapidly grows and differentiates into three layers. Brain develops from the outermost layer, the ectoderm; the other organs that develop from ectoderm are the sense organs, other parts of central and peripheral nervous system, the skin and appendages, which are often affected in the presence of ID.

The growth and maturation of the brain is under tight genetic control. However, the environmental factors are also known to affect this process. Under favourable circumstances, this continuous, orderly, and orchestrated process of growth (increase in size), maturation (emergence of functions). and development (continuous process of change/acquisition of skills and competencies) goes along the expected lines, leading to typical patterns of development. Such changes in growth, maturation, and development stretch into adolescence and early adulthood, but are maximal in their velocity in the prenatal period and in the first three years of life. During this period of explosive growth, maturation, and development, any adverse event or influence is likely to cause impairments in the development of intelligence, thereby leading to ID. There are thousands of such causes, both genetic and environmental, either acting singly or together. This section describes an approach to understanding these causes.

Historically, the two-group theory was proposed to account for the distribution of intelligence in the community; the biomedical group for more severe forms of ID, and the cultural-familial group for milder forms of ID (8). However, the current trend is to transcend this dichotomy and think of the causes in a multi-factorial framework, where both biomedical and psycho-social factors are considered important and often interacting (5). However, there may be a range of possibilities—some forms of ID solely determined by a particular genetic, biomedical, or environmental factor and others more through interaction of multiple factors. For instance, teenage pregnancy with maternal undernutrition and poor antenatal care is more often associated with prematurity and these babies are more prone for birth complication such as hypoxic-ischemic encephalopathy; when this is combined with poor postnatal care, and lack of opportunities for learning, ID may be the outcome. Similarly, babies with chromosomal disorders may have intra-uterine growth retardation with low birth weight and these babies are at greater risk for perinatal complications.

Current approaches to classification of causes of ID are based on both the timing of the insult (pre-, peri-, and postnatal), and the type of insult (genetic and environmental). The following section describes this classification and is summarized in Table 3.1.

Prenatal causes

These are causes operative during the first and second trimester of pregnancy, especially during the first 12 weeks. These causes could be intrinsic to the embryo (i.e. embryonic/genetic causes) or could be extrinsic (i.e., environmental) in origin. Most known causes of ID are prenatal and tend to produce delays in development that are noticeable from very early infancy. Most of these babies tend to improve with age, albeit at a slower pace. However, there are some genetic causes that have an onset later and lead to progressive cognitive decline—the so-called childhood onset neuro-degenerative disorders or progressive encephalopathies. Some examples are lysosomal storage disorders and adrenoleukodystrophy.

- Embryonic or genetic causes: These are group of disorders with either known or inferred genetic aetiology, and are dealt in a separate section below because of their emerging importance.
- Prenatal maternal/environmental: These include deficiencies, infections, certain maternal diseases, exposure to toxins and teratogens and substances such as alcohol and nicotine. These conditions are of importance because they are preventable in nature.

Perinatal causes

These include causes that are operative from the third trimester of pregnancy to the neonatal period and can be further sub-classified into the following periods:

- Third trimester complications: There are many late pregnancy complications such as placenta praevia, chronic infections, uncontrolled gestational diabetes, severe pre-eclampsia or

Table 3.1 Aetiological classification of ID

Category	Sub-category	Type	Examples
Prenatal	Embryonic	Chromosomal disorders	Down syndrome, Klinefelter syndrome, Turner syndrome, Cri-du-chat syndrome, Trisomy 18
		Microdeletions	Prader-Willi syndrome, Angelman syndrome, William syndrome, Smith Magenis syndrome
		Single gene disorders	Autosomal dominant: tuberous sclerosis, neurofibromatosis
			Autosomal recessive: primary microcephaly, classical phenylketonuria, metachromatic leukodystrophy, Bardet-Biedl syndrome
			X-linked recessive: Hunter syndrome, Duchenne muscular dystrophy, Lesch-Nyhan syndrome, Börjeson-Forssman-Lehmann syndrome, pyruvate dehydrogenase deficiency,
			X-linked dominant: Rett syndrome, Fragile X syndrome, Aicardi syndrome, Coffin-Lowry syndrome
		Copy Number Variations	17q21.31 microdeletion, 1q21.1 microdeletion
	Adverse maternal / environmental influences	**Deficiencies**	Iodine deficiency, folate deficiency
		Exposure to other harmful chemicals	Teratogenic medications (such as thalidomide, phenytoin and warfarin sodium in early pregnancy), heavy metals, pollutants, abortifacients
		Maternal infections	Toxoplasmosis, rubella, cytomegalovirus, Herpes (TORCH infections), syphilis, and HIV
		Using substances	Alcohol (foetal alcohol syndrome), nicotine, and cocaine during early pregnancy
		Maternal diseases	Chronic renal or cardiac disease
		Others	Severe malnutrition in pregnancy, excessive exposure to radiation, Rh iso-immunization, hyperthermia
	Brain malformations of uncertain/multiple aetiology		Lissencephaly, double cortex, heterotopias, polymicrogyria, schizencephaly, neural tube defects, congenital hydrocephalus
Perinatal		Third trimester	Complications of pregnancy: Eclampsia Maternal Diseases: cardiac, renal, diabetes Placental dysfunction /deprivation of supply
		Labour	Severe prematurity, very low birth weight, hypoxic ischemic encephalopathy (birth asphyxia), Difficult and/or complicated delivery, Birth trauma
		Neonatal	Septicaemia, severe prolonged jaundice, hypoglycaemia
Postnatal			Brain infections (tuberculosis, Japanese encephalitis, and bacterial meningo-encephalitis), head injury, chronic lead exposure, severe and prolonged malnutrition, gross under-stimulation and experiential deprivation

Source data from *International Classification of Diseases*, 11th edition. World Health Organization.

eclampsia and severe systemic diseases in mother (e.g. cardiac problems, renal disease etc.). These may adversely affect the developing foetus, most often through placental dysfunction or deprivation of supply, and thereby affect brain development resulting in ID.

- Labour/birth related: Difficult and complicated labour such as prolonged second stage of labour, cord round the neck, premature rupture of membranes, abnormal presentations, and meconium aspiration can lead to severe asphyxia and result in hypoxic ischaemic encephalopathy (HIE). Babies with milder forms of HIE may escape significant brain injury, but those with more severe forms of HIE are likely to present with global developmental delays that later evolve as ID and/or cerebral palsy. Severe HIE often damages brain parenchyma around the lateral ventricles, and shows up as periventricular leukomalacia in brain imaging. There may also be mechanical damage to brain because of inappropriate use of forceps. In addition, prematurity and low birth weight are also significant risk factors for developmental problems.
- Neonatal: These include neonatal septicaemia, severe hypoglycaemia and hyperbilirubinemia of any cause, and may put the baby at risk for ID. Rh-isoimmunization leading to severe, prolonged hyperbilirubinemia and deposition of bile pigments in basal ganglia (kernicterus) can also lead to ID as well as dyskinetic cerebral palsy.

Postnatal causes

Causes operative beyond the neonatal period probably account for less than 10 per cent of ID and include infective encephalopathies (viral, bacterial, tuberculous) as well as traumatic brain injury. Severe, prolonged undernutrition and experiential deprivation are the two other factors that are known to be associated with impairments in cognitive development.

Prevalence of etiological factors

In an earlier exhaustive review, McLaren and Bryson found that chromosomal disorders were present in 4–8 per cent of mild ID and

20–40 per cent of more severe forms. Similarly, single gene disorders were responsible for 0–8per cent of mild ID and 5–20 per cent of more severe forms. Overall, aetiology was unknown in up to 62 per cent of mild ID and 40 per cent of more severe forms (9).

The relative importance and prevalence of different aetiological factors varies widely across different regions and countries. For instance, environmental factors continue to be important causes of ID in low and mid-income countries because of gaps in optimal pre-, peri-, and postnatal care. A clear difference has also been noticed in the pattern of distribution of different aetiologies in mild ID vis-a-vis more severe forms of ID. A review of causes of ID in India found that at least 25 per cent were attributable to environmental factors (10). A recent study from Brazil found that around 40 per cent of causes were environmental in origin (11). In contrast, a recent birth cohort study from Finland reported that in all cases of ID less than 15 per cent of aetiology were attributable to environmental factors and around 35 per cent attributable to genetic causes (12).

Aetiology remains unknown in at least about a third of cases. This scenario could be changing, with more genetic causes being uncovered. A recent major review of the genetic basis of ID has reported that there has been an exponential increase in the diagnostic yield in moderate and severe ID in the last five years, and the yield in 2015 was around 60 per cent. (13)

Genetics

Due to the observed patterns of inheritance, a genetic basis for ID had been suspected for more than a century. However, it is only in the last five decades that rapid strides have been made in uncovering precise genetic aetiologies, and this progress has been most marked in the last decade.

Application of advances in genetic technology has led to massive expansion in our understanding of the aetiology of ID. Some of the landmarks include the discovery of chromosomal analysis in the 1950s, fluorescent *in situ* hybridization (FISH) in the 1980s, Sanger sequencing in the 1990s and chromosomal microarray (CMA) and whole genome sequencing (WGS) over the last decade. Novel pathogenic variations are being described with the availability of these technologies. Also, the role of genes in the process of neural development and functioning is being characterized by advances in cellular and molecular biology.

As noted earlier, the complex and intricate process of brain maturation is under tight genetic control. It is estimated that around one-third of the approximately 20,000 genes in the human genome are thought to be involved in this process (14). Hence, any pathological alteration in the human genome is likely to lead atypical brain development and lead to ID. To date, more than 2000 genetic causes for ID have been identified (15). Some of these are more common, whereas most are rare in their occurrence, but as a group they contribute to a large proportion of the occurrence of ID. It is beyond the scope of this chapter to go into depths of genetics of ID, but this section will focus on some basic concepts of genetics as relevant to ID with examples. Excellent reviews are available on this topic for more exhaustive information. (13,16,17).

The pathogenic changes in human genome can be as small as a change in a single nucleotide or base pair (e.g. Hunter syndrome) or as big as the presence of an extra chromosome (e.g. Down syndrome).

Classification based on the type of change in the genome

- Chromosomal disorders: These are conditions that are characterized by microscopically visible abnormal alterations in the form of structural or numerical changes in the 22 sets of autosomes and one set of sex chromosomes. Typically, these alterations are detected by G-banded karyotyping in metaphase cells. Numerical alterations (or aneuploidies) could be the absence of a whole chromosome as in Turner syndrome (XO), or presence of an extra chromosome as in Down syndrome (Trisomy 21). Structural alterations include deletions, duplications, unbalanced translocations, or other re-arrangements of parts of chromosomes.
- Microdeletions/duplications including sub-telomeric rearrangements: These are conditions that may not be microscopically visible, but can be detected by a technique called Fluorescent *in situ* hybridization (FISH), in which a region of interest in the chromosome is examined for alterations. Typical examples are Prader-Willi syndrome and Smith Magenis syndrome. One class of this disorder is the alterations in tips of chromosomes (sub-telomeric regions) that are rich in genes, detected either by FISH or by more advanced techniques.
- Copy number variations (CNVs): copy number variation is defined as a deletion or duplication of a stretch of DNA as compared with the reference human genome. (18) Though gross DNA alterations can be detected by karyotyping and FISH, subtle gains and losses in DNA are now discernible by newer techniques that examine the chromosomes for deletions and duplications at the molecular level. These techniques are called chromosomal micro-array (CMA). As a class, these molecular variations have emerged as causative in ID and other neuro developmental disorders (NDDs) in the last decade, and are estimated to be responsible for 12 per cent of cases of ID (17). CNVs can be alterations in just a few thousand base pairs (kilobase or kB) to million base pairs (mB's). Not all CNVs are of pathological significance; some may be benign or of unknown significance. Also, they may be *de novo* (new changes) or can be inherited in Mendelian fashion. The examples of CNVs that are known to result in ID are 1q21.1 microdeletion, 1q21.1 microduplication, 3q29 microduplication, and 12q14 and 17q21.31 microdeletion (18). CMA is now considered as the standard diagnostic test and is rapidly replacing cytogenetic chromosomal analysis (17).
- Single gene disorders: A large number of genetic causes belong to this class in which there is an alteration in a single gene, either in the form of a change in a single base pair or nucleotide (point mutation) or other mechanisms such as trinucleotide repeat mutation. The commonest mechanism that such mutations give rise to disease is through alteration in structure and function of proteins that are coded by the gene. Table 3.2 lists some of these conditions. Apart from the pattern of inheritance, there are other methods of classifying single gene disorders, for example, syndromic (with a distinctive phenotype) or non-syndromic (when the features are non-specific). Likewise when a single gene disorder affects a key metabolic pathway, it is called inherited metabolic disorder. Targeted gene sequencing or whole genome sequencing are the genetic approaches to diagnose these disorders. There is about 30 pre cent

Table 3.2 Single gene disorders

Category	Sub-category	Examples
Inborn errors of metabolism (neurometabolic disorders)	Carbohydrate metabolism	Galactosaemia, glycogen storage disease
	Amino acid disorders	Phenylketonuria, homocystinuria, maple syrup urine disease
	Organic acidemias	Propionic academia, Methylmalonic academia, Glutaric academia type I
	Urea cycle disorders	Arginase deficiency, ornithine transcarbamylase deficiency
	Peroxisomal disorders	Zellweger syndrome, Refsum disease
	Lysosomal storage disorders	Mucopolysaccharidoses (Hunter, Hurler, Sanfillipo), Tay-Sach's disease, Mucolipidoses, Metachromatic leukodystrophy, Krabbe's disease, neuronal ceroid lipofuscinosis
	Fatty acid oxidation disorders	Medium Chain Acyl Dehydrogenase deficiency (MCADD)
	Congenital disorders of glycosylation	Disorders of protein n-glycosylation
	Endocrine	Congenital hypothyroidism
	Purine/ pyrimidine	Lesch-Nyhan syndrome,
	Mineral metabolism	Wilson's disease, Menkes disease
	Respiratory chain disorders	Mitochondrial encephalomyopathy, lactic acidosis, and stroke-like episodes (MELAS), Leigh's syndrome
Neuro-cutaneous		Tuberous sclerosis, neurofibromatosis
Brain malformations		autosomal recessive primary microcephaly, lissencephaly due to PAFAH1B1 gene mutation
Other specific syndromes		Fragile X syndrome, Rett syndrome Bardet Biedl syndrome, Smith-Lemli-Opitz syndrome, Coffin Lowry syndrome
Non-specific syndromes		ATRX mutations

excess of prevalence of ID in males compared to females, and this has been attributed at least partly to X-linked disorders that cause ID (XLID). These may be syndromic or non-syndromic. More than 100 X-linked genes have been identified to be mutated in XLID (13). Typical examples of syndromic XLID are fragile X syndrome, Rett syndrome, Hunter syndrome, and Coffin-Lowry syndrome.

- *Mitochondrial disorders:* There is a small part of human genome that is outside the nucleus and located in the mitochondria. This is the extra-nuclear genome or mitochondrial genome. Genes that are present in this part of human genome are responsible for producing proteins that play a key role in intra-cellular energy production. Point mutations and other pathogenic alterations in this mitochondrial DNA also contribute to occurrence of ID. These have a distinctive pattern of maternal inheritance, because the entire mitochondrial DNA is of maternal origin.
- *Polygenic/multi-factorial basis:* There are some gene variants that confer a small risk for the impairment in cognitive development, but by themselves do not cause ID. When several such gene variants happen to come together in an individual they can cause ID, and this is called polygenic inheritance. A major characteristic of polygenic inheritance is that these tend to become expressed under specific environmental circumstances, in other words through adverse gene-environment interactions. The precise contribution of this mechanism to the prevalence of ID is not known but suspected to play a significant role in the occurrence of milder forms of ID.

Common syndromes and their manifestations

Though there are hundreds of genetic causes for ID, there are some conditions that are clinically recognizable by their typical features. This section describes some of these disorders. These descriptions are based on standard resources (15,19,20).

- *Down Syndrome (DS)* is the most common genetic cause of ID and responsible for around 8 per cent of cases of ID, with a population prevalence of 1 per 800–1000 live births. It is caused by triplicate state (trisomy) of all or critical parts of chromosome 21. Most individuals have three free copies of chromosome 21; in about 5 per cent of patients, one copy is translocated to another acrocentric chromosome, most often chromosome 14 or 21. In the remaining cases of around 1 per cent, there is mosaicism. Except in cases of translocation with parents having balanced translocation, DS has a low recurrence risk of around 1 per cent or maternal age related risk, whichever is higher. Milder forms of ID is seen in younger ages with more severe disability as they age, because of decrease in velocity of their development. In cases where there is mosaicism, the level of ID may vary depending on the percentage of cells with trisomy 21, with many of them having relatively higher levels of functioning. DS is clinically characterized by typical facies, hypotonia, a flat facial profile, up slanting palpebral fissures, small, cup-shaped low-set ears, short stature, clinodactyly, and simian crease. Refractive error, hearing impairment, thyroid disorders, and cardiac anomalies are also common. By 60 years of age, about 60 per cent of subjects with DS develop Alzheimer's dementia. Advanced maternal age is an established risk factor for the condition. Although psychiatric disorders like depression and externalizing disorders are seen at a higher rate in DS (18–23%) than subjects with normal intelligence, they appear to occur at lower rate than ID of mixed aetiologies (30–40%) (21, 22). The incidence of birth of a child with DS in women aged 45 years or above have been reported to be as high as one in every 25 live births. However, more babies with DS are born to younger women and may be screened prenatally by testing blood levels of human chorionic gonadotropin (hCG) and unconjugated estriol, alpha-fetoprotein, and inhibin A. Diagnosis can be made by karyotyping.

- *Fragile X syndrome* is the most common inherited cause of ID, with a prevalence of one in 4000 males, and is clinically characterized by ID, connective tissue dysplasia (joint laxity), characteristic facial appearance, and post pubertal macro-orchidism. Facial features include large head, prominent forehead and chin (triangular face), and protruding ears. A significant proportion of cases have mild to moderate ID. Poor eye contact and social relatedness, motor stereotypy, speech delay, and sensory issues leads to diagnosis of autism spectrum disorder in a significant proportion of subjects. Expansion of trinucleotide CGG repeats in the 5' untranslated region of *FMR1* gene located at Xp27.3 causes 99 per cent of cases of fragile X syndrome. This expansion of CGG repeats leads to DNA methylation and transcriptional silencing of gene product FMRP which is involved in synaptic function. The affected individuals have CGG repeats of more than 200 (full mutation). Females with premutation (54–200 CGG repeats) present with infertility (premature ovarian failure) while male premutation carriers present with tremor, ataxia, and dementia (fragile X associated tremor/ataxia syndrome). Both methylated/unmethylated mosaicism and permutation/mutation mosaicism are seen in a minor fraction. Molecular genetic testing (methylation analysis of *FMR1* gene promotor or targeted mutation analysis using polymerase chain reaction of CGG repeats), can detect more than 99 per cent of the mutations in this gene. The mutation is inherited in an X-linked dominant manner. In some families, this syndrome shows anticipation, in which a premutation expands into full mutation in successive generations. Targeted treatments with medications such as minocycline and lovastatin have shown some benefits and are currently undergoing trial (23,24).
- *Rett syndrome* is clinically characterized by normal psychomotor development until 6–18 months old followed by a short period of developmental plateauing, then rapid regression of language, motor skills, and followed by long term stability. During the period of rapid regression, midline stereotypic hand movements replace purposeful hand movements. Seizures, acquired microcephaly, gait ataxia, and episodic apnoea/hyperpnoea are additional features that are commonly associated. Most cases are associated with severe ID. Behaviourally, symptoms of autism and anxiety are commonly seen. The syndrome is primarily seen in girls, as the *MECP2* gene (Xp28) mutation/deletion causing this syndrome is lethal in males (neonatal encephalopathy and death). The mutation usually arises *de novo* and is inherited in an X-linked manner. The majority of the pathogenic variants in this gene are detected using sequence analysis/targeted gene deletion analysis.
- *Prader-Willi syndrome (PWS)* is clinically characterized by hypotonia, hypogonadism, obesity, as well as small hands and feet. Severe hypotonia as well as feeding difficulties in early infancy is followed in early childhood by excessive eating and gradual development of morbid obesity. Hypogonadism is present in both males and females and manifests as genital hypoplasia, incomplete pubertal development, and in most, infertility. The ID is mild to moderate. PWS has a characteristic behavioural phenotype, with obsessive-compulsive symptoms (hoarding, redoing, symmetry, cleanliness, and so on), skin picking, and emotional lability. Psychotic disorders have also been reported in young adults with PWS (25). PWS is caused by absence of Prader-Willi critical region (deletion), situated in long arm of chromosome 15 of paternal origin (15q11.2-q13). This can occur either because of deletion in the critical region or maternal uniparental disomy 15 (both copies of chromosome 15 of maternal origin). Recurrence risk is negligible, except in a minority of the cases, where there is either an imprinting defect or translocation of 15q. DNA methylation analysis is abnormal (only methylated sequence in 15q paternally expressed genes) in almost all cases of PWS and is used to establish diagnosis. Further tests like FISH (detects deletion at 15q) and DNA polymorphism analyses (to detect uniparental disomy 15q) are used to establish recurrence risk for genetic counselling.
- *Angelman syndrome (AS)* is clinically characterized by severe global developmental delay, gait ataxia, and a unique behaviour, with paroxysms of laughter accompanied by flapping movements of hands. Usually they have normal periods of early infancy, followed by developmental delay noted by late infancy, leading to severe ID. Speech impairment, where expressive speech is more affected than receptive speech is seen. Tremors, seizures, and microcephaly are other common features. Maternally imprinted gene *UBE3A* at the 15q region, expressed only in chromosome of maternal origin (due to differential methylation) is involved in AS. Deletion of maternally inherited 15q11.2-q13 locus, uniparental disomy of the paternal chromosome 15 or an imprinting defect of the maternal chromosome 15q11.2-q13 locus has been described in 80 per cent of cases of AS. DNA methylation analysis of this locus at 15q detects abnormal methylation in all these three genetic changes. Further tests like FISH (detect deletion at 15q) and DNA polymorphism analysis (to detect uniparental disomy 15q) are used to establish recurrence risk for genetic counselling purposes. In cases where DNA methylation analysis is normal, an additional 11 per cent of cases having pathogenic variant of maternally derived *UBE3A* gene can be detected by targeted sequencing analysis. Recurrence risk varies from <1 per cent (deletion and uniparental disomy) to 50 per cent (imprinting defect and variant).
- *Williams-Beuren syndrome (WS)* is clinically characterized by distinctive 'elfin' facies, hoarse voice, and cardiovascular anomalies. Facial features include broad forehead, long face, dental abnormalities, small jaws, thick lips, and a hypotonic face. Cardiovascular anomalies (arising due to elastin arteriopathy), lead to narrowing of most arteries, of which supravalvular aortic stenosis is the most common and clinically significant manifestation. Most subjects with WS have some degree of ID, ranging from mild to severe. They have poor visuospatial skills with intact verbal skills. Behaviourally, they are quite sociable despite their speech difficulties. Anxiety disorders and attention deficit hyperactivity disorders are common. Idiopathic hypercalcemia and hypothyroidism are also seen. In most cases, WS is caused by *de novo* deletion of 7q11.23 (Williams-Beuren Syndrome Critical Region) that encompasses elastin gene (*ELN*). This deletion shows complete penetrance, and can be detected using FISH
- *22q11.2 Deletion Syndrome (includes Velo-Cardio-Facial Syndrome and DiGeorge Syndrome),* is clinically characterized by congenital heart disease (conotruncal abnormalities like ventricular septal

defect, right aortic arch, and tetralogy of Fallot) and palatal abnormalities (velopharyngeal incompetence, cleft palate and bifid uvula). Even though variable in their expression, facial features including nasal abnormalities (prominent nasal root, hypoplastic alae nasi), ear abnormalities, and asymmetric crying facies are seen. Hypocalcaemia and immune deficiency have been noted. Learning difficulties and mild ID are common. Autism spectrum disorder, schizophrenia and attention deficit hyperactive disorder and anxiety disorder are seen in a significant of proportion of subjects. Cognitive phenotypes include problems with retrieval of contextual information, visual memory, executive control and focusing of attention.(26) This deletion can be diagnosed using FISH or CMA. Inheritance of this syndrome is in an autosomal dominant manner.

- *Tuberous sclerosis complex (TSC)* is clinically characterized by hamartomata's/tumorous lesions, seizures and ID. TSC is also commonly associated with autism spectrum disorders. Skin lesions include flame-shaped hypomelanotic macules (ash-leaf spots), angiofibroma, sub-ungual fibroma and Shagreen patches (pigmented 'orange peel' skin lesions). Other lesions occur in brain (cortical dysplasia, sub-ependymal nodules, giant cell astrocytoma), kidney (angiomyolipomas, cyst, renal cell carcinoma), heart (rhabdomyomas), and lungs (lymphangioleiomyomatosis). Brain tumours and renal abnormalities are the leading life-threatening conditions. Uncontrolled seizures contribute significantly to the severity of ID. Higher risk for development of autism spectrum disorders, attention deficit hyperactivity disorder, depression and anxiety disorders is seen. TSC is an autosomal dominant disorder, because of mutations in TSC1 (hamartin) and *TSC2* (tuberin) genes, both of which are tumour suppressor genes. The variants show compete penetrance. However, two-thirds of the mutation arise *de novo*. Variants of these two genes can be found in 85 per cent of cases by sequence analysis and gene targeted deletion/duplication analysis. Medications such as rapamycin and everolimus targeting mTOR pathways that are affected in this condition have shown some beneficial effects.
- *Cornelia De Lange syndrome (CdLS) or Brachmann–de Lange Syndrome* is clinically characterized by distinct facial features, limb reduction defects, and growth retardation. Facial features include synophrys, high arched eyebrows, long eyelashes, short nose with anteverted nares, long and smooth philtrum, and microcephaly. Limb reduction defects like micromelia, oligodactyly, and clinodactyly are common. Intellectual function ranges from average to severe disability. Many also show symptoms of autism spectrum disorder, attention deficit hyperactivity disorder, self-injurious behaviour, and internalizing disorders. Cardiac septal defects, refractive error, hearing loss, gastrointestinal disorders (reflux, malrotation), and hypogonadism are the other common associated features. Subjects with the milder phenotype have less growth retardation, cognitive, and limb involvement but have similar facial features. Variants of *NIPBL* gene located on 5p13 chromosome region (autosomal dominant inheritance) account for 60 per cent of cases. An additional 5 per cent (mainly the milder phenotype) are explained by variants in *SMC1A* gene located in Xp11.2 chromosome region (X-linked recessive inheritance). Other gene variants in *RAD21* (8q24.11), *SMC3* (10q25.2), *HDAC8* (Xq13.1) explain <10 per cent of cases. Sequence analysis and gene targeted deletion/duplication analysis are used to establish the presence of the described variants. Most cases are sporadic and there is marked variability in expression. Presence of parental germline mosaicism (in a minor proportion of cases) or carrier status will increase the recurrence risk in siblings.
- *Rubinstein Taybi syndrome* is clinically characterized by distinct facial features, broad thumb and toes, short stature, and moderate to severe ID. Facial features include slanted palpebral fissure, prominent beak shaped nose, and maxillary hypoplasia. Postnatal onset of growth retardation leads to short stature. Obesity may occur in childhood and adolescence. Congenital heart diseases, cryptorchidism, renal anomalies, and hirsutism are other common associations in this syndrome. Behavioural issues like hyperactivity, impulsivity, and symptoms of autism are also frequently seen. Targeted duplication/deletion analysis and sequence analysis can identify variants in *CREBBP* (16p13.3) and *EP300* (22q13.2) genes in 50 per cent and 3–8 percent of individuals with this syndrome respectively. The majority of the cases are of a sporadic nature, with negligible recurrence risk in siblings. Variants are inherited in an autosomal dominant manner.
- *Epileptic encephalopathies* are a group of disorders that are characterized by infantile presentation of multiple, difficult to control type of seizures (tonic-clonic, myoclonic, atonic, and absence), global developmental delay, and gross EEG abnormalities such as hypsarrhythmia. When they grow up they often have severe forms of ID and/or ASD. Examples are West syndrome, Lennaux-Gestaut syndrome, and Dravet syndrome. The genetic basis of many of these disorders ae being discovered in the recent years.
- *Autosomal recessive primary microcephaly* is a condition of severe congenital microcephaly because of a small brain and varying degrees of ID, with no other major anomalies. It is genetically heterogeneous, with at least 11 genes shown to be mutated giving rise to this condition. All mutated genes are known to have a role in mitotic division of neuronal progenitor cells.

Neural basis and molecular pathways: Beginning with neural stem cells, growth and maturation of the brain, or neurodevelopment, proceeds through neuronal proliferation by symmetric cell division followed by asymmetric cell division, and later neuronal migration, differentiation, and organization into neuronal circuits that take up specific functional roles. There is continuous remodelling of the brain in terms of inter-neuronal connections through dendrites and axons, and synaptic development and pruning. This process is largely complete by the end of adolescence, but stretches beyond that age in terms of further myelination. Any factor that adversely affects any of these stages is likely to impact on cognitive development, thereby leading to ID.

Structural changes in ID have been the focus of post-mortem studies historically, but in recent times studies have focused on brain imaging. In general, gross structural changes have been identified in 14 per cent to 40 per cent of patients with ID (27). These abnormalities range from mild cortical atrophy, ventricular dilatation, to gross changes such as lissencephaly, polymicrogyria, microcepahly, schizencephaly and heterotopias.

With the initial discovery of pheylketonuria several decades ago by Asbjørn Følling, hundreds of inherited metabolic disorders associated with ID have since been described, and the list is growing. The metabolic pathways have also been elucidated for many of these disorders. Over the years these disorders have become the focus of public health importance because many of them are preventable and treatable following early detection.

The precise mechanisms by which mutations lead to ID are being discovered and described with rapid advances in molecular and cellular biology and development genetics. Some of these are disturbances in neural proliferation (primary microcephaly), neuronal migration (lissencephaly), synaptogenesis and synaptic functioning (fragile X syndrome, PAK3 mutations), transmembrane protein functions (NLGN4 mutations), NMDA receptor signalling pathways (DLG3 mutations), inter and intra-cellular signalling pathways such as Ras-MAP Kinases pathway (neurofibromatosis 1, Rubinstein Taybi syndrome, Coffin-Lowry syndrome), and chromatin remodelling (MECP2 mutations) (28).

Genetics in clinical management: There are several reasons to identify the cause of ID. From a genetic viewpoint, identifying the genetic cause has significant implications in the clinical management of ID. This includes genetic counselling, prevention of genetic disorders through mass screening, and treatment of genetic disorders. Advanced techniques such as preimplantation genetic diagnosis and analysis of foetal DNA in maternal circulation are rapidly emerging as options in prevention and management.

Approach to identify aetiology

Identifying the cause or causative factors is integral part clinical evaluation and calls for specialized set of knowledge and skills. These are dealt with in some detail in this section.

- *Need to identify the cause:* There are many reasons as to why the cause of ID needs to be identified. These include: spotting a treatable or modifiable cause (e.g. hypothyroidism, PKU, etc.), screening and managing known complications of a genetic disorder (hypothyroidism and Alzheimer's dementia in Down syndrome), genetic counselling, and other preventive strategies, for prognostication, educating, and empowering the families, and for research and advancement of medical knowledge.
- Clinical evaluation to identify the causative factors involve the following steps:
  - Family, developmental, medical history and behavioural patterns, including three generation genetic diagrams.
  - *Detailed physical examination to identify clues to aetiology:* Head to toe examination to detect major and minor congenital anomalies, and systemic examination. Table 3.3 provides an approach to physical examination with examples. Presence of

Table 3.3 Physical examination in ID

Aspect of examination	Examples of anomalies
Facial appearance	Typical facies (Down, coarse, progeroid), elongated, triangular, mid-facial hypoplasia
Height	Short stature, tall stature, increased arm span, gigantism
Weight	Obesity, emaciation
Head circumference	Microcephaly, macrocephaly
Shape of skull:	Brachycephaly, scaphocephaly, trigonocephaly, oxycephaly, plagiocephaly
Ears	Low set, small, large, malformed, protruding, posteriorly rotated, pre-auricular tags, cup-shaped
Skin	Dry and coarse, café-au-lait spots, abnormal pigmentation, haemangioma, ichthyosis, eczema, absence of sweating
Nose	Depressed nasal bridge, short and stubby, beak shaped, bulbous tip, flaring or hypoplastic nostrils
Vision	Amblyopia, refractive error, nyctalopia
Hearing	Partial or complete loss
Neck	Short, webbed, torticollis
Eyes	Deeply set, proptosis, microphthalmia, upslanting/downslanting eyes, telecanthus, hypertelorism, epicanthal folds, strabismus, nystagmau, ptosis, bushy eyebrows, synophrys, microcornae, corneal clouding, Kayser-Fleischer rings, cataracts, coloboma of iris, blue sclera, telangiectasia
Palate	High arched, shallow, clefting, bifid uvula
Hair	Hirsutism, light-coloured, double whorl on scalp, easily breakable, low anterior/posterior hairline
Other facial features	Long/absent philtrum, micrognathia, sloping forehead
Hands	Simian crease, spade shaped, small
Fingers	Clinodactyly, camptodacyly, arachnodactyly, short little finger, syndactyly, polydactyly, broad thumb
Chest:	Pectus excavatum, pectus carinatum, nipple anomalies, gynaecomastia, inverted nipples, cardiac problems
Abdomen	Protuberant, umbilical hernia, hepato-splenomegaly, inguinal hernia
Spine:	Kyphosis, scoliosis, spina bifida
External genitalia	Hypogenitalism, macro-orchidism, undescended testis, ambiguous genitalia, hypospadias, absent secondary sexual characteristics, shawl scrotum
Feet	Pes planus, pes cavus, valgus/varus anomaly, broad hallux, increased distance between 1st & 2nd toe
Skeletal	Exostoses, increase carrying angle, joint hypermobility

Table 3.4 Physical investigations to determine the cause in ID

Category	Test	Examples of conditions detected
Biochemical and metabolic	Urine screen for abnormal metabolites	Phenyketonuria, homocysteinuria, galactosemia, MPS
	Thyroid function test	Hypothyroidism
	Advanced metabolic tests (Gas chromatographic Mass Spectroscopyc (GCMS), tandem mass spectroscopy (TMS)	Wide range of neuro-metabolic disorders such as fatty acid oxidation disorders, aminiacidopathies, urea cycle disorders and organic acidurias
	Enzyme studies	Tay-Sach disease, meatachromatic leukodystrophy
Genetic studies	Karyotyping	Down syndrome, other chromosomal disorders
	FISH	Prader-Willi syndrome, William syndrome, Sub-telomeric deletions
	Chromosomal micro-array	Copy number variations
	Targeted mutation testing	Fragile X syndrome (FMR1 mutation), Rett syndrome (MECP2 mutation),
	Exome sequencing	Point mutations
Brain imaging	MRI	Tuberous sclerosis, lissencepahly, other brain malformations
Electrophysiological	*EEG*	Epileptic encephalopathies such as West syndrome
Hearing tests	Hearing evaluation (BAER)	Sensory-neural hearing impairment
Ophthalmological tests	Visual evaluation	Wilson disease, cataract, Optic atrophy, cortical blindness, refractive error
Others	Blood group of child and parents	Rh iso-immunization
	Immunologic tests (Ig M antibodies)	TORCH infections

three or more minor congenital anomalies indicates a genetic aetiology (20).

- *Interpretation and synthesis:* Once the history and clinical examination has been completed there is a need to review, interpret and synthesize the available information so as to narrow down the possibilities. This will help in further planning, such as collecting further information, referral, and deciding the relevant investigations. It is always a good practice to write down the synthesis or formulation, ending with the diagnostic possibilities and further course of action. There are many electronic databases and online sources such as Online Mendelian Inheritance in Man (OMIM) and Gene Reviews that are useful in searching for genetic causes (15,19).
- *Investigation and referrals:* There are several recommendations by international expert groups about the range and utility of different investigations in ID and developmental delays (16,17,27). However, the list of investigations and referrals are often dictated by the unique characteristics of a given case. Table 3.4 lists some of the investigations and referrals that are commonly employed.

Conclusion

Over the years there has been better understanding and refinement of the concept of ID, and also major advances in understanding the aetiological basis of this condition, especially genetic causes. Uncovering the aetiology is an essential part of the clinical work-up of an individual with ID and leads to better management.

Glossary

Annealing refers to complementary sequences of single stranded DNA or RNA paring by hydrogen bonds to form a double stranded polynucleotide, usually used to describe the binding of a DNA probe to a DNA strand during a polymerase chain reaction.

Alleles are alternative forms of a gene or DNA sequence occurring at the same locus on homologous chromosomes.

Allelic association refers to the occurrence of two particular alleles at neighbouring loci on the same chromosome more commonly than would be expected by chance.

Allelic heterogeneity refers to the situation where a clinical condition can be caused by any of several different mutations within a certain gene.

Aneuploid (that is not euploid) refers to a chromosomal constitution having one or more missing or extra chromosomes.

Anticipation is the tendency of a disease to become more severe, more frequent, or to start at an earlier age, in successive generations of a family.

Association is the statistical tendency of two things to go together more often or less often than by random chance.

Balanced translocation refers to a chromosomal constitution, having no extra or missing chromosomal material.

cDNA or complimentary DNA is a single stranded DNA copy of messenger RNA, made using reverse transcriptase. Unlike genomic DNA, cDNA's are tissue specific.

Candidate gene is a gene identified as being a possible cause of a genetic disease usually when mutated.

Carrier refers to a non-affected person possessing a mutant gene in its heterozygous form.

Cascade screening is a method of ascertaining gene carriers by systematic testing of the extended family of the index patient affected.

Comparative genomic hybridization (CGH) is a technique for detecting genetic sequences anywhere in the genome that are present in an abnormal number of copies.

Concordance is the presence of the same character or trait in both members of a pair of twins.

Congenital refers to the condition being present at birth not necessarily genetic.

Copy number variant (CNV) is a form of DNA variation in which a certain sequence (which may be anything between a few to a million base-pairs) is present in differing numbers of copies in different individuals.

Deletion refers to the loss of genetic material.

Dominant is a character or trait if it manifests in a heterozygote. Dominance and recessiveness are properties of characters, not of genes or alleles.

Dosage sensitive refers to genes where different non-zero copy numbers have an effect on the phenotype.

Dysmorphology refers to the study of congenital malformations arising from abnormal embryogenesis.

Empirical risks refer to the risk of recurrence of multifactorial or polygenic disorders based on family studies survey data, unlike risks worked out by applying genetic theory.

ENCODE (Encyclopaedia of DNA elements) is an international collaborative project that aims to identify all functions of human DNA (www.genome.gov/10005107).

Epigenetic refers to the phenomenon of making heritable changes in gene expression from a cell to a daughter cell, or sometimes from generation to generation, without changing the nucleotide sequence, usually by the process of DNA methylation and changing structure of chromatin.

Epistasis refers to the phenomenon where the effect of one gene is dependent on the presence of one or more modifier genes in the genetic background. Epistatic mutations have different effects in combination than individually.

Euploid state of a cell or organism means the presence of a complete set of chromosomes with no extra or missing chromosomes.

Exome is the totality of all exons in a genome.

Exon is a segment of genomic DNA that corresponds to sequence in a mature mRNA. Exons include the 5' and 3' untranslated regions of a gene as well as the coding sequence.

Familial refers to the tendency to run in families not necessarily genetic.

Fluorescence in situ hybridization (FISH) is a technique of *in situ* hybridization, using a fluorescently labelled DNA or RNA probe, used to detect presence or absence of specific sequences in chromosome preparations.

Fragile site in a chromosome preparation is a region that appears relatively uncoiled and extended. Most fragile sites are non-pathogenic polymorphic variants. The FRAXA and FRAXE sites are pathogenic.

Functional genomics is the study of the functions of all the genes in a genome or all the genes expressed in a cell or tissue.

G-banding is a standard procedure in which chromosomes are treated so that they stain in a characteristic and reproducible pattern of dark and pale bands.

Gene tracking uses linked polymorphic markers to follow the segregation of a chromosomal segment for example pathogenic mutation through a pedigree if it is not possible to check for the mutation directly by sequencing.

Genome refers to the totality of the genetic material of an organism.

Genome-wide association study (GWAS) is a study in which single nucleotide polymorphisms spread across the genome are tested for association with a disease in a case-control study.

Haploid of a cell/organism means having only a single genome (23 chromosomes—human genome).

HapMap project is an international collaboration, aiming to catalogue all the conserved ancestral chromosome segments in several human populations (www.hapmap.org).

Hardy-Weinberg distribution is a mathematical relationship between gene frequencies and genotype frequencies observed when no distorting factors are present. In humans, it is seen rarely in recessive conditions where many cases are due to consanguinity.

Heritability refers to the influence of genetic as opposed to environmental factors contributing to phenotypic variance.

Heterozygous refers to possessing different alleles at the same locus on homologous chromosomes.

Homozygous refers to having both alleles at the same locus on homologous chromosomes.

Homologous chromosomes are chromosomes that pair at meiosis and contain the same set of gene loci.

Hybridization is the process by which single stranded DNA or RNA anneal to complementary DNA or RNA.

Intron is a segment of a gene that is part of the primary transcript but is excised by the splicing machinery and not included in the mature mRNA.

Inversion is a structural abnormality in which part of a chromosome is in the wrong orientation compared to the rest.

Karyotype is the chromosomal constitution of an individual. A karyogram is a display of the individual's chromosomes.

Linkage is a phenomenon whereby loci that are close together on a chromosome tend to segregate together in families.

Linkage equilibrium refers to the association of particular alleles at two or more loci in the population, seen when the loci are closely linked and the alleles are features of a shared ancestral chromosomal segment.

Locus is the specific position of a gene or DNA sequence on a chromosome.

Locus heterogeneity is a situation where a clinical phenotype can be caused by mutations at any one of several different loci.

Lod score is a statistical measure of the significance of evidence for or against a linkage and is the logarithm of the odds that the loci are linked. Positive Lod scores are evidence in favour of linkage, negative scores evidence against and the threshold for significance is a Lod score of +3.0.

Lyonization or X-inactivation is the process by which one copy of the X chromosome in mammalian females is inactivated at the blastocyst stage by epigenetic mechanisms.

Marker refers to a biochemical or DNA polymorphism occurring close to a gene and hence used in gene mapping.

Mendelian inheritance refers to the manner in which genes and traits are passed from parents to their offspring. The four modes of Mendelian inheritance are: autosomal dominant, autosomal recessive, X-linked dominant, and X-linked recessive.

Microdeletion is a very small deletion (<3–5 Mb) seen on a chromosome usually detected by fluorescence *in situ* hybridization, comparative genomic hybridization, or multiplex ligation-dependent probe amplification.

Missense mutation is a point mutation in which a single nucleotide change results in a codon producing a different amino acid.

Monosomy refers to a chromosomal constitution having one copy of one particular chromosome, but two of all the others (e.g. 45, XO syndrome).

Mosaic refers to having two or more genetically different cell lines, and an individual can be a mosaic for a chromosomal variant or single-gene change.

Multifactorial is an inclusive term used to describe a character that is determined by many factors including genetic and environmental factors.

Multiplex ligation-dependent probe amplification (MLPA) is a method used for simultaneously checking a large number (30–50) of short DNA sequences for copy number variations.

Mutation refers to the alteration of the normal sequences of nucleotides in a gene.

Next generation sequencing is a collective name for different technologies that conduct millions of sequencing reactions in parallel, thereby generating more sequence data than other techniques.

Odds ratio for a variant is the ratio of the odds, for people who do not have the variant of being a case rather than a control in a case-control study.

Penetrance refers to the probability of a character (not a gene or allele) to become manifest given a particular genotype.

Phenotype refers to the observable physical or biochemical characteristics of a person, reflecting genetic constitution and environmental influence.

Point mutation refers to the substitution, insertion, or deletion of a single nucleotide in a gene.

Polygenic refers to the effects of the combined action of a several susceptibility genes, each with a small effect.

Polymerase chain reaction is a technique used in molecular biology, using DNA polymerase to amplify a single or a few copies of a segment of DNA, by generating thousands of copies of a particular DNA sequence.

Polymorphism refers to a genetic variant present in a population, at a frequency too high to be maintained by recurrent mutation alone.

Positional candidate is a candidate gene located in a chromosomal region identified by linkage analysis as containing a disease gene.

Positional cloning helps in identifying a disease through linkage analysis followed by testing positional candidates for mutations.

Pre-mutation is seen in diseases caused by expanded nucleotide repeats, an expansion that is not long enough to cause the disease, but long enough to destabilize the repeat, so that later generations are affected (e.g. between 50–200 CGG repeats in the FMR1 gene in Fragile X syndrome).

Probe is a piece of single stranded nucleic acid labelled for example with a radioligand (^{32}P) or a fluorescent dye, that is used in hybridization assays to test for the presence of a complimentary sequence.

Recessive refers to a character that is not manifest in a heterozygote. Dominance and recessiveness are properties of characters, not of genes or alleles.

Restriction fragment length polymorphism (RFLP) is a DNA polymorphism due to a nucleotide change that creates or abolishes the recognition site for restriction endonucleases (that cleaves dsDNA), causing a variation in size of DNA fragments produced.

Robertsonian translocation refers to a translocation in which two acrocentric chromosomes (13, 14, 15, 21, 22) are joined close to their centromeres.

Sanger sequencing is a method of DNA sequencing, based on the selective incorporation of chain terminating dideoxynunucleotides by DNA polymerase during in vitro DNA replication.

Single nucleotide polymorphism (SNP, pronounced snips) refers to any polymorphic variation at a single nucleotide and is the most common type of genetic variation in people.

Southern blotting is a technique used in molecular biology, transferring DNA molecules, usually restriction fragments, from an electrophoresis gel to a nitrocellulose membrane in such a way that the DNA banding pattern present in the gel is reproduced on the membrane and then hybridized to a labelled probe.

Tandem repeats are any array of consecutive DNA sequence repeats that are adjacent to one another. They include three subclasses: satellites (100kb–1Mb), minisatellites (1kb–20kb), and microsatellites (short tandem repeats <150bp).

Translocation refers to a structural abnormality in which two chromosomes exchange non-homologous segments.

Trisomy refers to having three copies of one particular chromosome, but two of all the others.

MULTIPLE CHOICE QUESTIONS

Questions

Please select the single most appropriate answer.

1. Diagnosis of intellectual disability (ID) in an individual requires establishing the following features except:
A. Evidence of sub-average intellectual functioning
B. Significant impairment of adaptive functioning
C. Presence of a chromosomal or genetic disorder
D. Onset of the condition during the developmental period

2. Which one of the following statements about Fragile X syndrome is not correct?
A. The prevalence is reported to be 1/4000 males
B. The genetic abnormality is caused by abnormal trinucleotide CGG repeats at a fragile site on the X chromosome
C. Associated with microorchidism
D. Associated with mitral valve prolapse
E. Associated with reduced volume of cerebellar vermis

3. A 10-year-old girl presenting with ID, severe epilepsy, repetitive hand movements that are difficult to control and a history of rapid regression of skills, after a period of normal development until her first birthday, is likely to have the following condition
A. Down syndrome
B. Rett syndrome
B. Prader-Willi syndrome
B. Fragile X syndrome
B. Landau-Kleffner syndrome

4. Which one among the following is not a feature of Cornelia De Lange syndrome?
A. Self-injurious behaviour
B. Microcephaly
C. Limb reduction defects
D. Synophrys
E. Short philtrum

5. Which one among the following is not an example of a single gene disorder?
A. Tuberous sclerosis
B. Lesch-Nyhan syndrome
C. Williams-Beuren syndrome
D. Metachromatic leukodystrophy
E. Hunter syndrome

Answers

1. C. In 30–50 per cent of cases the cause of ID is idiopathic. Non-genetic factors prenatal, natal, and postnatal causes are also known to cause ID.
2. C. Fragile X syndrome is associated with macroorchidism not microorchidism. Hippocampal size may be increased in some patients, and the size of the cerebellar vermis is reduced.
3. B. Rett syndrome affects 1 in 12,000 girls born each year and rarely affects males. It is caused by a mutation in the MECP2 gene, which is found on the X chromosome. There's usually no family history of Rett syndrome, almost all cases (over 99%) are caused by *de novo* mutations. Landau-Kleffner syndrome, also called acquired epileptic aphasia is an epilepsy syndrome of childhood. It usually starts before the age of six years affecting twice as many males than females. The main clinical features are loss of acquired speech and language skills and seizures.
4. E. Children with Cornelia de Lange syndrome are reported to have a long and smooth philtrum. Cornelia de Lange syndrome is also characterized by self-injurious behaviour.

Other features include language delay, autism, stereotypic movements, sleep disturbance, and severe to profound ID.

5. C. Williams-Beuren syndrome is an example of contiguous gene deletion syndrome or microdeletion syndrome, and is caused by the deletion of 7q11.23; all other conditions listed are single gene disorders.

REFERENCES

1. Wechsler D. *The Measurement of Adult Intelligence*. Baltimore, MD, US: Williams & Wilkins Co; 1939. ix, 226.
2. Sternberg RJ. Beyond IQ: *A Triarchic Theory of Human Intelligence*. CUP Archive; 1985.
3. Cattell RB. Theory of fluid and crystallized intelligence: A critical experiment. *J Educ Psychol.*, 1963;54(1):1–22.
4. Wechsler D. *Wechsler Intelligence Scale for Children—Fourth Edition (WISC-IV)*. San Antonio TX Psychol Corp. 2003.
5. Schalock RL, Borthwick-Duffy SA, Bradley VJ, Buntinx WHE, Coulter DL, Craig EM, et al. *Intellectual Disability: Definition, Classification, and Systems of Supports.* Eleventh Edition. *American Association on Intellectual and Developmental Disabilities*;2010.
6. American Psychiatric Association. Diagnostic and statistical manual of mental disorders (DSM-5®). *American Psychiatric Pub.*, 2013.
7. ICD-11 Beta Draft [Internet]. [cited 2016 Oct 15]. Available from: http://apps.who.int/classifications/icd11/browse/f/en#/http%3a%2f%2fid.who.int%2ficd%2fentity%2f605267007.
8. Hodapp RM, Burack JA. *Issues in the Developmental Approach to Mental Retardation*. Cambridge University Press; 1995.
9. McLaren J, Bryson SE. Review of recent epidemiological studies of mental retardation: Prevalence, associated disorders, and etiology. *Am J Ment Retard.*, 1987;92(3):243–254.
10. Srinath S, Girimaji S. Epidemiology and child and adolescent mental health problems and mental retardation. 1999.
11. Karam SM, Barros AJD, Matijasevich A, dos Santos IS, Anselmi L, Barros F, et al. Intellectual disability in a birth cohort: Prevalence, etiology, and determinants at the age of 4 years. *Public Health Genomics*, 2016;19(5):290–297.
12. Heikura U, Linna S-L, Olsén P, Hartikainen A-L, Taanila A, Järvelin M-R, et al. Etiological survey on intellectual disability in the northern Finland birth cohort 1986. *Am J Ment Retard.*, 2005;110(3):171–180.
13. Vissers LELM, Gilissen C, Veltman JA. Genetic studies in intellectual disability and related disorders. *Nat Rev Genet*, 2015 Oct 27;17(1):9–18.
14. Brain Basics: Genes at work in the brain [Internet]. [cited 2016 Oct 15]. Available from: http://www.ninds.nih.gov/disorders/brain_basics/genes_at_work.htm
15. 'mental retardation'—OMIM—NCBI [Internet]. [cited 2016 Oct 15]. Available from: https://www.ncbi.nlm.nih.gov/omim/?term=%22mental+retardation%22.
16. Michelson DJ, Shevell MI, Sherr EH, Moeschler JB, Gropman AL, Ashwal S. Evidence Report: Genetic and metabolic testing on children with global developmental delay: Report of the Quality Standards Subcommittee of the American Academy of Neurology and the Practice Committee of the Child Neurology Society. *Neurology*, 2011 Oct 25;77(17):1629–1635.
17. Moeschler JB, Shevell M, Committee on genetics. Comprehensive evaluation of the child with intellectual disability or global developmental delays. *Pediatrics*, 2014 Sep 1;134(3):e903–e918.
18. Mefford HC, Batshaw ML, Hoffman EP. Genomics, intellectual disability, and autism. N Engl J Med. 2012;366(8):733–743.
19. GeneReviews®—NCBI Bookshelf [Internet]. [cited 2016 Oct 15]. Available from: https://www.ncbi.nlm.nih.gov/books/NBK1116/.
20. Jones KL, Jones MC, Del Campo M. *Smith's Recognizable Patterns of Human Malformation*. Elsevier Health Sciences; 2013. https://www.us.elsevierhealth.com/smiths-recognizable-patterns-of-human-malformation-9781455738113.html
21. Einfeld S, Tonge B. Population prevalence of psychopathology in children and adolescents with intellectual disability: II epidemiological findings. *J Intellect Disabil Res.*, 1996;40(2):99–109.
22. Dykens EM, Kasari C. Maladaptive behavior in children with Prader-Willi syndrome, Down syndrome, and nonspecific mental retardation. *Am J Ment Retard.*, 1997;102(3):228–237.
23. Leigh MJS, Nguyen DV, Mu Y, Winarni TI, Schneider A, Chechi T, et al. A randomized double-blind, placebo-controlled trial of minocycline in children and adolescents with fragile x syndrome. *J Dev Behav Pediatr JDBP.*, 2013;34(3):147–155.
24. Çaku A, Pellerin D, Bouvier P, Riou E, Corbin F. Effect of lovastatin on behavior in children and adults with fragile X syndrome: An open-label study. *Am J Med Genet A.*, 2014;164(11):2834–2842.
25. Dykens E, Shah B. Psychiatric disorders in Prader-Willi syndrome. *CNS Drugs.*, 2003;17(3):167–178.
26. Biswas AB, Furniss F. Cognitive phenotype and psychiatric disorder in 22q11. 2 deletion syndrome: A review. *Res Dev Disabil.*, 2016;53:242–257.
27. van Karnebeek CDM, Jansweijer MCE, Leenders AGE, Offringa M, Hennekam RCM. Diagnostic investigations in individuals with mental retardation: A systematic literature review of their usefulness. *Eur J Hum Genet.*, 2005 Jan;13(1):6–25.
28. Chelly J, Khelfaoui M, Francis F, Chérif B, Bienvenu T. Genetics and pathophysiology of mental retardation. *Eur J Hum Genet.*, 2006 Jun;14(6):701–713.

4

Children and Adolescents with Intellectual Disability

Tom Berney and Mark Lovell

Introduction

The psychiatry of young people with intellectual disability (ID) is a hybrid speciality which has emerged from the specialities of Intellectual Disability Psychiatry and Child, and Adolescent Psychiatry. Here we focus on how it differs from these, leaving aside issues such as the cause and effect of specific medical disorders, behavioural phenotypes, and neurodevelopmental conditions which are covered in other chapters.

It is characterized by:

1. The dependency of young people on others, particularly on their family members and carers. Their referral is usually at the behest of others, so that their cooperation cannot be assumed but must be won.
2. Disturbance which arises in the context of family relationships. Such is the emphasis on these in any assessment or intervention that, at times, the child's problems may seem peripheral.
3. The young person lives their life in parallel systems, notably in their home and at school, with substantial variation in their presentation in the different situations. The system for specialist education is complex, but it is also readily accessible and more intimately involved than in the mainstream schools. This means that it plays a greater part in any intervention and there is a greater emphasis on multiagency teamwork, community (as opposed to clinic) appointments, and information sharing. This brings some sacrifice of privacy by the person and their family which, coupled with limited comprehension, complicates the issues around confidentiality and its boundaries.
4. The overlay of ID blurs the distinction between child and adult pathology with a greater recognition of lifespan continuities softening, for example, the sharp demarcation between childhood neurodevelopmental disorder and adult personality disorder. The transition to adulthood is a matter of major importance.
5. The young person lives in a very distinct world, subject to specific legal constraints and firmly embedded in the complex network of children's services which includes education, child health, and social services.

Prevalence

Epidemiology depends on reliable classification which is subject to psychiatry's ever evolving concepts. At present, there is an arbitrary division into:

1. The Neurodevelopmental Disorders—notably autistism spectrum disorder (ASD) and attention deficit hyperactivity disorder (ADHD), as well as a more generalized ID. As we dissect their symptomatology, we start to recognize the overlapping presence of other disorders, such as motor tics and developmental coordination disorder. It is debatable whether these should be considered as disorders (an essential qualification for health funding in the USA), disabilities, or conditions (akin to personality types). Lacking definitive laboratory tests, their shape and identity is under constant review and our perception has shifted with the development of the behavioural phenotype. Habit disorders, expressed in problems with sleep, eating, continence, and behaviour, often arise from this substrate as it struggles to cope with an unsuitable environment. The personality disorders, a concept coming from general psychiatry, remain lodged in a classificatory limbo, although they also would seem to meet the requirements for a neurodevelopmental disorder.
2. The psychiatric disorders, which include psychosis, depression, bipolar disorder, and the emotional disorders. The old, clear distinctions are being eroded by a growing recognition that these too have neurodevelopmental characteristics and, at the same time as DSM and ICD define their characteristics with ever-greater precision, their very identity is being questioned. Their categories are undermined by shared symptomatology, an inconsistent response to treatment, and overlapping genetic predispositions, coupled with a comorbid association with the neurodevelopmental disorders.
3. Medical disorders. These include epilepsy which is present in about 3 per cent of those with ASD, 7 per cent of those with Mild ID, and 35 per cent of those with Severe ID (1). However, the greater the degree of ID, the more likely it is that, besides any

characteristic dysmorphism, there will be physical abnormalities which range from the immune system to the gastrointestinal.

In the context of ID, the emphasis in childhood is on neurodevelopmental conditions while psychiatric disorders tend to come to the fore only in adolescence but often pass unrecognized until adulthood. Neurodevelopmental conditions change with age, many, such as ASD and ADHD, tending to improve as the result of a combination of innate maturation, learned compensatory skills and a shift to a more accommodating environment. This trajectory means that symptoms are often starker in childhood although puberty, a process which may stretch over years, may bring deterioration. This does not reflect the complexity of change in coexistent psychiatric disorders (2) and it is only now that we are coming to appreciate how frequently a disorder, often subtly altered, may persist into adulthood. By contrast, the trajectory of other phenotypes, such as Fragile X and Williams syndrome, may show later deterioration and there is also the disconcerting suggestion that there may be late-onset variants, notably in ADHD (3).

Terminology and classifications change with time and place. For example, in the USA 'learning disability' is the equivalent of 'specific learning difficulty' in the UK and of 'developmental learning disorder' in ICD-11. The UK adopted 'learning disabilities' in place of 'mental handicap', unaware that 'learning difficulties' was an established educational category, let alone that 'moderate' learning difficulties identified those who had a 'mild' degree of 'learning disabilities/ID. The professionals in children's services, unaware of the distinction and the different grading of impairment, used the terms interchangeably and the term 'moderate' became so ambiguous as to be meaningless without amplification. This confusion looks to be resolved when we move on to 'intellectual disability'.

Where there is one neurodevelopmental disorder, there are likely to be others (the more so, the more numerous and severe its symptoms), and the tendency has been to identify co-occurring disorders. Their protean nature leads to the identification of new categories such as Pathological Demand Avoidance (PDA) and Multiple Complex Developmental Disorder, representing a merger of ASD with psychosis (4). Individual symptoms are common to different disorders and it is arguable that, rather than emphasize symptom clusters, we might see these disorders as the constituent elements of an ill-defined neurodevelopmental porridge. Categories persist though, as they allow us to plan services and individual treatments. However, whatever the conceptual framework, the discovery of some neurodevelopmental symptoms should encourage the clinician to seek others; thinking in categories risks the impetuous oversight of symptomatology thought to be unrelated.

Diagnostic consistency is also threatened by idiosyncratic clinical definitions of thresholds such as the points at which repetitive self-stimulation becomes self-injury, at which sexual activity is considered abusive, or at which a collection of traits becomes syndromic.

Any estimate of prevalence must take account of the nature of the population and its selection pressures. Specialist schools would seem to provide ready access to a clearly defined and representative population but, in practice, studies struggle to take account of the real nature of educational allocation. This can be distorted by the inclusion of children in mainstream provision, travel to specialist schools outside the study area, selective non-attendance and family disengagement. Surveillance studies are particularly prone to variations in the diagnostic process and fashion, producing, for example, the remarkable geographical variation in ASD prevalence across the USA (5).Childhood ID is closely associated with psychiatric disturbance (6). A study of UK children, aged 5–16 years, found 14 per cent of those who had a diagnosable psychiatric disorder, to have an ID. Conversely, the prevalence of psychiatric disorder (notably ASD, ADHD, and Conduct Disorder) was 36 per cent among children with ID compared to 8 per cent for those without (7). Different studies produce different results, often politicized in support of a campaign, making it essential to consult the original reports to understand how conditions and populations had been defined and selected and whether there had been appropriate allowance for age, ability, and gender.

Assessment

Any assessment of someone with ID, irrespective of age, must take into account their environment which, for a child, includes their family, teachers, and carers. Whether interviews are done in the home, school, or clinic depends on their purpose. For example, the school is convenient for a comparison of the child's performance across different settings or their presentation with a peer group whereas a home visit may be the only way to ensure privacy (something that is important where there are issues such as parental mental health or sexual problems) or to meet a key family member. Wherever it is, a community approach makes for flexibility. On the other hand, joint work with a multidisciplinary team or other departments (such as genetics, paediatrics, or neurology) may require the set format of a clinic.

The direction of the assessment is determined by its purpose; it must be clear who is driving the referral and what their expectations are. Disagreement about the referral, its nature, and necessity, requires careful negotiation if the clinician is to avoid being seen as aligned with one side and losing credibility with the other.

An assessment should aim to get a reasonably reliable, all-round view of:

1. The young person's presentation—their symptomatology and its development over time, including its changes with different people or circumstances. The significance of a symptom (such as inattentiveness or impulsivity) must be measured against the person's age, ability, and gender. Communication difficulties, particularly in identifying and describing internal states that include thoughts and feelings (alexithymia), can block access to a substantial element of subjective psychiatric symptomatology. Although emotional literacy may be learned later, but the barrier is particularly severe in childhood and much psychiatric disorder may pass unnoticed unless revealed by behaviour: depression may be recognized while anxiety can be difficult to spot and even harder to categorize.
2. Their background:
   (a) Their family, their relationships and any events that might have affected the person.
   (b) Their school and their staff—including how the child behaves in their unstructured free time, at meals, and in the classroom

3. Their development from early childhood, including such characteristics as their warmth and responsiveness, as well as the more standard milestones.
4. Their ability, both cognitive and functional, and including their self-help, social, communicative, and academic skills. Here, standard instruments such as the Kauffman Brief Intelligence Test (K-Bit) (8), Vineland Survey Scales (9), British Ability Scale (BAS) and the British Picture Vocabulary Scales (BPVS) (10) may be sufficient without the need to obtain more specialist psychometry such as the Wechsler Intelligence Scale for Children (WISC) or detailed language assessments. For many, school is the most demanding time that they will encounter. It can reveal disabilities that, although contributing to their difficulties, might otherwise remain unidentified.
5. Their medical history—physical problems are easily overlooked or misinterpreted because of limited communication, which prevents them from telling others how they feel and giving a history, let alone cooperating (11). Epilepsy is particularly frequent and, even when identified, more subtle, sensory, subclinical, or modified seizures may be missed in the desire not to ascribe every symptom to it—diagnostic overshadowing works both ways.
6. Their physical state—which includes genetic stigmata as well as evidence of physical disorder and illness. Fast-changing technologies mean that it is worth consulting the local service as to how far previous genetic testing precludes further and routine tests. The individual's difficulty with reporting symptoms, the risk that these will be overshadowed by behavioural signs and the likelihood of future medication make a case for a baseline series of routine medical investigations.

Given sufficient information, the clinician makes a summary diagnosis, a provisional hypothesis that will explain their plan of management. However, everything changes over time, and this diagnosis should be regularly reviewed and explicitly modified or discarded as it becomes inappropriate or no longer useful.

The process, multidisciplinary and multiagency, defines a community of people around the young person that includes family, carers, and professionals. The last may include psychologists (educational and clinical), teacher, support worker, speech and language therapist, occupational therapist, community nurses (the young person and the parents may each have their own), social worker, various doctors, as well as other key figures, such as people from the voluntary agencies and clergy. Someone, often the clinician, has to orchestrate and conduct this network.

Treatment

The family

Family work is fundamental, its nature depending on when the disability was recognized. Severe forms of ID may be identified in pregnancy or soon after birth, but it might not be until adolescence that mild ID is recognized when the child starts failing at school, or when a similar disability shows in a sibling. Its arrival can overturn a family's world, bringing a large number of appointments in varied places with multiple professionals and over a long time. It can alter access to the community and to work, make going to the shops a complicated adventure, isolate people from friends and dominate the family, sometimes to the detriment of siblings (12). Genetic investigation can intrude, dividing families and demanding difficult decisions about future pregnancy.

The response to discovering that your child has a disability varies, but a bereavement model has been helpful, provided it is recognized that it is not an inevitable process (13). Complicating this is the effect of psychosocial adversity, a frequent accompaniment to ID (14) which, coupled with disturbance in the child (15), contributes to increased levels of parental psychiatric disturbance. However, causality is not straightforward as exampled by the association of ASD with maternal depression which can predate her child's arrival (16).

The diagnostic assessment can be the start of planning to help the child and their family; the gateway to a range of special services from education, social services, and health as well as to the various associations dedicated to particular disorders. Close behind should come support for the family, taking many forms and delivered in the community by a multidisciplinary team. Whatever the treatment, its delivery must be consistent. This means that the initial focus is often on marital and family issues to ensure that the family are comfortable enough to put programmes into practice. Parental confidence is fundamental; the knowledge that they are in control of their child's circumstances, disorder, and future. In ID psychiatry, the placebo effect is a powerful element that can contribute usefully to a treatment programme (17, 18).

Much depends on the level of community support and the ability to help parents cope, not just with an unhappy child, but also difficult living circumstances, critical neighbours, siblings under stress, and each other (19).

The parental phenotypes may have elements that echo their child's disability and call for joint work between child and adult services. This can be very effective, provided it is recognized that it extends the network of people that the family have to cope with.

Medication

Given the increased frequency of medical disorder, particularly epilepsy, it is not easy to disentangle the extent to which psychotropic drugs are prescribed inappropriately. The same principles apply both to ID and to paediatric prescribing where consent is a recurrent difficulty, increasing the prescriber's responsibility to ensure that its benefits outweigh its risks. Medication is introduced at a low dose, gradually increased ('start low, go slow'), closely monitored with the expectation of the unexpected, and constantly reviewed with the intention of its eventual withdrawal (20). The better the available resources, including education, social care, and alternative treatments, the less medication is likely to be needed.

Neuroleptics and stimulants may be prescribed more frequently than for the mainstream population (11, 21, 22) but this may simply reflect the higher prevalence of disorder. There are no published audits of paediatric prescribing in this population but, given that psychiatric prescribing is usually long-term and its adverse effects may only emerge after some years, it has to be approached with caution. In February 2019, concern about misuse of medication led the Royal College of Paediatrics and NHS England to launch the STAMP (Supporting Treatment and Appropriate Medication in Paediatrics) programme.

Research is beginning to identify which drug is most likely to be effective for a specific disorder or symptom, suggesting, for example, that glutamate antagonists may be a starting point in Fragile-X or oxytocin in autism. However, the response by a specific individual to a specific drug is so idiosyncratic as to encourage experimental, off-licence and off-label prescribing.

Outcome measures

The measures developed for mainstream use may not be appropriate, relevant, or ethical, particularly where they influence funding. Any measure must be sensitive to the (sometimes small) changes that can be significant for a child or their family. Change may be hidden by a 'ceiling effect' related to the underlying disability. While there are some specific routine outcome measures for children and adolescents with ID, they are still unproven and norms have yet to be established.

Services and their boundaries

Disability brings entry into a service maze within which people have to navigate through the shifting responsibilities of a variety of agencies. Their evolution in England is a typical example: the care and education of people with a disability originally fell to health services with the emphasis on the physical leaving little room for mental health. Although dominated by hospital care, only 20 per cent of the ID population were admitted; most people remained at home with their parents in a system that worked while the population was substantially paediatric. In 1970, Social Services and Education began to take responsibility for their components with the intention of replacing segregated, specialist schooling with integration into mainstream education in line with the philosophy of normalization. The process, see-sawing with the rabid enthusiasm required for change, has arrived at a mix of provision, which ranges from the specialist and sometimes residential to the all-inclusive mainstream school, the latter using different forms of extra support in an effort to match the kaleidoscope of individual need (23). The original, discrete population, tidily grouped into special schools became diffused across a wider network along with the professionals serving it.

The voluntary bodies, many established by parents, played a prominent part. The Charity for the Asylum of Idiots established five large asylums across England in the 1850s. Camphill (a Rudolf Steiner school) started its first community in Aberdeen in 1940, the National Association of Parents of Backward Children (later to become Mencap) started in 1946 and the National Autistic Society in 1962. Other forms of disability led to the Royal National Institute for the Blind (1868), the National Deaf Society (1944) and the Spastics Society (1952), which has since become Scope. These and many others have developed services dedicated to specific disabilities, promoted research, the concept of neurodiversity, and a more tolerant society.

However, these categorical boundaries have been blurred by our better recognition of the overlaps in neurodevelopmental disability. In turn, this has coloured diagnostic practice and given us a jigsaw of services.

ID Psychiatry was established as a separate speciality, delivering a lifespan service to which the limited life expectancy lent a paediatric bias and the assumption that the demands of disability overrode those of age. However, improved survival, the move to community care, and the arrival of other psychiatric specialities all combined to change both the service's structure and the clinician's role. Increasing standards, expectations, and demands together with a different style of clinical practice, personnel, and specialist services led to the all-age ID Psychiatrist being replaced, first by the generic (all-ability) Child Psychiatrist and more recently, by the hybrid specialist in the Psychiatry of Child and Adolescent ID, although recruitment and training opportunities have limited the last. Besides the question as to how such a specialist might get the appropriate training and recognition, there is the question of how they should relate to other areas of the child mental health service; whether they should be a stand-alone service or be incorporated within the broader Child and Adolescent Mental Health Services (CAMHS) (24). This has been a long-running discussion, with the underlying ethos that people with ID should not be excluded from mainstream (generic) services (25). These shifts are reflected in the successive revisions of the advice published by the Royal College of Psychiatrists over the last 25 years (26). The style of the hybrid specialist service differs substantially from that of mainstream CAMHS in its emphasis on working in the community rather than the clinic, being part of the network of care around the child, largely within the home, schools, respite/short break units, and in coalition with a variety of statutory and independent agencies. In addition, there is the marked medical bias which helps knit it together with developmental paediatrics, community child health, and other specialities such as neurology and genetics which, in overstretched or informal services brings the risk of gaps in medical responsibility (19).

The downside of these changes has been a weakening of the links with adult ID services, affecting the process of that transition. The other effect, in line with the change in mainstream children's services, has been the reduction of inpatient resources and their replacement by intensive community provision. However, delay in this has led to a growth in residential admissions to schools as well as hospitals in far-flung places (19, 27).

The school

The basis for the management of much disorder, whether it is predominantly neurodevelopmental, emotional (e.g. anxiety and anger), or behavioural, is educational. Teaching is a blend of compensatory (to make up for the learning that most acquire informally) and remedial (to correct innate deficits, such as social skills, emotional literacy or language). This approach sits well with treatment derived from a more formal behavioural analysis with, for example, Rewards Based Learning, already familiar in the world of autism, which has translated into ID practice as Positive Behavioural Support.

Such teaching may be delivered across a wide range of circumstances from the child in a mainstream school with additional support (a class-room assistant or a withdrawal unit) through to separate specialist schools that deal with a certain category of disability. Understandably, the more specialist the school the more likely it is to take young people with psychiatric disorders and the more skilled its staff with those individuals. Such a school can become a cornerstone of the community psychiatric service and, where residential, may have much in common with a hospital unit. Consequently, a key attribute of the clinician is the ability to develop a sustained liaison with school staff and the wider educational system.

Transition

Transitions take many forms as the young person moves towards adulthood and increased autonomy, but change is inevitable, involving not just new personnel, places and bureaucracy, but a shift in style, usually with the emphasis moving from the family to the individual and from care to support. Discharge from hospital or a change to a more open ward brings changes in the degrees of supervision and structure. Geographical change, often to a very different setting may come with a move to a far-distant college or adult placement. Less obvious are administrative changes, for example in funding or the rationalization of a community team, which can be sufficient to unseat a family or, at least, to affect their relationships.

Adult Learning Disability services do not mirror those for younger people, particularly for those who have a mild ID or whose impaired functional ability is largely the result of some other disorder (such as ASD). Many of the elements of the young person's service, notably schools and colleges, do not have adult equivalents and, in particular, the very active part that can be played by the school health service, which includes not just paediatrician and nurse, but also the speech, occupational, and physiotherapists, who can form a longstanding team that includes a school's teachers and carers.

Therefore the change in people and place may be profound and must be managed carefully, safely and with sufficient time. It needs to include all the major agencies and be prepared far enough in advance to be a natural progression with little uncertainty. For example, once a child has been identified as having additional needs in England, an Education, Health, and Care Needs Plan is prepared and then revised annually until they are 25 years old (by which time they should have engaged successfully in their new, adult services) (28). Perhaps the most important element in this is the transparency that allows the individual and family to understand what is happening, where things are going, and to see that their worries are understood by all.

It is easy to underestimate the time required: the more complex a case is, the longer the required transition period. For example, if a young person is to move to a bespoke, residential placement (as against being fitted into an existing vacancy), it can take up to a year to find the accommodation, to recruit and train the staff, and to plan the actual move. Autism, in particular, can make an individual exquisitely sensitive to change so that a relatively seamless continuity may need to go beyond simple discussion to funding an overlap of existing staff with the new; something that can be cost-effective where it holds a tenuous gain, averting relapse or readmission.

However, no matter how good the intention, transition frequently turns into a dislocation for the young person and their family, destabilizes a hard-won mode of life and reveals unsuspected fragility.

Childhood's legal framework

Young people are subject to a range of legal frameworks which, while varying with jurisdiction, have common, underlying principles. The United Nations Convention on the Rights of the Child has shaped legislation to 'put children first' and has been important in encouraging services that minimize discrimination and encourage integration and inclusion. It has been incorporated into national legislation such as the Children and Social Work Act (2017), which is about the social care of vulnerable children; children with disabilities being of special concern in child protection.

Increasing awareness of the individual's capacity to give or withhold consent to a particular decision has led to a steady reduction in the required age for competence, exemplified by the decision in the case of Gillick (29). In this erosion of the extent of parental authority, it is noteworthy that the threshold for the acceptance of treatment is lower than for its refusal.

Legislative concepts are evolving as they are defined and clarified by statute and case law. In England, at present, the Mental Capacity Act (2005) and its safeguards only apply to those above 16-years-old while the Mental Health Act (2007) applies irrespective of age, Consequently, even where a young person is considered capacitous and they and their families desire hospital admission, they may well be detained if they need an intrusive level of supervision.

Consent for clinical research has always been a contentious issue and, historically, has been worked around by getting a proxy consent from a parent or the legal guardian. With the development of the concept of capacity, the inclusion of children in research has become more subject to scrutiny. It is relatively straightforward where it is in the individual's best interests to be included in a project if, for example, it allows access to a treatment that otherwise would be unavailable. However, where there is no direct benefit to the individual, for example where the child is only in the placebo arm of a therapeutic trial, it becomes more problematic. Where the project has little impact on the child, the same rules apply as to children of normal ability, research involvement requiring parental permission, an independent assessment of the balance of benefit against harm, and the child's assent (30). However, the presence of disability can affect the child's perception and make minor procedures, such as phlebotomy, intolerable.

Forensic issues

Common issues run through ID irrespective of age, including fitness to be interviewed, fitness to plead, and the reasonable adjustments to be made by the Criminal Justice System. However, young offenders are served by a separate system, balanced between education (e.g. residential schools and colleges with varying degrees of security), criminal justice settings (e.g. youth offender institutions), social services (e.g. secure children's homes), and mental health (e.g. community forensic services, and low and medium secure inpatient settings).

A number of disabilities appear to be associated with offending behaviour such as an association with genetic conditions or an environment that promotes impulsivity, irritability, or aggression. ADHD, particularly with conduct disorder appears a predictor of adult offending (31). The suggestion that autism might predispose someone to offending behaviour (32, 33) is controversial and there is a strong case for the protective effect that comes with a preference for rule-bound regularity.

Common threads are:

- A misinterpretation of rules and social situations which may be linked to a failure to foresee either the seriousness or the likely outcome of their actions.
- A failure to appreciate the need to change or a rigidity that makes change especially difficult.
- A sense of immunity, the result of being excused from the consequences of their previous actions because of their disability.
- A greater level of supervision keeps many out of trouble.

A maladroit response by the police may compound these issues, whether they hide the problem by failing to proceed or amplify it by an inflexibly standard response.

Child abuse

Children are open to abuse and those with disability even more so, even if the ID is mild in severity (34). Their intimate dependency on adults, their use of residential placements for respite, residential care or treatment, and their limited communication, combine to make them vulnerable. Children, the focus of paedophilic interest, are likely to be targeted by a group that differs from those who abuse adults with ID. Additionally, the experience of being a victim of abuse, particularly sexual abuse, is associated with later becoming a similar offender (35).

Case study 1: The contribution of developmental delay

A 6-year old boy has not settled into school. He is different to the other children and does not get involved in their play, but his comprehension and his self-help skills are within normal limits. He is always on the go, fidgety and restless; he is unable to concentrate on anything for more than a couple of minutes. He has an unusually strong interest in a children's TV character, a repetitive style of speech and, when excited, he flaps his hands.

Likely diagnoses: ASD and ADHD. While he is unlikely to have ID, he may well have one or more developmental learning disorders (specific learning difficulties) such as dyslexia, as well as other neurodevelopmental disorders such as developmental coordination disorder. His strong interest in the TV character, coupled with his repetitive communication and his hand flapping suggest that he may have ASD. His inattentiveness and hyperactivity probably indicate ADHD which, of itself, may interfere with his peer relationships. While ASD and ADHD often co-occur, it may require the treatment of the ADHD before it is clear whether ASD is present.

The same six-year-old as before but with a more pronounced, two year developmental delay. This was recognized when he was three years old and he is now about two years behind his peers.

Likely diagnoses: Mild ID, possibly ASD and ADHD. The important, clinical judgement is how far a Mild ID might be responsible for the symptoms of ADHD. A four-year-old should be able to sit still for periods of time and, when interested, can concentrate for longer than a few minutes. While ADHD is a possibility here, it is not normally diagnosed in a child below a developmental age of five years unless it is very clear. Hand flapping is not unusual with emotional overflow and a strong interest in a children's TV character may be less abnormal. However, the repetitive language suggests that ASD may also be present.

The same six-year-old child but developmentally four years behind.

Likely diagnoses: Moderate/Severe ID. At this degree of ID there is likely to be very limited vocabulary with all of the above symptomatology and, to consider ASD, there needs to be additional symptomatology (e.g. of social isolation and poor non-verbal language) to support an additional diagnosis of ASD.

Learning point: A knowledge of childhood development, normal and delayed, is essential in the diagnosis of neurodevelopmental disorder. This must take account of chronological age and intellectual ability in order to tease apart and interpret the significance of a symptom.

Case study 2: The multifactorial underlay to behavioural disturbance

Over the last year, a 15-year-old girl who has severe ID, ASD and no functional language, has had episodes lasting several hours, during which she will cry, hold her abdomen, bang her head repetitively, and lash out at others. Some of these episodes occur after shift changes in the residential unit where she has regular respite care and some appear to be in response to noise. Yet others occur at no particular time and for no obvious reason. Her sleep has been disturbed for several months.

Assessment: This requires a comprehensive history which includes her development, physical health and her social relationships and circumstances, as well as focusing on her symptoms and any potential triggers. She should have a physical examination and her behaviour should be observed in different situations. The aim is to come to a formulation which includes differential diagnoses and the potential function of her behaviour.

Additional information: Physically, she has poor dentition, constipation, and her abdominal holding appears to coincide with her menstrual cycle. Her urinalysis was clear but she was found to have chlamydia. Closer observation found that she appeared to become very anxious in response to a variety of events and that this was followed by anger and aggression. These events included unplanned changes of circumstance (transitions), certain noises (such as a vacuum cleaner), or simply a sudden, loud noise. She would also appear more distressed when certain male staff were on duty at the respite unit.

Formulation: She has ID which entails comprehension and communication difficulties. It seems likely that she might have discomfort from constipation, her menstrual periods and her teeth. Her ASD might account for her difficulties with change and a sensory intolerance of noise. In addition, the chlamydial infection suggests the possibility of sexual abuse.

Management: Her physical complaints should be treated appropriately. Speech and language therapy should be asked for help in improving communication and occupational therapy should be asked for advice on her sensory issues. She should have psychological work to assess and reduce her anxieties which may be helped by offering stability and predictability across her life. The possibility of sexual abuse should be investigated within her local authority's safeguarding process by social services and possibly the police.

Learning points: An ill-defined pattern of distress may be the result of a number of contributory factors and there should be a conscious consideration of the possible biological, psychological, and social factors that might be in play. Abuse should always be considered as a potential factor when exploring behavioural change in vulnerable young people.

MULTIPLE CHOICE QUESTIONS

Questions

Please select the most appropriate answers.

1. Epilepsy is present in approximately how much of the population?

A. 3 per cent of those with ASD
B. 50 per cent of those with Severe Intellectual Disability
C. 6 per cent of the general population
D. 7 per cent of those with Mild Intellectual Disability
E. 12 per cent of those with ADHD

2. What is the prevalence of psychiatric and behavioural disorder in children and young people (5–16 years old) with ID?

A. 24 per cent
B. 50 per cent
C. 16 per cent
D. 36 per cent

3. The UK term of *Mild Intellectual Disability* is the equivalent of what?

A. Mild Learning Disabilities in the USA
B. Mild Learning Difficulties in the UK
C. Mild Learning Disabilities in the UK
D. Moderate Learning Difficulties in the UK
E. Mild Mental retardation in ICD-10

4. Abuse of children with ID is:

A. Less frequent than in the general population because the children require constant supervision
B. Less often noticed because the child is isolated by difficulties with communication and peer relationships
C. More frequent because of the child's intimate dependency on adults.
D. Less frequent because the child has numerous professionals teaching/caring for them who might detect its occurrence.
E. Very unlikely in a well-managed residential school

5. Child and adolescent psychiatry of ID is characterized by working with (rank the following):

A. Very dependant young people, held in an unusual network of care, who are vulnerable to a variety of forms of abuse
B. Families that are coping with disability and the specialist world of disability
C. Specialist networks within health, education and social care
D. A series of transitions over time, from home, to school, to adult services
E. Psychiatric disorders which have a basis of physical disorder
F. Special educational provision

Answers

1. A and D. Epilepsy is present in approximately 3 per cent of those with ASD and 7 per cent of those with Mild Intellectual Disability
2. E. Psychiatric and behavioural disorders are present in about 36 per cent of 5–16 year olds with ID
3. C, D and E. ICD-11 has replaced *Mental retardation* with *Disorders of Intellectual Development* but the grading, from *Mild* through to *Profound*, remains the same. A *Mild Disorder of Intellectual Development* is equivalent to *Moderate Learning Difficulties.*
4. B & C. Child abuse is more common than in the general population because of the child's dependency, the opportunities with multiple carers and the isolating effect of its disabilities.
5. All these points are characteristic and different clinicians attach different weight to them in their contribution to their enjoyment of the speciality—so effectively a question to make people think (all answers are correct).

Conclusions

The complexity of this area, both of the conditions experienced by the individual and their family and of the services to support and treat them means that it is developing into a separate specialism working with a specialist network.

The skills required are a composite of those derived from both child and adolescent psychiatry and ID psychiatry. The psychiatrist has to assess, formulate/diagnose and treat children and adolescents with ID, using a framework that combines the medical, psychological and social elements and draws on a wide range of community resources, particularly education and social care.

This is an under-researched field, so that the evidence to support the treatments used is very limited, and there is a greater reliance on the therapeutic trial than in other areas of psychiatry.

REFERENCES

1. Airaksinen EM, Matilainen R, Mononen T, Mustonen K, Partanen J, Jokela V, et al. A population-based study on epilepsy in mentally retarded children. *Epilepsia*. 2000;41(9):1214–1220.
2. Simonoff E, Jones CR, Baird G, Pickles A, Happé F, Charman T. The persistence and stability of psychiatric problems in adolescents with autism spectrum disorders. *Journal of Child Psychology and Psychiatry*. 2013;54(2):186–194.
3. Faraone SV, Biederman J. Can attention-deficit/hyperactivity disorder onset occur in adulthood? *JAMA Psychiatry*. 2016;73(7):655–656.
4. Jansen LMC, Gispen de Wied CC, Van der Gaag RJ, ten Hove F, Willemsen Swinkels SWM, Harteveld E, et al. Unresponsiveness to psychosocial stress in a subgroup of autistic-like children, multiple complex developmental disorder. *Psychoneuroendocrinology*. 2000;25(8):753–764.
5. Centers for Disease Control and Prevention. Prevalence of autism spectrum disorder among children aged 8 years—Autism and developmental disabilities monitoring network, 11 Sites, United States, 2010. Morbidity and Mortality Weekly Report (MMWR). 2014;63(SS02):1–21.

6. Charman T, Pickles A, Simonoff E, Chandler S, Loucas T, Baird G. IQ in children with autism spectrum disorders: data from the Special Needs and Autism Project (SNAP). *Psychological Medicine*. 2011;41:619–627.
7. Emerson E, Hatton C. Mental health of children and adolescents with intellectual disabilities in Britain. *British Journal of Psychiatry*. 2007;191:493–499.
8. Kaufman AS, Kaufman NL. Kaufman *Brief Intelligence Test. Wiley Online Library*; 2004.
9. Sparrow SS, Cicchetti DV, Balla D. Vineland Adaptive Behavior Scales:(Vineland II), Survey Interview Form/Caregiver Rating Form. Livonia, MN: Pearson Assessments. 2005.
10. Dunn LM, Dunn DM. T*he British Picture Vocabulary Scale. GL Assessment Limited*; 2009.
11. Allerton LA, Welch V, Emerson E. Health inequalities experienced by children and young people with intellectual disabilities: A review of literature from the United Kingdom. *Journal of Intellectual Disabilities*. 2011;15(4):269–278.
12. Giallo R, Gavidia-Payne S. Child, parent and family factors as predictors of adjustment for siblings of children with a disability. *Journal of Intellectual Disability Research*. 2006;50(12):937–948.
13. Bicknell J. The psychopathology of handicap. *British Journal of Medical Psychology*. 1983;56:167–178.
14. Emerson E, McCulloch A, Graham H, Blacher J, Llwellyn GM, Hatton C. Socioeconomic circumstances and risk of psychiatric disorders among parents of children with early cognitive delay. *American Journal on Intellectual and Developmental Disabilities*. 2010;115(1):30–42.
15. Totsika V, Hastings RP, Emerson E, Berridge DM, Lancaster GA. Behavior problems at 5 years of age and maternal mental health in autism and intellectual disability. *Journal of Abnormal Child Psychology*. 2011;39(8):1137–1147.
16. Rai D, Lee BK, Dalman C, Golding J, Lewis G, Magnusson C. Parental depression, maternal antidepressant use during pregnancy, and risk of autism spectrum disorders: Population-based case-control study. *BMJ*. 2013;346:f2059.
17. Weimer K, Colloca L, Enck P. Placebo effects in psychiatry: Mediators and moderators. *The Lancet Psychiatry*. 2015;2(3):246–257.
18. Sandler A. Placebo effects in developmental disabilities: Implications for research and practice. *Mental Retardation and Developmental Disabilities Research Reviews*. 2005;11(2):164–170.
19. Lenehan DC. These are our children. Independant review. London: Council for Disabled Children; 2017 26 January 2017.
20. Turk J. Use of medication in children and young people with intellectual disability and challenging behaviours. In: Lovell M, Udwin O, eds. Intellectual disabilities and challenging behaviour. Occasional Papers. London: *Association for Child and Adolescent Mental Health*; 2014. pp. 36–44.
21. Osunsanmi S, Turk J. Influence of age, gender, and living circumstances on patterns of attention-deficit/hyperactivity disorder medication use in children and adolescents with or without intellectual disabilities. *Journal of Child and Adolescent Psychopharmacology*. 2016;26(9):828–834.
22. Tobi H, Scheers T, Netjes KA, Mulder EJ, de Bildt A, Minderaa RB. Drug utilisation by children and adolescents with mental retardation: A population study. *European Journal of Clinical Pharmacology*. 2005;61(4):297–302.
23. Mittler P. Educating pupils with intellectual disabilities in England: Thirty years on. *International Journal of Disability, Development and Education*. 2002;49(2):145–160.
24. Wright B, Williams C, Sykes M. A child and adolescent mental health service for children with intellectual disabilities—8 years on. *The Psychiatrist*. 2010;34(5):195–199.
25. World Health Organisation. The case for change. Better health, Better lives: Children and young people with intellectual disabilities and their families; 26–27 November 2010; Bucharest. Copenhagen: WHO Regional Office for Europe; 2010.
26. Royal College of Psychiatrists. *Psychiatric Services for Young People with Intellectual Disabilities*. Council Report. London: Royal College of Psychiatrists; 2016. Report No.: CR200.
27. Lenehan C, Geraghty M. Good intentions, good enough?: A review of the experiences and outcomes of children and young people in residential special schools and colleges. November 2017.
28. Department for Education; Department of Health. Special educational needs and disability code of practice: 0–25 years. London: HMSO; 2014 (updated 2015).
29. Cave E. Goodbye Gillick? Identifying and resolving problems with the concept of child competence. *Legal Studies*. 2014;34(1):103–122.
30. Kodish E. Informed consent for pediatric research: Is it really possible? *The Journal of Pediatrics*. 2003;142(2):89–90.
31. Lindsay WR, Carson D, Holland AJ, Taylor JL, O'Brien G, Wheeler JR. The impact of known criminogenic factors on offenders with intellectual disability: Previous findings and new results on ADHD. *Journal of Applied Research in Intellectual Disabilities*. 2013;26(1):71–80.
32. Geluk CAML, Jansen LMC, Vermeiren R, Doreleijers TAH, van Domburgh L, de Bildt A, et al. Autistic symptoms in childhood arrestees: Longitudinal association with delinquent behavior. *Journal of Child Psychology and Psychiatry*. 2012;53(2): 160–167.
33. Siponmaa L, Kristiansson M, Jonson C, Nyden A, Gillberg C. Juvenile and young adult mentally disordered offenders: The role of child neuropsychiatric disorders. *The Journal of the American Academy of Psychiatry and the Law*. 2001;29(4):420–426.
34. Euser S, Alink LR, Tharner A, IJzendoorn MH, Bakermans-Kranenburg MJ. The prevalence of child sexual abuse in out-of-home care: Increased risk for children with a mild intellectual disability. *Journal of Applied Research in Intellectual Disabilities*. 2016;29(1):83–92.
35. van der Put CE, Asscher JJ, Wissink IB, Stams GJJM. The relationship between maltreatment victimisation and sexual and violent offending: Differences between adolescent offenders with and without intellectual disability. *Journal of Intellectual Disability Research*. 2014;58(11):979–991.

5

Measuring Outcomes Including Use of Rating Scales and Instruments in People with Intellectual Disability

Peter Tyrer, Freya Tyrer, Marisa Hanney, and Stephen Tyrer

Introduction

In this chapter, we describe commonly used rating scales and instruments to measure outcomes of children and adults with intellectual disability (ID). This is not an easy task, as the assessment of outcomes in ID poses much greater problems than measuring outcomes in those without ID. For most assessments of outcome it is traditional to include both self-ratings and observer ones. It is also sensible to do this, because clearly many symptoms such as depression and anxiety are best rated by the person who is suffering from them. For those with profound ID self-ratings are precluded, and so other assessments have to do their best to compensate for this.

There has been a tendency for those involved in research in this area to generate outcome measures of their own rather than use standard accepted ones. Ideally one needs to have common outcomes with standard instruments if data are to be combined in systematic reviews and meta-analyses. In this chapter we are confining discussion to those measures that are both psychometrically validated and also used frequently in research studies. Those instruments that have not been cited since their publication are not included unless they are extremely recent and naturally do not yet have the opportunity to be cited even though they may be novel. Because it is important for the discipline of ID to have standard outcome scales we have also taken the liberty of giving our 'best buy' recommendations in each area of outcome. We realize that there is an element of subjectivity in making such recommendations and so we have tried to justify the choices wherever possible.

We have decided to exclude some instruments that are less commonly used and relatively outdated, such as the Reiss Screen for Maladaptive Behaviour (1) and the Psychopathology Instrument for the Mentally Retarded (PIMRA) (2). 'Every scale has its day', but when new knowledge is gained even the best of scales have to make way for new ones.

The decision on which scales to include a minimum degree of psychometric measurement has been set by us. The essential requirements are internal consistency (often measured by Cronbach's alpha [α]), inter-rater reliability (agreement) (using a variety of correlation measures) and, in some cases, test retest reliability. The interpretation of the statistical measures used are based on standard guidelines (3–5).

Challenging behaviours

We start with challenging behaviour (often described as 'behaviour that challenges') because, arguably, it presents one of the most difficult aspects for clinicians, families, and other caregivers. These behaviours may include physical abuse, self-injury, destruction, verbal aggression and sexual behaviours. They are not considered to constitute a diagnosis (although this is currently a matter of dispute), but they can have devastating effects on the individual, caregivers and, for those in institutions or care homes, other residents.

As well as being mindful of known factors that increase the risk of displaying challenging behaviour, such as mental ill-health, visual impairment, or restrictive social environments, there are many rating scales and instruments in the public domain, some of which are recommended in general guidance (6–8), to help with screening, monitoring, and management strategies. Rating scales to assess behaviours provide a more objective means of establishing what triggers the individual's behaviour, helping to put suitable management strategies in place and also to assess whether these strategies have been successful. They are particularly important in applied health and social care research, given the need for research studies to use robust, objective methodology that can be replicated.

As with all of the rating scales and instruments to which we refer in this chapter, the degree of personal reflection required to assess one's own behaviour often precludes the use of self-report instruments in this population. Instead, many of the measures are designed to be completed by caregivers which, of course, can be problematic since challenging behaviour is a social construct and one person's interpretation of behaviour that is 'challenging' differs from another's.

Aberrant Behaviour Checklist (ABC)

The Aberrant Behaviour Checklist (ABC) (9, 10) is probably the most widely used instrument (currently cited in Scopus 632 times) to assess challenging behaviour among children and adults with intellectual disability. It is completed by an informant and has components for both community and residential settings. The checklist contains 58 items with five sub-scales for agitation; lethargy, social withdrawal, stereotypies, hyperactivity/non-compliance and inappropriate speech. Behaviour ratings are scored from 0 (not a problem) to 3 (severe) and include measures of frequency and disruption of the behaviour to daily activities and people concerned. The ABC has been found to have good to excellent internal consistency ($\alpha = 0.86–0.95$) across the sub-scales, excellent test-retest reliability (Spearman-Rank correlation; rho = 0.96–0.99) and moderate inter-rater reliability (rho = 0.63) (10).

This is a good instrument for screening for challenging behaviours and monitoring their worsening or improvement over time; it can also assess changes in outcomes after introducing an intervention. However, it is lengthy and may not always be suitable for clinical trials that require repeated measures or are linked to a range of other assessment tools. There are also only a few items for each 'behaviour cluster' which may compromise reliability.

AAMD Adaptive Behaviour Scales–Residential and community

The Adaptive Behavior Scales (ABS:RC2), developed by the American Association on Mental Retardation (AAMD), are also commonly used to measure how individuals with intellectual disability cope with the demands of their environment (11). The scales are designed to be completed by an informant (either independently or via interview) and have versions for school and community/residential settings. The second part of the instrument relates to challenging behaviours. This contains 41 items (each with up to 12 items) and eight sub-domains: social behaviours (including verbal and physical aggression), conformity (including rebellious behaviours), trustworthiness (including destructive behaviours), stereotypies and hyperactive behaviours, sexual behaviour, self-abusive behaviour, social engagement, and disturbing interpersonal behaviours. Behaviour ratings are scored by frequency ('never', 'occasionally', 'frequently'). The instrument has good to excellent test-retest reliability (intraclass correlation coefficient; ICC = 0.81–0.94 across the domains).

The ABS:RC2 covers a range of behaviours so is a good outcome measure to assess the efficacy and effectiveness of interventions. However, it may not be a good screening tool (12) and, like the ABC, has only a few items for each 'behaviour cluster' so may not be as reliable as some other measures.

Behaviour Problems Inventory

The most recent version of the Behaviour Problems Inventory (BPI-01) (13) is designed to be rated by an informant and contains 52 items. There are three sub-scales: self-injurious behaviours, stereotypic behaviour, and aggressive/destructive behaviour. Items are rated on a 5-point frequency scale and a 4-point severity scale. There is also a short form (14). The instrument has good internal consistency, excellent inter-rater reliability (Pearson's product-moment correlation; r = 0.91), and good test-retest reliability (r = 0.76).

The instrument is purported to be useful as a clinical assessment for people who are 'at risk' of challenging behaviour, as an outcome for intervention studies, and to explore the epidemiology of specific behaviours. Moreover, by focusing in more depth on specific behaviours, the instrument is likely to be more reliable than the two previous instruments (as shown by the high inter-reliability correlation). However, it cannot be used as an overall assessment of challenging behaviours.

Challenging Behaviour Interview

The Challenging Behaviour Interview (CBI) was developed in 2003 by Oliver et al. (15) to assess the severity of challenging behaviour in children and adults with ID who are already displaying some of these behaviours. The instrument involves an interview with an informant (member of staff), has 14 items and two parts relating to self-injury, verbal aggression, disruption of the environment, and inappropriate vocalization. Behaviours are measured by their severity and frequency in the previous month. The instrument also incorporates measures on the duration of episodes, effect on the individual and the caregiver, and the management strategies undertaken. Each item is coded on a Likert scale. Test-retest reliability has been found to be moderate to excellent (kappa = 0.70–0.91) across the sub-scales for Part 1 and moderate to good (r = 0.66–0.85) for Part 2. Inter-rater reliability is variable for Part 1 and Part 2 (kappa = 0.50–0.80) and again for Part 2 (r = 0.02–0.77) (15).

The developers' rationale for the instrument is that the identification of challenging behaviour varies between settings and those who are more able to manage severe behaviours will not find the behaviours 'challenging'. As a consequence, this scale is good for assessing the significance of challenging behaviours to services and the individuals themselves. The downside is that it cannot be used as a screening instrument as it is designed for people who already display some behaviours (regardless of whether or not they are deemed to be challenging). It is also unlikely to be adequately sensitive to allow for differences in identification of challenging behaviour within settings, such as where staff members' views differ.

Diagnostic Assessment for the Severely Handicapped scale

The Diagnostic Assessment for the Severely Handicapped (DASH-II) scale is a revised version of the DASH (16, 17) and measures mental ill-health and challenging behaviours in people with severe and profound ID. It is informant-based, has 84 items and 13 subscales. Items on behaviour are scored on a 3-point scale, according to severity, frequency, and duration of the identified behaviour. Test-retest reliability of the DASH-II (proportion agreement) has been found to range from 0.84 to 0.95 for the subscales (18), but the scale has only poor to moderate internal consistency ($\alpha = 0.53–0.84$) (19).

The DASH-II is perceived to be a good measure for screening and diagnosis of overall mental ill-health, but only challenging behaviours that are related to anxiety can be assessed and the DASH-II has been found to be inferior to the ABC in terms of monitoring changes in challenging behavior (20).

Health of the Nation Outcome Scales-LD

The Health of the Nation Outcome Scales-LD (HoNOS-LD) (21) are modified versions of the HoNOS (22). The scales are clinician-led and are designed to measure areas of behaviour and functioning that are relatively stable to enable the assessment of treatment effects. The scales comprise 18 items which are graded on severity on a 5-point scale. The behaviour components of the scale include behaviour towards others, self-injurious behaviours, destructive behaviours, problems with personal behaviours, stereotypies, panic, phobias, obsessive or compulsive behaviours, other behaviours, problems with sleeping, and problems with eating or drinking. Moderate to good inter-rater reliability has been found across items and time points (kappa = 0.58–0.86) (21).

The HoNOS-LD is perceived to be a good screening and diagnostic instrument to identify challenging behaviour and to monitor changes in challenging behaviour over time. However, it has not been subject to the same reliability and validity testing as some of the other measures and is probably inferior to them.

Modified Overt Aggression Scale (MOAS)

The Modified Overt Aggression Scale (MOAS) (23, 24) is a short and simple to use informant-related scale comprising four items on the frequency and severity of verbal aggression, aggression towards property, 'auto aggression' (self-injury) and physical aggression occurring during the past week. The scores range from 0 (no aggression) to 4 (severe aggression) and responses are weighted for behaviours that are more likely to affect the physical and social environment or the quality of life of the individual and the caregivers (i.e. most for physical aggression, least for verbal aggression). The inter-rater reliability of the MOAS in adults with intellectual disability ranges from fair to excellent (ICC = 0.49–0.90; kappa = 0.65–0.90) (25).

The MOAS is particularly useful in clinical trials and other research studies where it is important to assess outcomes without overly burdening the caregivers. However, it is restricted to specific behaviours and requires an understanding of what these mean (e.g. verbal aggression might encompass a range of behaviours) which compromises reliability.

Motivation Assessment Scale (MAS)

The Motivation Assessment Scale (MAS) (26) is a functional informant-rated assessment scale, designed for children and adults with ID to identify situations where an individual is likely to behave in a certain way. It requires the informant to identify a specific behaviour and to rate this behaviour on 16 items according to their own observations. The scale comprises 16 items with four sub-scales: attention (seeking positive or negative reactions from others), sensory (self-stimulation), tangible (trying to acquire/reacting to the loss of a physical object), and escape (avoiding tasks or demands). Behaviours are rated by frequency on a 7-point Likert scale from 0 (never) to 6 (always). Among children (teacher-informed), test-retest reliability of self-injurious behaviours was good (rho = 0.82–0.89) and inter-rater reliability was moderate to excellent (rho = 0.66–0.92).

This scale is useful as an initial screening assessment. It can also be used to monitor changes in challenging behaviours once new management strategies have been introduced. However, the reliability of this scale appears to vary across studies,(12, 27–29).

Questions About Behavioural Function scale (QABF)

The Questions About Behavioural Function scale (QABF) (30–31) is another informant-rated functional assessment used to identify functions important in maintaining behaviour among children and adults with ID. The scale has 25 items and five sub-scales: attention, escape, non-social, physical, and tangible. Behaviours are rated on a 4-point Likert frequency scale from 0 (never) to 3 (often). Internal consistency has been found to be excellent for the individual subscales (α = 0.90–0.93) and reliability measures vary from good to excellent (rho = 0.80–1.00) for test-retest reliability and fair to excellent (rho = 0.64–1.00) for inter-rater reliability.

The scale is relatively short, taking approximately 20 minutes to complete. The developers also suggest that the QABF can be used in a hierarchical model of functional analysis and this has been supported in more recent research (32). However, as with the MAS, which appears to measure similar constructs, other researchers have failed to replicate the reliability findings in different populations (29, 33–35).

Problem Behaviour Check List (PBCL)

The Problem Behaviour Check List (PBCL) is a new scale (36) developed to identify the severity of challenging behaviours over a longer period with frequent assessments. It identifies seven behaviours—personal violence, violence against property, self-harm, sexually inappropriate, contrary, demanding, and disappearing behaviour—and these are all scored on a five-point scale. It takes only five minutes to complete in most cases. Although it covers all aspects of challenging behaviours, factor analysis has shown that demanding, violent, and contrary behaviour account for most of the variance. The tool has excellent inter-rater reliability (weighted kappa = 0.91) and validity testing against the MOAS has also shown high sensitivity (97%) and specificity (85%).

It is too early to assess the usefulness of this scale but it does have the major advantage of speed.

Best buys

On the basis of comprehensiveness and extent of use, the Aberrant Behaviour Checklist and the ABS:RC2 are the two preferred choices, together with the Challenging Behaviour Interview when children with already manifest challenging behaviour are being assessed.

Mental ill-health

There are a range of assessments for mental ill-health designed for adults with ID, but we have narrowed the list down substantially for this chapter. It is worth noting that the DASH-II scale (17) described in the previous chapter is also perceived to be a good measure for screening and diagnosis of overall mental ill-health, although it perhaps not as well validated as some of the measures described.

Overall mental ill-health

Mini Psychiatric Assessment Schedule for Adults with a Developmental Disability (Mini PAS-ADD)

The Mini Psychiatric Assessment Schedule for Adults with a Developmental Disability (Mini PAS-ADD) (37) is derived from the PAS-ADD semi-structured interview for caregivers to observe possible psychiatric symptoms in adults with ID. It has 86 psychiatric symptoms and seven subscales for: depression, anxiety, expansive mood (bipolar disorder), obsessive-compulsive disorders, psychosis, unspecified disorder (including dementia), and autism spectrum disorder. Psychometric properties of the instrument reveal good to excellent internal consistency ($\alpha \geq 0.80$) for depression, expansive mood, psychosis and autism, fair internal consistency ($\alpha = 0.73$) for anxiety, but unacceptable internal consistency ($\alpha < 0.70$) for obsessive compulsive disorder and unspecified disorder (38). The depression ($r = 0.62$), obsessive-compulsive disorder ($r = 0.52$), psychosis ($r = 0.61$) and autism ($r = 0.65$) sub-scales have moderate inter-rater reliability. However, the anxiety ($r = 0.36$), expansive mood ($r = 0.37$) and unspecified disorder ($r = 0.32$) have relatively poor inter-rater reliability. The schedule is also relatively lengthy such that the PAS-ADD Checklist (below) has been found to be more favourable for adults with ID when administered with other assessments (39).

PAS-ADD Checklist

The PAS-ADD Checklist (40) can be used by untrained healthcare professionals and consists of 29 symptoms of psychiatric disorders scored on a four point scale that combine to produce three scores for affective/neurotic disorder, possible organic disorder and psychotic disorders. The internal consistency of the affective/neurotic disorder score is good ($\alpha = 0.84$), but the remaining two scores have unacceptable internal consistency ($\alpha = 0.63$ for organic disorder and $\alpha = 0.51$ for psychotic disorders). The inter-rater reliability varies from moderate ($r = 0.55$ for organic disorder; $r = 0.60$ for psychotic disorders) to good ($r = 0.76$; affective/neurotic disorder).

Depression

Glasgow Depression Scale for people with a Learning Disability (GSD-LD)

The Glasgow Depression Scale for people with a Learning Disability (GSD-LD) (41)[41] is a self-report instrument that measures depressive symptoms among people with mild or moderate ID. The GDS-LD comprises 20 items, with 16 of these observable via the caregiver version (GDS-CS). The tool is short to administer and has excellent internal consistency ($\alpha = 0.90$). Test-retest reliability is also excellent ($r = 0.97$). The carer version has good internal consistency ($\alpha = 0.88$) and excellent test-retest ($r = 0.98$) and inter-rater reliability ($r = 0.98$)

Personality disorders

There are no really good accepted measures for assessing personality disorder and as a consequence the range of prevalence levels is unacceptably large (42). One of the main difficulties of assessment is the degree of allowance that is made for intellectual impairment. Severe and profound ID is very frequently associated with challenging behaviours that overlap with personality disturbance but have a very different cause.

Standardized Assessment of Personality (SAP)

One of the most frequently used instruments which determine personality disorders is the Standardized Assessment of Personality (SAP) (43)[43]. The SAP is a semi-structured informant-based interview conducted face-to-face or via telephone and has been found to have good inter-rater reliability (kappa = 0.76) and moderate to good test-retest reliability (kappa = 0.54–0.75) (44, 45). It has been used in samples of adults with ID (46), but has not been formally validated.

Revised NEO Personality Inventory (NEO PI-R)

The revised NEO Personality Inventory (NEO PI-R) (47) is a commonly used measure of the 'Big Five' personality traits, or the five factor model (FFM). The observer-report version (Form R) comprises 240 questions, each one rated on a five-point scale. It produces scores for the five factors, or domains, of general personality functioning: neuroticism/emotional instability, extraversion, openness to experience, agreeableness, and conscientiousness. Each domain has six facets, and the instrument can provide scores for all 30 facets (such as 'angry hostility, altruism', self-discipline, 'openness to aesthetics' and 'gregariousness'). The NEO PI-R has good to excellent internal consistency ($\alpha = 0.86$–0.92) across the domains. Inter-rater reliability of the NEO PI-R observer rating is also good to excellent at both the facet (ICC = 0.71–0.98) and domain levels (ICC = 0.94–0.97).

Reiss Profile of Fundamental Goals and Motivational Sensitivities Mental Retardation Version

The Reiss Profile of Fundamental Goals and Motivational Sensitivities Mental Retardation Version is a relatively widely-used observer rating scale instrument based upon Reiss's theory of fundamental motives (48). This theory emphasizes the role of intrinsic, universal motives in human behaviour. It is noteworthy that the theoretical conceptualization of motives and their role in behaviour is the same for people with and without intellectual disabilities.

Reiss Profile Mental Retardation/Developmental Disability (MR/DD) Version

The Reiss Profile MR/DD is an informant-rated instrument developed for use with adults with intellectual and/or developmental disabilities, based upon the Reiss Profile of Fundamental Goals and Motivational Sensitivities (for adults of typical intellectual functioning, It constitutes 100 items across 15 scales (e.g. food, helping others, frustration, acceptance). Ratings are based on a five-point Likert scale. Internal consistency is good (average $\alpha = 0.84$) and inter-rater reliability evidence is fair (average ICC = 0.52) (49). The Reiss Profile MR/DD has been used in person-centred planning interventions and crisis planning as well as roommate-matching (50).

The forthcoming ICD-11 classification of personality disorders is a radical departure from former classifications (51), but is planned to have strong clinical utility and be helpful in assessing those with ID. The simplest format (52) has been found to be useful in identifying personality disorder in those with challenging behavior (53).

Autism spectrum disorders

Diagnostic Interview for Social and Communication Disorders (DISCO)

The Diagnostic Interview for Social and Communication Disorders (DISCO) (54) is a clinician-led, semi-structured interview with a caregiver or subject that focuses on level of development, behaviours, disabilities, and needs. The interviews are lengthy, containing more than 300 items (90–180 minute administration time), but there is an abbreviated version containing 68 items (55). Evidence suggests (ninth version) that inter-rater reliability is good to excellent (kappa or ICC ≥ 0.75) for more than 80 per cent of the items.

Autism Diagnostic Interview-Revised (ADI-R)

Like the DISCO, the ADI-R (56) is a clinician-led semi-structured interview. However, the interview is informant-based only and focuses more fully on current behaviours, primarily in the three domains of social interaction, language, and communication, and repetitive or stereotyped interests or behaviours. The interview comprises 93 items and takes approximately 90 minutes to administer. Test-retest and inter-rater reliability are generally excellent (most ICC > 0.90).

Social Communication Questionnaire (SCQ)

The SCQ questionnaire is a short, 40-item screening questionnaire for caregivers to identify children and adults who require further assessment with the ADI-R or DISCO (57). It was originally developed to accompany the ADI-R and focuses on reciprocal social interaction, language, and communication, and stereotyped patterns of behaviour, taking approximately 10 minutes to administer. The unacceptable levels of internal consistency ($\alpha < 0.50$) in the language and communication domain (58, 59) preclude its use as a diagnostic instrument, but it is likely to be useful for screening those whose early developmental history is uncertain.

Autism Diagnostic Observation Schedules 2nd Version (ADOS-2)

The ADOS-2 (60) is a direct observation measure to determine whether participants demonstrate 'autistic-like' behaviour during a series of rated tasks that evaluate communication, social functioning, creativity, imagination, stereotyped, and restricted interests. Validity of the first version of the ADOS (Module 1) with the DISCO and ADI-R has shown promising results among adults with ID, when compared with the DISCO and ADI-R (sensitivity 0.67, specificity 0.88) (61). However, the ADOS-2 does not consider sensory symptoms, so clinicians may need to supplement the tool with additional information to align with DSM-5 (62) and future ICD-11 criteria.

Best buys

The Mini PAS-ADD appears to be the best tool for screening for the presence of overall mental ill-health, rather than a specific disorder. However, given the difficulties in diagnosing psychotic disorders in people with ID owing to its complex, varied, and subjective symptoms, this tool may also provide the best option for identifying these disorders in the absence of other clinical investigation. For more specific disorders, we recommend the GDS-LD for self-reported depression, the SAP for personality disorders, and the ADOS-2 or DISCO for autism spectrum disorders.

Dementia

Dementia is a clinical diagnosis that requires evidence of cognitive decline sufficient to impair function in daily life over a period of at least six months (62). When diagnosing dementia in adults with ID, the focus should be to recognize change and decline in relation to premorbid level of functioning. There are no agreed reliable screening instruments but there are valid and reliable tools that aid diagnosis, which are either administered to informants or rely on direct assessment of the subject.

Informant-based assessments

Informant-based reporting has been shown to be effective in facilitating dementia diagnosis (63). In studies comparing informant reports to direct cognitive tests, informant reports have been shown to be more effective than cognitive assessments (64–66).

Dementia questionnaire for people with learning disabilities (DLD)

The Dementia Questionnaire for People with Learning Disabilities (DLD) (67) has been suggested as the most promising informant-rated screening tool in most adults with ID (68). It contains 50 items divided into eight subscales (working memory, long-term memory, orientation, speech, practical skills, mood, activities, and behavioural disturbance) and takes between 15–20 minutes to administer. Overall inter-rater reliability is excellent (r = 0.94), but is low for the subscale 'behavioural disturbance' (r = 0.44); there is also a floor effect on more severe ID. The sensitivity and specificity for detecting Alzheimer's Disease (AD) in Down syndrome was 92 per cent.

Dementia scale for Down syndrome (DSDS)

The Dementia Scale for Down Syndrome (DSDS) (69) is one of four instruments suggested by NICE for assessing severity of dementia in people with ID (70). It is designed to detect cognitive decline in people with ID, especially at the lower range of functioning, and contains 60 questions divided into three categories to indicate the stage of dementia. Behaviours (present for at least six months) are rated as 'present', 'absent', 'not applicable' or' typical', with only those marked 'present' contributing to the score. The scoring system is not simple. The DSDS has a specificity of 89 per cent and a sensitivity of 85 per cent in identifying dementia in people with ID. Restrictions on its use apply but it has been used by other mental health professionals.

Dementia Screening Questionnaire for Individuals with Intellectual Disabilities (DSQIID)

The 53 items of the Dementia Screening Questionnaire for Individuals with Intellectual Disabilities (DSQIID)[71] cover areas such as loss of memory, confusion, loss of skills, social withdrawal, behavioural changes, psychological symptoms, physical symptoms, sleep disturbance, and speech abnormalities. The questionnaire has three parts related to the person's 'best' ability, behavior, or symptoms and comparative questions (such as 'speaks (signs) less' and 'seems generally more tired'). Scores from part two and three are added to provide a total score. The questionnaire takes 10–15 minutes to administer and has a fixed cut off of 20. It has excellent internal consistency (average α = 0.91), inter-rater (ICC = 0.90) and test-retest reliability (ICC = 0.95). However, its fixed cut-off may compromise its usefulness in people with more severe ID or advanced dementia (72).

Subject-based assessments

The opinions and views of informants and family members sometimes affect the ratings that are used in informant-based schedules. The advantage of testing subjects directly is that assessments are more accurate and not influenced by others' memories and perceptions. For an accurate assessment the subject being tested needs to be in a cooperative mood and able to engage with the assessor.

The Prudhoe Cognitive Function Test (PCFT)

The Prudhoe Cognitive Function Test (65) is designed for the direct assessment of cognitive abilities in people with Down syndrome and is used serially to detect cognitive decline over time. It takes no more than 45 minutes to administer, but its two shorter versions only take 10 minutes to administer and have excellent correlations (more than 0.97) with the longer version, so are preferable (73). The instrument covers the major domains of cognitive functioning including orientation, recall, language, praxis and calculation.

The PCFT has been validated against The Kaufman Brief Intelligence Test (K-BIT) (74) and shown good correlations between the verbal and performance sections (r = 0.85 and r = 0.78 respectively)(73). Inter-rater and test-retest reliability are both excellent (ICC = 0.99 for both) (75), but there is a floor effect in the more intellectually disabled.

The Test for Severe Impairment (TSI)

The Test for Severe Impairment (TSI) (76) was originally designed to assess people with severe dementia in the general population. It has particular value for those with more severe levels of ID. The test takes approximately 10 minutes and has no significant ceiling or floor effect (77). It includes assessment of motor performance, language production and comprehension, memory, conceptualization, and general knowledge. Only eight out of the 24 items available require the person to answer a question verbally. The test has good internal consistency (α = 0.89) and excellent inter-rater and test-retest reliability (rho = 0.97 and rho = 0.98 respectively). Inter-rater and test-retest reliability are also good among those with severe ID (rho = 0.81 and rho = 0.84 respectively) (78).

Cambridge Cognitive Examination-Down Syndrome (CAMCOG-DS)

The Cambridge Cognitive Examination-Down Syndrome (CAMCOG-DS) (79) is a modified version of the CAMCOG, the neuropsychological component of the Cambridge Examination for Mental Disorders in the Elderly (CAMDEX) (80) and has been validated in people with Down syndrome (81, 82). CAMCOG-DS consists of a group of neuropsychological tests covering all areas of cognitive function that characteristically decline with the onset of dementia. The domains assessed include orientation, language, memory, praxis, attention/calculation, abstract thinking, and perception. There are few floor effects (83). Inter-rater reliability is good (kappa >0.8) for 91 per cent of the items and fair (kappa >0.6) for the remaining items.

Best buys

The DLD is recommended on the basis of the extent of its use and coverage of both cognitive and behaviour symptoms. The TSI is also recommended for its lack of ceiling and floor effects for people with moderate and severe ID.

Quality of life

The promotion of positive well-being among people with ID is crucial to global policies (84). It is also an indicator of the quality of service provision and can be used as an outcome measure to evaluate changes in service provision or to evaluate the impact of new interventions. Well-being is most commonly measured using 'quality of life' assessments, but they are all subject to the same challenges as the other measures collected in adults with ID in that they can only be self-reported in people with mild or moderate ID and thus rely on proxy report which, although believed to have some merit (85), is sometimes unreliable (86, 87). Whilst there have been attempts to develop subjective quality of life measures specifically for people with profound ID (e.g. Lyons et al. (88)), we have focused on those instruments that are commonly used and have been validated.

Comprehensive Quality of Life Scale–Intellectual Disability Form (ComQol-I5)

The Comprehensive Quality of Life Scale—Intellectual Disability Form (ComQol-I5) (86) was designed for people with ID or some other form of cognitive impairment. It contains both objective and subjective measures. The subjective sub-scale is designed for the interviewee alone or with one close friend, while the objective sub-scale is designed to be completed by both the interviewee and a non-disabled friend, family member, or staff member. There is also a scale for proxy interviews (subjective interview from the primary carer). Each objective and subjective axis comprises seven domains which cover the quality of life components: material wellbeing, health, productivity, intimacy, safety, place in the community, and emotional wellbeing. The subjective internal consistency and test-retest reliability are good (α = 0.81; test-retest 'correlation' 0.82–0.87 for the sub-scales), but the proxy response is less reliable (86).

Quality of Life Questionnaire (QoLQ)

Similar to the ComQol-I5, the Quality of Life Questionnaire (QoLQ) (89) can be completed by the client with or without assistance or by proxy by someone who knows the person well. It is designed to measure self-perceived quality of life and has 40 items and four subscales measuring satisfaction, competence/productivity, empowerment/independence, and social belonging/community. Items are rated on a three-point scale from one (poor quality of life) to three (good quality of life). The instrument has good internal consistency (α = 0.83) and good inter-rater reliability (r = 0.83), but there is little agreement between client and proxy measures with regard to the empowerment/independence domain which tends to be overestimated by carers (87).

Personal Wellbeing Index–Intellectual Disability (PWI-ID)

One disadvantage with the ComQol-I5 and the QoLQ is that they cannot be used in the general population so the scores cannot be compared with the general population. Cummins et al. (90) have attempted to address this gap by developing the Personal Wellbeing Index—Intellectual Disability (PWI–ID), a parallel version of the Personal Wellbeing Index for adults in the general population (91), but with more concretely worded questions. The tool begins with pre-testing to determine whether the individual can reliably respond to questions and understand more abstract concepts. There are then questions on eight life domains: standard of living, personal health, life achievement, personal relationships, personal safety, community connectedness, future security, and spirituality/religion (added more recently). Evidence suggests that the tool has good internal consistency (α = 0.76) and moderate test-retest reliability (ICC = 0.57; r = 0.58) (92).

EuroQol Five Dimensions Questionnaire (EQ-5D)

The EuroQol Five Dimensions Questionnaire (EQ-5D) (93) is a widely used generic health-related quality of measure that is recommended for economic evaluations that use Quality-Adjusted Life Years (QALYs) (e.g. NICE (94)). It is a short and simple measure that contains five items and three levels relating to mobility, self-care, usual activities, pain/discomfort, and anxiety/depression. To date, the EQ-5D has not been validated in people with ID, but validation work is current being undertaken (95). In the meantime, the youth version of the EQ-5D (EQ-5D-Y) (96) is sometimes deemed to be more suitable for this population.

36-item Short Form Survey (SF-36)

As with the EQ-5D, the 36-item Short Form Survey (SF-36) is a generic health-related quality of life measure that is often used for economic evaluations in the general population (97). The survey has eight subscales that measure: physical functioning, the effect of physical health on work or other daily activities, bodily pain, general health, vitality, social functioning, the effect of mental health on work or other daily activities, and mental health. Jones et al. (98) conducted pilot work on the SF-36 using 'minimal adaptation' to make it suitable for adults with ID who were living in small community homes. Internal consistency was good (α = 0.92) and inter-rater reliability was moderate (r = 0.63; range 0.31–0.89).

Best buys

For subjective quality of life measures, we would recommend the ComQol-I5, based on its extensive use, and the PW-ID where general population comparisons are required. More work is needed to assess the validity of informant-based measures in this population.

Lifestyle

To date, there are no validated lifestyle and health behaviour questionnaires that are suitable for people with ID. Therefore, we have not included any scales in this section.

MULTIPLE CHOICE QUESTIONS

Questions

Please select the single most appropriate answer.

1. What is a good assessment tool to assess overall mental ill-health in people with intellectual disabilities?

A. Mini Psychiatric Assessment Schedule for Adults with a Developmental Disability (Mini PAS-ADD)

B. Diagnostic Interview for Social and Communication Disorders (DISCO)
C. Glasgow Depression Scale for people with a Learning Disability (GSD-LD)

2. Why is it important to have standardized instruments to measure outcomes in people with ID?
A. To enable researchers to decide on an agreed outcome that effectively measures improvement
B. To be able to combine and compare research findings
C. To improve the skills and techniques of the assessors using them
D. To ensure that all assessors using the same standard
E. So that observer and self-rating scales can be compared mathematically

3. Which of the following psychometric properties are not important when evaluating the value of self-reported instruments?
A. Measures of internal consistency
B. Test-retest reliability
C. Content validity
D. Inter-rater reliability
E. Acceptability of instrument to those being tested

4. Why are standardized adult psychiatric rating scales not generally suitable for assessing people with intellectual disabilities?
A. People with intellectual disabilities have different mental conditions from those without intellectual disabilities
B. Scales for assessing adults without intellectual disabilities do not compensate for the difficulties in rating behaviour in those with intellectual disabilities
C. They use different norms from those instruments developed in assessing intellectual disabilities
D. They use language that is too complicated for those with intellectual disabilities to understand
E. Standardized scales are only appropriate in a specific population and cannot be generalized to others

5. Which self-report instrument is considered to be the most appropriate for assessing the presence and severity of dementia in those with severe intellectual disabilities
A. Cambridge Cognitive Examination (CAMCOG-DS)
B. Dementia Screening Questionnaire for Individual with Intellectual Disability (DSQIID)
C. Dementia Questionnaire for People with Learning Disabilities (DLD)
D. Test for Severe Impairment
E. Prudhoe Cognitive Function Test

Answers

1. A. The Mini PAS-ADD. The DISCO and GSD-LD are to assess specific mental health disorders (autism and depression).
2. B. Although assessors who use standardized instruments may be technically more competent, this is not the main reason that they are employed.
3. D. Inter-rater reliability cannot be carried out when a self-report instrument is being developed. There is only one person completing a self-report scale and it is not possible for another person to rate responses.
4. E. Standardized rating scales are developed in a particular defined population and are not suitable when outside this specific group as they have not been applied in a different setting.
5. D. The CAMCOG-DS, DSQIID and the DLD are all schedules that rely on an informant. The Test for Severe Impairment has little to no floor effect and can be administered successfully to individuals with severe and profound intellectual disabilities

REFERENCES

1. Reiss S. *Test Manual for the Reiss Screen for Maladaptive Behavior.* Orland Park, IL: International Diagnostic Systems; 1998.
2. Matson JL, Kazdin AE, Senatore V. Psychometric properties of the psychopathology instrument for mentally retarded adults. *Applied Research in Mental Retardation*, 1984;5:81–89.
3. Cicchetti DV, Sparrow SA. Developing criteria for establishing interrater reliability of specific items: Applications to assessment of adaptive behaviour. *American Journal of Mental Deficiency*, 1981;86:127–137.
4. Cicchetti DV, Sparrow SA. *Assessment in adaptive behavior in young children.* In: J.J. Johnson, J. Goldman (eds.). Developmental assessment in clinical child psychology: A handbook. New York: Pergamon Press, 1990.
5. Hinkle D, Wiersma W, Jurs S. *Applied statistics for the behavioural sciences (5th edition).* Boston: Houghton Mifflin, 2002.
6. Aman MG, Crismon ML, Frances A, King BH, Rojahn J. *Treatment of Psychiatric and Behavioral Problems in Individuals with Mental Retardation: An Update of the Expert Consensus Guidelines.* White Plains, NY: Expert Knowledge Systems, 2004.
7. Deb S, Matthews T, Holt G, Bouras N. *Practice Guidelines for the Assessment and Diagnosis of Mental Health Problems in Adults with Intellectual Disability.* Brighton: *Pavillion*, 2001.
8. NICE. *Challenging Behaviour and Learning Disabilities: Prevention and Interventions for People with Learning Disabilities whose Behaviour Challenges. NICE Guideline [NG11].* London: National Institute for Health and Care Excellence, 2015.
9. Aman MG, Singh NN, Steward AW. The aberrant behavior bhecklist: A behavior rating scale for the assessment of treatment effects. *American Journal of Mental Deficiency* 1985;89:485–491.
10. Aman MG, Singh NN. *Aberrant Behavior Checklist Manual.* East Aurora, NY: Slosson Educational Publications, 1986.
11. Nihira K, Leland H. Lambert N. *AAMR Adaptive Behaviour Scales—Residential and Community (ABS:RC-2).* Austin, Texas: Pro-Ed, 1993.
12. O'Brien G, Pearson J, Berney T, Barnard, L. Measuring behaviour in developmental disability: A review of existing schedules. *Developmental Medicine and Child Neurology Supplement.* 2001;S87:1–72.
13. Rojahn J, Matson JL, Lott D, Esbebsen AJ, Smalls Y. The behavior problems inventory: An instrument for the assessment of self-injury, Stereotyped behavior, and aggression/destruction

in individuals with developmental disabilities. *Journal of Autism and Developmental Disorders*. 2001;31:577–588.
14. Rojahn J, Rowe EW, Sharber AC, Hastings R, Matson JL, et al. The behavior problems inventory-short form for individuals with intellectual disabilities: Part I: development and provisional clinical reference data. *Journal of Intellectual Disability Research*. 2012;56:527–545.
15. Oliver C, McClintock K, Hall S, Smith M, Dagnan D, Stenfert-Kroese B. Assessing the severity of challenging behaviour: Psychometric properties of the challenging behaviour interview. *Journal of Applied Research in Intellectual Disability*. 2003;16:53–61.
16. Matson JL, Gardner WI, Coe DA, Sovner R. A scale for evaluating emotional disorders in severely and profoundly mentally retarded persons: Development of the Diagnostic Assessment for the Severely Handicapped (DASH) Scale. *British Journal of Psychiatry*. 1991;159:404–409.
17. Matson JL, Rush KS, Hamilton M, Anderson SJ, Bamburg JW, Baglio S. Characteristics of depression as assessed by the Diagnostic Assessment for the Severely Handicapped-II (DASH-II). *Research in Developmental Disabilities*. 1999;20:305–313.
18. Sevin JA, Matson JL, Williams D, Kirkpatrick-Sanchez S. Reliability of emotional problems with the Diagnostic Assessment for the Severely Handicapped (DASH). *British Journal of Clinical Psychology*. 1995;34:93–94.
19. Paclawskyj TR, Matson JL, Bamburg JW, Baglio CS. A comparison of the Diagnostic Assessment for the Severely Handicapped-II (DASH-II) and the Aberrant Behavior Checklist (ABC). *Research in Developmental Disabilities*. 1997;18:289–298
20. Valdovinos MG, Zarcone J, Hellings JA, Schroeder S. Using the diagnostic assessment of the severely handicapped-II (DASH-II) to measure the therapeutic effects of risperidone. *Journal of Intellectual Disability Research*. 2004;48:53–59.
21. Roy A, Matthews H, Clifford P, Fowler V, Martin DM. Health of the Nation Outcome Scales for People with Learning Disabilities (HoNOS-LD). *British Journal of Psychiatry*. 2002;180:61–66.
22. Wing JK, Beevor AS, Curtis RH, Park SB, Hadden S, Burns A. Health of the Nation Outcome Scales (HoNOS). Research and development. *British Journal of Psychiatry*. 1998;172:11–18.
23. Kay SR, Wolkenfelf F, Murrill LM. Profiles of aggression among psychiatric patients: I. Nature and prevalence. *Journal of Nervous and Mental Disease*. 1998;176:539–554.
24. Ratey JJ, Gutheil CM. The measurement of aggressive behavior: Reflections on the use of the Overt Aggression Scale and the Modified Overt Aggression Scale. *Journal of Neuropsychiatry and Clinical Neuroscience*. 1991;3:S57–S60.
25. Oliver PC, Crawford MJ, Rao B, Reece B, Tyrer P. Modified Overt Aggression Scale (MOAS) for people with intellectual disability and aggressive challenging behaviour: A reliability study. *Journal of Applied Research in Intellectual Disabilities*. 2007;20:368–372.
26. Durrand VM, Crimmins DB. *The Motivation Assessment Scale*. Topeka, KS: Monaco and Associates. 1998.
27. Thompson S, Emerson E. Inter-informant agreement on the motivation assessment scale: another failure to replicate. *Mental Handicap Research*. 1995;8:203–208.
28. Conroy MA, Fox JF, Bucklin A, Good W. An analysis of the reliability and stability of the motivation assessment scale in assessing the challenging behaviors of persons with developmental disabilities. *Education and Training in Mental Retardation and Developmental Disabilities*. 1996;31:243–250.
29. Shrogen KA, Rojahn J. Convergent reliability and validity of the Questions About Behavioral Function and the Motivation Assessment Scale: A replication study. *Journal of Developmental and Physical Disabilities*. 2003;15:367–375.
30. Matson JL, Vollmer TR. *Users Guide: Questions about Behavioral Function (QABF)*. Baton Rouge LA: Scientific Publishers, Inc.; 1995.
31. Paclawskyj TR, Matson JL, Rush KS, Smalls Y, Vollmer TR. Questions about behavioral function (QABF): A behavioral checklist for functional assessment of aberrant behavior. *Research in Developmental Disabilities*. 2000;21:223–229.
32. Watkins N, Rapp JT. The convergent validity of the Questions About Behavioral Function scale and functional analysis for problem behaviour displayed by individuals with autism spectrum disorder. *Research in Developmental Disabilities*. 2013;34:11–16.
33. Nicholson J, Konstantinidi E, Furniss F. On some psychometric properties of the Questions About Behavioral Function (QABF) scale. *Research in Developmental Disabilities*. 2006;27:337–352.
34. Freeman KA, Walker M, Kauffman J. Psychometric properties of the questions about behavioral function scale in a child sample. *American Journal on Mental Retardation*. 2007;112:122–129.
35. May ME, Yanyan S, Chitiyo M, Howe AP. Internal consistency and inter-rater reliability of the questions about behavioral function (QABF) rating scale when used by teachers and paraprofessionals. *Education and Treatment of Children*. 2014;37:347–364.
36. Tyrer P, Nagar J, Evans R, Oliver P, Bassett P, et al. The Problem Behaviour Checklist: Short scale to assess challenging behaviours. *BJPsych Open*. 2016;2:45–49.
37. Prosser H, Moss S, Costello H, Simpson N, Patel P. *The Mini PAS-ADD: An Assessment Schedule for the Detection of Mental Health Needs in Adults with Learning Disability (Mental Retardation)*. Manchester, UK: Hester Adrian Research Centre; 1997.
38. Prosser H, Moss S, Costello H, Simpson N, Patel, P, Rowe, S. Reliability and validity of the Mini PAS-ADD for assessing psychiatric disorders in adults with intellectual disability. *Journal of Intellectual Disability Research*. 1998;42:264–272.
39. Tyrer F, Dunkley AJ, Spong R, Gangadharan SK, Bhaumik S, Khunti K. Involving service users with intellectual disability in research: experiences from the STOP Diabetes Study. *Journal of Policy and Practice in Intellectual Disabilities*. 2016;DOI: 10.1111/jppi.12176
40. Moss SC, Prosser H, Costello H, Simpson N, Patel P, et al. Reliability and validity of the PAS-ADD checklist for detecting disorders in adults with intellectual disability. *Journal of Intellectual Disability Research*. 1998;42:173–183.
41. Cuthill FM, Espie CA, Cooper SA. Development and psychometric properties of the Glasgow Depression Scale for people with a learning disability. Individual and carer supplement versions. *British Journal of Psychiatry*. 2003;182:347–353.
42. Alexander R, Cooray S. Diagnosis of personality disorders in learning disability. *British Journal of Psychiatry*. 2003;S44:S28–S31.
43. Mann AH, Jenkins R, Cutting JC, Cowen PJ. The development and use of standardized assessment of normal personality. *Psychological Medicine*. 1981;11:839–847.
44. McKeon J, Roa B, Mann A. Life events and personality traits in obsessive compulsive neurosis. *British Journal of Psychiatry*. 1984;144:185–189.
45. Pilgrim JA, Mellers JD, Boothby HA, Mann AH. Interrater and temporal reliability of the Standardized Assessment of Personality and the influence of informant characteristics. *Psychological Medicine*. 1993;23:779–786.

46. Flynn A, Matthews H, Hollins S. Validity of the diagnosis of personality disorder in adults with learning disability and severe behavioural problems. Preliminary study. *British Journal of Psychiatry*. 2002;180:543–546.
47. Costa PT, McCrae RR. *NEO PI-R Professional Manual*. Odessa, FL: Psychological Assessment Resources, Inc; 1992.
48. Reiss S, Havercamp SM. Toward a comprehensive assessment of fundamental motivation: Factor structure of the Reiss Profiles. *Psychological Assessment*. 1998;10:97–106.
49. Lecavalier L, Havercamp SM. Are caregivers' reports of motivation valid? Reliability and validity of the Reiss Profile MR/DD. *Journal of Intellectual Disability Research*. 2004;48:217–224.
50. Wiltz J, Reiss S. Compatibility of housemates with mental retardation. *American Journal on Mental Retardation*. 2003;108:173–180.
51. Tyrer P, Reed GM, Crawford MJ. Classification, assessment, prevalence and effect of personality disorder. *Lancet*. 2015;385:717–726.
52. Tyrer P, Crawford M, Mulder R, Blashfield R, Farnam A, Fossati A, Kim Y-R, Koldobsky N, Lecic-Tosevski D, Ndetei D, Swales M, Clark LA, Reed GM. The rationale for the reclassification of personality disorder in the 11th Revision of the International Classification of Diseases. *Personality and Mental Health*. 2011;5:246–259.
53. Tyrer P, Oliver P, Turabi A. Prevalence of aggressive challenging behaviours in intellectual disability and its relationship to personality status: Jamaican study, *Journal of Intellectual Disability Research*. 2014;58:1083–1089.
54. Wing L, Leekam SR, Libby SJ, Gould J, Larcombe M. The diagnostic interview for social and communication disorders: Background, inter-rater reliability and clinical use. *Journal of Child Psychology and Psychiatry*. 2002;43:307–325.
55. Carrington SJ, Kent RG, Maljaars J, Le Couteur A, Gould J, et al. DSM-5 Autism Spectrum Disorder: In search of essential behaviours for diagnosis. *Research in Autism Spectrum Disorders*. 2014;8:701–715.
56. Lord C, Rutter M, Le Couteur A. Autism Diagnostic Interview-Revised: A revised version of a diagnostic interview for caregivers of individuals with possible pervasive developmental disorders. *Journal of Autism and Developmental Disorders*. 1994;24:659–685.
57. Rutter M, Bailey A, Lord C. *Social Communication Questionnaire (SCQ)*. Los Angeles, CA: Western Psychological Services, 2003.
58. Snow AN, Lecavalier L. Sensitivity and specificity of the modified checklist for autism in toddlers and the social communication questionnaire in preschoolers suspected of having pervasive developmental disorders. *Autism*. 2008;12:627–644.
59. Brooks WT, Benson BA. The validity of the Social Communication Questionnaire in adults with intellectual disability. *Research in Autism Spectrum Disorders*. 2013;7:247–255.
60. Lord C, Risi S, Lambrecht L, Cooke EH, Leventhal BL, et al. The autism diagnostic observations schedule—generic: A standard measure of social and communication deficits associated with the spectrum of autism. *Journal of Autism and Developmental Disorders*. 2002;30:205–223.
61. Brugha T, Cooper SA, McManus S, Purdon S, Smith J. et al. *Estimating the Prevalence of Autism Spectrum Conditions in Adults: Extending the 2007 Adult Psychiatric Morbidity Survey*. Leeds: Health and Social Care Information Centre, 2012.
62. American Psychiatric Association. *Diagnostic and Statistical Manual of Mental Disorders (5th edition)*. Arlington, VA: American Psychiatric Publishing; 2013.
63. Elliott-King J, Shaw S, Bandelow S, Devshi R, Kassam S, Hogervorst E. A critical literature review of the effectiveness of various instruments in the diagnosis of dementia in adults with intellectual disabilities. *Alzheimer's and Dementia: Diagnosis, Assessment and Disease Monitoring*. 2016;4:126–148.
64. Deb S, Braganza J. Comparison of rating scales for the diagnosis of dementia in adults with Down's syndrome. *Journal of Intellectual Disability Research*. 1999;43:400–407.
65. Kay DWK, Tyrer SP, Margallo-Lana M-L, Moore PB, Fletcher R, et al. Preliminary evaluation of a Scale to Assess Cognitive Function in Adults with Down's Syndrome: The Prudhoe Cognitive Function Test. *Journal of Intellectual Disability Research*. 2003;47:155–168.
66. McCarron M, McCallion P, Reilly E, Mulryan N. A prospective 14-year longitudinal follow-up of dementia in persons with Down syndrome. *Journal of Intellectual Disability Research*. 2014;8:61–70.
67. Evenhuis H, Kengen MM, Eurlings HA. *Dementia Questionnaire for People with Learning Disabilities (DLD)*. San Antonio: Pearson; 2007.
68. Strydom A, Hassiotis A. Diagnostic instruments for dementia in older people with intellectual disability in clinical practice. *Aging and Mental Health* 2003;7:431–437.
69. Gedye A. *Dementia Scale for Down Syndrome*. Vancouver, BC: Gedye Research and Consulting; 1995.
70. NICE. *Dementia: Supporting People with Dementia and their Carers in Health and Social Care [CG42]*. London: National Institute for Health and Care Excellence; 2006.
71. Deb S, Hare M, Prior L, Bhaumik S. Dementia screening questionnaire for individuals with intellectual disabilities. *British Journal of Psychiatry*. 2007;190:440–444.
72. O'Caoimh R, Clune Y, Molloy DW. Screening for Alzheimer's disease in Downs Syndrome. *Journal of Alzheimer and Parkinsonism*. 2013;S7:001.
73. Tyrer SP, Wigham A, Cicchetti D, Margallo-Lana M-L, Moore PB, Reid BE. Comparison of short and long versions of the Prudhoe Cognitive Function Test and the K-BIT in participants with intellectual impairment. *Journal of Autism and Developmental Disorders*. 2010;40:1000–1005.
74. Kaufman AS, Kaufman NL. *Kaufman Brief Intelligence Test (2nd ed.)*. Bloomington, MN: Pearson; 2004.
75. Margallo-Lana ML, Moore PB, Tyrer SP, Dawson H, Jenkins K, Kay DW. The Prudhoe Cognitive Function Test, a scale to assess cognitive function in adults with Down's syndrome: Inter-rater and test-retest reliability. *Journal of Intellectual Disability Research*. 2003;47:488–492.
76. Albert M, Cohen C. The Test for Severe Impairment: An instrument for the assessment of patients with severe cognitive dysfunction. *Journal of the American Geriatrics Society*. 1992;40:449–453.
77. Tyrrell J, Cosgrave M, McCarron M, McPherson J, Calvert J, et al. Dementia in people with Down's syndrome. *International Journal of Geriatric Psychiatry*. 2001;16:1168–1174.
78. Cosgrave MP, McCarron M, Anderson M, Tyrrell, J, Gill M, Lawlor BA. Cognitive decline in Down syndrome: a validity/reliability study of the test for severe impairment. *American Journal on Mental Retardation*. 1998;103:193–197.
79. Ball SL, Holland AJ, Huppert FA, Treppner P, Watson P, et al. The modified CAMDEX informant interview is a valid and reliable tool for use in the diagnosis of dementia in adults with Down's syndrome. *Journal of Intellectual Disability Research*. 2004;48:611–620.

80. Roth M, Huppert F, Mountjoy C, Tym E. *CAMDEX-R: The Cambridge Examination for Mental Disorder of the Elderly.* Cambridge University Press: Cambridge; 1998.
81. Ball SL, Holland AJ, Hon J, Huppert FA, Treppner P, et al. Personality and behaviour changes mark the early stages of Alzheimer's disease in adults with Down's syndrome: Findings from a prospective population-based study. *International Journal of Geriatric Psychiatry* 2006;21:661–673.
82. Maatta T, Tervo-Maatta T, Taanila, A, Kaski M, Iivanainen M. Mental health, behaviour and intellectual abilities of people with Down syndrome. *Down Syndrome Research and Practice* 2006;11:37–43.
83. Hon J, Huppert FA, Holland AJ, Watson P. Neuropsychological assessment of older adults with Down's syndrome: An epidemiological study using the Cambridge Examination (CAMCOG). *British Journal of Clinical Psychology.* 1999;38:155–165.
84. World Health Organization. *World Report on Disability.* Geneva: World Health Organization; 2011.
85. Perry J, Felce D. Subjective and objective quality of life assessment: Responsiveness, response bias and residence: Proxy concordance. *Mental Retardation.* 2002;40:445–456.
86. Cummins RA. *Comprehensive Quality of Life Scale—Intellectual/Cognitive Disability: Manual 5th edition.* Australia: School of Psychology, Deakin University; 1997.
87. Rapley M, Ridgway J, Beyer S. Staff:staff and staff:client reliability of the Schalock & Keith (1993) Quality of Life Questionnaire. *Journal of Intellectual Disability Research.* 1998;42:37–42.
88. Lyons G. The Life Satisfaction Matrix: An instrument and procedure for assessing the subjective quality of life of individuals with profound multiple disabilities. *Journal of Intellectual Disability Research.* 2005;49:766–769.
89. Schalock R, Keith K. *Quality of Life Questionnaire.* Worthington, OH: IDS Publishing; 1993.
90. Cummins RA, Lau A. *Personal Wellbeing Index—Intellectual Disability (English).* Manual 3rd Edition. Melbourne: Deakin University; 2005.
91. Cummins RA, Lau ALD. *An Introduction to the International Wellbeing Group and the International Wellbeing Index.* Fifth Conference of the International Society for Quality-of-Life Studies, Frankfurt, Germany, July, 2003.
92. McGillivray JA, Lau ALD, Cummins RA, Davey G. The utility of the Personal Wellbeing Index Intellectual Disability Scale (PWI-ID) in an Australian sample. *Journal of Applied Research in Intellectual Disability.* 2009;22:276–286.
93. EuroQoL Group. EuroQoL—A new facility for the measurement of health-related quality of life. *Health Policy.* 1990;16: 199–208.
94. NICE. *Guide to the Methods of Technology Appraisal 2013 NICE Process [PMG9].* London: National Institute for Health and Care Excellence, 2013.
95. Beeken RJ, Spanos D, Fovargue S, Hunter R, Omar R, et al. Piloting a manualised weight management programme (Shape Up-LD) for overweight and obese persons with mild-moderate learning disabilities: Study protocol for a pilot randomised controlled trial. *Trials.* 2013;14:71
96. Wille N, Badia X, Bonsel G, Burstrom K, Cavrini G, et al. Development of the EQ-5D-Y: A child-friendly version of the EQ-5D. *Quality Life Research* 2010;19:875–886.
97. Ware JE, Snow KK, Kosinski M. Gandek MS. *SF-36 Health Survey: Manual and Interpretation Guide.* MA: New England Medical Center; 1993.
98. Jones J, Dagnan D, Ruddick L. Pilot study of the use of the SF-36 to assess health status of adults with learning disabilities living in small community based homes. *British Journal of Developmental Disabilities.* 1997;84:27–35.

6

Types of Mental Disorders in People with Intellectual Disability

Sally-Ann Cooper

Introduction

Mental disorders are common in people with intellectual disability (ID). People with ID can experience the full range of mental disorders that occur in the general population, though presentations can differ from those found in the general population, and hence diagnostic classification manuals have been developed specifically for people with ID (1, 2). Additionally, people with ID experience some mental disorders that are infrequent in the general population, such as self-injurious behaviour, pica, and other problem behaviours. The aetiology of mental disorders in this population is typically multi-factorial, though some specific causes of ID are associated with specific types of mental disorders ('behavioural phenotypes'); other factors can also influence presentations of behavioural phenotypes.

Mental disorders are not usually isolated conditions; multimorbidity is the norm in this population. A range of neuro-developmental conditions tend to co-occur, for which the term ESSENCE has been coined (Early Symptomatic Syndromes Eliciting Neurodevelopmental Clinical Examination) (3). ESSENCE includes major problems in motor skills, general development, speech and language, social interaction and communication, behaviour, hyperactivity or impulsivity, hypoactivity, inattention, sleep or feeding difficulties (3). Genetic data also increasingly supports the clustering of neuro-developmental (including epilepsy) and mental disorders (4). Physical health disorders and disabilities, and sensory impairments are also common in people with ID, and important for mental health clinicians to be aware of, as they impact on mental disorder presentations and treatment decisions, and differential diagnosis is always important to carefully consider.

Views differ as to whether or not challenging behaviours should be considered as mental disorders. In this chapter they are considered as such. This is because they have multi-factorial aetiology which includes biological factors (as seen in some of the behavioural phenotypes, see Chapters 2, 3, and 23 for more detail), and are influenced in their precipitation and maintenance by psychological and social factors such as life events (5), and by their physical environments and social interactions (5). They also can remit and relapse. In these regards they have characteristics that are very similar to other mental disorders such as depression. Statistical investigation also supports this approach; a study using exploratory and confirmatory factor analyses on two large datasets of psychopathology in adults with mild-profound ID (n = 457; n = 274) extracted a model of psychopathology with five factors: depressive, anxiety, cognitive decline, psychosis, and affect dysregulation-problem behaviour (6, 7). The affect dysregulation-problem behaviour factor had good discriminate validity, face validity, and predictive validity (over a five-year follow-up period).

Prevalence and incidence

Mental disorders are more common in children and young people with ID than in children and young people within the general population (8). Mental disorders are also common in adults with ID (9). This is perhaps not surprising, given the complex mix of biological factors, psychological and social disadvantages, and additional developmental factors that people with ID have and are exposed to (10).

Reported rates of mental disorders in children and young people (including problem behaviours) range from 30 per cent (11, 12) to 50 per cent (13). Robust UK private household surveys reported a prevalence of 36 per cent in 641 children and young people (aged 5–16 years) with ID compared with 8 per cent of 17,774 children without ID, which reveals that the children and young people with ID accounted for 14 per cent of all children with mental disorders (14).

The largest adult population-based prevalence study in which each person (aged 16 years and over) was individually assessed included 1,023 adults with ID (15). It reported a point prevalence of mental disorders of 40.9 per cent, or 28.3 per cent when excluding challenging behaviours. Its methods were more robust than previous smaller population-based studies (16–19), which had reported rates from 14.5 per cent (excluding problem behaviours, attention-deficit hyperactivity disorder (ADHD), autism, dementia, personality disorder, people aged 65 and over, and people with severe ID (16)) to 43.8 per cent (adults with moderate to profound ID only (17)).

Prevalence of mental disorders in children and young people with ID is reported to be higher than for other children and young people for 27 out of 28 International Classification of Diseases version 10 Classification of Mental and Behavioural Disorders (ICD-10) (20) categories (14).

Some types of mental disorders are more common in adults with ID than in the general population, including schizophrenia (21, 22), bipolar disorder (23), dementia (particularly in adults with Down syndrome (24, 25), but also in people with ID not due to Down syndrome (26, 27)), autism (14, 28, 29), and ADHD (14). Challenging behaviours, which do not have an obvious general population comparator, are also common. A population-based study of 1,023 adults aged 16 years and over reported 22.5 per cent had challenging behaviours (15); 10 per cent had aggressive behaviour (including physically aggressive behaviour to others, verbally aggressive behaviour, and destructive behaviour to property) (30)); and 5 per cent had self-injurious behaviour (31). Depression and anxiety are common in people with ID; maybe not more so than in the general population (23, 32), though longitudinal studies suggest they may be more enduring conditions in people with ID, albeit with there being small numbers of people with ID within these longitudinal studies (33–35).

Regarding the course of mental disorders in childhood, an Australian cohort followed children and young people with ID, aged 4–19.5 years, over 14 years. Hyperactivity was more prominent at younger ages and persisted for longer in children and young people with more severe degrees of ID. Emotional disorders emerged later in childhood (36–38). Similar findings have been reported from longitudinal studies with children in the Netherlands (39, 40).

Regarding the course of mental disorders in adults, the incidence of mental disorders, excluding challenging behaviours, has been reported to be 12.6 per cent over a two-year period; 8.3 per cent for affective disorders, 1.7 per cent for anxiety disorders, and 1.4 per cent for psychotic disorders (5, 22). The incidence of challenging behaviours is reported to be 4.6 per cent (5); 1.8 per cent specifically for aggressive behaviour (30) and 0.6 per cent specifically for self-injurious behaviour (31). At age 65 years or older, the standardized incidence ratio for dementia is reported to be 4.98 (41), showing it is much higher in adults with ID—it is even higher still in adults with Down syndrome. Full remission of psychosis after two years was reported to be only 14.3 per cent (22), for aggression it was 27.7 per cent, and self-injury 38.2 per cent (30, 31). These findings suggest that whilst incidences are higher than those found in the general population, much of the current high prevalence of mental ill-health is due to enduring disorders rather than new episodes; though the evidence-base is limited in quantity.

Differences are found between reported rates in different studies. These are largely accounted for by the types of mental disorders included in the studies (particularly whether or not challenging behaviours and autism are included); the methods used to identify mental disorders; the classification system used for mental disorders; whether rates reported are point prevalence, period prevalence, or lifetime prevalence; and the population that the samples are drawn from including their ages, level of ID, and whether the sample is population-based or a clinical population.

Different study methodologies have different advantages. For example, the study of 1,023 adults quoted above has the advantage of being both population-based and that detailed mental health assessments were undertaken. However, it did not have a direct general population comparison. Scotland's Census, 2011 provides information on a much larger population (believed to be 97% of all Scotland's population) and allows direct comparison between people with ID and the rest of the population. However, it relies on self/proxy reports of mental disorders, and hence reports lower rates. It found that 5,038/21,115 (23.9%) of adults with ID were reported to have mental disorders compared with 224,584/4,357,930 (5.2%) of all other adults (42).

Aetiology

Mental disorders experienced by people with ID typically have multi-factorial aetiology, and this can be considered on biological, psychological, social, and developmental dimensions; and in terms of predisposing, precipitating, and maintaining factors. Aetiology of mental disorders has been represented in detail graphically across the life course by 'ACORNS' (Accessible Cause-Outcome Representation and Notation System) (43). Some of the multiple, interacting aetiologies are transactional; and linear cause and effect directions cannot usually be inferred. Considering aetiology is helpful in finding ways to prevent or reduce mental disorders, or to aid recovery.

Consideration of aetiology of mental disorders is therefore similar to that for the general population, but with additional complexity. This includes the addition of the developmental dimension, with parental bonding and development of attachments at early age, impairments in attentional control, and communication limitations. There are transactional effects of the person with ID and carers (mental disorder in the person with ID affecting the carer-person with ID interaction, and carer stress and health, in turn further affecting the mental health of the person with ID; a spiralling vicious circle can be established). Being dependent on others in daily tasks can be restrictive upon what one can achieve and aspire to, which may impact upon health.

Further complexity stems from people with ID having a greater burden in all of the dimensions, such as the behavioural phenotypes of some causes of ID; additional physical disorders and disabilities; psychological factors associated with ID; and multiple social disadvantages. Abuse, neglect, or exploitation has been shown to predict mental disorders in adults with ID. Life events are more common for people with ID, and when they do occur they tend to be multiple, for example, the death of a parent-carer leading to multiple changes in the person's life and care, moving their home, and dislocation from former environment, family friends, and occupations. Lone parent family, poor family functioning, lack of parental educational qualifications, income poverty, and households with no paid employment have been shown to be associated with mental disorders in children and young people with ID. Social disadvantages experienced by people with ID also include lack of paid employment, poverty of environment and recreational opportunities, social exclusion, and experience of bullying, harassment, stigma, and hate crimes.

Multi-morbidity

Whilst this text book is focused on the psychiatry of ID, it is neither possible nor desirable to consider mental disorders in isolation of physical disorders, because physical disorders are very common, and coexistence of mental and physical disorders is therefore typical in people with ID. This renders assessments for mental disorders more complex, as mental disorders, physical disorders, and drug side effects can mimic each other, and mental disorders may therefore be misattributed. It also results in people with ID having problems with polypharmacy, and also potential problems with disease-disease, disease-drug, and drug-drug interactions. People with ID may not be able to self-report drug side effects, and are reliant on others observing these, hence pharmacovigilance is essential. Anticholinergic burden due to polypharmacy can be an issue for people with ID, with potential negative side effects such as further impairments of cognition (44).

Physical disorders that are more common in children, young people, and adults with ID than in the general population include epilepsy (25% (45)), visual impairments (50%), hearing impairments (40%), impacted cerumen, gastro-oesophageal reflux disorder (50% (46)), dysphagia (47), constipation, diabetes, thyroid dysfunction, osteoporosis, contractures, mobility and balance impairments, injuries, eczema, xerosis, obesity, heart failure, and possibly asthma (48–51). Some physical disorders relate to the person's underlying cause of ID (e.g. thyroid dysfunction and Down syndrome), but lifestyle and environmental factors, sub-optimal support and health care are also important contributors. Some problems predispose to others; for example, psychotropic drugs (prescribed to about 20% of adults with ID (52)) can increase diabetes risk, as can obesity which is common (53), and sedentary lifestyles, which are also more common in people with ID than in the general population (54).

Assessment and classification; DC-LD and DM-ID2

Distinguishing between types of mental disorders, co-occurring mental disorders, physical disorders, and drug side effects requires careful assessment. Communication is a two-way process, and it is important for the professional conducting the assessment to optimize this, and also to adjust for hearing and visual impairments. It is essential to involve carers in assessments, as well as the person with ID. This may include paid carers for details on current symptoms, or several paid carers depending upon how well information is shared within and across staff teams (e.g. day carers, night carers, carers at the person's home and in day opportunity provisions), and family carers for the background information needed to conduct a developmental assessment, and to ensure that state symptoms can be distinguished from long-standing traits.

When assessing psychopathology, it is important to consider that paid carers may spontaneously report the psychopathology that is most challenging for them, such as aggressive behaviour. Hence after the person with ID (if they are able to) and their carers have described the symptoms they are experiencing, it is important to specifically enquire about all other possible psychopathology. Psychopathology and course of the mental disorder is classified using standard manuals; in the general population, typically the ICD-10 (21) is used in the UK and the *Diagnostic and Statistical Manual of Mental Disorders, fifth edition* (DSM-5) (55) in the USA. ICD-10 and DSM-5 do not provide clear categories for challenging behaviours and also include some symptoms within required symptom counts that are not experienced by people with ID due to the developmental level of their cognitive functioning, and in some categories require developmental history details that might no longer be available for adults with ID. For these reasons, strict application of ICD-10 or DSM-5 criteria under-reports mental disorders in people with ID. Consequently, diagnostic manuals for mental disorders have been designed specifically for use with people with ID. DC-LD (Diagnostic Criteria for Psychiatric Disorders for Use with Adults with Learning Disabilities/Mental Retardation) (1) was designed to be used to complement ICD-10, and the Diagnostic Manual-Intellectual Disability 2 (DM-ID 2) (2) was designed to interpret how to apply DSM-5 criteria.

DC-LD provides three axes: I. Severity of ID, II. Cause of ID, and III. Psychiatric disorders. Axis III is divided into five levels: A. Developmental disorders, B. Psychiatric illness, C. Personality disorders, D. Problem behaviours, and E. Other disorders. It also provides information on behavioural phenotypes, other associated medical conditions (ICD-10 chapters other than V), and factors influencing health status and contact with health services (ICD-10 chapter XXI). It provides instruction on how to use the manual and its hierarchical approach to diagnosis, provides diagnostic approaches to 'organic' disorders and behavioural phenotypes, cross-references between DC-LD, ICD-10, and DSM; and provides additional information on the stages of psychiatric diagnosis, and additional diagnostic considerations that are needed for people with ID. Further information about the concepts and evidence behind DC-LD were provided in a special edition of the *Journal of Intellectual Disabilities Research*, in September 2003, volume 47, supplement 1.

The structure of DM-ID 2 adheres to that of DSM-5, with background information relevant to people with ID provided for each diagnostic category, and additional tables provided to interpret the DSM-5 criteria of use for people with ID. It additionally provides chapters on assessment and diagnostic procedures with people with ID, and on behavioural phenotypes. There are two versions, one also being a textbook, providing updated information on each of the types of mental disorders. The previous edition of DM-ID 2 was field-tested and found to have good clinical utility (56).

Final considerations

Children, young people, and adults with ID have high rates of mental disorders, and working with them and their carers is complex, interesting, and highly rewarding. People with ID experience considerable health and health care inequalities compared with other people, and knowledgeable practitioners who work carefully and empathically can make important differences in the lives of individuals and their families.

REFERENCES

1. Royal College of Psychiatrists. *DC-LD (Diagnostic Criteria for Psychiatric Disorders for Use with Adults with Learning Disabilities/ Mental Retardation)*. London: Gaskell Press; 2001.

2. Fletcher R, Barnhill J, Cooper S-A. *The Diagnostic Manual—Intellectual Disability 2.* eds. R. Fletcher, J. Barnhill and S-A. Cooper. New York: NADD Press; 2016.
3. Gillberg C. The ESSENCE in child psychiatry: Early symptomatic syndromes eliciting neurodevelopmental clinical examinations. *Research in Developmental Disabilities*, 2010;31:1543–1551.
4. Moreno-De-Luca A, Myers SM, Challman TD, Moreno-De-Luca D, Evans DW, Ledbetter DH. Developmental brain dysfunction: Revival and expansion of old concepts based on new genetic evidence. *Lancet Neurology*, 2013;12:406–414.
5. Smiley E, Cooper S-A, Finlayson J, et al. The incidence, and predictors of mental ill-health in adults with intellectual disabilities. Prospective study. *British Journal of Psychiatry*, 2007;191:313–319.
6. Melville C, McConnachie A, Johnson P, et al. Problem behaviours and symptom dimensions of psychiatric disorders in adults with intellectual disabilities: An exploratory and confirmatory factor analysis. *Research in Developmental Disabilities*, 2016;55:1–13.
7. Melville CA, Smiley E, Simpson N, et al. Statistical modelling studies examining the dimensional structure of psychopathology experienced by adults with intellectual disabilities. Systematic review. *Research in Developmental Disabilities*, 2016;53–54:1–10.
8. Einfeld SL, Ellis LA, Emerson E. Comorbidity of intellectual disability and mental disorder in children and adolescents: A systematic review. *Journal of Intellectual and Developmental Disabilities*, 2011;36:137–143.
9. Buckles J, Luckasson R, Keefe, E. A systematic review of the prevalence of psychiatric disorders in adults with intellectual disability, 2003–2010. *Journal of Mental Health Research in Intellectual Disabilities*, 2013;6:181–207.
10. Simpson N, Mizen L, Cooper S-A. Intellectual disabilities. *Medicine*, 2016;44:679–682.
11. Rutter M, Tizard J, Whitmore K. *Education, Health and Behaviour.* London, UK: Longman; 1970.
12. Birch HG, Richardson SA, Baird D, Horobin G, Illsley R. *Mental Subnormality in the Community: A Clinical and Epidemiological Study.* Baltimore, MD: Williams and Wilkins; 1970.
13. Dekker MC, Koot HM, van der Ende J, Verhulst FC. Emotional and behavioural problems in children and adolescents with and without intellectual disabilities. *Journal of Child Psychology and Psychiatry*, 2002;43:1087–1098.
14. Emerson E, Hatton C. Mental health of children and adolescents with intellectual disabilities in Britain. *British Journal of Psychiatry*, 2007;191:493–499.
15. Cooper S-A, Smiley E, Morrison J, Allan L, Williamson A. Prevalence of and associations with mental ill-health in adults with intellectual disabilities. *British Journal of Psychiatry*, 2007;190:27–35.
16. Deb S, Thomas M, Bright, C. Mental disorder in adults with intellectual disability. 1: Prevalence of functional psychiatric illness among a community-based population aged between 16 and 64 years. *Journal of Intellectual Disability Research*, 2001;45:495–505.
17. Bailey N. Prevalence of psychiatric disorders in adults with moderate to profound learning disabilities, *Advances in Mental Health and Learning Disabilities*, 2007;1:36–44.
18. Cooper S-A, Bailey NM. Psychiatric disorders amongst adults with learning disabilities: Prevalence and relationship to ability level. *Irish Journal of Psychological Medicine*, 2001;18:45–53.
19. Corbett JA. Psychiatric morbidity and mental retardation. In *Psychiatric Illness and Mental Handicap* (eds. F. E. James and R. P. Snaith), pp. 11–25. London: Gaskell Press; 1979.
20. World Health Organisation. *The ICD-10 Classification of Mental and Behavioural Disorders.* Geneva: WHO; 1990.
21. Turner TH. Schizophrenia and mental handicap: an historical review, with implications for further research. *Psychological Medicine*, 1989;19:301–314.
22. Cooper S-A, Smiley E, Morrison J, et al. Psychosis and adults with intellectual disabilities. Prevalence, incidence, and related factors. *Social Psychiatry and Psychiatric Epidemiology*, 2007;42:530–536.
23. Cooper S-A, Smiley E, Allan L, Morrison J. The incidence of unipolar and bipolar depression and mania in adults with intellectual disabilities. Prospective cohort study. *British Journal of Psychiatry*, 2018;212:295–300.
24. Oliver C, Holland AJ. Down's syndrome and Alzheimer's disease: A review. *Psychological Medicine*, 1986;16:307–322.
25. Prasher VP. Age-specific prevalence, thyroid dysfunction and depressive symptomatology in adults with Down syndrome and dementia. *International Journal of Geriatric Psychiatry*, 1995;10:25–31.
26. Cooper S-A. High prevalence of dementia amongst people with learning disabilities not attributed to Down's syndrome. *Psychological Medicine*, 1997;27:609–616.
27. Strydom A, Livingston G, King M, Hassiotis A. Prevalence of dementia in intellectual disability using different diagnostic criteria. *British Journal of Psychiatry*, 2007;191:150–157.
28. Baird G, Simonoff E, Pickles A, et al. Prevalence of disorders of the autism spectrum in a population cohort of children in South Thames: The Special Needs and Autism Project (SNAP). *The Lancet*, 2006;368(9531):210–215.
29. Brugha TS, Spiers N, Bankart J, et al. Epidemiology of autism in adults across age groups and ability levels. *British Journal of Psychiatry*, 2016;209:498–503.
30. Cooper S-A, Smiley E, Jackson A, et al. Adults with intellectual disabilities. Prevalence, incidence, and remission of aggressive behaviour, and related factors. *Journal of Intellectual Disability Research*, 2009;53:217–232.
31. Cooper S-A, Smiley E, Allan L, et al. Adults with intellectual disabilities. Prevalence, incidence and remission of self-injurious behaviour, and related factors. *Journal of Intellectual Disability Research*, 2009;53:200–216.
32. Reid K, Smiley E, Cooper S-A. Prevalence and associations with anxiety disorders in adults with intellectual disabilities. *Journal of Intellectual Disability Research*, 2011;55:172–181.
33. Maughan B, Collishaw S, Pickles A. Mild mental retardation: Psychosocial functioning in adulthood. *Psychological Medicine*, 1999;29:351–366.
34. Collishaw S, Maughan B, Pickles A. Affective problems in adults with mild learning disability: The roles of social disadvantage and ill health. *British Journal of Psychiatry*, 2004;185:350–351.
35. Richards M, Maughan B, Hardy R, Hall I, Strydom A, Wadsworth M. Long-term affective disorder in people with learning disability. *British Journal of Psychiatry*, 2001;170:523–527.
36. Einfeld SL, Tonge, BJ. Population prevalence of psychopathology in children and adolescents with intellectual disability: II Epidemiological findings. *Journal of Intellectual Disability Research*, 1996;40:99–109.
37. Tonge BJ, Einfeld SL. Psychopathology and Intellectual Disability: The Australian child to adult longitudinal study. *International Review of Research in Mental Retardation*, 2003;26:61–91.

38. Einfeld SL, Piccinin AM, Mackinnon A, et al. Psychopathology in young people with intellectual disability. *Journal of the American Medical Association*, 2006;296:1981–1989.
39. Wallander JL, Dekker MC, Koot HM. Risk factors for psychopathology in children with intellectual disability: A prospective longitudinal population-based study. *Journal of Intellectual Disability Research*, 2006;50:259–268.
40. De Ruiter KP, Dekker MC, Frank C, Verhulst FC, Koot HM. Developmental course of psychopathology in youths with and without intellectual disabilities. *Journal of Child Psychology and Psychiatry*, 2007;48:498–507.
41. Strydom A, Chan T, King M, Hassiotis A, Livingston G. Incidence of dementia in older adults with intellectual disabilities. *Research in Developmental Disabilities*, 2013;34:1881–1885.
42. Hughes-McCormack, L.A., Rydzewska, E., Henderson, A., Rintoul, J., Macintyre, C., Cooper, S-A. Prevalence of mental ill-health and relationship with physical health in a whole country population of 26,349 people with intellectual disabilities, compared with the general population. *British Journal of Psychiatry Open*, 2017, **3**, Issue 5, http://bjpo.rcpsych.org/content/3/5/243.
43. Moore DG, George R. ACORNS: A tool for the visualisation and modelling of atypical development. *Journal of Intellectual Disability Research*, 2011;55:956–972.
44. O'Dwyer M, Peklar J, McCallion P, McCarron M, Henman MC. Factors associated with polypharmacy and excessive polypharmacy in older people with intellectual disability differ from the general population: A cross-sectional observational nationwide study. *BMJ Open*, 2016; http://bmjopen.bmj.com/content/6/4/e010505.
45. Bowley C, Kerr M. Epilepsy and intellectual disability: Invited review. *Journal of Intellectual Disability Research*, 2000;44:529–543.
46. Böhmer CJ, Niezen-de Boer MC, Klinkenberg-Knol EC, Deville WL, Nadorp JH, Meuwissen SG. The prevalence of gastroesophageal reflux disease in institutionalized intellectually disabled individuals. *American Journal of Gastroenterology*, 1999;94:804–810.
47. Robertson J, Chadwick D, Baines S, Emerson E, Hatton C. People with intellectual disabilities and dysphagia. *Disability Rehabilitation*, 2017;12:1–16.
48. Cooper S-A, McLean G, Guthrie B, et al. Multiple physical and mental health comorbidity in adults with intellectual disabilities: Population-based cross-sectional analysis. *BMC Family Practice*, 2015; DOI: 10.1186/s12875-015-0329-3.
49. Carey IM, Shah SM, Hosking FJ, et al. Health characteristics and consultation patterns of people with intellectual disability: A cross-sectional database study in English general practice. *British Journal of General Practice*, 2016;66(645):e264–e270.
50. McCarron M, Swinburne J, Burke E, McGlinchey E, Carroll R, McCallion P. Patterns of multimorbidity in an older population of persons with an intellectual disability: results from the intellectual disability supplement to the Irish longitudinal study on aging (IDS-TILDA). *Research in Developmental Disabilities*, 2013;34:521–527.
51. Hermans H, Evenhuis HM. Multimorbidity in older adults with intellectual disabilities. *Research in Developmental Disabilities*, 2014;35:776–783.
52. Sheehan R, Hassiotis A, Walters K, Osborn D, Strydom A, Horsfall L. Mental illness, challenging behaviour, and psychotropic drug prescribing in people with intellectual disability: UK population based cohort study. *British Medical Journal*, 2015;35 631:h4326.
53. Melville CA, Cooper S-A, Morrison J, Allan L, Smiley E, Williamson A. The prevalence and determinants of obesity in adults with intellectual disabilities. *Journal of Applied Research in Intellectual Disabilities*, 2008;21:425–437.
54. Finlayson J, Jackson A, Cooper S-A, et al. Understanding predictors of low physical activity in adults with intellectual disabilities. *Journal of Applied Research in Intellectual Disabilities*, 2009;22:236–247.
55. American Psychiatric Association. *Diagnostic and Statistical Manual of Mental Disorders; Fifth Edition*. Arlington, VA: American Psychiatric Association; 2013.
56. Fletcher R, Havercamp S, Ruedrich S, et al. (2009) Clinical usefulness of the diagnostic manual-intellectual disability for mental disorders in persons with intellectual disability. *Journal of Clinical Psychiatry*, 2009;70:967–974.

7
Autism Spectrum Disorder

Mary Barrett and Traolach S. Brugha

Definitions

Intellectual Disability (ID) requires an IQ below 70 associated with impairment in two or more areas of adaptive functioning which began in the developmental period (i.e. before 18 years of age). Autism Spectrum Disorder (ASD) refers to the triad of impairments described by Lorna Wing (1) encompassing differences in social interaction, social communication, social imagination, and difficulties adjusting the behavioural repertoire to the changing demands of new social situations. Again, the importance of impairment in functioning must be acknowledged. Both these conditions represent part of the neurodevelopmental spectrum and overlap in features can occur. A diagnosis of ASD is therefore only appropriate in ID practice if the features seen are out of keeping with the person's developmental stage.

Background

Descriptions of individuals who appear to manifest the features of ASD are scattered through the literature dating back centuries, for example Victor of Aveyron (c1788--1828), a French feral child. Descriptions by Kanner (2) and Asperger (3) heralded the start of modern-day awareness and thinking, albeit only being brought to wider attention and rigorous study by the efforts of Lorna Wing and Judith Gould (4). Further important developments in understanding were the recognition of ASD as a lifelong condition (5, 6, 7) and awareness of the variety of its presentations, the latter reflected in changes in classification systems, most recently with the merging of social interaction and social communication domains in DSM-5 (8).

Terminology

The term Autism Spectrum Disorder is here used to encompass a range of conditions including Childhood Autism, High Functioning Autism and Asperger Syndrome and will be used here in that context, albeit many patients still wish to use the terms Autism and Asperger Syndrome, finding these labels more meaningful. A move towards a unitary term is in line with the recent publication of DSM-5 (8), ICD 11 still being awaited.

A further debate centres on the utility of diagnosing 'Autistic traits', that is, presence of certain features in the absence of a 'full house' of symptoms. We often ape medicine too thoughtlessly (diagnosis = cause = treatment): the issue, some say, is surely to identify what impact Autistic traits (whether or not they cross some arbitrary diagnostic threshold) have on functioning, well-being and mental health, and what can be done about it. For example, being unable to express affection to the degree that it distresses the person's partner sufficiently to jeopardize that vital supportive relationship does matter (and could be addressed) regardless of whether full criteria are met. The ICD-10 (9) coding 'Atypical Autism' can be used for individuals who fail to fulfil the full diagnostic criteria or the age of onset criteria. It is argued in ICD-10 that this is a useful concept in its own right, particularly for individuals with more significant levels of ID who necessarily may not have the behavioural repertoire to demonstrate abnormalities across all domains, or who may not have early developmental history available. In clinical practice, it can also be a useful concept for more able individuals who experience significant impairment(s) in one or two of the core aspects of ASD but do not meet full criteria, albeit the label can also be a cause of frustration if it is deemed to fall below the 'threshold' for receipt of Statutory Services. Clinical judgement and a discussion with the person and their family is therefore required when any diagnostic label is applied, as making a diagnosis that is helpful to the person, fairly reflects their difficulties and allows them access to much needed support are all important considerations.

Aetiology

There is increasing evidence for ASD being a familial condition but with incomplete penetrance, with the X chromosome having the strongest association, as well as links to 15q and 7q. In many cases, the 'full blown' condition is not seen passing through the generations, rather it appears that traits will pass down the generations and enquiry as to whether other family members display any of the features can often prove fruitful. Alongside the genetic propensity, the importance of environmental factors must be considered (See Box 7.1), with researchers favouring an interaction between an early environmental insult and a genetic predisposition. Care should be taken when considering some of the below causations, for example

Box 7.1 Environmental factors implicated in ASD

- Advanced parental age (M>F)
- Gestational diabetes
- Shorter gestation
- Bleeding prepartum
- Maternal stress
- Insufficient dietary folate pre-conception
- Infections e.g. rubella, CMV
- Valproic acid
- Foetal alcohol syndrome
- Low birth weight
- Birth hypoxia

a difficult birth could be the cause of brain damage, but equally an abnormal foetus may be more prone to a difficult birth.

Well-publicized proposed causations which have subsequently been discredited include the 'Refrigerator Mother' hypothesis championed by Bruno Bettelheim in the 1950s and 1960s, or more recently the MMR vaccine. Research evidence has not supported the efficacy of secretin treatment, or of gluten and casein-free dietary regimes.

Prevalence

Debate continues as to whether there has been a true increase in prevalence of ASD over time, or whether this is a product of increasing awareness and change in diagnostic criteria. Miller et al (10) recently re-examined the Utah child cohort (11) and found that when DSM-IV-TR criteria were applied to the previous records, more individuals met diagnostic criteria for Autism than at original assessment using DSM-III. One of the most reliable sources of data in recent years is Brugha et al.'s population-based study (12) which estimated the overall prevalence of Autism in England to be 1.1 per cent (95% CI 3–19/1000). Male gender was only a strong predictor of Autism for those with no or Mild ID (Adjusted OR = 8.5, 95 per cent CI 2.0–34.9; interaction with gender, $P = 0.03$).

Many studies have shown frequent coexistence of Autism and ID—more commonly than is formally documented in clinical practice—suggesting a degree of under-recognition and/or labelling by services. Interestingly, Miller et al (10) in the study detailed above, found that the later diagnostic criteria better identified cases of ASD with ID, with 84 per cent of the newly-identified cases having intellectual impairment. Recent population-based work by Brugha et al. (12) has found the prevalence of ASD in adults with moderate to profound ID living in communal care establishments to be 31 per cent and in private households to be 35.4 per cent. Clinicans should clearly be mindful of this high degree of comorbidity whenever they assessing an individual with ID.

Autism has not been found to be causal for ID, nor ID for Autism and it is thought that the high rate of co-occurrance is due to both conditions arising from a common cause (13). This notwithstanding, Brugha et al. (12) found the prevalence of ASD to increase as IQ decreases and particularly as verbal IQ decreases. Interestingly, reduced verbal IQ has also been found to be strongly associated with Autism in more able adults in the general population (14). It is also notable that sex differences are less marked in adults with ID, with the divide closing as IQ goes down (60% males vs 43% females with Profound ID), likely due to increasing influence from the greater degree of cognitive impairment.

Even when a full clinical diagnosis is not possible, autistic traits are commonly seen in people with ID and important to recognize in their own right due to the impact they have on the person's functioning as well as the adjustments needed in management strategies. Bhaumik and colleagues (15) looked at the prevalence of autistic traits amongst adults with ID in Leicestershire. They looked at five different traits, namely lack of empathy, poor social interaction, marked stereotypies, elaborate routines and minimal speech/echolalia. 46.2 per cent of the population had one or more of these traits, with lack of empathy being the most common. The study found an association between autistic traits and severe to profound ID, younger age, living apart from the family, use of additional medication, presence, and severity of challenging behaviour, causing physical hurt to others and hurt to the extent of needing attention and use of constant or close supervision.

Core cognitive difficulties

In order to understand the presenting features in ASD, it is helpful to first consider what are currently thought to be the underlying cognitive difficulties, namely impaired theory of mind, lack of central coherence, and difficulties in executive functioning.

Theory of mind

Theory of mind refers to the ability to attribute mental states (including beliefs, intents, desires, knowledge, and pretence) to both oneself and other people, and to understand that others have beliefs, desires, and intentions that are different from one's own. The most well-known test used to demonstrate difficulties in this area is the 'Sally Ann Test' (16), however a note of caution must be used here, as more able individuals with ASD can learn how to intellectually 'pass the test'. Difficulties in this area are better demonstrated by enquiring how a person functions in real-life social situations, where they are required to apply their understanding in an uncontrolled and unrehearsed setting, noting the degree of extra effort this costs the person.

Central coherence

Central coherence is the ability to assimilate all the information at hand, along with using relevant prior knowledge, to see the 'bigger picture'. It is a necessary process to allow information to be taken in context. Difficulties in this domain mean that people with ASD naturally tend to focus in on minor details and think about things in the smallest possible parts but 'cannot see the wood for the trees' (17). Consequently, they may miss important information or misinterpret situations due to failing to understand the full circumstance, however it can also prove a useful skill, for example, the occasionally seen individual with ID with an ability to draw highly detailed and accurate scenes from memory, play a musical instrument or retain detailed factual information at a much higher ability level than would be expected by their IQ.

Executive functioning

Executive functioning is employed for activities such as sequencing, organising and planning ahead. Lack of awareness and internal monitoring of time and space in people with ASD can render them less likely to think in a sequential framework and thus understand and predict the world. As a consequence, even those who are highly intellectually able can struggle to attend to their 'day to day' functions such as scheduling, keeping up with household chores and managing money, as well as more major challenges.

Clinical presentation

Core features

Each individual who meets diagnostic criteria for an ASD will display differences across the domains of social communication, social interaction, social imagination, and fixed repetitive behaviours. In turn, within each domain there a spectrum of impairment (Figure 7.1) which present in different combinations in different individuals. Generally, a person with ID is more likely to present with those features at the more severe end of each spectrum domain, and more intellectually-able individuals with the less severe features. Lorna Wing (18) described three subtypes of social impairment which appear to correlate to different levels of functioning. The aloof group are the most impaired, showing no interest in social interaction aside from getting their needs met; in addition there is usually severe impairment in or absence of verbal and non-verbal communication. The passive group generally has a higher level of skills than the aloof group—they may copy peers and assume everyone who speaks to them is a friend, putting them at risk of exploitation by others. The 'active but odd' group demand social attention in inappropriate ways and their physical touching and clinging can become physically aggressive if demands are not met. They have more skills, however their behaviour interferes with their achievements, in addition their apparent sociability and talkativeness can lead to an overestimation of abilities and underestimation of handicaps. Volkmar et al (19) suggested that these subtypes may be mainly related to IQ, with the aloof group being mainly lower functioning, the passive group

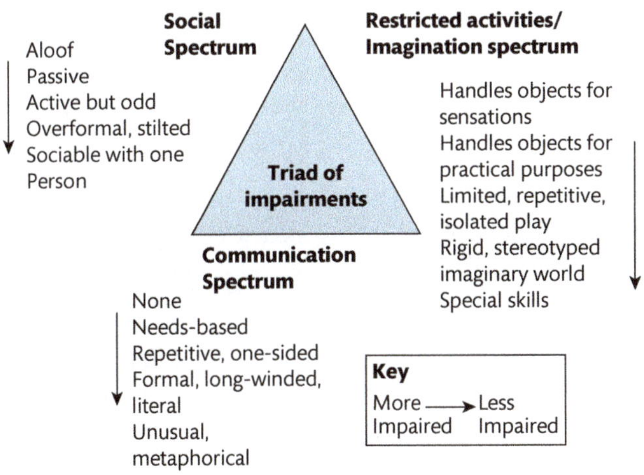

Figure 7.1 A spectrum perspective

at an intermediate level and the active but odd group having the highest level of functioning. However, Wing and Gould's study in Camberwell (4) found some individuals with Profound ID who clearly fell into the sociable category, therefore IQ cannot be the only factor involved.

Social interaction and social communication

The integration of these domains within DSM-5 has been helpful, as they are clearly inter-related concepts that hard to tease out. In line with this approach, the following differences may be commonly observed:

Social-emotional reciprocity

- Difficulties initiating/responding appropriately to social interaction.
- Problems with two-way social conversation, particularly 'small talk'.
- Problems recognizing/responding appropriately to social and emotional cues from others—for example that they are upset or bored—resulting in the person appearing rude or insensitive.

Nonverbal communicative behaviours used for social interaction

- Difficulties with eye contact—often reduced or avoided, also staring
- Limited/odd use of gesture and facial expression.
- Difficulty reading and understanding others' facial expressions and body language.

Developing, maintaining, and understanding relationships

- Difficulties in this area range from lack of interest in forming friendships and/or relationships, through to problems making and/or keeping them going.
- Failing to understand the social hierarchy and adjust behaviour according to the social context (e.g. pub vs church) is common and becomes an increasing issue with age as social expectations on the person increase.

Social imagination and fixed, repetitive behaviours

Difficulty reading and understanding other people's thoughts and emotions and thus empathy problems are a likely consequence of the differences observed in social imagination. In addition it presents challenges in 'thinking outside the box', which can be manifest as difficulties in predicting what will or could happen next, preparing for and coping with change or new/unfamiliar situations. Generalizing learning from theory to practice, or between situations is difficult, as is engaging in imaginative activities/play that is spontaneous or requires novel creativity. More intellectually-able individuals may have an elaborate and complex fantasy world/engage in play, but it is likely to be set and repetitive in content, or may be directed by others, including participating in drama.

Fixed, repetitive behaviours are often a way to help the person make sense of the world in which they live; the need to deviate from the planned behaviour—even in a minor way—can be a source of extreme anxiety. Conversely, the person can gain a sense of pleasure and satisfaction from fulfilling the behaviours; that is to say they are egosyntonic, differentiating them from the rituals seen in Obsessive Compulsive Disorder (OCD) which are egodystonic with the person feeling compelled to undertake them to ward off negative consequences.

Activities are usually limited to one or a few circumscribed themes which may persist or change over time, but always have the quality of being all-consuming of the person's interest and time. Examples are sticking to a strict daily routine, or alternatively not planning or organizing anything even when there is a requirement to do so, keeping belongs arranged 'just so', arranging objects in a set way, for example in lines, and complex rituals with no clear practical purpose (e.g. series of movements carried out before crossing a threshold). Collecting objects or facts, potentially resulting in large storage problems, is common; more able individuals may have Special Interests which are all-consuming and 'more than just a hobby', for example space, trains, tigers, history, computer coding.

Common additional features

Sensory sensitivities

Recent years have seen a growing awareness of the frequency and importance of sensory differences in people with ASD, to the extent that they are now included in the core diagnostic features in DSM-5. Differences can be of under (hypo) sensitivity or over (hyper) sensitivity, in any modality. In general, individuals with a greater degree of ID are more likely to be hyposensitive, whilst those with normal or higher IQ levels tend to be hypersensitive, however any combination of differences can be seen. These differences are more commonly reported in children, however, if questioned, many adults still experience difficulties, albeit they may have learned ways to cope/mask the problem, for example, wearing headphones when in a noisy environment or actively avoiding situations where they know they will be exposed to the stimulus. Table 7.1 lists common presentations of sensory differences in each modality.

In addition to sensitivities, sensory likes and dislikes can occur, for example sparkly lights, furry fabrics, tumble dryer vibrations, and the smell/feel of hair. Management problems can occur if the person vigorously pursues or avoids the stimulus, especially once they reach teenage and adult years.

Table 7.1 Signs of sensory difference

Modality	Hyposensitive	Hypersensitive
Vision	Touches everything Repeatedly moving objects before eyes	Looking down most of time Focus on detail
Hearing	Enjoying loud noises Screeches, claps	Fear of sudden sounds Dislike of high-pitched sounds Covering ears
Touch	Likes firm pressure High pain threshold	Clothing/shoes Personal care difficult
Balance	Spinning, swinging, rocking Lying on ledges	Difficulty with uneven surfaces/stairs Fear of feet leaving ground
Smell/Taste	Licking objects May eat anything	Restricted food choices Dislike of certain smells Toileting problems

Sleep problems

Difficulty settling, poor quality sleep, frequent awakenings, and day-night reversal are all seen and often a major cause of stress for carers. Establishing a consistent end of day routine and regular bedtime is vital, along with strategies such as blackout blinds. Increasingly, consideration is being given to the use of Melatonin for difficulty settling, albeit this remains off-licence in the UK, aside for short term treatment in the over-55 age group.

Dietary preferences

Marked preferences are common, with the person restricting their food choices, for example to certain flavours (e.g. very bland or very spicy), food types or brands; dislike of certain textures and refusal to try new foods. This commonly requires adaptations within the living environment, for example the person being prepared separate meals, and in its extreme form to concerns about low BMI and malnutrition. Other specifications may be foods not touching on the plate and only using specific crockery and cutlery which no-one else can touch.

Motor abnormalities

Repetitive movements such as hand flapping, rocking, bouncing up and down, screeching and/or gyration are seen, most commonly in children but also can continue in adult life particularly if there is a situation of high emotion. The movements may have a comforting quality for the person, and/or be done for sensory purposes ('stimming').

Comorbidities

In clinical literature and practice, ASD is commonly comorbid with a wide range of conditions which will inevitably impact on both its presentation and outcome; indeed, it has been stated that comorbidity is to be expected and occurs both directly and indirectly (20). To date, comorbidity has not been studied in general population samples in adulthood, only in those who present to clinical services, so the reported associations may be partly due to this being a self-selected population.

Whatever the ability level of the individual being seen, there is the potential for diagnostic overshadowing, with all symptoms being attributed to the ASD. Clinicians must therefore remember the high chances of comorbidity and screen thoroughly for additional conditions, particularly if there has been a change in functioning/behaviour. The value of an initial assessment by a clinician with a wide range of experience cannot be underestimated, particularly with the ASD population where communication difficulties impact on the person's ability to understand and express their emotional state and experience.

Conversely, a neurodevelopmental or psychiatric disorder that does not respond to treatment as expected should lead to consideration of an underlying comorbidity, including ASD.

ID

ID has been reported to influence the nature of ASD (21). Certainly the presence of ID will make it more difficult for an individual to learn new skills and overcome problems and in addition there may be associated physical impairments, such as speech or sensory impairments and physical disabilities, which are likely to have a multiplicative rather than additive effect on the ASD. These difficulties all impact on learning and thus the presence of a ID may result in an individual remaining 'more autistic' than would otherwise be the case (22).

The level of ID should always be taken into account when considering whether suspected ASD features are significant, for example behaviours such as rocking, jumping, and flapping of hands can be seen during routine child development; if the person with ID is functioning at that developmental level then the behaviour may be judged to be in keeping with that expected for ID. When ASD is being considered in the context of ID, the clinician should therefore be confident the features represent 'difference not just delay'.

Other neurodevelopmental disorders

Studies have found a number of other neurodevelopmental disorders to occur comorbidly with ASD and to show considerable overlap in symptomatology; a review of the literature by Gillberg and Billstedt (20) reported evidence for Attention Deficit Hyperactivity Disorder (ADHD), DAMP and Tourette's syndrome in children and adolescents, while Wing and Shah (23) described catatonia in adolescents and adults with ASD. Clinicians are well aware of the challenges presented when trying to untangle the significance of overlapping symptomatology, for example whether a tendency to social gaffes and bluntness are due to a lack of social understanding with its origins in ASD, as opposed to the wandering attention and 'lack of filter' more likely due to ADHD. Management of dual diagnosis also presents additional challenges, for example, treatment of ADHD then allowing the person with ASD to pursue their routines and rituals with increased focus.

Specific learning difficulties (dyslexia, dyspraxia, and dyscalculia) all occur in clinical practice more commonly than would be expected by chance in individuals with ASD and should not be missed due to the significant additional burden they place on the individual trying to negotiate everyday activities, whether it be coping in the classroom environment, filling in paperwork or even tying shoelaces. Conversely, consideration of the possibility of ASD may be wise in an individual with a specific learning difficulty whose problems spread more widely, for example problems socializing with peers or communicative misunderstandings. The practitioner needs to be mindful however that the features of the specific learning difficulty can have wider-reaching effects in their own right, for example the slower cognitive processing speed and difficulty holding information in working memory seen in dyslexia may impact on social functioning, for example, keeping up with a group conversation, particularly in a busy environment.

Psychiatric disorders including challenging behaviour

It is notable that Kanner described mood symptoms in his first report of autism in 1943 (2); more recently Abramson et al's (24) preliminary study of adults identified through specialist ASD clinics found that the rates of affective disorder may be as high as 33 per cent. A wide range of other disorders have been reported in association with ASD in such settings, including schizophrenia, paranoia, delusional disorder, catatonia, obsessive-compulsive disorder, Tourette syndrome and anorexia nervosa (20, 25), but in clinical practice, anxiety and mood symptoms are the most commonly encountered and should always be enquired about.

The relationship between ASD and personality disorder (PD) is an interesting and under-researched one, given the commonalities seen, for example impaired relating to others and affective regulation. Anckrsäter et al. (26) examined the impact of ASD and ADHD on personality development and concluded that both conditions were associated with an increased risk of PD. In clinical practice ASD and PD are rarely diagnosed together: the reasons for this are unclear, whether it be diagnostic overshadowing, lack of clinician awareness, or other factors. This notwithstanding, the presence of the combination—particularly with Emotionally Unstable or Antisocial PD—presents a major management challenge for services, with such individuals potentially requiring involvement from other branches of Psychiatry such as Forensic Services.

Most studies of psychiatric illness in ASD to date have looked at relatively high functioning individuals. It is widely acknowledged that a different approach is needed for the detection of psychiatric disorder in low functioning individuals, for example increased aggression, irritability, self-injury, and challenging behaviour or reduction in communication can all indicate psychiatric illness in this group (27).

A wide range of behavioural difficulties has been reported in association with ASD, including suicidal acts, hyperactivity, aggression, temper outbursts, antisocial behaviour, unusual fantasy, preoccupation with weapons and violence, firesetting, inappropriate sexual behaviours, school refusal, enuresis and encopresis, elective mutism, illicit substance use, and appetite and sleep disturbances (25).

Individuals with ASD and ID are reported to have particularly high rates of challenging behaviour (28); aggression and self-injury have been found to be particularly common in those with an aloof social interactional style and low ability levels and in those with severe expressive communication difficulties (29). Those with severe ID, ASD, and little speech have been reported to develop behavioural swings in adolescence consisting of periods of excitement and overactivity alternating with apathy. These can also have a profound impact on a person's social life, with both extremes interfering with social interaction however, they do tend to become less intense with age (28).

In general, behavioural difficulties have been shown to cause a range of problems, including limiting the level of independence achieved (22), limiting community integration and being a major reason for institutional care (30), as well as being offputting to others, further exacurbating problems with social relationships (28).

Studies suggest a striking similarity in psychiatric and behavioural symptom patterns in children/adolescents and adults with ASD, suggesting a continuity of clinical disorders across the lifespan. It is likely that adults with ASD present for psychiatric attention more frequently than previously recognized and some patients with resistant chronic psychiatric illness may actually have an undiagnosed ASD (31). Clinical evidence suggests that the presence of psychiatric disorder, especially depression, may affect the long-term outcome of ASD in its own right, with symptoms leading to social withdrawal and oppositional/aggressive behaviour; this can interfere with community placements, impact on families, and depression has even resulted in moves to institutional care (32).

Medical disorders

ASD have been associated with a wide range of medical conditions including epilepsy, Fragile X Syndrome, Tuberous Sclerosis, untreated Phenylketonuria, maternal rubella infection, Rett Syndrome and sensory impairments (4, 20, 33). Each of these conditions may change the presentation of ASD, influence health and mortality, and have a lifelong impact on the individual (33). Rai et al (34), using data from the 2007 APMS study, found epilepsy was strongly associated with ASD (odds ratio [OR] 7.4, 95% CI 1.5-35.5). Fragile X Syndrome has been reported in up to 10 per cent of the population with Autism and usually occurs in association with ID and up to 25 per cent of those with Tuberous Sclerosis have Autism. People with Rubella Syndrome are reported to become 'less autistic' over time and some of the resemblence to ASD is felt to be related to sensory impairments and the presence of severe ID.

Both visual and hearing impairments occur at higher rates than would be expected in the general population, in particular it has been reported that 10–20 per cent of people with autism have at least a moderate hearing deficit (20). Awareness of these issues is important in two respects, firstly because of the impact that they may have on a person's development, for example, further hindering social interactional opportunities, and secondly because their presentation may overlap with symptoms of ASD, potentially contributing to misdiagnosis (35).

Assessment and diagnosis

NICE guidelines CG128 (36) 'Autism spectrum disorder in under 19s: recognition, referral and diagnosis' and CG142 (37) 'Autism spectrum disorder in adults: diagnosis and management' set out current guidance and standards for the assessment process across the lifespan and should be referred to by the reader in conjunction with this text. The importance of a comprehensive, team-based assessment by trained professionals, assessment of developmental status, and screening for comorbidities is highlighted in both documents. CG128 (36) and CG142 (37) fully list the elements to be included in the assessment process for children and adults respectively and should be referred to if the reader is unfamiliar with the process.

Box 7.2 Testing for ASD in adults with moderate to severe ID

- difficulties in reciprocal social interaction including:
  - limited interaction with others (e.g. being aloof, indifferent or unusual)
  - interaction to fulfil needs only
  - interaction that is naïve or one-sided
- lack of responsiveness to others
- little or no change in behaviour in response to different social situations
- limited social demonstration of empathy
- rigid routines and resistance to change
- marked repetitive activities (for example, rocking and hand or finger flapping), especially when under stress or expressing emotion.

If two or more of the above categories of behaviour are present, offer a comprehensive assessment for autism.

Assessing ASD in ID

Assessing ASD can prove challenging at times for even the most experienced clinicians, especially when faced with disentangling the features from other comorbidities. The presence of ID means that there will necessarily be developmental delay; therefore a diagnosis of ASD will require the clinician to be satisfied that there is in addition developmental difference across the core domains of social interaction, social communication, social imagination, and fixed/repetitive behaviours that cannot be better explained by that underlying delay.

Screening

Autism is not included in national and NHS recommendations for screening. CG142 (37) provides some helpful pointers when testing for possible ASD in an adult with at least moderate ID.

Diagnosis

The clinician needs to consider what adaptations need to be made to the assessment process. Practicalities such as the location of the assessment, suitability of the assessment room, impact of disrupting the person's usual routine to attend the appointment, difficulty coping with a new situation, difficulty waiting, length of the appointment, communication difficulties, and challenging behaviours—to name but a few—must be considered and reasonable adjustments made. Awareness of sensory sensitivities (e.g. dislike of bright lights) and obsessions (e.g. collecting anything plastic) can allow simple adjustments to be made, which allow the assessment to proceed as smoothly as possible.

Assessment should take account of all the key areas listed above, including core and additional features, as well as common comorbidities, risk, and capacity issues. It must include those elements relevant to both ASD and ID, for example, presence of epilepsy, sensory impairment, challenging behavior, and communication level including ability to communicate pain and make choices, all of which will impact on level of functioning and outcome.

Diagnosis is usually possible on the basis of a good developmental history and observations, using ICD-10 (9) or DSM-5 (8) criteria. Appendix C (pp. 40–50) of CG128 (36) helpfully sets out features suggestive of possible ASD at three different key developmental stages in their equivalent mental ages (Preschool; Primary 5–11 years; Secondary i.e. older than 11 years) to guide clinicians in the context of 'normal' development. Clinicians assessing individuals with ID may find this helpful to reference when making diagnostic judgements in the context of developmental delay.

In more complex cases the use of formal assessment tools should be considered. The PDD-MRS (38) is a simple diagnostic aid which is easy to administer and can be used to inform clinical judgement. Structured history taking tools such as the Diagnostic Interview for Social and Communication Disorders (DISCO) (39) and Autism Diagnostic Interview—Revised (ADI-R) (40) which both require a detailed interview with a parent or carer who has known the person over their lifespan, are suitable for use in ID, as is the Autism Diagnostic Observation Schedule 2 (ADOS-2) (41) which is a practical tool involving a series of tasks designed to elicit features of ASD in the clinic setting and has a range of modules for different levels of communicative ability. The DISCO, ADI-R and ADOS-2 all require specific training before the clinician is accredited in their use, therefore are necessarily reserved for the more complex cases, not least because of the time-intense nature of their completion. A further note of caution is that assessment in the clinic setting does not necessarily represent how a person will perform in a 'real life' setting, indeed the quiet and ordered setting of a clinic where engagement takes place on a one to one basis may allow the person to perform at a higher level than they would do as a rule. The importance of observations carried out in the person's natural setting—or failing that collateral information gathered from those who support the person day to day—should not be underestimated.

One of the most challenging areas to accurately assess is that of imaginative ability, however this is key when considering issues of risk and capacity. A thorough developmental history can provide useful evidence of whether the person engaged in imaginative play as a child; checking the person's ability to predict consequences of actions and to cope with the unexpected (e.g. what would you do if the bus didn't come?) is also helpful. Tasks requiring novel creativity, such as the 'creating a story' task in the ADOS assessment can provide valuable evidence of how more able individuals actually function when put 'on the spot'.

Differential diagnosis

Earlier in the chapter we discussed commonly occurring comorbid conditions, many of which also now need to be considered here as part of differential diagnosis. The approach here, however, is to establish whether the features seen better fit an alternative diagnostic picture and in this instance an ASD can then be discounted.

Common differentials include the following:

ID

Abnormalities of social interaction, language development and stereotyped behaviour can be found in some children with ID, especially those with an IQ < 50 (4), which can lead to diagnostic confusion, especially in older individuals where early developmental information is incomplete, making it difficult to ascertain whether social and communicative abnormalities are out of keeping with developmental age (35).

Anxiety disorders

Social anxiety is an important differential, where the root of the difficulty is a fear of scrutiny, whereas in ASD the anxiety stems from difficulty understanding the social situation.

OCD

Is marked by recurrent obsessional thoughts or compulsive acts: these occur in a stereotyped fashion that the person resists finding them unpleasant and are differentiated from the rigidity and repetitive behaviours of ASD that the person finds consoling and prefers not to give up.

Psychosis

Odd ideas and difficult to follow trains of thought, catatonic behaviours, social withdrawal and apathy/self-absorption can be seen in both Schizophrenia and ASD. A key differential is age of onset, highlighting the importance of the early childhood developmental history.

PD

The pattern of pervasive difficulty engaging and interacting with the world, abnormal maladaptive behaviour patterns that impact on social situations and problems in occupational and social performance seen in PD can be mistaken for ASD. Deficits in non-verbal communication described in ASD are absent in PD, not do repetitive, routine bound behaviours form part of the clinical picture. Age of onset may not be a useful differentiator, because such individuals often report a difficult early upbringing with poor attachments and social difficulties and, consequent to this, may be unable or unwilling to provide an informant history, making differentiating the two conditions challenging.

ADHD

Attention and concentration difficulties along with impulse control problems all can lead to social difficulties, with the person failing to pick up social cues, follow the thread of conversation, and make inappropriate comments. This can lead to social isolation from peers, which further compounds the problem.

Management

It is vital that the needs of adults with a dual diagnosis of ID and ASD are recognized and appropriately managed, both because of the complexity of their presentation and also because it is likely there will be heightened vulnerability and risk.

CG142 (37) and CG170 (42) provide guidance on management of ASD in adults and children respectively and should be referred to by the reader. In addition, the reader is referred to two recently published specialist ID texts: 'The Frith Prescribing Guidelines for People with Intellectual Disabilities' (43), Chapter 10, reviews the evidence base around medication and provides practical advice on prescribing for ASD in association with ID, and 'Clinical Topics in Disorders of Intellectual Development (44) in Chapters 10 and 11 detail the research and evidence base around pharmacological and psychological strategies in ASD respectively. The focus here will be more on the practicalities of day to day issues for the person with ID and ASD.

Social interventions

This is the key management domain, forming the basis of the person's support system and often the 'make or break' factor when crises occur. Appropriate education, training, or work is important for providing structure, routine, and meaningful activity: support to obtain and maintain this is usually required.

Suitable accommodation (location, resident mix, noise levels, etc) with the right level of support is key to maximizing the person's independence. Social support and networks need to be put in place, if not already present, with opportunities to engage in activities in the wider community. For more able individuals, opportunity to engage with others through a club or society in line with their special interest may open doors to friendship and satisfying occupation.

Understanding the value of money and wider financial management such as budgeting may require ongoing support and guidance, while vulnerability to exploitation must be monitored in individuals who are managing their own money. Support may be needed to obtain benefits, with traditional assessment methods failing to highlight the hidden needs of those with ASD, for example the need for repeated prompting to follow a daily routine to get out of the house in the morning.

Carer support is vital to prevent burnout and crises, including assessment of entitlement to benefits and often access to respite and suitable activities or occupation for the person. CG142 highlights the importance of offering both an assessment to carers in their own right and offering/signposting them to appropriate help, support, and training. Respite care should be considered to allow a break for family carers, and may also provide the opportunity to gently start transitioning out of the family home.

Within the UK, the growing awareness of ASD through lobbying has led to legislation requiring services to adapt how they support people with ASD. The Disability Discrimination Act 1995, Autism Act 2009, Adult Autism Strategy 2014, and recently published Statutory Guidance (45) are of particular relevance here. Within the UK NHS local authority social services departments and planning and commissioning teams are the local NHS lead for supporting adults with ASD, however any care provided is subject to the same access to care eligibility rules that apply to disability in any individual seeking support from services.

The language of 'Reasonable Adjustments' is becoming more widespread, from simple measures such as offering early appointments to avoid waiting, through cinemas offering autism friendly screenings and on to environments being designed in an 'Autism friendly' way (e.g. plain walls and low lighting). A key area of difficulty for people with ASD highlighted in the literature is coping with transitions between life stages (46). Problems such as loneliness and communication difficulties can compound the challenge of negotiating life experiences such as puberty, the menopause and old age in this group (33). Due to the difficulties people with ASD experience around change it is essential to plan transitions further in advance than typically would be the case, whatever the developmental stage (46). The transition period of 16 to 25 years of age is a high-risk period for mental disorders in the general population and the risks are further increased in people with developmental disabilities. A particular stressor noted at this time is the move from education to adult services and the related life changes this brings (47).

Psychological interventions

Use of psychological interventions in people with ASD has grown over the years but unfortunately the evidence base remains limited; most studies focus on children with normal IQ, with adults and those with ID receiving limited attention. Reitzel et al in Woodbury-Smith (Ed) (44) summarize the current evidence base for well-known techniques such as Applied Behaviour Analysis (ABA), and Cognitive Behaviour Therapy (CBT) in ASD, and www.researchautism.net is a good up to date source for evidence of what works (and also what does not work).

The literature also contains reports of interventions in individuals with ASD plus ID including anxiety management, relaxation, and desensitization, as well as individual psychotherapy for higher-functioning individuals for insight-related understanding, low mood, anxiety, and obsessive-compulsive symptoms (48). The need to modify the content and delivery of therapy such as CBT is widely acknowledged in ID, and also now in ASD, for example using 'Easy Read' formats, shorter sessions incorporating breaks, simplifying language, and regularly checking understanding.

Functional analysis of challenging behaviour is highlighted as an integral part of ASD assessment in adults (37), with guidance on psychosocial approaches to its management as first line. Simple strategies widely used in clinical practice include providing clear structure and boundaries, use of timetables and communication support systems.

Social Stories™ (49) are a further technique worthy of consideration, helping individuals to understand a social situation and act appropriately. Again, the evidence base is primarily in children with ASD, in some cases with associated ID, however recent work has started to look at the role of the technique in adults with ID (50).

Pharmacological interventions

It is important to begin this section by acknowledging the clear lack of RCT-based evidence for the risk-benefit of pharmacological treatments that have been tested in the non-ID, non-ASD adult population. Therefore recommendations are necessarily based on collective clinical experience, rather than the levels of evidence demanded in the general population. Given this, it is vital that the practitioner always considers how to prescribe as safely as possible and also remains in dialogue with patients, carers, and colleagues to ensure they are engaging in shared clinical decision-making and not working in isolation.

Useful key principles whenever medication is considered in this population are (i) assess mental capacity and follow the best interests process if found to lack capacity, (ii) use medication as a last resort, when other techniques have failed/proved insufficient, (iii) obtain baseline parameters before commencing, both any necessary physical monitoring and also recording of the targeted symptoms, (iv) use only in conjunction with other approaches, for example, psychological treatment, (v) apply a 'start low and go slow' dosage regime, closely monitoring for side effects and (vi) monitor and review regularly, including considering dose reduction/withdrawal at each meeting.

NICE guidance for both children and adults deems the role of medication to be in the treatment of associated diagnoses, such as depression, and should not be used for the core features described above. Barrett and Bradley in (43) discuss the current evidence base for individual medications, which again is limited for this population, highlighting the pragmatics of management of this challenging patient population, including the difficulties of limited communication and understanding of emotional states. In day to day clinical practice, melatonin for sleep latency, SSRIs for mood and anxiety and in some cases low-dose risperidone (Or increasingly certain other antipsychotics e.g. Aripirazole) for agitation and aggressive behaviour most commonly form the mainstay of the psychotropic treatment armoury. It should be noted that due to lack of trial data to date, much of prescribing practice is done off-licence and based on best clinical consensus among practitioners specializing in this area; however, the importance of using medication to support effective management of ASD-associated anxiety in this patient population should not be underestimated.

There has been relatively little work on the drug treatment of psychiatric disturbance in adults with ASD, with or without ID. Drug treatment tends to play a central role in managing psychotic and affective disorders (33) and there is some evidence for the efficacy of antidepressants, including SSRIs, in heightening mood in depression. In addition, beta blockers have been shown to help with panic attacks in some individuals (51). More recently there has been growing interest in treating ADHD in ASD, with some evidence emerging for the use of Immediate Release (IR) methylphenidate, although caution should be exerted as there is a higher reported incidence of side effects and lower rate of efficacy than in the general population (see Elvins and Green in 44). The interplay of ASD and ADHD should also be considered here—once ASD is treated the person may be in a better position to engage in social interaction and learn more skills in this area, however on the flip side they may develop better focus on their obsessions and actually appear 'more autistic' as a consequence.

Capacity and risk issues

The impact of ASD on a person's ability to make everyday decisions—as well as more complex judgements—should not be underestimated. When ID with its limited cognitive reserve is added into the mix, the difficulties are further compounded. Careful assessment of both the person's theoretical understanding and also their ability to translate this into 'real life' situations is equally essential for any clinician faced with such a dilemma. Box 7.3 highlights some of the common difficulties encountered in everyday clinical practice and management suggestions:

Box 7.3 Capacity and risk issues in ASD

- Level of understanding
  - Assumptions cannot be made from the person's general ability level or performance in other situations
  - A specific assessment of the situation in question must be made
- Predicting consequences of actions
  - The person may struggle to think of alternatives outside a known—and potentially pre-rehearsed—set of circumstances
  - Support to think through the possible alternatives may be required
- Translating theory into practice
  - Understanding a situation on paper is different to experiencing it in 'real life' where unexpected occurrences and unplanned interactions may occur
  - Assessment of the person in 'real life' situations may be required to fully determine capacity
- Problem solving
  - The ability to 'think outside the box' may be challenging due to the above issues
  - In addition, problems prioritizing and focusing on the whole task at hand (rather than certain minor details) may occur
  - Specific support and teaching may be needed to help with these issues
- Decision-making ability
  - This may be impacted by the above factors, as well as others such as anxiety levels
  - Time, support and specific teaching may be required
- Vulnerability and risk
  - The person may be naïve to others' social intentions or alternatively prioritize the need for social approval over any potential risks to himself/herself
  - Formal assessment of risk and capacity may therefore be needed
  - The person may be unaware of the needs/sensibilities of others and pursue their own interests to the detriment of others
  - Social skills training and use of Social Stories™ may be helpful
  - Again, assessment of risk and capacity may be required if the person is placing others/or his/herself at risk as a consequence of the behaviour

Prognosis

There have been few studies to date looking specifically at the course of ASD over time and the work done has been based on clinic populations: a group whom, by virtue of their being in need of specialist services, are more likely to have a greater level of impairment. Rutter et al (52) conducted a five to 15 year follow up study of 63 children with a mean IQ of 62 and a diagnosis of 'infantile psychosis'. Seventeen per cent achieved a good level of adaptation, a further 17 per cent showed fair adaptation while 64 per cent had an outcome was classed as poor to very poor. Two key factors were predictive of a good outcome in adulthood, namely higher IQ and the presence of spoken language at age five. More recent work by Howlin et al (53) has found that individuals with a childhood performance IQ of 70 and above had a significantly better outcome than those with an IQ below 70, however within the normal IQ range outcome was very variable and neither verbal nor performance IQ proved to be consistent prognostic indicators.

Looking next at the course of the core triad of impairments in ASD over time,Rutter et al (52) found that most subjects showed some decrease in features and increase in flexibility over time, but social impairment, in particular, tended to persist. Rumsey et al. (54) reported a similar picture. More recently, Beadle-Brown et al. (55) reported on the Camberwell Cohort 25 years on; repetitive behaviours, steretypies, and insistence on sameness all improved with time, however social impairment was ongoing. Shattuck et al. (56) conducted a prospective study which echoed these findings, but also reported improvements in verbal communication in 51 per cent of those with speech. The scenario of an individual who becomes 'less autistic' over time is recognized in clinical practice: often due to the person learning strategies to manage and mask their difficulties, which latterly may only manifest at times of particular stress. In contrast, other individuals are seen whose difficulties become more marked over time: here the consequence of increasing social demands exceeding the person's limited capacities.

Puberty is a particularly significant time in development for people with ASD and often the most difficult stage of life for the individual to negotiate (13). The onset of puberty is not usually delayed (18) and many of the physical and psychological changes of adolescence will affect the person's social and interpersonal behaviour (28). There may be an increased self-awareness, bringing with it a desire for independence and a reluctance to accept authority, although manifestations in people with ASD may be odd or unexpected (28). In individuals with limited abilities, feelings of frustration may result in a return to former behavioural problems such as temper tantrums and aggressive outbursts but these are now more difficult to manage as the individual is older and stronger. A further major difficulty for adolescents with ASD is that as they mature, like their counterparts without ASD, they tend to lose interest in childhood activities, however unlike their peers they may not have the skills to develop new interests or to occupy themselves constructively, increasing the chances of inappropriate behaviours. The concerns of adolescence are reported to continue long into adult life for people with ASD, compounded by the fact that adults tend to look and behave much younger than their years, however increasing age eventually brings with it calmer and more appropriate behaviour (18).

Moving on to cognitive abilities, adolescence brings a mixed picture with some children making major gains but slightly more reported to undergo significant developmental losses (35).

The move into adulthood tends to be characterized by a slowing down in the capacity to learn, but this needs to be taken in the context of difficulties with transferring skills and the need to develop new attachments (33). Studies have shown that a subgroup of individuals with ASD will show a decline in intellectual ability during or after adolescence and that these individuals usually have low IQ (13).

Overall it appears that long term outcome in ASD is to a great extent dependent on the person's innate cognitive, linguistic, and social abilities; in addition, outcome can be improved by the presence of additional skills and interests to assist in a person's social integration (27). On a related note, the onset of epilepsy during puberty may be a poor prognostic sign, possibly through an impact on social adaptation, but this is not such a clear indicator (13).

One particularly under-researched area is that of the effects of maturation and ageing in autism and little is known about the function and development of people with autism as they reach old age (13). To date there have been no longitudinal studies following people through into old age, however a study looking at the prevalence of ASD in the elderly population with ID found no decline in the 65-plus age group compared to a control group aged 20 to 64, suggesting that autism is likely to persist throughout life (57).

Case study 1

Bill is a 68-year-old man with mild ID living with his elderly mother. He and his mother support each other and attend bingo with a neighbour twice a week at the local community centre. Bill was not known to health or social care services until his mother fell ill and was taken into hospital. The neighbour becomes concerned when Bill starts attending the bingo sessions in an agitated and dishevelled state and contacts Bill's GP, who makes a referral to the mental health team.

Bill is seen by his local mental health team. He makes poor eye contact and talks at length about the numbers he likes on the bingo cards. He is very anxious about coming to the clinic, complains that the lights are too bright and insists he needs to leave after 25 minutes to get home in time to watch his usual TV programme schedule.

He accepts a worker visiting him at home the next day. Bill shows the worker his considerable collection of bingo cards and memorabilia. He then stands rocking on the spot and humming to himself. The worker finds that Bill has run out of fresh food and milk and has not been shopping as 'Mum always told me not to go out on my own'. He has not changed his clothes or had a shower in the last week as 'Mum always reminds me to do it'.

The worker, in discussion with Bill's mother, arranges a package of care to support him with activities of daily living. The allocated carer reports Bill is uncooperative with personal care and becomes agitated when asked to help with household chores. The mental health worker has developed a good rapport with Bill, so visits to try and assess the problem. Bill says that the carer arrives late and 'doesn't understand the routine' and this makes him stressed. The worker spends time with Bill and the carer talking through Bill's usual pattern of activities and the need to stick to time. Two weeks later Bill is engaging well with his support, attends bingo in good spirits and tells his neighbour 'Things are good'.

Case study 2

Anne is 18 and has moderate ID and ASD. She is in her last year at school and plans to move to the local college to study life skills. At the start of the last term at school she becomes increasingly anxious and starts hitting and biting her hand. She also pushes another pupil over and hits her teacher when he intervenes. She is also unsettled at home and her parents report she is not sleeping or eating as well as usual and sometimes becomes tearful.

Anne is referred to the ID psychiatry team and is allocated a psychiatrist and a nurse. The nurse observes Anne at school and home and notices there have been a number of changes in the staff team at school. She also observes that Anne is more unsettled in the busy communal areas. The nurse works with the school to establish a consistent staff team for Anne and advises them on her sensory difficulties. The nurse also attends the transition planning meetings, looking at how to prepare Anne for the move to college, and seeks help from the ID team speech therapist to create accessible information about the move for Anne.

The psychiatrist meets with Anne and her parents, with the nurse present, to discuss the concerns around mood, anxiety, and behaviour and it is noticed that the problems are usually worse just before Anne's menstrual period. Anne goes to see the GP for review of her menstrual cycle and also a general health check to rule out any other underlying physical issues.

Despite all these interventions, Anne continues to display challenging behaviour, tearfulness, and sleep disturbance and the ID team suspect underlying depression and anxiety. A trial of an SSRI is agreed under best interests principles. After some initial irritability, Anne shows a steady improvement and within three months is back to her usual self. She attends all the end of term activities without any problem and is looking forward to starting college in the autumn.

MULTIPLE CHOICE QUESTIONS

Questions

Please select the single most appropriate answer

1. Which one of these statements is correct regarding the core cognitive difficulties in ASD?

A. People with ASD have strong central coherence
B. Theory of mind refers to the ability to attribute mental states to self and others
C. The Sally Ann test is good for demonstrating theory of mind difficulties in people with ASD of all ability levels
D. People with ASD find it easy to keep track of the passage of time
E. Special skills (sometimes referred to as 'savant') do not occur in people with ASD who also have ID

2. With regard to mental health and behaviour in people with ASD, which one of these statements is correct?

A. Psychiatric disorders are less common in people with ASD compared to the general population
B. Mood symptoms are rarely seen in ASD
C. Anxiety in ASD is based in a fear of scrutiny by others
D. Anxiety should be considered as an underlying cause for aggression in ASD

E. ASD is less common in people with Down syndrome (Trisomy 21)

3. When carrying out an assessment of ASD, which one of the following is correct?

A. Diagnosis can be made on the basis of a good historical account
B. The detailed schedules recommended in clinical practice, for example, DISCO, ADI-R are not suitable for assessing ASD in a person with ID
C. Informant history and observation of the person are both required for assessment
D. When assessing the person, reasonable adjustments can not be made as this will invalidate the findings
E. The DISCO, ADI-R or similar schedule must be used for all assessments

4. When considering sensory differences in ASD, which one of the following is correct?

A. People with ASD plus ID are more likely to be oversensitive to sensory stimuli than those with ASD and normal range/high IQ
B. Are uncommon in ASD
C. Usually disappear by adulthood
D. Spinning and rocking can indicate balance hypersensitivity
E. Are included in the core DSM-5 diagnostic criteria

5. Management and outcome

Please select the single most appropriate answer.

A. Pharmacological treatment is not recommended for the core features of ASD
B. There is a strong evidence base for psychological treatment in adults with ASD
C. Social support needs are likely to reduce during times of transition
D. 'Reasonable adjustments' to support attendance for treatment are good practice but not recognized in law
E. IQ is not an important predictor of outcome

Answers

1. A. People with ASD have weak central coherence, tending to focus on the detail, rather than seeing the picture 'as a whole'

B. Correct

C. More able people with ASD can 'learn to pass the test' intellectually, despite still having profound underlying difficulties with perspective taking

D. Time is an abstract concept and its passing is therefore difficult for people for ASD to naturally process

E. Special skills can occur in people with ASD who are within the ID range, usually those with mild ID and less commonly in those with moderate ID

2. A. Psychiatric disorders are more common in the ASD population.

B. Mood symptoms are common and should always be asked about, albeit the person may have difficulty understanding and articulating their mood state. A change in behaviour could indicate an altered mood state.

C. This refers clinically to social anxiety. People with ASD with some insight into their difficulties may however worry about getting things wrong in a social situation.

D. Correct.

E. ASD is more common in people with Down syndrome but can be missed due to public perception of the Down syndrome personality as 'happy go lucky' and sociable.

3. A. This is important but insufficient—the clinician also needs to ascertain current functional difficulties and have observational evidence to corroborate the history.

B. These schedules are all valid for assessing ASD in people with ID.

C. Correct

D. Reasonable adjustments should be made to allow the person maximum chance to participate. These adjustments should be noted in the assessment report, and any potential impact on the process considered in the diagnostic discussion and formulation, for example, use of an interpreter when assessing social communication.

E. These are detailed, gold-standard tools which can be used to support clinical judgement in complex cases, but may not be required—or practicable—in all cases.

4. A. As a general rule, people with ID and ASD are more likely to be undersensitive, but equally some such individuals are oversensitive in one or more modalities, or there may be a mix of the two.

B. Sensory differences are common and may be missed unless specifically considered during assessment. Behavioural reactions may be linked to a sensory stimulus.

C. Sensory differences often persist into adulthood; more able adults may find ways of masking the impact of these, for example, wearing headphones to cut out background noise.

D. These can indicate balance undersensitivity.

E. Correct

5. A. Correct

B. There is very little evidence for either psychological or pharmacological treatment in adults with ASD and much of the evidence used is extrapolated from studies in children.

C. Transition is a time of increased change and stress, so support needs are likely to increase.

D. The Equality Act (2010) has made it a legal requirement for organizations to make reasonable adjustments, if an individual declares that they have a disability.

E. IQ and presence of spoken language by age 5 are both important factors in predicting outcome.

REFERENCES

1. Wing L. Language social and cognitive impairments in autism and severe mental retardation. *Journal of Autism and Developmental Disorders*. 1981;11:31–44.
2. Kanner L. Autistic disturbances of affective contact. *Nervous Child*. 1943; 2:217–250.
3. Asperger H. Die 'Autistischen psychopathen' im kindesalter. *Arch Psychiatr Nervenkr*. 1944;117:76–136.
4. Wing L, Gould J. Severe impairments of social interaction and associated abnormalities in children: Epidemiology and classification. *Journal of Autism and Developmental Disorders* (1979) 9(1):11–29.
5. Kanner L. Follow-up study of 11 autistic children originally reported in 1943. *Journal of Autism and Childhood Schizophrenia*. 1971;1:119–145.
6. Rutter M. Autistic children: Infancy to adulthood. *Seminars in Psychiatry* 1970;2:435–450.
7. Gillberg C, Steffenburg S. Outcome and prognostic factors in infantile autism and similar conditions: a population-based study of 46 cases followed through puberty. *Journal of Autism and Developmental Disorders*. 1987;17:273–287.
8. APA. *Diagnostic and Statistical Manual of Mental Disorders, 5th Edition*. Arlington: APA; 2013.
9. WHO. *The ICD-10 Classification of Mental and Behavioural Disorders*. Geneva: WHO; 1992.
10. Miller J, Bilder D, Farley M, Coon H, Pinborough-Zimmerman J, Jenson W, Rice C, Fombonne E, Pingree C, Ritvo E, Ritvo R-A, McMahon, W. Autism spectrum disorder reclassified: A second look at the 1980s Utah/UCLA autism epidemiologic study. *Journal of Autism and Developmental Disorders*. 2013;43(1):200–210.
11. Ritvo E, Freeman B, Pingree C, Mason-Brothers A, Jorde L, Jenson W et al. The UCLA-University of Utah epidemiologic survey of sutism: Revalence. *The American Journal of Psychiatry*. 1989;146:194–199.
12. Brugha TS, Spiers N, Bankart J, Cooper S-A, McManus S, Scott FJ, Smith J, Tyrer F. Epidemiology of autism in adults across age groups and ability levels. *The British Journal of Psychiatry*. 2016. Available from: http://bjp.rcpsych.org/content/early/2016/06/27/bjp.bp.115.174649 [Accessed 16th October 2016].
13. Akerstrom B. *Adults with Autism and Mental Retardation*. Stockholm: Elanders Gotab; 2001.
14. Brugha T, Cooper SA, McManus S, Purdon S, Smith J, Scott F, Spiers N, and Tyrer F. *Extending the 2007 Adult Psychiatric Morbidity Survey*. 2012. Available from: http://content.digital.nhs.uk/catalogue/PUB05061/esti-prev-auti-ext-07-psyc-morb-surv-rep.pdf [Accessed 10th August 2017].
15. Bhaumik S, Branford D, McGrother C, Thorp, T. Autistic traits in adults with learning disabilities. *British Journal of Psychiatry*. 1997;170:502–506.
16. Baron-Cohen S, Leslie A, Frith U. Does the autistic child have a 'theory of mind'?. *Cognition*. 1985;21:37–46.
17. Happé F, Frith U. The weak coherence account: Detail-focused cognitive style in autism spectrum disorders. *Journal of Autism and Developmental Disorders*. 2006;36:5–25.
18. Wing L. *The Autistic Spectrum*. London: Constable; 1996.
19. Volkmar F, Cohen D, Bregman J, Hooks M, Stevenson, J. An examination of social typologies in autism. *Journal of the American Academy of Child and Adolescent Psychiatry*. 1989;28:82–86.
20. Gillberg C, Billstedt E. Autism and Asperger syndrome: Coexistence with other clinical disorders. *Acta Psychiatrica Scandinavica*. 2000;102:321–330.
21. Bartak L, Rutter, M. Differences between mentally retarded and normally intelligent autistic children. *Journal of Autism and Childhood Schizophrenia*. 1976;6:109–120.
22. Jordan R. *Autism with Severe Learning Difficulties*. London: Souvenir Press; 2001.
23. Wing L, Shah A. Catatonia in autistic spectrum disorders. *The British Journal of Psychiatry*. 2000;176(4):357–362.
24. Abramson R, Wright H, Cuccaro M, Laurence L, Babb S, Pencarinha, D et al. Biological liability in families with Autism. *Journal of American Academy of Child and Adolescent Psychiatry*. 1992;31:370–371.
25. Sverd J. Psychiatric disorders in individuals with pervasive developmental disorder. *Journal of Psychiatric Practice*. 2003;9(2):111–127.
26. Anckrsäter H, Stahlberg O, Larson T, Hakansson C, Jutblad S, Niklasson L, Nydén A, Wentz E, Westergren S, Cloninger C, Gillberg C, Rastam M. The impact of ADHD and autism spectrum disorders on temperament, character, and personality development. *American Journal of Psychiatry*. 2006;163:1239–1244.
27. Howlin P. *Autism, Preparing for Adulthood*. London: Routledge; 1997.
28. Schopler E, Mesibov, G (eds). *Autism in Adolescents and Adults*. New York: Plenum Press; 1983.
29. Poustka F, Lisch S. Autistic behaviour domains and their relation to self-injurious behaviour. *Acta Paedopsychiatrica*. 1993;56:69–73.
30. Smith S, Branford D, Collacott R, Cooper S, McGrother C. Prevalence and cluster typology of maladaptive behaviours in a geographically defined population of adults with learning disabilities. *British Journal of Psychiatry*. 1996;169:219–227.
31. Ryan R. Treatment resistant illness: Is it Asperger's syndrome? *Hospital and Community Psychiatry*. 1992;43:807–811.
32. Ghaziuddin M, Ghaziuddin N, Greden J. Depression in persons with autism: Implications for research and clinical care. *Journal of Autism and Developmental Disorders*. 2002;32(4):299–306.
33. Morgan H. *Adults with Autism*. Cambridge: Cambridge University Press; 1996.
34. Rai D, Kerr MP, McManus S, Jordanova V, Lewis G, Brugha TS. Epilepsy and psychiatric comorbidity: A nationally representative population-based study. *Epilepsia*. 2012;**53**:1095–1103.
35. Volkmar F, Cook E, Pomeroy J, Realmuto G, Tanguay P. Practice parameters for the assessment and treatment of children, adolescents and adults with autism and other pervasive developmental disorders. *Journal of the American Academy of Child and Adolescent Psychiatry*. 1999;38(12):32s–54s.
36. NICE. *CG128: Autism spectrum disorder in under 19s: Recognition, referral and diagnosis*. 2011. Available from: nice.org.uk/guidance/cg128 [Accessed 16th October 2016].
37. NICE. *CG142: Autism spectrum disorder in adults: Diagnosis and management*. 2012. Available from: nice.org.uk/guidance/cg142 [Accessed 16 October 2016].
38. Kraijer D. *Pervasive Developmental Disorder in Mental Retardation Scale (PDD-MRS)*. Leiden: PITS; 2006.
39. Leekham S, Libby S, Wing L, Gould J, Taylor C. The Diagnostic Interviewfor Social and Communication disorders (DISCO): Algorithms for ICD 10 childhood autism. *Journal of Child Psychology, Psychiatry and Allied Disciplines*. 2002;43:327–342.

40. LeCouteur A, Lord C, Rutter M. *Autism Diagnostic Interview, Revised (ADI-R)*. California: WPS; 2003.
41. Lord C, Rutter M, DiLavore P, Risi S, Gotham K, Bishop S, Luyster R, Guthrie W. *Autism Diagnostic Observation Schedule, 2nd Edition (ADOS-2)*. California: WPS; 2012.
42. NICE. *CG170: Autism spectrum disorder in under 19s: Support and management*. 2013. Available from: nice.org.uk/guidance/cg170 [Accessed 16th October 2016].
43. Bhaumik S, Branford D, Barrett M, Gangadharan S (eds). *The Frith Prescribing Guidelines for People with Intellectual Disability, 3rd Edition*. Oxford: Wiley; 2015.
44. Woodbury-Smith M (ed.). (2015) *Clinical Topics in Disorders of Intellectual Development*. London: Royal College of Psychiatrists; 2015.
45. Department of Health. *Statutory guidance for Local Authorities and NHS organisations to support implementation of the adult autism strategy*. Available from: www.gov.uk/government/uploads/system/uploads/attachment_data/file/422338/autism-guidance.pdf [Accessed 16th October 2016].
46. Schroeder S, LeBlanc J, Mayo L. Brief report: A lifespan perspective on the development of individuals with autism. *Journal of Autism and Developmental Disorders*. 1996;26(2):251–255.
47. Mclntyre L, Blacher J, Baker B. Behaviour/mental health problems in young adults with intellectual disability: The impact on families. *Journal of Intellectual Disability Research*. 2002;46(3):239–249.
48. Campbell M, Schopler E, Cueva J, and Hallin A. Treatment of autistic disorder. *Journal of the American Academy of Child and Adolescent Psychiatry*. 1996;35(2):134–143.
49. Gray C. *The New Social Story Book*. Texas: Future Horizons; 2000.
50. Aphale N. *Using a social story with an adult diagnosed with a learning disability and autism spectrum disorder*. 2015. Available from: https://lra.le.ac.uk/bitstream/2381/33300/1/Thesis%20FINAL.pdf [Accessed 16th October 2016].
51. Morgan H, Jones G, Jordan R. *Autistic Spectrum Disorders. A Guide to Services for Adults with Autistic Spectrum Disorders for Commissioners and Providers*. London: The Mental Health Foundation; 2001.
52. Rutter M, Greenfield D, and Lockyer L. A five to fifteen year follow-up study of infantile psychosis: II. Social and behavioral outcome. *British Journal of Psychiatry*. 1967;113:1183–1199.
53. Howlin H, Goode S, Hutton J, Rutter M. Adult outcome for children with autism. *Journal of Child Psychology and Psychiatry*. 2004;45(2):212–229.
54. Rumsey J, Rapoport L, Sceery W. Autistic children as adults: Psychiatric, social and behavioral outcomes. *Journal of the American Academy of Child Psychiatry*. 1985;24:465–473.
55. Beadle-Brown J, Murphy G, Wing, L. The Camberwell cohort 25 years on: Characteristics and changes in skills over time. *Journal of Applied Research in Intellectual Disability*. 2006;19(4):317–329.
56. Shattuck P, Seltzer M, Greenberg J, Orsmond G, Bolt D, Kring S, Lounds J, Lord C. Change in autism symptoms and maladaptive behaviors in adolescents and adults with an autism spectrum disorder. *Journal of Autism and Developmental Disorders*. 2007;37(9):1735–1747.
57. Cooper S. Epidemiology of psychiatric disorders in elderly compared with younger adults with learning disabilities. *British Journal of Psychiatry*. 1997;170:375–380.

8

Attention Deficit Hyperactivity Disorder (ADHD) in People with Intellectual Disability

Kiriakos Xenitidis, Shazia Zahid, and Caryl Marshall

Introduction

Attention Deficit Hyperactivity Disorder (ADHD) is a common condition and its clinical significance has long been established in the paediatric population. More recently it has been acknowledged that, in a large proportion of cases, ADHD symptomatology persists into adulthood, causing significant impairment (1–2). The association between ADHD and intellectual disability (ID) is well established (3–7), however, partially due to the difficulties in applying established rating scales in this population, it is only recently that recognition and management of the condition in individuals with an ID, especially when considering adults, has attracted clinical and academic attention (6–8). The validity of the diagnosis of ADHD in individuals with ID has thus been the focus of research (5–7). Similarly, the co-existence of ADHD and autism spectrum disorders, as well as other psychiatric comorbidities, has been extensively studied (5, 9--11). It has been established that children, and adults, with ID are more likely to have ADHD and the combination may be associated with a poorer prognosis overall (12–13).

Epidemiology

It is difficult to be exact about how frequently ADHD occurs in individuals with ID. Prevalence rates of ADHD in both children and adults with ID vary; a number of factors contribute to this finding. Variance in ADHD rates in the general population can be explained by differences in operational criteria and the cut-off points of symptoms, for example, full syndromal ADHD vs. partial remission. When considering adult epidemiology, uncertainty about the diagnostic criteria of ADHD beyond childhood and adolescence remains problematic. The current classification systems offer very limited guidance on making this diagnosis in the adult population with ID [14, 15]. In addition to the factors contributing to the general variability of ADHD prevalence, differences in diagnostic criteria and cut off points of intellectual functioning used to establish a diagnosis of ID, along with other methodological differences between studies, compound the variance. There exists little guidance about diagnosing ADHD in children and adults with an ID. A significant attempt to bridge this gap has been made in the United Kingdom by establishing diagnostic criteria for a range of mental disorders, including ADHD, as presented in individuals with ID, namely the DC-LD: Diagnostic Criteria Learning Disabilities (16).

In the general paediatric population a prevalence of ADHD between 4–5 per cent is often quoted. This prevalence rate has been found to be eight-fold increased in children with ID (17). In a longitudinal study of ADHD in children, with and without ID, ADHD was found to be over three times as prevalent in the ID group compared to the non-ID children (12). A further study, utilizing a screening tool for neurodevelopmental-neuropsychiatric disorders, the five to fifteen questionnaire, found approximately 50 per cent of children with mild ID had clinically relevant diagnosis of ADHD (8). One US study suggested that, at the very least, 15 per cent of children with severe and profound levels of ID may meet diagnostic criteria for ADHD, even when mental age has been taken into account (18).

In adults epidemiological studies are limited. A meta-analysis, regarding the persistence of ADHD into adulthood, in the general population, established a prevalence of 4.5 per cent. (19) A further meta-analysis showed the persistence of ADHD from childhood into adulthood to be 15 per cent, 65 per cent when partial residual symptoms were taken into account (20).

When considering adults with ID prevalence rates of 15% for ADHD are commonly quoted. A study of a modest sample of adults with ID, with varying degrees of severity, quoted an 'ADHD positive' rate of 16.9% (21). Prevalence rates are significantly higher, exceeding 50%, from studies, which only measure target symptoms, such as hyperactivity, poor concentration and impulsivity. (18)

Assessment and diagnosis

Validity of ADHD diagnosis in intellectual disabilities

The validity of the diagnosis of ADHD in children and adults has been established (2). The clinical presentation of ADHD in people with an ID is less well established and diagnostic disagreement amongst clinicians is common (22). Although mental health problems in general often have an atypical presentation in individuals with ID, the clinical presentation of ADHD is actually similar across individuals with different intellectual levels in childhood. This holds true for individuals with high IQ (23) and children with an ID. (24) It has been demonstrated that children with ID and ADHD show a characteristic pattern of symptoms, similar to those observed in children without ID diagnosed with the disorder (24). Additionally, no statistically significant difference has been found in the presentation of DSM-IV symptoms of ADHD in children with ID, compared with children without ID (10). Furthermore, a case control study established a negative linear relationship between ADHD symptoms and IQ in adolescents with mild ID (25). Neither the profiles of ADHD symptoms, nor the comorbidity with emotional and behavioural problems, differed according to the presence of ID.

There is evidence that children with ID and ADHD exhibit the characteristic symptoms of ADHD, such as poor selective attention (26), off-task behaviour and fidgeting, when compared to their ID peers without ADHD symptoms (27). An analysis of data of three samples of children with ID found a small, but significant, negative association of mental age and ADHD symptom ratings. These findings supported the diagnosis of ADHD in children with ID (28). A study comparing two groups of children, ID and non-ID, who met criteria for ADHD at age five, found that there was no significant difference in the number of inattentive, hyperactive/impulsive or total ADHD symptoms endorsed (13).

A study examining the clinical presentation, developmental course and functional impairment of adolescents with ID, compared to a group without ID, found similar presentations of ADHD in the two groups (4), thus further supporting the validity of ADHD diagnosis in children with ID group.

Comorbidities

Conditions associated with ADHD include mental illnesses, for example, mood disorders, as well as substance use disorders and personality disorders in addition to other developmental disorders, including autism (5). Both ADHD and ID are independently associated with increased lifelong rates of psychiatric morbidity, for example, adults with ID have increased rates of schizophrenia (29), and adults with ADHD experience higher rates of affective, anxiety, and substance use disorders (30). The fact that neurodevelopmental disorders tend to cluster together is also well established. The available data indicates that the co-occurrence of ID and ADHD further increases the risk of other psychiatric morbidity, particularly behavioural disorders. When compared to peers with ADHD and normal intellectual ability, children with ADHD and ID have similar, if not increased, risk for persistence of ADHD from childhood into adolescence (31). Additionally, comorbid anxiety disorder is found more often in this group, and they are more likely to have more restrictive educational placements (32). The comorbidity of ADHD and ID is associated with challenging behaviour; a cross sectional study found increased rates of oppositional defiant disorder in children with both conditions (33). A study following up 51 people with ADHD and moderate to borderline ID found that many continued to have behavioural problems, and take prescribed medication, at 1 to 5 years follow-up (34). A study of medication for disruptive behaviour in children with ID also reported high rates of comorbid ADHD (32).

Diagnostic evaluation

The diagnostic evaluation of ADHD symptoms is based on both cognitive and behavioural symptoms. Both these categories of symptoms are often present in individuals with ID without ADHD. This is not surprising, given that ID is often accompanied by deficits in attention and executive functioning; these abilities are highly correlated with intelligence. It is known that in childhood a decreasing IQ is associated with a reduced capacity for impulse control and an increase in mental health problems (12, 13). Some evidence exists of a negative correlation of IQ with ADHD symptoms severity in adults across the intellectual ability range (28, 35).

A comprehensive diagnostic evaluation is based on *detailed history*, including developmental history, and *mental state examination*. The former aims to establish a childhood diagnosis of ADHD and, where appropriate, the persistence of symptoms and impairment into adulthood. The accuracy and utility of historical information is increased by gathering both written and oral information from multiple sources. It is greatly assisted by educational records, previous health records and psychiatric and behavioural history. The mental state examination may be unremarkable or may reveal symptoms of inattention, hyperactivity and/or impulsivity. This should be complimented by symptom and impairment rating scales, of both childhood and adulthood. In cases where doubt still exists a structured diagnostic interview may be necessary to reach a diagnostic conclusion. Neuropsychology may be of some value in the diagnostic assessment process. This is more likely to be in its contribution to the formulation of symptomatic and impairment dimensions for the individual affected.

Studies have shown individuals with ID and comorbid ADHD exhibit more severe neuropsychological deficits in comparison to those who have ADHD without ID, particularly with regard to executive impairment (36–38). Other studies, which have focused more directly on aspects of attention, including selective and sustained, suggest that the combined effects of ADHD and ID have a greater detriment on these domains than either condition alone (39–41). A study of adults with ADHD found that general intellectual functioning has a substantial effect on attentional and response inhibition functioning. The effect was greater in ADHD/ID patients compared with ADHD/non-ID. Moreover, this effect remained significant when the analysis specifically controlled for the contribution of intelligence (35).

Treatment and management

With regards to the context of management, although treatment should be tailored to the individual's needs, multiagency-multidisciplinary involvement is typically necessary. The general principle of the management of individuals with ADHD and ID starts with the collection of detailed information concerning the nature and outcome of previous interventions. Outpatient treatment is the norm, although in some complex cases inpatient assessment and treatment may be necessary; some rare cases may, perhaps, necessitate use of the legal framework of the Mental Health Act, if the legal criteria for its use are met.

With regards to specific treatment approaches, NICE guidelines provide detailed guidance for the management of ADHD in children and adults in the general population. Although no specific guidance exists some references are made within the NICE guidelines to people with ID (42). Whilst the clinical team may combine treatment modalities, only one treatment should be introduced at a time, so that its implementation and effectiveness/safety can be evaluated.

Pharmacological

There is some evidence that ADHD can be successfully treated with medication in individuals, mainly children, with ID (43-44). A recent literature review recognized that the majority of the ID research focuses on children with ADHD. It found, although ADHD medication can be helpful, response rates are lower and adverse side effects increased in individuals with ID/ADHD comorbidity (45). Medication used includes stimulants, for example, methylphenidate and dexamfetamine, and non-stimulants, including atomoxetine and risperidone.

Similar to ADHD in the general population, methylphenidate is considered an efficacious treatment for both cognitive and behavioural symptoms in ADHD in people with ID. A randomized controlled trial (RCT), conducted in children, suggests methylphenidate performs favourably compared with placebo in terms of symptom improvement. Typical side effects, seen in the general population, were observed (46). There is limited research examining ADHD treatment outcome in adults with ID. One retrospective study of patients treated with stimulants in a clinic specializing in developmental disabilities has shown good results (47).

A meta-analysis has shown that amphetamine, prescribed either as the D-isomer (dexamfetamine) or as a mixture of L- and D-isomers (mixed amphetamine salts), has been shown to be moderately more effective than methylphenidate in the treatment of ADHD in children and adolescents (48). When considering its efficacy in people with ID and comorbid ADHD, however, a RCT studying 15 children with ADHD and ID or Fragile X Syndrome found this treatment had no significant effect on symptoms compared to placebo. The amphetamine was also associated with increased reports of adverse effects, predominantly mood lability and irritability (49).

In terms of non-stimulant medication, atomoxetine is a noradrenaline reuptake inhibitor which, according to NICE guidelines, is the recommended second line treatment for ADHD. Studies regarding atomoxetine use in children, or adults, with ID and ADHD, are lacking. A review of studies of the use of this treatment in young people with developmental disabilities, predominantly focused on individuals with comorbid autism spectrum disorder (ASD) and ADHD, found improvement in symptoms overall but, as with stimulants, adverse effects were reported more commonly (50). Until there exists RCTs in children, or adults, with ID and ADHD for atomoxetine, its use as a treatment in this population lacks supportive research based data.

It is estimated that just under one-third of people with ID are prescribed antipsychotic medication; this is commonly for psychiatric disorders or challenging behaviours such as aggression and self-injury (51). A prescribing survey, conducted in the USA, reported far greater rates of antipsychotic prescribing compared to stimulants in children with intellectual and developmental disabilities (52). Risperidone is an atypical antipsychotic drug that has been associated with greater reductions in ADHD symptoms than methylphenidate in children with ADHD and ID. A four-week, single-blind, parallel-group trial in this group showed that risperidone was associated with greater reductions in ADHD symptoms. Of note there was a significant weight reduction in the methylphenidate group and a weight gain in the risperidone cohort (53). There exists a poverty of randomized controlled trials investigating the efficacy of risperidone for the treatment of ADHD in individuals with ID (54).

The fact that available clinical evidence is mostly based on small, open-label trials or retrospective studies is an obstacle in developing specific guidelines for the pharmacological management of ADHD in this population. Good quality, independent research is required to determine the efficacy and safety of pharmacological treatments of ADHD in people with ID. The comorbidities present in people with ID represent a further diagnostic challenge and may influence both the types of treatment offered and its efficacy.

Psychosocial interventions

Psychosocial interventions are recommended by NICE either as a first line treatment in children or an adjunct to pharmacotherapy in adults. In some cases, for example, patient expressed preference or unacceptable risk of side effects, psychosocial interventions may be considered first line treatment for adults.

A wide range of approaches have been used for the treatment of ADHD in the general population. These mainly focus on behavioural therapy, psychoeducation, cognitive behavioural therapy (CBT) and coaching approaches. In terms of their therapeutic targets they commonly include anger management, social skills training, and anxiety management. Most of these interventions are delivered in a group or individual setting.

Although research evidence is largely limited to management of children and adolescents some evidence relating to the effectiveness of psychosocial interventions in adults, but not specifically with ID, exists (55). Such approaches, appropriately modified, may be suitable for application in people with ID. Current UK guidance supports the efforts of mainstream psychological services, for example Improving Access to Psychological Therapies (IAPT), to make 'reasonable adjustments' to accommodate the therapeutic needs of people with ID (56).Whilst mainstream (generic mental health or specialist ADHD) services should be considered, where appropriate, there is still a role for specialist ID, community based services in the management of those individuals with comorbid ADHD and ID. This option should be considered when it is felt that despite reasonable adjustments use of mainstream services would not be adequate to meet the person's needs. This is typical in cases where systemic ID specific issues form part of the management plan and are not available in mainstream services. For example, when working with the wider educational or residential network is considered necessary. In this context, positive behavioural support teams often have a role in the symptom modification and support of individuals with ADHD and ID and their families/care network (57–58).

Although psychosocial interventions are available for adults with ADHD, there is a poverty of research evidence regarding these treatments for the population of adults with co-existing ID (59-60).

Prognosis

Although it has become increasingly established that ADHD symptoms often persist into adulthood, it remains true that the severity of symptoms, and associated impairment, tend to improve over time. This, in part, is unrelated to treatment and attributed to a combination of brain and psychosocial maturation processes. People with ID have a poorer prognosis when they present with mental health problems in general (61). In the case of ADHD, people with ID may present with a decreased ability to develop coping strategies because of their cognitive deficits; as a result ADHD symptoms may manifest more severely and persist longer. This is supported by a longitudinal, case control study, and cross sectional analysis, which concluded that ADHD persistence into adulthood is related to lower IQ (31, 62).

Regarding ADHD symptom trajectory within childhood a study observed similar changes in both ID and non-ID children with ADHD. In both groups, hyperactive/impulsive symptoms decreased significantly from age 5–8 years, while inattentive symptoms remained relatively stable (12).

However, a retrospective study based on informant-rated symptom scales, looking at the trajectory of symptoms from childhood into adulthood, found that the improvement of symptoms in adulthood was less pronounced in the ADHD/ID group compared to the ADHD/non ID group (35). This indicates that, not only do people with ID may have more severe symptoms but these symptoms show a lower tendency to improve over time when compared with non-ID peers.

Case study 1

Kate is a 20-year-old woman with mild ID and a history of having had a traumatic childhood, where she had lived in a variety of institutions from her early adolescence, following a number of short-lived foster placements. This was due to aggressive and disruptive behaviour. In her late teenage years she was placed in a secure accommodation, following an incident during which she set a fire, in the context of an impulsive reaction to being bullied. She was prescribed antipsychotic medication and when she became 18 she was admitted to an adult ID secure unit. She was offered, and to an extent engaged in, a wide range of psychosocial interventions, including social skills training, anger and anxiety management, and psychoeducation around fire setting. During this period a diagnosis of ADHD and emerging emotionally unstable personality disorder (borderline subtype), were made. Treatment with stimulant medication was started. This was followed by a significant decrease in her impulsivity, improved adherence to psychological treatments and a dramatic reduction of behavioural disorder. Although the direct stimulant effect is likely to have exerted a therapeutic effect, it is also possible that the diagnostic formulation itself (and associated care plan) played a role in her own behaviour and the professionals' responses to it.

Case study 2

Henry is a 19-year-old man with a moderate ID and severe autism. Disruptive behaviour at school, and later college, triggered a referral to the ID psychiatry team. Careful collateral history taking, from his parents and school, combined with behavioural observations in both settings, provided evidence of extreme hyperactivity/impulsivity together with life-long inattention. It is likely that the autism was deemed an exclusionary criterion, and the severity of his impairment due to autism and the ID had overshadowed the symptoms of ADHD in childhood, thus impeding diagnosis. The prescription of a stimulant medication was followed by a modest, but noticeable, improvement in his hyperactivity and attention span, with a consequent increased ability to sustain his attendance at educational and therapeutic activities at college. The monitoring of physiological side effects, blood pressure, and pulse, on a regular basis presented a challenge. The implementation of a sensory programme, and incorporation of the vital signs monitoring in this programme, allowed for better cooperation and facilitated the continuation of treatment.

Clinical implications

Current research findings support the notion that individuals with ADHD and ID face 'double vulnerability'; they experience both the deficits imposed by ADHD and those associated with ID (63). People with ID are at increased risk for ADHD and they may experience a greater symptom severity than non-ID individuals with the condition. Moreover, it is likely that the course of the disorder will be longer, and more persistent, and associated with increased impairment.

Despite these findings ADHD is underdiagnosed in both children and adults with ID. There is a risk that hyperactivity and inattentive behaviour are automatically attributed to ID, through the process of 'diagnostic overshadowing', rather than the co-existing problems in need of targeted intervention. Identification of the contribution of ADHD and any comorbidities to the overall impairment is important as ADHD symptoms can be managed, with both pharmacological and non-pharmacological treatments, leading to everyday life improvement. With regards to pharmacotherapy and psychosocial interventions, more outcome research is required, specifically in people with ID.

It is clinically important to consider a diagnosis of ADHD in individuals with ID when the relevant symptoms are present. This is because ADHD is commoner amongst people with ID than the general population, is associated with challenging and potentially offending behaviour, carries a high risk of psychiatric comorbidity, is a source of financial burden and stress to families, but is a potentially treatable condition.

Key points

- ADHD is more prevalent in both children and adults with ID.
- Diagnostic overshadowing is a barrier to effective diagnosis and treatment of individuals with an ID and ADHD symptoms.

- Although atypical presentation is possible, the clinical symptomatology of ADHD is similar in individuals across different intellectual abilities. Individuals with ADHD and ID have a decreased ability to develop coping strategies, and ADHD symptoms can be more severe and persist longer.
- Pharmacological treatment may be helpful for individuals with comorbid ADHD/ID, however, response rates may be low and adverse side effects increased.
- Psychosocial interventions have a significant role in management of individuals with ADHD/ID, especially in the event of lack of response, or sensitivity, to medication.
- More research evidence is needed for both pharmacological and psychosocial interventions, specifically within the ID population.

MULTIPLE CHOICE QUESTIONS

Questions

Please select the single most appropriate answer.

1. What are the approximate prevalence rates of ADHD in non-ID adults and ADHD in ID adults?

A. Non-ID—15-65 per cent ID—50 per cent
B. Non-ID—4.5 per cent ID—50 per cent
C. Non-ID—4.5 per cent ID—15 per cent
D. Non-ID—4.5 per cent ID—50 per cent
E. Non-ID—15-65 per cent ID—15 per cent

2. ADHD in non-ID individuals is typically associated with which co-morbid conditions?

A. Schizophrenia and anxiety
B. Anxiety disorders, affective disorders, and substance misuse
C. Behavioural disturbances and eating disorders
D. Schizophrenia, behavioural disturbances, and affective disorders
E. Substance misuse and schizophrenia

3. Which of the following medications are classed as stimulants?

A. Atomoxetine and risperidone
B. Methylphenidate and risperidone
C. Methylphenidate and clonidine
D. Methylphenidate, dexamphetamine, lisdexamfetamine
E. Atomoxetine, dexamphetamine and lisdexamfetamine

4. Which of the following statements is false?

A. Individuals with comorbid ADHD/ID are more likely to have restrictive educational placements
B. Prognosis for individuals with comorbid ADHD/ID is better than their non-ID peers
C. Stimulants can be used in the treatment of ADHD in ID
D. Co-morbid ADHD/ID has a greater detriment on selective and sustained attention than either condition alone
E. Individuals with ADHD/ID comorbidity have less pronounced improvement of symptoms in adulthood compared to their ADHD/non ID peers

5. Which of the following statements is true?

A. ADHD cannot be diagnosed in individuals with a severe ID
B. Presentation of ADHD symptoms varies significantly according to the level of IQ of the individual
C. Stimulant medication is not helpful in individuals with comorbid ADHD/ID
D. The LD-DC does not provide diagnostic criteria for ADHD
E. Untreated ADHD in individuals with an ID is associated with challenging behaviour, family financial burden and stress

Answers

1. C. Prevalence rates of comorbid ADHD/ID in children are significantly higher when compared to the non-ID paediatric population. This heightened risk extends into adulthood with individuals with comorbid ADHD/ID occurring *at least* 3 times more frequently compared to non-ID peers.
2. B. Individuals with adult ADHD in the general population are at increased risk of developing comorbid anxiety, substance misuse, affective disorders, and personality disorders; this is also applicable to adults with comorbid ADHD/ID. Intellectual disability additionally carries the increased risk of schizophrenia and behavioural disturbance; these are not as commonly found in non-ID adults with ADHD. The best answer from the options is, therefore, B.
3. D. Only methylphenidate, dexamfetamine and lisdexamfetamine are stimulant medications. Risperidone is an antipsychotic medication, atomoxetine a noradrenaline reuptake inhibitor, and clonidine is an alpha-2 adrenergic receptor agonist.
4. B. Whilst adult ADHD is an established condition in the general population for individuals with comorbid ADHD/ID the symptoms are found to be more severe and pervasive. Severity of adult ADHD symptoms is correlated with decreasing IQ, likely related to difficulties in the development of strategies to manage symptoms in those with cognitive deficits.
5. E. Despite individuals with comorbid ID/ADHD carrying the risk of more severe and pervasive symptoms treatment can be effective. Untreated ADHD in individuals with ID is associated with psycho-social inequality including challenging behaviour and family financial burden and stress.

REFERENCES

1. Biederman J. The course and persistence of ADHD throughout the life cycle. In: Buitelaar JK, Kan CC, Asherson P. editors. *ADHD in Adults. Characterisation, Diagnosis and Treatment*. Cambridge University Press. 2011.
2. Spencer T, Biederman J, Willens T, Faraone SV. Is ADHD in adults a valid disorder? *Harvard Review of Psychiatry*. 2009 1: 326–335.

3. Antshel KM, Phillips MH, Gordon M, Barkley R, Faraone SV. Is ADHD a valid disorder in children with intellectual delays? *Clin Psychol Rev.* 2006, Sep; 26(5):555–572.
4. Neece CL, Baker B, Crnic K, Blacher J. Examining the validity of ADHD as a diagnosis for adolescents with intellectual disabilities: clinical presentation. *J Abnorm Child Psychol.* 2013, 41(4): 597–612.
5. Frazier JA, Biederman J, Bellordre CA, Garfield SB, Geller DA, Coffey BJ, Faraone SV. Should the diagnosis of ADHD be considered in children with Pervasive Developmental Disorder? *J. of Atten. Disorders.* 2001, 4(4): 203–211.
6. Buckley S, Dodd P, Burke A, Guerin S, Evoy JM, Hillery J. Diagnosis and management of attention-deficit hyperactivity disorder in children and adults with and without learning disability. *Psychiatric Bulletin.* 2006,30:251–253.
7. Xenitidis K, Paliokosta E, Pappas V, Bramham J. ADHD in adults with intellectual disabilities in *ADHD.* In: Buitelaar JK, Kan CC, Asherson P. eds. *ADHD in Adults. Characterisation, Diagnosis and Treatment.* Cambridge University Press. 2011.
8. Lindblad I, Gillberg C, Fernell E. ADHD and other associated developmental problems in children with mild mental retardation. The use of the "Five-To-Fifteen" questionnaire in a population-based sample. *Res Dev Disabil. 2011,* Nov;32(6):2805–2809.
9. Antshel KM, Zhang-James Y, Wagner KE, Ledesma A, Faraone SV. An update on the comorbidity of ADHD and ASD: A focus on clinical management. *Exp. Rev. of Neurotherapeutics.* 2016 Mar 3;16(3):279–293.
10. Ishii T, Takahashi O, Kawamura Y, Ohta T. Comorbidity in attention deficit-hyperactivity disorder. *Psychiatry Clin Neurosci.* 2003 Oct;57(5):457–463.
11. Xenitidis K, Maltezos S, Asherson P. Attention Deficit Hyperactivity Disorder (ADHD). In: Tsakanikos E, McCarthy J. eds. *Handbook of Psychopathology in Intellectual Disability. Research, Practice and Policy.* Springer. 2014.
12. Neece CL, Baker BL, Blacher J, Crnic KA. Attention-deficit/hyperactivity disorder among children with and without intellectual disability: An examination across time. *J Intellect Disabil Res.2011 Jul;* 55(7):623–635.
13. Baker BL, Neece CL, Fenning RM, Crnic KA, Blacher J. Mental disorders in five-year-old children with or without developmental delay: Focus on ADHD. *J Clin Child Adolesc Psychol 2010;* 39(4):492–505.
14. World Health Organization. *The ICD-10 Classification of Mental and Behavioural Disorders: Clinical Descriptions and Diagnostic Guidelines.* Geneva, 1992 Available from: http://www.who.int/classifications/icd/en/bluebook.pdf.
15. American Psychiatric Association. *Diagnostic and Statistical Manual of Mental Disorders* (5th ed.). Washington, DC: 2013.
16. Szymanski LS. DC-LD: Diagnostic criteria for psychiatric disorders for use with adults with learning disabilities. Royal College of Psychiatrists. *Occasional Paper OP 48, Gaskell, London.* 2001. 128 pp.
17. Emerson E. Prevalence of psychiatric disorders in children and adolescents with and without intellectual disability. *J Intellect Disabil Res.* 2003 Jan; 47(1):51–58.
18. Fox RA, Wade EJ. Attention Deficit Hyperactivity Disorder among adults with severe and profound mental retardation. *Res. in Dev. Disabilities.* 1998 May–Jun;19(3):275–280.
19. Simon V, Czobor P, Bálint S, Mészáros A, Bitter I. Prevalence and correlates of adult attention-deficit hyperactivity disorder: Meta-analysis. *Bri. J. of Psychiatry.* 2009 Feb; 194 (3) 204–211.
20. Faraone S, Biederman J, Mick E. The age-dependent decline of attention deficit hyperactivity disorder: A meta-analysis of follow-up studies. *Psychol Medicine.* 2006 Feb;36(2):159–65.
21. La Malfa G, Lassi S, Bertelli M, Pallanti S, Albertini G. Detecting attention deficit/hyperactivity disorder (ADHD) in adults with intellectual disability: The use of Conners' Adult ADHD Rating Scales (CAARS). *Res Dev Disabil.* 2008 Mar-Apr;29(2):158–164.
22. Sevin JA, Bowers-Stephens C, Crafton CG. Psychiatric disorders in adolescents with developmental disabilities: Longitudinal data on diagnostic disagreement in 150 clients. *Child Psychiatry Hum Dev.* 2003;34(2):147–163.
23. Antshel KM, Faraone SV, Maglione K, Doyle A, Seidman L, Biederman J. Is adult ADHD a valid diagnosis in the presence of high IQ? *Psychol Med.* 2009 Aug;39(8):1325–1335.
24. Fee VE, Matson JL, Benavidez DA. Attention deficit-hyperactivity disorder among mentally retarded children. *Res Dev Disabil.* 1994 Jan-Feb;15(1):67–79.
25. Simonoff E, Pickles A, Wood N, Gringras P,Chadwick O. ADHD symptoms in children with mild intellectual disability. *J Am Acad Child Adolesc Psychiatry.* 2007 May;46(5):591–600.
26. Pearson DA, Yaffee LS, Loveland KA, Lewis KR. Comparison of sustained and selective attention in children who have mental retardation with and without attention deficit hyperactivity disorder. *Am J Ment Retard.* May 1996;100(6):592–607.
27. Handen BL, McAuliffe S, Janosky J, Feldman H, Breaux AM. A playroom observation procedure to assess children with mental retardation and ADHD. *J Abnorm Child Psychol.* 1998 Aug;26(4):269–277.
28. Hastings RP, Beck A, Daley D, Hill C. Symptoms of ADHD and their correlates in children with intellectual disabilities. *Res Dev Disabil.* 2005 Sep-Oct;26(5):456–68.
29. Emerson E, Baines S, Allerton L, Welch V. Health inequalities and people with learning disabilities in the UK: Improving health and lives. 2012: Available from: https://www.improvinghealthandlives.org.uk/securefiles/170403_1120//IHAL%202012-11%20Health%20Inequalities_r1.pdf.
30. Kessler RC, Adler L, Barkley R et al. The prevalence and correlates of adult ADHD in the United States: Results from the national comorbidity survey replication. *Am J Psychiatry.* 2006 Apr;163(4):716–723.
31. Lambert NM, Hartsough CS, Sassone D, Sandoval J. Persistence of hyperactivity symptoms from childhood to adolescence and associated outcomes. *Am J Orthopsychiatry.* 1987 Jan;57(1):22–32.
32. Aman MG, Armstrong S, Buican B, Sillick T. Four-year follow-up of children with low intelligence and ADHD: A replication. *Res Dev Disabil.* 2002 Mar-Apr;23(2):119–134.
33. Ahuja A, Martin J, Langley K, Thapar A. Intellectual disability in children with Attention Deficit Hyperactivity Disorder. *J of Pediatrics.* 2013 Sept; 163(3):890–895.
34. Handen BL, Janosky J, McAuliffe S. Long-term follow-up of children with mental retardation/borderline intellectual functioning and ADHD. *Journal of Abnormal Child Psychology.* 1997 Aug;25(4):287–295.
35. Xenitidis K, Paliokosta E, Rose E, Maltezos S, Bramham J. ADHD symptom presentation and trajectory in adults with borderline and mild intellectual disability. *J Intellect Disabil Res.* 2010 Jul;54(7):668–677.
36. Seidman LJ, Biederman J, Monuteaux MC, Doyle AE, Faraone SV. Learning disabilities and executive dysfunction in boys with attention-deficit/hyperactivity disorder. *Neuropsychology.* 2001 Oct;15(4):544–556.

37. Seidman LJ, Biederman J, Valera EM, Monuteaux MC, Doyle AE, Faraone SV. Neuropsychological functioning in girls with attention-deficit/hyperactivity disorder with and without learning disabilities. *Neuropsychology.* 2006 Mar;20(2):166–177.
38. Lazar JW, Frank Y. Frontal systems dysfunction in children with attention-deficit/hyperactivity disorder and learning disabilities. *J Neuropsychiatry Clin Neurosci.* 1998;10(2):160–167.
39. Tarnowski KJ, Prinz RJ, Nay SM. Comparative analysis of attentional deficits in hyperactive and learning-disabled children. *J Abnorm Psychol.* 1986 Nov;95(4):341–345.
40. Robins PM. A comparison of behavioural and attentional functioning in children diagnosed as hyperactive or learning-disabled. *J Abnorm Child Psychol.* 1992 Feb;20(1):65–82.
41. Pearson DA, Santos CW, Roache JD, et al. Treatment effects of methylphenidate on behavioural adjustment in children with mental retardation and ADHD. *J Am Acad Child Adolesc Psychiatry.* 2003 Feb;42(2):209–216.
42. National Institute for Health and Clinical Excellence. Attention deficit hyperactivity disorder: Diagnosis and management. CG72. 2008. Available From: https://www.nice.org.uk/guidance/CG72.
43. Handen BL, Feldman HM, Lurier A, Murray PJ. Efficacy of methylphenidate among preschool children with developmental disabilities and ADHD. *J Am Acad Child Adolesc Psychiatry.* 1999 Jul;38(7):805–812.
44. Pearson DA, Santos CW, Roache JD, et al. Treatment effects of methylphenidate on behavioural adjustment in children with mental retardation and ADHD. *J Am Acad Child Adolesc Psychiatry.* 2003 Feb;42(2):209–216.
45. Courtenay K, Elstner S, Drug therapy in ADHD in people with intellectual disabilities. *Adv in Men Health and Int Disabilities.* 2016 10(1):27–35.
46. Simonoff E, Taylor E, Baird G et al. Randomized controlled double-blind trial of optimal dose methylphenidate in children and adolescents with severe attention deficit hyperactivity disorder and intellectual disability *J Child Psychol Psychiatry.* 2013 May;54(5):527–535.
47. Jou R, Handen B, Hardan A. Psychostimulant treatment of adults with mental retardation and attention-deficit hyperactivity disorder. *Australas Psychiatry.* 2004 Dec;12(4):376–379.
48. Faraone SV, Buitelaar J. Comparing the efficacy of stimulants for ADHD in children and adolescents using meta-analysis. *J. Eur Child Adolesc Psychiatry* 2010 Apr; 19(4):353–364.
49. Hagerman RJ, Murphy MA, Wittenberger MD. A controlled trial of stimulant medication in children with the fragile X syndrome. *Am J Med Genet.* 1988 May-Jun;30(1-2):377–392.
50. Aman MG, Smith T, Arnold LE, et al. A review of atomoxetine effects in young people with developmental disabilities. *Research in Developmental Disabilities.* 2014 Jun;35(6): 1412–1424.
51. Valdovinos MG, Napolitano DA, Zarcone JR, Hellings JA, Williams DC, Schroeder SR. Multimodal evaluation of risperidone for destructive behaviour: Functional analysis, direct observations, rating scales, and psychiatric impressions. *Exp Clin Psychopharmacol.* 2002 Aug;10(3):268–275.
52. Lott IT, McGregor M, Engelman L, et al. Longitudinal prescribing patterns for psychoactive medications in community-based individuals with developmental disabilities: Utilization of pharmacy records. *J Intellect Disabil Res.* 2004 Sep;48(6):563–571.
53. Correia Filho AG, Bodanese R, Silva TL, Alvares JP, Aman M, Rohde LA. Comparison of risperidone and methylphenidate for peducing ADHD symptoms in children and adolescents with moderate mental retardation. *J. of the Am Acad of Child and Adolesc Psychiatry.* 2005 Aug; 44(8):748.
54. Thomson A, Maltezos S, Paliokosta E, Xenitidis K. Risperidone for attention-deficit hyperactivity disorder in people with intellectual disabilities. *Cochrane Database Syst Rev.* 2009 Apr; 15(2):CD007011.
55. Bramham J, Young S, Bickerdicke A, Spain D, McCartan D, Xenitidis K. Evaluation of group cognitive behavioural therapy for adults with ADHD. *J of Atten Disord.* 2009 Mar; 12(5):434–441.
56. *Reasonably Adjusted?* Mental health services for people with autism and people with learning disabilities NDTi July 2012. Available From: http://www.ndti.org.uk/major-projects/reasonably-adjusted/.
57. Fabiano GA, Pelham WE Jr, Coles EK, Gnagy EM, Chronis-Tuscano A, O'Connor BC. A meta-analysis of behavioural treatments for attention-deficit/hyperactivity disorder. *Clin Psychology Rev.* 2009 Mar:29(2):129–140.
58. Sonuga-Barke EJS, Brandeis D, Cortese S et al. Non-pharmacological interventions for ADHD: Systematic review and meta-analyses of randomized controlled trials of dietary and psychological treatments. *Am J Psychiatry.* 2013 Jan:170(3).
59. Knouse LE, Cooper-Vince C, Sprich S, Safren SA. Recent developments in the psychosocial treatment of adult ADHD. *Expert Rev Neurother.* 2008 Oct;8(10):1537–1548.
60. Safren SA. Cognitive-behavioural approaches to ADHD treatment in adulthood. *J Clin Psychiatry.* 2006;67(8):46–50.
61. Tonge B, Einfeld S. The trajectory of psychiatric disorders in young people with intellectual disabilities. *Aust N Z J Psychiatry.* 2000 Feb;34(1):80–84.
62. Peterson BS, Pine DS, Cohen P, Brook JS. Prospective, longitudinal study of tic, obsessive-compulsive, and attention-deficit/hyperactivity disorders in an epidemiological sample. *J Am Acad Child Adolesc Psychiatry.* 2001 Jun;40(6):685–695.
63. Hardan A, Sahl R. Psychopathology in children and adolescents with developmental disorders. *Res Dev Disabil.* 1997 Sep-Oct;18(5):369–382.

9

Dementia and Other Disorders Associated with Ageing in People with Intellectual Disability

Andre Strydom, Karen Dodd, Nwamaka Uchendu, and Suzanne Wilson

Ageing in individuals with Intellectual disabilities

In keeping with improvements in medical and social care, people with intellectual disabilities now have a substantially increased mean life-expectancy compared to the earlier part of the twentieth century (1). It is predicted that over a third of this growing and ageing population will be over 50 years of age by 2020 (2), and 40 per cent of those with Down syndrome in the UK are now aged 40 and older (3). However, while individuals with mild intellectual disability have life expectancies approaching those of the general population, people with more severe intellectual disabilities continue to die at relatively young ages (4).

Older people with intellectual disabilities may develop age-related problems at a younger age and at a higher rate than their peers in the general population because of syndrome-specific conditions in addition to exposure to the same age-related risks as the general population (5). The causes for health problems are likely multi-factorial and in addition to genetic factors in some individuals, social factors such as poor housing, diet, and a sedentary lifestyle are also implicated (5). Furthermore, people with intellectual disabilities continue to have difficulties accessing equitable healthcare, and are more likely to have treatable conditions undiagnosed (6, 7).

The prevalence of cataracts and visual problems, hearing problems, diabetes, and musculoskeletal conditions increases with age in those with intellectual disabilities and impacts on pre-existing functional impairments. Rates of cardiovascular diseases on the other hand are similar or possibly lower to those in the general population (5, 7) and rates of smoking and alcohol use were lower than in the general population in a recent European survey of older individuals with intellectual disabilities (8). Clinical recognition of all health conditions can be complicated by atypical presentations influenced by poorly managed pain, sensory impairments, mental health problems, and side effects of medication.

All those working with adults with intellectual disability should therefore be aware of their needs related to the ageing process and also be aware of current recommendations and developments concerning maximizing access to health care and treatment. Person-centred support that is responsive to needs that change with age and any progressive illnesses, the quality of family and other support, communication needs, life events including any history of trauma and abuse, and suitability of the home environment are all important considerations when providing health and social care for older individuals with intellectual disabilities (9).

Epidemiology of dementia in older people with intellectual disability

Dementia is defined as a chronic, progressive brain disorder which particularly affects higher cortical functions such as memory, language, and orientation and is associated with considerable morbidity and mortality (10). Age is a strong risk factor, and dementia rates are therefore expected to increase with improved life expectancy in people with intellectual disabilities.

Alzheimer's pathology is probably universal in older individuals with Down syndrome (trisomy of chromosome 21) due to their having three copies of the amyloid precursor protein (APP) gene resulting in overproduction of the toxic amyloid-β, which eventually forms amyloid plaques (11). The consequence is that dementia is exceptionally common in older adults with Down syndrome, with a sharp increase in prevalence rates between ages 40 and 60, from less than 10 per cent by age 49 to more than 30 per cent by age 60 (10). Prevalence rates are however likely to underestimate overall risk because dementia is now a common cause of death in people with Down syndrome (12), and the cumulative incidence for Alzheimer's dementia in people with Down syndrome has been estimated to be more than 90 per cent by age 65 (13).

Though less common than in individuals with Down syndrome, increased rates for dementia have also been found in other elderly people with intellectual disability in the UK (14, 15). Dementia prevalence was estimated to be approximately 13 per cent among people with intellectual disabilities aged 60 and older, and 18 per cent among those aged 65 and older. Alzheimer's disease was the most common type of dementia found and three times more common than comparable general older adult population rates, with a prevalence of 12 per cent (7.1–18.5%) among those aged 65 and older. Other dementia subtypes such as Lewy body and fronto-temporal dementias can also be identified in individuals with intellectual disabilities (15). Incidence rates were also found to be increased compared with those in the general population (16).

Assessment of dementia

Assessment of dementia in people with intellectual disabilities is complex, and requires the clinician to undertake 3 functions: 1) gather a detailed clinical history; 2) establish that the person has had a change in function from a known baseline; and 3) undertake a differential diagnosis and exclude other conditions or issues that may mimic dementia (9). People with intellectual disabilities cannot be assessed using mainstream norm-based assessment tools such as the mini-mental state examination (MMSE) as they assume the premorbid level of functioning to have been within the average range (17). To overcome this, the functioning of each person with an intellectual disability must preferably be compared to their own baseline level taken when the person was healthy (18). It is therefore suggested that baseline assessments for people with Down syndrome should be in place before the onset of decline (9), which often occurs after 35 years of age (19).

Assessing people with intellectual disabilities for dementia requires specialist skills and expertise and should therefore preferably take place within specialist intellectual disability services or clinics rather than in mainstream services (9). A dementia care pathway which identifies the sequence of events required from referral and the professionals who are required to undertake the steps in the process may be useful (20). Careful consideration should be given to where assessments are carried out to maximize performance and inclusion of the person with intellectual disabilities and to minimize anxiety and distress. This should include how the assessment process is explained to the person and consent obtained (9).

Assessment process

The assessment process should include:

- File review and systematic history gathering from the person and key people who support them who have known the person for a significant time. This will include an exploration of the nature of the presenting issues, medical and mental health history, and psycho-social issues. Establishing a significant change in cognitive abilities such as memory and day-to-day functioning is an important aspect of dementia diagnosis.
- Mental state examination, to exclude other mental disorders such as depression—which may include use of specific measures to aid diagnosis (21–23).
- Evaluation of memory and other cognitive functions: although there is currently no agreed battery of assessments, direct cognitive testing with the person using tools suitable for individuals with intellectual disabilities is recommended wherever possible, to aid diagnosis and demonstrate change over time. Information can also be gathered from informants using standardized questionnaires to elicit changes in memory functioning and other cognitive abilities (24–29).
- Physical examination and investigations to exclude other causes of decline (such as hypothyroidism in individuals with Down syndrome) is essential. This should include cardiovascular, endocrine, and neurological investigations and, optionally, neuroimaging, electroencephalograms, and electrocardiograms (9).
- Environmental assessment including suitability of the physical and social environment, staffing levels, and competencies, as well as of the current support package.

Only once causes of decline other than dementia have been excluded can a formulation and diagnosis of dementia be made. Sequential assessment will usually be required to establish change in function and cognitive abilities, and its underlying causes. Under certain circumstances it may be possible to establish the diagnosis from a single assessment when there is good historical data and a very clear clinical picture.

Dementia criteria and diagnosis

Early diagnosis helps to ensure that people get the right treatment and support and an adequate plan is made for their future. Several diagnostic systems are currently in use. The International Statistical Classification of Diseases and Related Health Problems (ICD)-10 criteria include decline in memory, together with decline in other cognitive abilities such as organization, judgement and information processing and decline of emotional control and social behaviour such as emotional lability and apathy; all present for at least six months (30). The ICD-10 was modified in 2001 by the Royal College of Psychiatrists for use with people with intellectual disabilities (31), but will soon be replaced by the ICD-11 criteria.

The Diagnostic and Statistical Manual (DSM) system is an alternative to ICD-10 criteria, currently in its fifth version (DSM-5) (32). The previous version (DSM-IV-TR) was found to be more inclusive than ICD-10 or DC-LD when used in individuals with intellectual disability (15). Although both ICD10 and DSMIV-TR criteria were found to be reliable, predictive validity were less good when used in individuals with more severe intellectual disability and sensory deficits than in the general population (16).

The DSM-5 has renamed dementia as 'major neuro-cognitive disorder' (major NCD) and there is recognition of early cognitive change using new diagnostic criteria for 'mild NCD'. Diagnosis of dementia is based on presence of significant (major NCD) or modest deficit (mild NCD) in one or more of the following six domains—complex attention such as sustained attention and information processing speed; executive function such as planning and decision-making; learning and memory such as semantic and autobiographical long-term memory; language such as object naming and fluency; and perceptual-motor function such as visual perception and social cognition. Additionally for major NCD symptoms are sufficient to affect functional ability, and other mental disorders need to be considered (33).

Dementia subtypes

Diagnosis of dementia is followed by investigation of potential causes to assign a subtype. Common subtypes include Alzheimer's disease, frontotemporal dementia, dementia with Lewy bodies, and vascular dementia.

An area of future research being considered is the use of biomarkers for earlier diagnosis and subtyping. This could have important implications for treatment and prevention.

Sharing the diagnosis

Careful consideration needs to be given on how to share any diagnoses with the person and their families and /or staff support (20). The patient has a right to know their diagnosis but explaining the diagnosis and care plan can be difficult given cognitive difficulties, hence the need to use appropriate communication tools, and plan it carefully. It may be particularly difficult to share dementia diagnoses with individuals with severe impairments.

Pharmacological management

Pharmacological management is part of a range of interventions available to meet the needs of a person with intellectual disability and dementia. In dementia there is degeneration of nerve cells in the brain with resulting loss of neurotransmitters. The neurotransmitter acetylcholine that plays a role in information processing and consolidation in the brain is particularly affected in Alzheimer's disease (34). Anti-dementia medication with the exception of memantine prevents the breakdown of acetylcholine by blocking the action of acetylcholinesterase or butylcholinesterase (34). Existing medications do not cure Alzheimer's disease and cannot significantly affect the pathological process, however symptoms are alleviated and the early stages of clinical progression can be slowed. Medication is mainly used in Alzheimer's disease however improvements have also been seen in other types of dementia, particularly Lewy body dementia.

Available evidence for the use of medication in dementia is from research in the general population. There is no conclusive result from studies in people with intellectual disability (35–37) however there could be initial improvement in global functioning in people with Down syndrome and dementia (38). Acetylcholinesterase inhibitors include donepezil, galantamine, and rivastigmine, (39, 40). They are used for mild to moderate stages of dementia. Side effects may include unwanted dose-related cholinergic effects and include: nausea, vomiting, hallucinations, sleep disturbance, dizziness, and agitation. Acetylcholinesterase inhibitors are well tolerated in individuals with Down syndrome, though lower doses may be required (38).

Memantine is a glutamate receptor antagonist, which is approved in the UK for use in moderate Alzheimer's dementia in patients who are unable to take acetylcholinesterase inhibitors and in severe disease. Side effects include constipation, headache, dizziness, and hypertension. Memantine was found not to be beneficial in a trial for the treatment of dementia in older adults with Down syndrome (35).

Medication for dementia in individuals with intellectual disabilities is to be initiated by specialists. Once started, treatment should be carefully monitored to assess benefit in relation to side effects. Medication may need to be stopped when tolerability decreases as dementia progresses. Combination of acetylcholinesterase inhibitor and memantine is not recommended.

Non-pharmacological and behaviour management approaches

Non-pharmacological management of dementia or possible dementia should commence immediately after diagnosis (see Box 9.1). All interventions should be individualized and focused on supporting the person to live well and maintain their skills and interests as the dementia progresses (9). Interventions and support may be undertaken directly with the person, or through the family or staff who support the person. A social model holds that people with dementia are further disabled by the way they are treated or excluded from society (39). Caregivers should therefore be supported to understand that symptoms associated with dementia is not the fault of the individual and encouraged to focus support on remaining skills as well as on compensating for functional impairments. Ensuring that the psychosocial environment is supportive and providing professionals, families and staff with a person-centred philosophy of care ensures that the person is understood and responded to appropriately (41).

It is also essential that families and staff understand that dementia is a progressive disease. This means that the person's functional abilities and therefore their care needs will be constantly changing. As

Box 9.1 Non-pharmacological approaches for each stage of dementia

Early stages of dementia

- Support should be aimed at retaining abilities through prompts, aids, and simplification of routines and activities, for example, picture timetables to stay oriented in time, place and person
- A life story book with photos may improve communication, self-esteem, and help to delivering person-centred care while assisting with reminiscence (41).
- Cognitive and functional skills can be maintained through ongoing engagement in regular activities, for example, continuing attendance at day centres
- Cognitive stimulation and reminiscence therapy could be adapted for use in individuals with ID (42)

Later stages of dementia

- Preserve elements of abilities and functioning for as long as possible
- Over time memories 'roll back' and activities and objects from earlier parts of life become prominent. Families and staff need to then use reassurance and distraction rather than challenge the person's beliefs to avoid distress
- Ensure complications such as dysphagia, falls due to mobility issues are monitored and prevented
- Manage additional physical health issues, for example, chest infections and seizures as they occur (43).
- As the dementia advances towards end of life, the focus on health and supportive care becomes more prominent, but even at this stage families and staff should interact with the person throughout the day (44).

the person's cognitive and functional abilities decline, the level of support will need to be adapted to enable the person to continue to live well with dementia (20). Ongoing training and support for families and staff is essential so that they can adapt their approach as the dementia progresses (20, 41).

Management of behavioural problems associated with dementia

In those presenting with behavioural issues, management should begin with a review of the person's physical and mental health needs (including pain) and a medication review to eliminate treatable causes. Positive behaviour support approaches (or applied behaviour analysis) is recommended as the first line approach to guide the prevention, understanding, and management of behaviours in people with dementia. This approach places the emphasis on proactive and preventative approaches rather than reactive strategies. This will include simplifying activities/skills, ensuring that people are not stressed by being asked to do things above their current level of capability and enhancing functioning as far as possible (39, 41, 42). The behaviour should be viewed as a form of communication, and often only simple solutions are needed to resolve or manage problems (42).

Psychotropic medications have a very limited role as a last resort when the risk from symptoms such as agitation or psychosis is assessed as high, or causing significant distress. Treatment with an anti-psychotic drug may be offered, as long as target symptoms are identified and monitored and treatment is time limited (9). In general, starting doses should be low, and increased slowly (38). Carbamazepine or Valproate can be used for significant mood fluctuations (34). People with Lewy body dementia may be more susceptible to side effects of antipsychotic medication.

Environmental issues

A 'dementia-enabled' physical environment refers to the adaptations that need to be made to meet the needs of individuals with dementia. Noise and disturbance should be reduced while maintaining suitable stimulation. Routines should be predictable and familiarity of the environment is advantageous. Safety is an important consideration to avoid falls and other accidents, and facilities such as bathrooms should be clearly signposted with pictures, while toilets and furniture should contrast with the background colour to aid those with visual problems. Many individuals with dementia tend to wander; safe wandering can be encouraged using uncluttered corridors in the building and circular paths in a garden (45).

Course and prognosis

Understanding the progression of dementia and its consequences offers an important framework for understanding and appropriately responding to a person's experience and to inform adequate provision of care and support (9); (Boxes 9.1 and 9.2). In the early stages of dementia, there are subtle changes in level of function, cognition, behaviour and mood (46, 47). In the middle stages, there is more pronounced decline in cognitive domains along with severe impairment in functional abilities, and increasing severity of behavioural and psychiatric symptoms such as personality changes, disinhibition, apathy or agitation, wandering, sleep problems, and occasionally hallucinations or delusions (48). In late stage, there is worsening of above difficulties, problems with eating and drinking and increasing incontinence, myoclonus, or seizures (particularly in individuals with Down syndrome), increased risk of infections, difficulties with mobility, and the person may become bed-ridden and need 24-hour support.

End of life care

Knowing the prognosis in dementia is important in facilitating good end of life care (52). Generic breaking-bad-news models do not meet the needs of an individual with intellectual disability and diagnostic information may need to be broken down and communicated over time appropriate to the person's current framework of knowledge, and understanding (52).

Good practice requires working with the individual with dementia, their families and carers to ensure that all those involved understand the diagnosis and the associated decisions, issues, and care needs from the time of diagnosis onwards (41). Decision-making capacity issues, and dealing with these within the Mental Capacity Act 2005, need to be considered as the dementia progresses. Wherever possible, the person's views about current and future care

Box 9.2 Common health conditions associated with advancing dementia in people with intellectual disability

Epilepsy—occurs frequently in people with Down syndrome and dementia, and onset of seizures in older age should trigger assessment for dementia. Seizures are commonly myoclonic or tonic-clonic types and can be a presenting symptom in this population in contrast with the general population where it tends to occur in late stages of dementia. Sodium valproate, topiramate, or lamotrigine can be used to manage seizures associated with dementia in Down syndrome (49).

Pain—poor recognition and treatment of pain is common in this population for a variety of factors including diagnostic overshadowing and staff attitude to behaviours that challenge (50).

Sleep disorders—reversal of sleep-wake cycle is typical in dementia (9) and can be associated with challenging behaviour, respiratory disease such as sleep apnoea (a common comorbidity in Down syndrome), sensory impairments, psychiatric conditions and use of some types of psychotropic medication (47). Management involves understanding the problem, offering appropriate intervention and monitoring progress.

Depression is common in people with dementia including those with intellectual disabilities, and can be treated with antidepressants.

Gastrointestinal disorders—Dementia is associated with dysphagia and swallowing difficulties and active screening for swallowing difficulties is indicated to avoid aspiration pneumonia. If dysphagia develops, input from a speech and language therapist is required to assess risk and develop eating guidelines that may include a soft food diet and thickening of liquids to prevent aspiration. Percutaneous Endoscopic Gastrostomy (PEG) feeding was not found to improve outcomes in dementia (51).

Infections—People with dementia have higher rates of infection and any sudden change in presentation should prompt assessment particularly for urinary tract or respiratory infections.

should be established before their illness progresses, including how and where they will be supported at the end of life and when dying. In discussion with the person, their family and carers, consideration needs to be given to the person's preference with respect to use of invasive treatments in the advanced stages of dementia, future management of financial affairs, and the making of a will, and funeral arrangements. This can be summarized in an advanced care 'When I Die' document (9).

People with intellectual disabilities still underuse palliative care services and may not receive effective and coordinated end of life care (53). Joint and informed working and training in palliative care across services is beneficial to both the individual and staff (52).

Palliative and end of life care should aim to support quality of life, addressing psychological and physical needs, as well as social, cultural, and spiritual needs in addition to symptom management (54, 55). Areas that may require particular attention towards the end of the person's life include eating and drinking, pain relief, and posture. Essential services need to be available at all times within the care setting so that unnecessary hospital admissions can be avoided (55). When best interest decisions about resuscitation are required these should be formulated in partnership with palliative care services.

Key points

- Older adults with intellectual disabilities face obstacles in accessing health services.
- Some health problems (such as hearing problems, cataracts, and diabetes) are more common than in the ageing general population
- Individuals with Down syndrome are all potentially at risk for Alzheimer's disease due to triplication of the amyloid precursor gene on chromosome 21. Dementia prevalence and incidence is also more common in individuals with intellectual disability compared to the general population
- Baseline ability assessments by age 35 are recommended in individuals with Down syndrome. Comprehensive assessments (including consideration of health comorbidities and social factors) are necessary to aid the clinician in eliminating other causes of decline
- Management of dementia should take a person-centred and holistic approach. Polypharmacy should be avoided and non-pharmacological management should involve both the individual and their carers and family members
- All staff working with older adults with intellectual disabilities must be aware of important issues relevant to ageing and end-of-life care.

MULTIPLE CHOICE QUESTIONS

Questions

Please select the single most appropriate answer.

1. The point prevalence for dementia in adults with Down syndrome in their fifth decade is estimated to be:

A. <5
B. 5-10 per cent
C. 11-20 per cent
D. 21-40 per cent
E. >40 per cent

2. With regards to the incidence rate for dementia in older adults with Down syndrome it:

A. Continues to increase with age
B. Remains static with age
C. Is comparable to their age-matched peers in the general population
D. Increases to age 60, then becomes static
E. Increases to age 60, then reduces

3. A dementia care pathway for individuals with intellectual disabilities should be based upon key principles?

A. Transfer to a nursing home as soon as possible after diagnosis
B. Support that is aimed at improving abilities
C. Dementia information aimed at carers rather than patients
D. Access to palliative care in later stages
E. Focus on home-based activities to reduce risk of falls

4. A 52-year-old man with Down syndrome has an eight month history of memory problems and decline in abilities suggestive of dementia.

A. Sleep apnoea is an unlikely differential diagnosis
B. Treatment with acetyl cholinesterase inhibitors will be less effective than usual
C. Heart block is a potential side effect if treated with an acetyl cholinesterase inhibitor
D. Memantine is the first line medication treatment option
E. He has a 15 per cent chance of developing seizures

5. Looking at Dementia criteria according to current classifications in older individuals with intellectual disabilities:

A. They have poor inter-rater reliability
B. They have less good predictive validity compared to the general population
C. They are not useful because dementia presentation tends to be very different
D. ICD-10 dementia criteria will diagnose more cases than DSM criteria
E. DSM 5 has retained the term dementia

Answers

1. B. Individuals with Down syndrome develop dementia at much younger ages that their peers in the general population, with mean age of diagnosis of approx. 54, IQR 50–59. Lifetime risk has been estimated to be >90 per cent by age 65. However, dementia rates are relatively low in their 40's, and other causes for cognitive decline should be considered in this age range.
2. A. Just as in other individuals, dementia rates continue to increase with age in individuals with Down syndrome.
3. D. This is the most appropriate answer because a dementia care pathway will always adhere to the principles of being person-centred, involving the individual and their family in all significant decisions in a way that is consistent with the Mental Capacity Act, sensitively sharing the diagnosis and prognosis in a way that maximizes understanding, providing

medical interventions and physical, environmental, and personal support that minimizes distress and maximizes functioning at every stage, planning for the future and providing palliative and end-of-life care consistent with personal wishes and culture and religion.

a. This is unlikely to be person-centred and does not maximise function
b. This is not consistent with the diagnosis and is likely to stress the individual leading to challenging behavior.
c. This goes against all national guidance concerning involving individuals as well as carers. It is not person-centred
d. This goes against person-centred support, it is restrictive and risk-adverse.

4. C. Individuals with Down syndrome and dementia should not be excluded from treatment with anti-dementia drugs, which are recommended by the current NICE guidance. Acetyl-choline esterase inhibitors is the first option, and likely to be as effective as in other individuals with dementia, but memantine has been shown to be ineffective in an RCT.
5. B. Dementia criteria (ICD-10, DSM-IV and others) have been shown to have good inter-rater reliability, but somewhat less good predictive validity compared to their performance in the general population as severity of intellectual disabilities or comorbid sensory impairment may have an impact on the validity of diagnoses.

REFERENCES

1. Bittles AH, Petterson BA, Sullivan SG, Hussain R, Glasson EJ, Montgomery PD. The influence of intellectual disability on life expectancy. *J Gerontol A Biol Sci Med Sci*. 2002 Jul; 57 (7): M470–472.
2. Janicki MP, Dalton AJ. Dementia, aging, and intellectual iisabilities: A handbook. *Psychology Press*; 1999. 524 p.
3. Wu J, Morris JK. The population prevalence of Down's syndrome in England and Wales in 2011. *Eur J Hum Genet EJHG*. 2013 Sep;21(9):1016–1019.
4. Emerson E, Hatton, C. Estimating future need for social sare among adults with learning disabilities in England: An update [Internet]. 2011 [cited 2016 Feb 11]. Available from: http://www.improvinghealthandlives.org.uk/uploads/doc/vid_10673_IHaL2011-05FutureNeed.pdf.
5. Haveman M, Heller T, Lee L, Maaskant M, Shooshtari S, Strydom A. Major health risks in aging persons with intellectual disabilities: An overview of recent studies. *J Policy Pract Intellect Disabil.* 2010 Mar 1;7(1):59–69.
6. Heslop P, Blair PS, Fleming P, Hoghton M, Marriott A, Russ L. The confidential inquiry into premature deaths of people with intellectual disabilities in the UK: A population-based study. *The Lancet*. 2014 Mar 14;383(9920):889–895.
7. Jansen J, Rozeboom W, Penning C, Evenhuis HM. Prevalence and incidence of myocardial infarction and cerebrovascular accident in ageing persons with intellectual disability. *J Intellect Disabil Res JIDR*. 2013 Jul;57(7):681–685.
8. Haveman M, Perry J, Salvador-Carulla L, Walsh PN, Kerr M, Van Schrojenstein Lantman-de Valk H, et al. Ageing and health status in adults with intellectual disabilities: results of the European POMONA II study. *J Intellect Dev Disabil*. 2011 Mar;36(1):49–60.
9. Dodd, K, Coles, S, Finnamore, T, Holland, T, Gangadharan, S, Scheepers, M, et al. Dementia and people with intellectual disabilities: Guidance on the assessment, diagnosis, intervention and support of people with intellectual disabilities who develop dementia [Internet]. 2015 [cited 2016 Nov 7]. Available from: http://www.bps.org.uk/system/files/Public%20files/rep77_dementia_ and_id.pdf.
10. Strydom A, Shooshtari S, Lee L, Raykar V, Torr J, Tsiouris J, et al. Dementia in older adults with intellectual disabilities—Epidemiology, presentation, and diagnosis. *J Policy Pract Intellect Disabil.* 2010 Jun 1;7(2):96–110.
11. Wiseman FK, Al-Janabi T, Hardy J, Karmiloff-Smith A, Nizetic D, Tybulewicz VLJ, et al. A genetic cause of Alzheimer disease: Mechanistic insights from Down syndrome. *Nat Rev Neurosci*. 2015 Sep;16(9):564–574.
12. Englund A, Jonsson B, Zander CS, Gustafsson J, Annerén G. Changes in mortality and causes of death in the Swedish Down syndrome population. *Am J Med Genet A*. 2013 Apr;161A(4): 642–649.
13. McCarron M, McCallion P, Reilly E, Mulryan N. A prospective 14-year longitudinal follow-up of dementia in persons with Down syndrome. *J Intellect Disabil Res*. 2014 Jan 1;58(1):61–70.
14. Cooper S-A. High prevalence of dementia among people with learning disabilities not attributable to Down's syndrome. *Psychol Med*. 1997;27(3):609–616.
15. Strydom A, Livingston G, King M, Hassiotis A. Prevalence of dementia in intellectual disability using different diagnostic criteria. *Br J Psychiatry J Ment Sci*. 2007 Aug;191:150–157.
16. Strydom A, Chan T, King M, Hassiotis A, Livingston G. Incidence of dementia in older adults with intellectual disabilities. *Res Dev Disabil*. 2013 Jun;34(6):1881–1885.
17. Strydom A, Hassiotis A. Diagnostic instruments for dementia in older people with intellectual disability in clinical practice. *Aging Ment Health*. 2003 Nov;7(6):431–437.
18. Bush A, Beail N. Risk factors for dementia in people with Down syndrome: Issues in assessment and diagnosis. *Am J Ment Retard AJMR*. 2004 Mar;109(2):83–97.
19. Startin CM, Hamburg S, Hithersay R, Rodger E, Al-Janabi T, Strydom A. The LonDownS adult cognitive assessment to study cognitive abilities and decline in Down syndrome [version 1; peer review: 2 approved]. Wellcome Open Res 2016, 1:11 (https://doi.org/10.12688/wellcomeopenres.9961.1).
20. Strydom A, Al-Janabi T, Houston M, Ridley J. Best practice in caring for adults with dementia and learning disabilities. *Nurs Stand*. 2016 Oct 5;31(6):42–51.
21. Cuthill FM, Espie CA, Cooper S-A. Development and psychometric properties of the Glasgow Depression Scale for people with a learning disability. Individual and carer supplement versions. *Br J Psychiatry J Ment Sci*. 2003 Apr;182:347–353.
22. Mindham J, Espie CA. Glasgow Anxiety Scale for people with an Intellectual Disability (GAS-ID): Development and psychometric properties of a new measure for use with people with mild intellectual disability. *J Intellect Disabil Res JIDR*. 2003 Jan;47(Pt 1):22–30.
23. Taylor JL, Hatton C, Dixon L, Douglas C. Screening for psychiatric symptoms: PAS-ADD Checklist norms for adults with intellectual disabilities. *J Intellect Disabil Res JIDR*. 2004 Jan;48(1):37–41.

24. Crayton L, Oliver C, Holland A, Bradbury J, Hall S. The neuropsychological assessment of age related cognitive deficits in adults with Down's syndrome. *J Appl Res Intellect Disabil.* 1998 Sep 1;11(3):255–272.
25. Startin CM, Rodger E, Fodor-Wynne L, Hamburg S, Strydom A. Developing an informant questionnaire for cognitive abilities in Down syndrome: The Cognitive Scale for Down Syndrome (CS-DS). *PloS One.* 2016;11(5):e0154596.
26. Ball SL, Holland AJ, Huppert F, Treppner P, Dodd K. *The Cambridge Examination for Mental Disorders of Older People with Down's Syndrome and others with Intellectual Disabilities* (CAMDEX-DS). Cambridge University Press; 2016.
27. Deb S, Hare M, Prior L, Bhaumik S. Dementia screening questionnaire for individuals with intellectual disabilities. *Br J Psychiatry.* 2007 May 1;190(5):440–444.
28. Evenhuis HM. Further evaluation of the Dementia Questionnaire for Persons with Mental Retardation (DMR). *J Intellect Disabil Res.* 1996 Aug 1;40(4):369–373.
29. Sparrow SS, Cicchetti DV. Diagnostic uses of the vineland adaptive behavior scales. *J Pediatr Psychol.* 1985 Jun;10(2):215–225.
30. World Health Organisation. *The ICD-10 Classification of Mental and Behavioural Disorders: Clinical Descriptions and Diagnostic Guidelines.* World Health Organisation: Geneva; 1992.
31. Szymanski LS. DC-LD (Diagnostic Criteria for Psychiatric Disorders for Use with Adults with Learning Disabilities/Mental Retardation). *J Intellect Disabil Res.* 2002 Sep 1;46(6):525–527.
32. American Psychiatric Association. American Psychiatric Association: *Diagnostic and Statistical Manual of Mental Disorders.* 5th ed. Arlington: American Psychiatric Association; 2013.
33. Fletcher RJ, Barnhill J, McCarthy J, Strydom A. From DSM to DM-ID. *J Ment Health Res Intellect Disabil.* 2016 Jul 2;9(3):189–204.
34. Livingstone N, Hanratty J, McShane R, Macdonald G. Pharmacological interventions for cognitive decline in people with Down syndrome. *Cochrane Database Syst Rev.* 2015 Oct 29;(10):CD011546.
35. Hanney M, Prasher V, Williams N, Jones EL, Aarsland D, Corbett A, et al. Memantine for dementia in adults older than 40 years with Down's syndrome (MEADOWS): A randomised, double-blind, placebo-controlled trial. *Lancet Lond Engl.* 2012 Feb 11;379(9815):528–536.
36. Lott IT, Osann K, Doran E, Nelson L. Down syndrome and Alzheimer disease: Response to donepezil. *Arch Neurol.* 2002 Jul;59(7):1133–1136.
37. Prasher VP, Huxley A, Haque MS, Down syndrome ageing study group. A 24-week, double-blind, placebo-controlled trial of donepezil in patients with Down syndrome and Alzheimer's disease—pilot study. *Int J Geriatr Psychiatry.* 2002 Mar;17(3): 270–278.
38. Eady N, Courtenay K, Strydom A. Pharmacological management of behavioral and psychiatric symptoms in older adults with intellectual disability. *Drugs Aging.* 2015 Feb 1;32(2):95–102.
39. NICE and SCIE. Dementia: Supporting people with dementia and their carers in health and social care [Internet]. 2006 [cited 2016 Mar 11]. Available from: www.nice.org.uk/CG42.
40. Pharmaceutical Press—British National Formulary (BNF) 72 (September 2016) [Internet]. [cited 2016 Nov 3]. Available from: http://www.pharmpress.com/product/9780857112736/bnf72.
41. Dodd KD. Care considerations for dementia in people with Down's syndrome: a management perspective. *Neurodegener Dis Manag.* 2015 Aug;5(4):293–304.
42. Courtenay K, Jokinen NS, Strydom A. Caregiving and adults with intellectual disabilities affected by dementia. *J Policy Pract Intellect Disabil.* 2010 Mar 1;7(1):26–33.
43. Kalsy-Lillico, S. *Living Life with Dementia: Enhancing Psychological Wellbeing.* In: *Intellectual Disability and Dementia: Research into Practice.* Jessica Kingsley Publishers: London; 2014.
44. Bauer M. Collaboration and control: Nurses' constructions of the role of family in nursing home care. *J Adv Nurs.* 2006 Apr;54(1):45–52.
45. Jokinen N, Janicki MP, Keller SM, McCallion P, Force LT, National task group on intellectual disabilities and dementia practices. Guidelines for structuring community care and supports for people with intellectual disabilities affected by dementia. *J Policy Pract Intellect Disabil.* 2013 Mar 1;10(1):1–24.
46. Adams D, Oliver C. The relationship between acquired impairments of executive function and behaviour change in adults with Down syndrome. *J Intellect Disabil Res.* 2010 May 1;54(5):393–405.
47. Ball SL, Holland AJ, Hon J, Huppert FA, Treppner P, Watson PC. Personality and behaviour changes mark the early stages of Alzheimer's disease in adults with Down's syndrome: Findings from a prospective population-based study. *Int J Geriatr Psychiatry.* 2006 Jul;21(7):661–73.
48. Dekker AD, Strydom A, Coppus AMW, Nizetic D, Vermeiren Y, Naudé PJW, et al. Behavioural and psychological symptoms of dementia in Down syndrome: Early indicators of clinical Alzheimer's disease? *Cortex J Devoted Study Nerv Syst Behav.* 2015 Aug 13;73:36–61.
49. Simone RD, Puig XS, Gélisse P, Crespel A, Genton P. Senile myoclonic epilepsy: Delineation of a common condition associated with Alzheimer's disease in Down syndrome. Seizure—*Eur J Epilepsy.* 2010 Sep 1;19(7):383–389.
50. Kerr D. *Responding to the Pain Needs of People with a Learning Disability.* York Publishing Services; 2006.
51. Sampson EL, Candy B, Jones L. Enteral tube feeding for older people with advanced dementia. *Cochrane Database Syst Rev.* 2009 Apr 15;(2):CD007209.
52. Tuffrey-Wijne I, Watchman K. Breaking bad news to people with learning disabilities and dementia. *Learn Disabil Pract.* 2015 Sep 2;18(7):16–23.
53. NICE. Quality standard for end of life care. Quality standard 13. [Internet]. 2012. Available from: https://www.nice.org.uk/guidance/QS13.
54. Department of Health. End of life strategy. Promoting high quality care for all adults at the end of life [Internet]. *TSO* (The Stationery Office); 2008. Available from: https://www.gov.uk/government/publications/end-of-life-care-strategy-promoting-high-quality-care-for-adults-at-the-end-of-their-life.
55. Tuffrey-Wijne I, McLaughlin D, Curfs L, Dusart A, Hoenger C, McEnhill L, et al. Defining consensus norms for palliative care of people with intellectual disabilities in Europe, using Delphi methods: A White Paper from the European Association of Palliative Care. Palliat Med. 2016 May 1;30(5):446–55.

10

Schizophrenia and Related Psychoses in People with Intellectual Disability

Laura Humphries, Dasari Michael, and Angela Hassiotis

Introduction

Schizophrenia is one of the top 10 illnesses contributing to the global burden of disease (1) and can be extremely disruptive to a person's functioning and quality of life (2). Schizophrenia spectrum disorders (SSD) are generally considered to be more prevalent in people with intellectual disabilities ID (3) and although study estimates vary, consensus tends to converge around 3 per cent, three times that in the general population. There is even a suggestion that like other psychopathology in ID this may well be an underestimate, due to the problems of diagnostic overshadowing (4).

Until more recently, studies on schizophrenia in people with ID have been relatively sparse, and the bulk of established literature on psychotic disorders often explicitly excludes the ID population. The reasons for this are manifold, not least due to the challenges and limitations inherent in conducting and interpreting research in people with ID. There is considerable heterogeneity, not only in the cause and degree of underlying disability and comorbid conditions, but also variation in communication ability and adaptive behaviour. Different countries have divergent concepts of what constitutes ID, and terminology used in research can also differ. This is notwithstanding problems with sample size and ethical considerations.

Due to its relatively high prevalence and societal burden the majority of the literature on psychotic disorders in the general population has historically focused on schizophrenia; in light of this we will focus the content of this chapter on schizophrenia with broader reference to SSDs, which present in a similar manner to schizophrenia. We will be discussing diagnosis and classification, aetiology, assessment, epidemiology, and the link between ID and schizophrenia. The chapter ends by looking at the current thinking on management and service provision.

Diagnosis and classification

There has been a longstanding debate about the diagnosis and classification of schizophrenia, but current consensus is reflected in the operational criteria of the diagnostic manuals most widely used: International Classification of Diseases Tenth version (ICD-10) in the UK (4) and Diagnostic and Statistical Manual 5th Edition (DSM-5) (5). The current direction of classification is slowly moving away from distinct categorical constructs to a more dimensional approach; defining disorders along a spectrum, with a gradient of symptoms and continuum of severity (6). Therefore, some of the subtypes of schizophrenia in DSM-5 have been removed due to limited diagnostic stability, low reliability, and poor validity.

Schizophrenia can be difficult to diagnose, particularly in people with ID, where there may be additional communication challenges. Despite advances in the field of genetics and neuroimaging there is yet to be a definitive test to confirm schizophrenia. It therefore remains a clinical diagnosis, based on clinical interview and observation. Despite some criticisms around interview bias, research suggests that there is good inter-rater reliability amongst experienced clinicians diagnosing in psychosis in people with mild to moderate ID (7).

SSDs are disorders whose predominant feature is psychosis (e.g. hallucinations, delusions) and they include schizophrenia, schizoaffective disorder, persistent delusional disorder, and schizotypal disorders.

The manifestations of SSDs are diverse but they generally have one or more of the following core features: delusions, hallucination, disorganized thinking, motor disturbance (sometimes conceptualized as 'positive' symptoms) emotional blunting, avolition, anhedonia, and poverty of speech ('negative' symptoms). Positive symptoms generally represent changes in behaviour and thought. Negative symptoms represent withdrawal or loss of function. As clinicians, the terms 'positive and negative' help to define the condition and aid with diagnosis and management approaches. However, in practice, the terms can be confusing and easily misinterpreted by the patient (is a 'positive symptom' a good thing?) and so use of that terminology is best avoided if possible (8).

ICD-10 (Table 10.1) and DSM-5 classification can be used in people with ID, but their reliability and validity is best in those with mild ID and reasonable verbal ability, as their presentation is broadly similar to their peers of average intelligence (10).

Table 10.1 Schizophrenia spectrum disorders defined in ICD-10

Schizophrenia	As the archetypal psychotic illness, schizophrenia is a disorder of markedly distorted thinking, perception, and affect. Main symptoms include thought disorder, delusions, hallucinations, and negative symptoms. Cognitive deficits develop over time. Subtypes have been delineated by course and major features. • Paranoid schizophrenia The most common subtype. Paranoid or persecutory delusions and auditory hallucinations dominate. • Hebephrenic schizophrenia Delusions and hallucinations are less prominent. Behaviour is grossly disorganized and emotional response is lacking or inappropriate. • Catatonic schizophrenia Bizarre motor manifestations are the hallmark of catatonia. These include, but are not limited to, posturing, waxy flexibility, stupor, and mutism. • Residual (and simple) schizophrenia A slow but progressive decline in functioning accompanies social withdrawal and the appearance and deepening of negative symptoms.
Schizotypal disorder	Sometimes considered a form of personality disorder, schizotypal disorder is characterized by social and interpersonal deficits. There may be suspiciousness, odd beliefs, eccentric behaviour, and unusual perceptual experiences, though no single feature predominates. The disorder runs a chronic course.
Persistent delusional disorder	Chronic, frequently lifelong delusions occurring in the absence of other psychotic symptoms.
Acute and transient psychotic disorder	Psychotic symptoms develop rapidly and are not due to intoxication or an organic condition. There is an equally rapid and usually spontaneous recovery.
Induced delusional disorder	Occurs when a delusional belief, and sometimes other psychotic symptoms, are shared by two or more people with close emotional links. The sufferers are typically socially or physically isolated from others. Symptoms resolve in at least one of the sufferers following geographical separation. The illness is also known by the French term *folie à deux* (9).
Schizoaffective disorders	A disorder with prominent, persistent mood (affective) symptoms and episodic psychotic symptoms, not clearly coinciding with periods of extremes of mood.

Reproduced from *Journal of Applied Research in Intellectual Disabilities*, 7, 4, Clarke DJ, Cumella S, Corbett J et al., Use of ICD-10 Research Diagnostic Criteria to Categorise Psychiatric and Behaviourial Abnormalities Among People with Learning Disabilities: The West Midlands Field Trial, pp. 273–285. Copyright (1994) John Wiley & Sons Ltd. DOI: https://doi.org/10.1111/j.1468-3148.1994.tb00131.x.

Those criteria are less generalizable to those with the greatest degree of disability (severe/profound ID), in which it is not possible to make a diagnosis of SSD (10). Diagnostic manuals have been developed to better serve the population with severe and profound ID, namely the Diagnostic Manual-ID (DM-ID) (11) and Diagnostic Criteria-LD (DC-LD) (12), which are adaptations of the DSM and ICD manuals respectively.

DC-LD criteria suggest that early signs of psychotic illness could be a new challenging behaviour, especially if odd/bizarre/uncharacteristic for that person or increased frequency/severity of pre-existing behaviour. It gives less significance to negative symptoms than criteria in the general population.

Definitions within DC-LD include:

- Schizophrenic/delusional episode or disorder (Box 10.1)
- Schizoaffective episode or disorder
- Other non-affective psychotic disorders.

Epidemiology

Incidence

In one of the biggest epidemiological studies, the two-year incidence for psychotic disorders has been reported to be 1.4 per cent, and for first episode of psychosis, 0.5 per cent, giving a standardized incidence ratio for first episode psychosis of 10.0 (13).

There is some evidence to suggest that the onset of schizophrenia tends to be somewhat earlier in people with ID than in the peers with average intelligence. Bouras reported an increased incidence of psychosis in mild ID compared to more severe ID (14).

Prevalence

A recent systematic review and meta-analysis of 25 cross-sectional studies estimated the prevalence for all psychotic disorders in this population was 3.46 per cent (15). This confirmed results of previous studies, implying the higher prevalence rate in ID is a true finding. There was observed to be a variation in prevalence depending on the severity of ID, with higher rates reported in mild compared to severe ID (5.55% in mild vs 0.88% respectively).

In line with the general population, prevalence estimates were broadly similar in male and female patients, in contrast with a previous study (16) which suggested that it was more common in women. One study, looking at the population of prison inmates with ID, showed that they were twice as likely to have psychosis as the inmates of average intellectual ability (17).

However, the literature is subject to some limitations due to omitting populations from low and middle income (LAMI) countries, containing significant variation in service delivery and therefore ascertainment and variation in sampling frames between the studies. Further research is required to delineate whether this reflects a common underlying genetic aetiology, only affecting those with mild/moderate ID and schizophrenia, or whether the difference can be accounted for by the inherent difficulties in making a diagnosis of schizophrenia in severe ID.

Aetiology

There is no one clear underlying cause of schizophrenia, with increasing evidence in support of an interaction between genetic

Box 10.1 Summary of DC-LD criteria for Schizophrenic/delusional episode

A A disorder with prominent, persistent mood (affective) symptoms and episodic psychotic symptoms, not clearly coinciding with periods of extremes of mood. The symptoms/signs are not a result of any other psychiatric or physical disorder or a result of prescribed or illegal drugs.

B The criteria for schizoaffective episode are not met. (In DC-LD,unlike ICD-10, a diagnosis of schizoaffective disorder trumps a diagnosis of schizophrenic/delusional episode)

C One item of groups 1, 2, or 3 are met:

1 One of the following symptoms present on most days for at least two weeks:
 a. Third person auditory hallucinations discussing the person amongst themselves
 b. Hallucinatory voices coming from some part of the body
 c. Impossible/fantastic delusions
 d. Thought insertion or withdrawal or broadcasting, or thought echo or delusions of control, influence or passivity, or delusional perception or hallucinatory voices giving a running commentary

2 One of the following present for most of the time during one month:
 a. Delusions which are not mood congruent
 b. Hallucinations (in any sensory modality) which are not mood congruent

3 Two of the following present on most days for at least two weeks:
 a. Delusions which are not mood congruent
 b. Hallucinations which are not mood congruent
 c. Catatonic symptoms
 d. Negative symptoms
 e. Disordered form of thought, where there is evidence that this is a change from the individual's premorbid state

and environmental components (18). The leading hypothesis is that schizophrenia represents a disorder of neurodevelopment. Other theories include the aberrant connectivity hypothesis and the stress-vulnerability diathesis (19).

The relationship between cognition and schizophrenia remains complex and to an extent unclear. Various hypotheses have been postulated such as:

1. A common underlying aetiology (20)
2. Deficits related to ID increase the risk of psychosis (21)
3. A combination of ID and schizophrenia represents a severe form of schizophrenia (22)

Evidence from epidemiological studies supports a shared genetic risk for lower IQ and schizophrenia, with the strength of the genetic effect increasing with decreased IQ (23). A similar complexity underlies the association between ID, autism, and SSD (24, 25). Historical attempts to separate them may have been premature (26, 27).

Possible reasons behind an overlap:

1. ASD and psychoses could be on the same spectrum with a common origin. For example, childhood onset schizophrenia is comorbid with ASD in 30-50 per cent with common family genetic imaging findings (28). Recent molecular genetic studies strongly indicate that the genetic predisposition to schizophrenia is also shared with autism and ID (29).
2. ASD could be a risk factor for achizophrenia.
3. Diagnostic confusion because definitions or symptoms overlap (e.g. negative symptoms, social interaction/communication difficulties and repetitive stereotyped behaviours).

Biological

Familial

In the general population it is estimated that about 80 per cent liability for schizophrenia is due to inherited factors (29), though the mode of transmission is not well understood. Rigorous studies of SSDs suggest that the genetic risk for schizophrenia is more likely to be continuous rather than categorical and does not follow a Mendelian pattern of inheritance (30). Recent years have seen increasingly convincing evidence from genome-wide association study (GWAS) that genetic risk for schizophrenia is largely polygenic (23). This may well be a promising field for future research in people with ID.

Genetic

There are a number of rare inherited or arising *de novo* gene variants (Copy Number Variants, CNV) that have been implicated in schizophrenia and confer significant risk (odds ratios 2–60) (31). Mounting evidence suggests that such genes do not operate independently but interact with each other in biologically meaningful ways (epistasis).

There is strong evidence from a meta-analysis of 32 genome-wide linkage studies (32) for the involvement of chromosomes 1q, 5q, 6p, 6q, 8p, 10p, 13q, 15q, and 22q. There is also evidence of involvement of genes associated with dopamine D2/3 receptors, NMDA receptor signalling complex and the MHC locus (33).

Many CNVs also increase the risk for other neurodevelopmental disorders. In a study of 39,000 people referred to a diagnostic laboratory, about 1000 had a CNV at one of the loci identified in schizophrenia. Main clinical presentation included psychiatric disorders, developmental delay, ID and autism related disorders. Examples of neurodevelopmental genes implicated in schizophrenia include genes that regulate cell growth and behaviour, such as DISC1, NRG1, DTNBP1, KCNH2, AKT1, PAK7, and RGS4.

Genetic syndromes

VCFS on chromosome 22 has been implicated as a locus for genes important in schizophrenia following studies on people with Velo-Cardio-Facial Syndrome (also known as DiGeorge Syndrome) (34, 35). VCF Syndrome is a relatively common genetic disorder (1:4000) and one of the strongest known risk factors for psychosis. Schizophrenia develops in about 40 per cent of cases (36). It is often associated with ID (usually mild-moderate) and other clinical features.

There are a number of other genetic syndromes linked with ID that have been associated with SSDs, including fragile X syndrome (37), Klinefelter syndrome (38), Prader-Willi syndrome (39, 40), Dandy Walker (41, 42), Nieman Pick disease (43), Usher syndrome (44), Williams syndrome (45) and Charlexois ARSACS (46). A recent study reported a higher rate of psychosis reported in adolescents and young adults with Down syndrome (47), though further research in this area is needed.

Neuroanatomical

There is some evidence from imaging studies in the general population of structural brain abnormalities that correlate with genetic predisposition to schizophrenia. First degree relatives of those with schizophrenia show changes in regional brain volumes that are intermediate between those affected with schizophrenia and unrelated healthy controls (48).

Imaging studies are sparse in people with ID and SSDs, but those that are available appear to support the neurodevelopmental model. Many of the changes in gross brain morphology demonstrated in schizophrenia in the general population (enlarged ventricles, dilatation of cortical sulci and reduction in brain volume with proportionately greater loss in amygdala and hippocampus) are also seen in people with ID. However, imaging studies appear to show that the brains of people with ID and schizophrenia are more similar to the brains of those with schizophrenia in the general population than those with ID alone, suggesting a common pathophysiological process at work (49).

Histological

Alteration in synapses and dendrites have been observed in specific populations of neurons and glia in the cerebral cortex, hippocampus, and thalamus, suggesting differences in synaptic connection, in keeping with the aberrant connectivity hypothesis (50).

Neurochemical

Multiple biochemical pathways are likely to contribute to schizophrenia, so identifying a single abnormality is difficult. A number of key neurotransmitters have been linked to schizophrenia, including dopamine, glutamate, serotonin, noradrenaline, GABA, and glutamate. Some abnormalities in these pathways are also associated with ID (51) and comorbid conditions such as autism (52).

Neurophysiological

EEG studies demonstrate decreased synchronization/coherence of electrical activity in the pre-frontal cortex, reflecting noisy/inefficient cortical processing. Individuals with schizophrenia consistently demonstrate reduced sensory gating ability in the auditory evoked potentials P50 and P300 (53). Deficits in eye tracking have also been consistently observed. Evidence from functional neuroimaging shows a pattern of hypofrontality (a decrease in the cerebral blood flow) in the prefrontal cortex, seen in chronic medicated patients with schizophrenia (54).

Perinatal factors

Numerous perinatal factors are associated with an increased risk of neuropsychiatric outcomes that can involve both ID and schizophrenia (55). These include nutrition deficiencies (56) or viral illness in pregnancy (57), being born in winter months, changes in intrauterine environment (such as increased maternal cytokines resulting from hypoxia or infections), being born under 36 weeks gestation and with a low birth weight (58).

Stress

There is preliminary evidence that people with ID have higher rates of inflammatory cytokines and increased levels of oxidative stress, suggesting that allostatic load may be an underpinning mechanism for poor mental health (59). Current research in schizophrenia in the general population is focusing on the role of inflammation, oxidative stress, neuroimmune, and autoimmune influences.

Cannabis misuse

Research suggests that heavy cannabis use between the ages of 15–17 years may hasten onset of psychosis in those at high risk (60).

Ethnic minority status

There is an association between ethnic minority status and higher rates of schizophrenia but the relationship is complex (61).

Psychological

Increased vulnerability in terms of cognitive deficits (difficulty processing information, poorer problem solving, and planning skills), as well as emotional and social deficits, combined with increased levels of stressors can be an explanation for the association between ID and schizophrenia (62).

Social/environmental

Life events may occur more frequently for people with ID and are more likely to be multiple due to the numerous disadvantages they experience (63). These include birth trauma, stressful family circumstances, social exclusion, unemployment, deprivation, lack of self-determination and lack of supportive friendships and intimate relationships (64). People with ID may be victims of bullying, harassment, and hate crimes.

Assessment

The assessment of someone with ID suspected to be suffering with a psychotic illness is similar to that in those without ID. It involves taking a thorough history from the patient and collecting detailed collateral information from those who know the person well. It is important to gain an understanding of the person's pre-morbid state in order to make an assessment of how things have changed. In people with mild ID the symptoms and clinical features of schizophrenia are broadly the same as the general population (17). For those with more severe ID, information from collateral sources including recent behavioural changes is especially important.

A full physical examination should be performed, including heart rate, blood pressure, temperature, and blood tests, looking for common causes of infection or chronic disease that may be associated with abnormal mental states.

Relevant investigations should be considered to exclude important differential diagnoses that may present with psychotic symptoms. This might include performing a septic screen to look for evidence of infection underpinning a presentation of delirium. If there are suspicions of intracranial pathology (which may be particularly important in cases of first episode psychosis), computer tomography (CT), or magnetic resonance imaging (MRI) of the brain may be indicated. If there is a suspicion of epilepsy an electroencephalogram (EEG) may prove helpful. Urine toxicology may be needed if use of illicit substances is suspected.

When choosing investigations it is important to consider the risk versus benefit and how likely the person with ID is to tolerate them. There are several easy read guides to help people with ID understand investigations and medical consultations, and such materials should be available in all primary and secondary health services.

Table 10.2 Challenges in diagnosing SSD in people with ID

Challenge	Why
Severe or profound ID	Lack of verbal skills and general ability to report internal thinking processes or emotional states
Developmental age	Symptoms may be appropriate for level of development (e.g. mention of imaginary friend, talking about TV series plots as if real)
ASD	Stereotypies, rigid patterns of thinking, strange interests and ideas, suspiciousness, and inability to engage during interview can be seen as negative symptoms
Symptom presentation	Possibly explained by physical illness or other stress (e.g. trauma)
Low self-esteem or inability to understand others' actions	May be shown as increased sensitivity towards others bordering on paranoid thinking; may be a response to perceived stigma

The input of family or paid carers who know the person well is invaluable in the assessment. A description of behaviours that are outside the person's repertoire is important, including any changes observed in a variety of different contexts and settings.

When making a diagnostic formulation it is imperative to consider the developmental level of the patient (certain symptoms may be developmentally appropriate). It is also important to consider underlying cause of ID (if known) (65) (Table 10.2). Knowledge of past treatments and the individual's current life circumstances, including any change or other psychosocial stressors is vital.

There needs to be a thorough risk assessment to identify intentional or unintentional risks to the person or others. This will help to identify where treatment may be most safely given in the least restrictive manner.

Important considerations

Differentiating psychosis from the baseline features of ID can be difficult. Some of the difficulties relating to ascertaining mental illness and psychosis in particular are shown below.

Diagnostic overshadowing

This is a tendency to attribute all presentations to the ID, thereby leaving other co-existing conditions undiagnosed. Individuals with ID can have problems understanding and self-reporting psychiatric symptoms, and the resulting distress may result in behaviour which may be the only presentation of psychotic illness.

Confounders

ID is frequently associated with difficulties in communication, working memory, and insight, all of which are necessary to respond accurately to detailed questioning about inner emotional states and thoughts.

Developmentally appropriate behaviour (e.g. self-talk, fantasy, and talking to an imaginary friend), may be hard to distinguish from true delusional beliefs and hallucinations. Thoughts expressed simply and concretely can sound like hallucinations.

Apparent negative symptoms can be misattributed to a psychotic disorder but could in fact be due to other factors (e.g. autism), which shows the importance of obtaining a detailed developmental history (66).

Previous negative experiences of being bullied/rejected can result in hypersensitivity to how one is perceived by others, and this can present as paranoia.

Often people with ID express their thoughts in a way that appears jumbled, and this can be misattributed as disordered thinking in psychosis.

Cognitive and functional decline can present in schizophrenia as it can also be a feature of ID. Time of onset and course are important in differentiating long term traits from onset or relapse of illness.

Atypical presentation

There is some evidence to suggest that the onset of schizophrenia in people with ID is earlier than in the general population (67).

One particular study showed that people with SSDs or schizophrenia and ID have more observable psychopathology and negative symptoms when compared to a group without ID, and be less likely to have complex systematized delusions or report complex subjective symptoms (e.g. passivity) (68). Another showed that first rank symptoms are difficult to reliably assess in ID (69).

There is some evidence to show that people with ID and schizophrenia may present with social withdrawal, fearfulness, and sleep disturbance and appear frightened, worried, or perplexed. People with ID are more likely to be persuaded of the falseness of their beliefs, but will then continue to restate such beliefs (70, 71).

Some authors have suggested that dissociative symptoms may be more frequent in ID with psychosis (e.g. over breathing, pseudo seizures, gait disturbance, and Ganser state) (9).

Further details of the clinical presentation of schizophrenia in ID can be found in a systematic review by Welch et al. 2011 (72).

Behavioural observations

Early signs of psychotic illness could be the onset of new challenging behaviour, especially when odd or uncharacteristic, or an increase in frequency or severity. Behavioural disorganization has been found to be an especially reliable and valid indicator of schizophrenia in people with ID. Examples include staring to the side or blankly into space, nodding, glaring with anger, running in circles, and hiding from previously trusted others.

Assessment scales

Problems of diagnosis have improved in recent years with the development of standardized assessment instruments (73, 74). Emphasis remains on clinical interpretation of the results. Below, we report on some of the most established and validated instruments developed or adapted for people with ID and mental disorders.

1. Psychopathology Instrument for Mentally Retarded Adults (PIIMRA) is a screening instrument to aid in the

differential diagnosis of people with ID. It is an observer rating scale of psychopathology based on DSM III criteria, including schizophrenia (75).

2. Psychopathology Assessment Schedule—Adults with Developmental Disabilities (PASADD). Clinical interview is a comprehensive semi-structured diagnostic interview suitable for direct use with people with ID and separately with informants to aid diagnosis aligned to diagnostic criteria specified in the ICD or DSM. PASADD has two other shorter versions; a 25-item questionnaire, PAS-ADD checklist, designed for use by carers/family members and an informant-based semi-structured interview aimed at case identification, Mini PASADD.
3. Diagnostic Assessment for the Severely Handicapped-Revised (DASH-II) is an 84-item scale for use in people with severe and profound ID. It has been demonstrated to be useful in screening for schizophrenia in this group (76).

Differential diagnosis

It is important to rule out any potentially reversible causes in a presentation of psychosis. One must always consider first whether there might be an underlying physical health problem (77).

1. Delirium—can be differentiated from functional illness by the speed of change in mental state, a fluctuating course, coincident presentation with physical illness.
2. Epilepsy—is more common in people with ID, with a prevalence of about 22 per cent (40% if mild ID is excluded). It can be difficult to differentiate temporal lobe epilepsy from schizophrenia. Ictal changes can be mistaken for psychosis (78).
3. Migraine—for example, visual aura in complex migraine.
4. Medication (side effects and polypharmacy)—examples include corticosteroids, dopamine agonists, ketamine, some anticonvulsants including vigabatrin.
5. Psychoactive Substances—for example, cannabis, cocaine, amphetamine, LSD.
6. Alcohol—intoxication or withdrawal
7. Other mental illness: psychotic symptoms may also be seen in affective disorders (severe depressive or manic episode which are often mood congruent) severe anxiety, flashbacks in post-traumatic stress disorder, personality disorder. Apparent negative symptoms may be explained by depression or medication side effects.
8. ASD—recent research suggests that the presentation of SSD in people with autism is more atypical, with a different phenotype of psychosis compared to schizophrenia in people without ASD (79).
9. Pain, which may present as behavioural disturbance, for example, toothache, earache, sinusitis, gastro-oesophageal reflux disease, constipation, menstrual pain.
10. Sensory issues—for example, visual impairment, hearing impairment, impacted cerumen.

Management

The approach to management generally follows a bio-psycho-social format with care planning tailored to the individual. The best results are generally obtained by combining medication and psychosocial treatments. Treatment of the acute phase of illness and longer term management address different priorities.

In the acute phase the priority is often accessing appropriate services, adequate risk assessment, and ensuring safety of the patient and others. This is where the initiation of medication would be considered. Admission to hospital may be needed if risks are too high and symptoms florid, impacting the quality of life of the person and his/her family. Occasionally, inpatient admissions may need to be under the Mental Health Act 1983 (amended 2007) (80). It is generally believed that prompt treatment may well improve long-term prognosis. After the resolution of the acute phase, longer-term management including insight related work and relapse prevention planning can begin.

Clinicians should explain the treatment options to the patient in a format and language suited to the patient's needs. Capacity to consent to treatment should always be assessed and clearly documented. An independent advocate can be offered and families and carers consulted where appropriate. Patients should be supported by independent mental health advocates and empowered to make their own decisions where possible.

Medication

Guidelines for pharmacological management of schizophrenia are based on the NICE guidelines for the general population (81) but with adaptations for those with ID (82). Given the genetic deficits likely to be present in people with ID, additional care to titrate and monitor psychotropic medication and side-effects is needed. Therefore, whilst the guidelines may provide the overall treatment principles, reasonable adjustments relating to communication and cognitive deficits in people with ID must be made. When deciding the initial dose and subsequent increases, aim for the lowest effective dose. Take account of both potential side effects and difficulties the person may have in reporting them, and the need to avoid sub-therapeutic doses that may not treat the mental health problem effectively.

Typical antipsychotics include haloperidol, chlorpromazine, and flupentixol. Atypical antipsychotics include risperidone, olanzapine, quetiapine, amisulpiride, and clozapine amongst others. Atypical antipsychotics have largely replaced older antipsychotics as the first line treatment and seem to be better tolerated (83). They can be categorized into typical (first generation) and atypical (second generation) classes. The exact mechanism of action of antipsychotics is incompletely understood, but the effects of the second generation antipsychotics appear to be mediated by different subtypes of the dopamine and serotonin receptors, with varying affinities for other receptor subtypes, accounting for the variation in side effects. Long acting injectable (depot) medication is available if non-adherence is an issue.

Side effects

Antipsychotics are associated with a number of side effects, such as QTc interval prolongation associated with potentially fatal arrhythmias. It should also be noted that antipsychotics may produce gastric side effects, especially those with inherent muscarinic activity. A number of antipsychotics can cause an increase in the serum prolactin levels, which can lead to sexual dysfunction, which is one of the main causes of non-adherence to antipsychotic medication.

Typical antipsychotics are more associated with extrapyramidal side effects (EPSEs), which include parkinsonism, acute dystonia, akathisia, and tardive dyskinesia, thought to be a result of blockade of dopamine receptors in the striatal system. Such side-effects can be persistent, impair quality of life, and may be mistaken for core symptoms of ID. One study shows that people with brain pathology are more likely to develop tardive dyskinesia than people in the general population (84). A rare but potentially fatal side effect is neuroleptic malignant syndrome (presenting as hyperthermia, fluctuating consciousness, muscle rigidity, and autonomic dysfunction), for which urgent medical treatment is required. There is some evidence that the risk of NMS may be increased in people with ID on antipsychotics (85).

Atypical antipsychotics are not as strongly associated with EPSEs, although there is evidence that those with ID who take atypical antipsychotic drugs remain at increased risk of developing abnormal movement disorder (86). An important side-effect of atypical antipsychotics is the metabolic syndrome, comprising obesity, insulin resistance, impaired glucose tolerance, and dyslipidaemia (87). A long-term perspective on atypical antipsychotic use in people with ID is still not yet possible in the same way as it is with typicals (88).

The Matson Evaluation of Drug Side-Effects (MEDS) has been developed as a comprehensive informant-based measure that can be used to assess side-effects of psychotropic medication in people with ID (89).

Clozapine

The atypical antipsychotic clozapine is effective in improving symptoms in treatment-resistant schizophrenia. It is licensed where there has been no response to two adequate trials of alternative antipsychotics. Studies suggest that clozapine is safe and efficacious in people with ID (90). However, due to the risk of serious side-effects, including potentially fatal agranulocytosis, and the necessity of regular blood tests, clinicians can be hesitant to prescribe.

ECT

There is little published data for ECT in SSDs in people with ID and SSDs (91, 92).

Interactions

The risk of drug/drug interactions must be considered, as many individuals with an ID are likely to be on other medications for associated health comorbidities. Important interactions include lithium, antiepileptic drugs, and antidepressants.

Physical health recommendations

Monitoring of certain biological indices is important and includes measuring of blood pressure, ECG at initiation of medication, weight and BMI, cholesterol and a documented care plan in the preceding 12 months.

There are indications that people with ID frequently do not receive such investigations (92, 93, 94). The role of community ID teams to facilitate access to care is crucial in this respect. Those with schizophrenia and SSD on antipsychotic medication should be offered a programme of healthy eating and physical activity by their mental health provider. They also should be given help to stop smoking (even if previous attempts have failed). Nicotine affects the metabolism of other drugs, especially olanzapine and clozapine.

Medication should be prescribed at the smallest effective dose. If the clinical response is not satisfactory within a reasonable timescale (4–6 weeks of optimum dosage) or if unacceptable side effects emerge consider switching antipsychotic medication or reviewing the diagnosis.

Duration of treatment for psychosis depends on the response to medication. After the first episode the consensus is to treat for at least a two-year symptom-free period.

Psychosocial interventions

There is limited evidence so far on the use of psychological interventions in schizophrenia and SSD in people with ID (95). Therapy should be tailored to the developmental level of the individual and appropriate adaptations to the therapeutic environment and treatment framework should be considered. The involvement of family members (if they are not in conflict) may be particularly important to facilitate engagement. For people with severe or profound ID it may be particularly useful to help manage the person's environment to reduce stressors or help them manage change.

Research from the general population has shown some positive results for CBT therapy in psychosis. A case series of CBT in mild ID and psychosis showed positive improvements in symptoms and behaviour (96). A study of a psychoeducation group for dual diagnosis in adults with mild/borderline ID and psychosis was found to be helpful in the participants' understanding of their condition and helped prepare them to cope better (97). Other promising areas of psychological intervention in the general population include insight related work, adherence therapy, family/carer work, and relapse prevention (98). It is likely that similar approaches will be beneficial in people with ID with appropriate modifications.

In addition to psychological interventions, assessment of social care needs are important regarding accommodation, daytime activities, and occupational opportunities. Family carer assessment and support should also be offered. Provision of care under the Care Programme Approach (CPA) may be needed for those with severe mental illness and complex needs requiring long-term support.

People with ID and schizophrenia/SSD should also be protected from abuse and neglect via safeguarding and risk management.

Services

People with ID have the right to access the same health services as the general population (99). Compared to other people with ID alone, those with a comorbid diagnosis of SSD are likely to be heavy consumers of resources (100), and one study showed they are 15 times more likely to be admitted to hospital (101). There is evidence to show that compared to the general population hospital admissions for this group cost more (102) and last longer, although are fewer in frequency. At discharge they are likely to need more support than those without a diagnosis of ID.

Mental health services are required to make reasonable adjustments to accommodate the needs of this group of patients. When a patient with ID is in crisis, it is accepted that crisis and home treatment teams are likely to be involved in joint assessments and shared decision-making about management.

The policy direction in the UK is to maintain and support care in the community to avoid unnecessary hospital admissions. However, there is as yet a lack of high quality evidence about clinically and cost effective service models for people with ID and mental illness

(103). A study of consensus building on service elements important in treating schizophrenia in adults with ID showed that need for local integrated care pathways, strong leadership, and collaborative working were central to delivering good care (104).

Outcome/Prognosis

Schizophrenia is a major cause of functional disability worldwide, and tends to run a chronic course which can impair relationships, functioning, and quality of life. As with the challenges of diagnosis in the ID population it can be similarly difficult to define outcomes; predictors of outcomes can be remarkably heterogeneous. Available evidence in the ID population shows that people with comorbid ID and schizophrenia may have worse long-term outcomes, which are associated with lower quality of life, more severe psychotic symptoms and reduced functioning compared to those with schizophrenia and higher IQ (105).

There is some evidence that outcomes may be better when people with ID and psychosis are treated by specialist rather than generic services (106). A study in British Colombia noted that three factors improved prognosis in youths with ID and SDD: low rates of alcohol and substance misuse, increased compliance with medication and good psychosocial supports (107). More longitudinal data is needed to further substantiate our understanding of outcomes in those with ID and schizophrenia.

International perspective

Available research suggests that the prevalence of SSDs in ID is uniformly high across the world (108, 109). The WHO survey (110) suggests that inpatient care, primary care, and specialist services are now available in most nations. However, ensuring their availability and accessibility for individuals with ID should be an international priority. There is a vast variation in the provision of mental health care, with low income countries having a lower provision and access to care. This discrepancy highlights the importance of initiatives such as the WHO Mental Health GAP Action Programme (mhGAP) (110) in improving awareness and reducing stigma of mental illness in LAMI countries.

Case study 1

Angela is a 22-year-old lady with a mild ID. She lives with her mother, her parents having recently separated. She works as a cleaner at a local pub, which she enjoyed very much until approximately two months ago. She was referred to the ID service by the GP following concerns from her mother regarding a change in her behaviour. The history suggested that she had fallen out with most of her work colleagues as she was accusing them of talking about her, passing rude remarks about her and that they were 'out to get her'. She further felt her thoughts and actions were being controlled by the landlord of the pub. She stopped going to work which her mother put down to stress at work and that a break would do her good. However, once at home the situation deteriorated further, with Angela becoming suspicious of the neighbours talking about her, and that she could hear them through the walls planning to hurt her and calling her names. She would draw the curtains to her room and refuse to leave the room. Things came to a head one evening when she went across to the neighbour's home and challenged them. Her mother also noticed that she was not sleeping at night and would stay awake in her room talking to herself and appearing to be apparently responding to voices. She stopped eating food cooked by her mother, becoming suspicious of her, eating only cereals from the boxes, and in the process lost significant weight. On mental state examination she was a tall young lady who looked underweight. She looked suspiciously at the doctor and the accompanying community nurse, and became distressed when asked about her experiences. She had thought disturbances in the form of thought insertion, for which she blamed the landlord, and also delusions of control regarding him. She had persecutory delusions about her neighbours and workmates, and this recently had also extended to her mother. She had auditory hallucinations of the neighbours talking ill about her. She lacked insight into her illness. Given her presentation and mental state a diagnosis of paranoid schizophrenia was made and she was commenced on antipsychotic medication. She responded remarkably well and was soon able to return to her job.

Case study 2

Colin is a 56-year-old gentleman with moderate ID. He has been residing in a care home for the past six years. He had regular contact with his elderly parents whom he visited during the weekends. Six months ago his father suddenly passed away and his mother was taken into care, due to her inability to care for herself. His contact with her reduced and eventually ceased, as his mother felt distressed whenever he visited her. Since then the staff at Colin's care home noticed a gradual change in his presentation. Four months ago he began to isolate himself, avoiding contact with other residents, not communicating with the staff as he normally did and refusing activities such as the day centre and social outings. Over a period of time the staff noticed that his sleep gradually deteriorated and he would stay awake all night. He would also complain of a bad smell, but the staff did not take much notice of this. One night the staff noticed that he was in a fellow patient's bedroom, stood over him with a rod in his hand. The staff were able to intervene in time and sought an urgent referral to the ID service. He was seen in outpatient clinic as an emergency the following day. He presented as a middle-aged man of medium build and dressed appropriately. Further questioning revealed that he believed the other residents and staff were against him and were plotting to kill him. He also started believing that a foul smelling poisonous gas was being sent in through the vents in order to suffocate him. He said he had meant to attack the resident next door in order to protect himself. He had no other delusional beliefs. He also had olfactory hallucination of poisonous gas, which was of a more recent origin. Given the presentation a diagnosis of delusional disorder was made, and in order to manage the risks he was presenting with he was admitted to the inpatient unit. He was started on antipsychotic medication on admission. He made a gradual uneventful recovery and was able to be discharged back to the care home with an enhanced package of care.

MULTIPLE CHOICE QUESTIONS

Questions

Please select the single most appropriate answer.

1. When considering a diagnosis of a schizophrenia spectrum disorder (SSD), which of the following statements is true?

A. A diagnosis of SSD can never be made in people with intellectual disability (ID)
B. A diagnosis of SSD can be made in people with autism spectrum disorders
C. A diagnosis of SSD can be made in up to 10 per cent of people with ID
D. A diagnosis of SSD is not compatible with attention deficit hyperactivity disorder
E. It is easy to make a diagnosis of SSD in people with severe to profound ID

2. Which of the following statements regarding SSD is true?
A. SSD always present with changes in EEG in people with ID
B. SSD are not associated with cannabis use in people with ID
C. SSD do not have genetic causes in people with ID
D. SSD may share a common pathway with ID
E. SSD present in the same way in people with ID as in the non-ID population

3. In assessing a person with ID and SSD which of the following steps is essential?
A. You must always carry out an IQ test
B. You must ask about his/her physical health status
C. You must admit him/her into hospital to avoid a crisis
D. You must carry out an autism diagnostic interview
E. You must differentiate the symptoms from those of dementia

4. When treating a person with ID and SSD, which statement below is the most appropriate?
A. Always prescribe low doses of antipsychotic medication in order to avoid side effects
B. Consider the ease of reporting of medication side effects by the person and carers
C. Only review medication once a year
D. Prescribe high dosage antipsychotics to help control symptoms
E. Use clozapine

5. Which of the following statements is true regarding antipsychotic treatment of SSD in people with ID?
A. They always suffer with epilepsy as a result of antipsychotic medication side-effects
B. They are unlikely to recover from an episode of SSD
C. They do not have capacity to consent to treatment with antipsychotic medication
D. They must stop antipsychotic medication two years after initiation of treatment
E. They suffer higher rates of motor side effects than the population with SSD without ID

Answers

1. B. Schizophrenia Spectrum Disorders (SSD) are generally considered to be more prevalent in people with ID: approximately three times of that in the general population. Evidence is accumulating that individuals with ASD are at greater risk of developing psychotic illnesses than those in the general population. ADHD is a common condition and likely a common comorbidity with schizophrenia. There is some evidence to suggest that people with ADHD are more likely to develop psychotic disorders. Patients with severe and profound ID and autism cannot report their symptoms when they experience a psychotic condition so assessment and treatment must be based on thorough observations of behavioural characteristics.
2. D. The clinical significance of EEG changes in patients with functional psychoses is not yet clearly defined and EEGs do not form a routine part of assessment of SSD. Research suggests that heavy cannabis use between the ages of 15–17 years may hasten onset of psychosis in those at high risk. There is no evidence to suggest that people with ID are protected from this risk. There are a number of genetic syndromes linked with ID that have been associated with SSDs, including Velofacial cardio syndrome fragile X syndrome, Klinefelter syndrome and others. The leading hypothesis is that schizophrenia represents a disorder of neurodevelopment and there is evidence that there may be a common pathogenesis in intellectual disability co-occurring with schizophrenia. Reliability and validity of ICD-10 and DSM5 classification is best with those with mild ID and reasonable verbal ability as the presentation is broadly similar to average intelligence peers. Modified diagnostic manuals for ID (DM-ID/DC-LD) suggest other behavioural indicators used to diagnosis psychosis including new challenging behaviour, especially if odd/bizarre/uncharacteristic for that person.
3. B. Undertaking an IQ test or autism diagnostic interview would not be appropriate for someone presenting with acute psychosis as this would affect the accuracy of the test. It is important to rule out any potentially reversible causes in a presentation of psychosis. For example one must always consider first whether there might be an underlying physical health problem. Admission to hospital to avoid crisis would usually be considered a last resort. Dementia can be associated with psychotic symptoms but assessment for dementia would depend on a clinical suspicion in the presentation and would not be considered routine.
4. B. When deciding the initial dose of antipsychotic medication and subsequent increases, aim for the lowest effective dose. Take account of both potential side effects and difficulties the person may have in reporting them, and the need to avoid sub-therapeutic doses that may not treat the mental health problem effectively. When starting antipsychotic medication, evaluate response from two weeks, and ensure optimum duration of four to six weeks before switching unless adverse effects occur. The atypical antipsychotic clozapine is effective in improving symptoms in treatment-resistant schizophrenia which is licensed where there has been no response to two adequate trials of alternative anti-psychotics.
5. E. All antipsychotic medications decrease the seizure threshold to varying degrees but do not in themselves cause epilepsy, which is neurological in origin. In those with a comorbid diagnosis of epilepsy seizure potential is dose-related, so high-dose therapy and rapid upward dose titration should be avoided. Prophylactic use of an anticonvulsant may be necessary. Traditionally it is believed that the course and prognosis of schizophrenia is divided into three

categories: 25 per cent achieve full response to treatment leading to recovery from first episode; 50 per cent have recurrent illnesses in the form of exacerbations and remissions; 25 per cent have an unfavourable course with incomplete response and recovery from first episode. Having an intellectual disability does not automatically preclude an individual from having capacity to consent to medication. A person is not to be treated as unable to make a decision unless all practicable steps to help him do so have been taken without success. After one psychotic episode treatment is often continued for 1–2 years after recovery. After another psychotic episode antipsychotic treatment may be needed for longer, up to 5 years. After several psychotic episodes antipsychotic medication may be required long term. There is evidence that people with intellectual disability are more susceptible to movement side effects of antipsychotic drugs. Assessment for movement side effects should be integral to antipsychotic drug monitoring in people with intellectual disability.

REFERENCES

1. Murray CJL, Lopez AD. Global burden of disease—Harvard University Press [Internet]. [cited 31 Oct 2016]. Available from: http://www.hup.harvard.edu/catalog.php?isbn=9780674354487.
2. Galuppi A, Turola MC, Nanni MG, Mazzoni P, Grassi L. Schizophrenia and quality of life: How important are symptoms and functioning? *Int J Ment Health Syst.* 2010 Dec 8;4:31.
3. Carvill S, Marston G. People with intellectual disability, sensory impairments and behaviour disorder: a case series. *J Intellect Disabil Res.* 2002 1 Mar;46(3):264–272.
4. World Health Organisation. The ICD-10 classification of mental and behavioural disorders: Clinical descriptions and diagnostic guidelines. World Health Organization; 1992. 380 pp.
5. American Psychiatric Association. Diagnostic and statistical manual of mental disorders [Internet]. Fifth Edition. American Psychiatric Association; 2013 [cited 2016 Oct 31]. Available from: http://psychiatryonline.org/doi/book/10.1176/appi.books.9780890425596.
6. Bhati MT. Defining psychosis: the evolution of DSM-5 schizophrenia spectrum disorders. *Curr Psychiatry Rep.* 2013 Nov;15(11):409.
7. Einfeld S, Tonge B, Chapman L, Mohr C, Taffe J, Horstead S. Inter-rater reliability of the diagnoses of psychosis and depression in individuals with intellectual disabilities. *J Appl Res Intellect Disabil JARID.* 2007 Sep;20(5):384–390.
8. Clarke DJ, Cumella S, Corbett J, Baxter M, Langton J, Prasher V, et al. Use of Icd-10 research diagnostic criteria to categorise psychiatric and behavioural abnormalities among people with learning disabilities: The West Midlands field trial. *Ment Handicap Res.* 1994 Dec 1;7(4):273–85.
9. Shimizu M, Kubota Y, Toichi M, Baba H. Folie à deux and shared psychotic disorder. *Curr Psychiatry Rep.* 2007;9(3):200–205.
10. Dosen A., Day K. (2001) Epidemiology, aetiology and presentation of mental illness and behaviour disorders in persons with intellectual disabilities. In: *Treating Mental Illness and Behavior Disorders in Children and Adults with Intellectual Disabilities* (eds A. Dosen & K. Day), pp. 3–24. American Association Books, London.
11. Fletcher R, Loschen E, Stavrakaki C, First M (eds.). (2007). *Diagnostic Manual—Intellectual Disability (DM-ID): A Textbook of Diagnosis of Mental Disorders in Persons with Intellectual Disability.* Kingston, NY: NADD Press.
12. Psychiatrists RC of. DC-LD: *Diagnostic Criteria for Psychiatric Disorders for Use with Adults with Learning Disabilities/Mental Retardation.* 1 edition. London: *RCPsych Publications*; 2001. 144 pp.
13. Cooper S-A, Smiley E, Morrison J, Allan L, Williamson A, Finlayson J, et al. Psychosis and adults with intellectual disabilities. Prevalence, incidence, and related factors. *Soc Psychiatry Psychiatr Epidemiol.* 2007 Jul;42(7):530–536.
14. Bouras N, Drummond C. Behaviour and psychiatric disorders of people with mental handicaps living in the community. *J Intellect Disabil Res JIDR.* 1992 Aug;36 (Pt 4):349–357.
15. Aman H, Naeem F, Farooq S, Ayub M. Prevalence of nonaffective psychosis in intellectually disabled clients: systematic review and meta-analysis. *Psychiatr Genet.* 2016 Aug;26(4):145–155.
16. Bhaumik S, Tyrer FC, McGrother C, Ganghadaran SK. Psychiatric service use and psychiatric disorders in adults with intellectual disability. *J Intellect Disabil Res.* 2008 Nov 1;52(11):986–995.
17. Hassiotis A, Gazizova D, Akinlonu L, Bebbington P, Meltzer H, Strydom A. Psychiatric morbidity in prisoners with intellectual disabilities: Analysis of prison survey data for England and Wales. *Br J Psychiatry J Ment Sci.* 2011 Aug;199(2):156–157.
18. van Os J, Rutten BP, Poulton R. Gene-environment interactions in schizophrenia: Review of epidemiological findings and future directions. *Schizophr Bull.* 2008 Aug 20;34(6):1066–1082.
19. Cowen P, Harrison PJ, Burns T. Shorter Oxford textbook of psychiatry. 2012.
20. Gunnell D, Harrison G, Rasmussen F, Fouskakis D, Tynelius P. Associations between premorbid intellectual performance, early-life exposures and early-onset schizophrenia. Cohort study. *Br J Psychiatry J Ment Sci.* 2002 Oct;181:298–305.
21. David AS, Malmberg A, Brandt L, Allebeck P, Lewis G. IQ and risk for schizophrenia: A population-based cohort study. *Psychol Med.* 1997 Nov;27(6):1311–1323.
22. Doody GA, Johnstone EC, Sanderson TL, Owens DG, Muir WJ. 'Pfropfschizophrenie' revisited. Schizophrenia in people with mild learning disability. *Br J Psychiatry J Ment Sci.* 1998 Aug;173:145–153.
23. Kendler KS. A joint history of the nature of genetic variation and the nature of schizophrenia. *Mol Psychiatry.* 2015 Feb;20(1):77–83.
24. Bertelli MO, Piva Merli M, Bradley E, Keller R, Varrucciu N, Del Furia C, et al. The diagnostic boundary between autism spectrum disorder, intellectual developmental disorder and schizophrenia spectrum disorders. Marco O. Bertelli D, editor. *Adv Ment Health Intellect Disabil.* 2015 Sep 7;9(5):243–264.
25. Matson JL, Shoemaker M. Intellectual disability and its relationship to autism spectrum disorders. *Res Dev Disabil.* 2009 Dec;30(6):1107–1114.
26. Solomon M, Olsen E, Niendam T, Ragland JD, Yoon J, Minzenberg M, et al. From lumping to splitting and back again: atypical social and language development in individuals with clinical-high-risk for psychosis, first episode schizophrenia, and autism spectrum disorders. *Schizophr Res.* 2011 Sep;131(1–3):146–151.
27. Rapoport J, Chavez A, Greenstein D, Addington A, Gogtay N. Autism spectrum disorders and childhood-onset schizophrenia: Clinical and biological contributions to a relation

revisited. *J Am Acad Child Adolesc Psychiatry*. 2009 Jan;48(1): 10–18.
28. Shorter E, Wachtel LE. Childhood catatonia, autism and psychosis past and present: is there an 'iron triangle'? *Acta Psychiatr Scand*. 2013 Jul;128(1):21–33.
29. Sullivan PF, Kendler KS, Neale MC. Schizophrenia as a complex trait: Evidence from a meta-analysis of twin studies. *Arch Gen Psychiatry*. 2003 Dec;60(12):1187–1192.
30. Levinson DF, Duan J, Oh S, Wang K, Sanders AR, Shi J, et al. Copy number variants in schizophrenia: Confirmation of five previous findings and new evidence for 3q29 microdeletions and VIPR2 duplications. *Am J Psychiatry*. 2011 Mar;168(3):302–316.
31. Gejman PV, Sanders AR, Duan J. The role of genetics in the etiology of schizophrenia. *Psychiatr Clin North Am*. 2010 Mar;33(1):35–66.
32. Ng MYM, Levinson DF, Faraone SV, Suarez BK, DeLisi LE, Arinami T, et al. Meta-analysis of 32 genome-wide linkage studies of schizophrenia. *Mol Psychiatry*. 2009 Aug;14(8):774–785.
33. Harrison PJ, Weinberger DR. Schizophrenia genes, gene expression, and neuropathology: On the matter of their convergence. *Mol Psychiatry*. 2005 Jan;10(1):40–68; image 5.
34. Horowitz A, Shifman S, Rivlin N, Pisanté A, Darvasi A. A survey of the 22q11 microdeletion in a large cohort of schizophrenia patients. *Schizophr Res*. 2005 Mar 1;73(2–3):263–267.
35. Murphy KC. Schizophrenia and velo-cardio-facial syndrome. *Lancet Lond Engl*. 2002 Feb 2;359(9304):426–430.
36. Shprintzen RJ. Velo-cardio-facial syndrome: 30 years of study. *Dev Disabil Res Rev*. 2008;14(1):3–10.
37. Stoll G, Pietiläinen OPH, Linder B, Suvisaari J, Brosi C, Hennah W, et al. Deletion of TOP3β, a component of FMRP-containing mRNPs, contributes to neurodevelopmental disorders. *Nat Neurosci*. 2013 Aug 4;16(9):1228–1237.
38. Cederlöf M, Ohlsson GA, Larsson H, Serlachius E, Boman M, Långström N, et al. Klinefelter syndrome and risk of psychosis, autism and ADHD. *J Psychiatr Res*. 2014 Jan;48(1):128–130.
39. Boer H, Holland A, Whittington J, Butler J, Webb T, Clarke D. Psychotic illness in people with Prader Willi syndrome due to chromosome 15 maternal uniparental disomy. *Lancet Lond Engl*. 2002 Jan 12;359(9301):135–136.
40. Sinnema M, Einfeld SL, Schrander-Stumpel CTRM, Maaskant MA, Boer H, Curfs LMG. Behavioral phenotype in adults with Prader-Willi syndrome. *Res Dev Disabil*. 2011 Apr;32(2):604–612.
41. Bozkurt Zincir S, Kıvılcım Y, İzci F, Semiz UB. Schizophrenia-like psychosis and Dandy-Walker variant comorbidity: Case report. *Psychiatry Investig*. 2014;11(1):102.
42. Ryan M, Grenier E, Castro A, Nemeroff CB. New-onset psychosis associated with Dandy-Walker variant in an adolescent female patient. *J Neuropsychiatry Clin Neurosci*. 2012;24(2):241–246.
43. Maubert A, Hanon C, Metton JP. [Niemann-Pick type C disease and psychosis: Two siblings]. *L'Encephale*. 2015 Jun;41(3):238–243.
44. Domanico D, Fragiotta S, Trabucco P, Nebbioso M, Vingolo EM. Genetic analysis for two Italian siblings with Usher syndrome and schizophrenia. *Case Rep Ophthalmol Med*. 2012;2012:1–6.
45. Salgado H, Martins-Correia L. Williams syndrome and psychosis: A case report. *J Med Case Reports*. 2014 Feb 12;8:49.
46. Mignarri A, Tessa A, Carluccio MA, Rufa A, Storti E, Bonelli G, et al. Cerebellum and neuropsychiatric disorders: insights from ARSACS. *Neurol Sci Off J Ital Neurol Soc Ital Soc Clin Neurophysiol*. 2014 Jan;35(1):95–97.
47. Dykens EM, Shah B, Davis B, Baker C, Fife T, Fitzpatrick J. Psychiatric disorders in adolescents and young adults with Down syndrome and other intellectual disabilities. *J Neurodev Disord*. 2015;7(1):9.
48. Boos HBM, Aleman A, Cahn W, Hulshoff Pol H, Kahn RS. Brain volumes in relatives of patients with schizophrenia: A meta-analysis. Arch Gen *Psychiatry*. 2007 Mar;64(3):297–304.
49. Sanderson T, Best J, Doody G, Owens DC, Johnstone E. Neuroanatomy of comorbid schizophrenia and learning disability: A controlled study. *The Lancet*. 1999 Nov;354(9193):1867–1871.
50. PowerPoint presentation—neurobio_class_11.pdf [Internet]. [cited 2016 Nov 5]. Available from: http://www.hopkinsmedicine.org/gynecology_obstetrics/pdfs/medstudent/neurobio_class_11.pdf.
51. Verpelli C, Montani C, Vicidomini C, Heise C, Sala C. Mutations of the synapse genes and intellectual disability syndromes. *Eur J Pharmacol*. 2013 Nov;719(1–3):112–116.
52. Emanuele E. Does reverse transport of dopamine play a role in autism? *EBioMedicine*. 2015 Feb;2(2):98–99.
53. Bramon E, Rabe-Hesketh S, Sham P, Murray RM, Frangou S. Meta-analysis of the P300 and P50 waveforms in schizophrenia. *Schizophr Res*. 2004 Oct 1;70(2–3):315–329.
54. Hill K, Mann L, Laws KR, Stephenson CME, Nimmo-Smith I, McKenna PJ. Hypofrontality in schizophrenia: a meta-analysis of functional imaging studies. *Acta Psychiatr Scand*. 2004 Oct;110(4):243–256.
55. McNeil TF, Cantor-Graae E, Weinberger DR. Relationship of obstetric complications and differences in size of brain structures in monozygotic twin pairs discordant for schizophrenia. *Am J Psychiatry*. 2000 Feb;157(2):203–212.
56. Brown AS, Susser ES. Prenatal nutritional deficiency and risk of adult schizophrenia. *Schizophr Bull*. 2008 Nov;34(6):1054–1063.
57. Brown AS, Begg MD, Gravenstein S, Schaefer CA, Wyatt RJ, Bresnahan M, et al. Serologic evidence of prenatal influenza in the etiology of schizophrenia. *Arch Gen Psychiatry*. 2004 Aug;61(8):774–780.
58. Sussmann JE, McIntosh AM, Lawrie SM, Johnstone EC. Obstetric complications and mild to moderate intellectual disability. *Br J Psychiatry*. 2009 Mar 1;194(3):224–228.
59. Carmeli E, Imam B, Bachar A, Merrick J. Inflammation and oxidative stress as biomarkers of premature aging in persons with intellectual disability. *Res Dev Disabil*. 2012 Apr;33(2): 369–375.
60. Moore THM, Zammit S, Lingford-Hughes A, Barnes TRE, Jones PB, Burke M, et al. Cannabis use and risk of psychotic or affective mental health outcomes: A systematic review. *Lancet Lond Engl*. 2007 Jul 28;370(9584):319–328.
61. Fearon P, Kirkbride JB, Morgan C, Dazzan P, Morgan K, Lloyd T, et al. Incidence of schizophrenia and other psychoses in ethnic minority groups: results from the MRC AESOP Study. *Psychol Med*. 2006 Nov;36(11):1541–1550.
62. Schulz J, Sundin J, Leask S, Done DJ. Risk of adult schizophrenia and its relationship to childhood IQ in the 1958 British birth cohort. *Schizophr Bull*. 2012 Dec 30;sbs157.
63. Hulbert-Williams L, Hastings R, Owen DM, Burns L, Day J, Mulligan J, et al. Exposure to life events as a risk factor for psychological problems in adults with intellectual disabilities—a longitudinal design: Life events and psychological problems. *J Intellect Disabil Res*. 2014 Jan;58(1):48–60.
64. Ali A, King M, Strydom A, Hassiotis A. Self-reported stigma and its association with socio-demographic factors and physical disability in people with intellectual disabilities: results from a cross-sectional study in England. *Soc Psychiatry Psychiatr Epidemiol*. 2016 Mar;51(3):465–474.

65. Philip N, Bassett A. Cognitive, behavioural and psychiatric phenotype in 22q11.2 deletion syndrome. *Behav Genet.* 2011 May;41(3):403–412.
66. Pickard M, Paschos D. Pseudohallucinations in people with intellectual disabilities: Two case reports. *ResearchGate.* 2005 Jul 1;8(3):91–93.
67. Heaton-Ward A. Psychosis in mental handicap. The tenth Blake Marsh lecture delivered before the Royal College of Psychiatrists, 2 February 2 1976. *Br J Psychiatry.* 1977 Jun 1;130(6):525–533.
68. Meadows G, Turner T, Campbell L, Lewis SW, Reveley MA, Murray RM. Assessing schizophrenia in adults with mental retardation. A comparative study. *Br J Psychiatry J Ment Sci.* 1991 Jan;158:103–105.
69. Bouras N, Martin G, Leese M, Vanstraelen M, Holt G, Thomas C, et al. Schizophrenia-spectrum psychoses in people with and without intellectual disability. *J Intellect Disabil Res JIDR.* 2004 Sep;48(Pt 6):548–555.
70. Moss S, Prosser H, Goldberg D. Validity of the schizophrenia diagnosis of the psychiatric assessment schedule for adults with developmental disability (PAS-ADD). *Br J Psychiatry J Ment Sci.* 1996 Mar;168(3):359–367.
71. Eaton LF, Menolascino FJ. Psychiatric disorders in the mentally retarded: Types, problems, and challenges. *Am J Psychiatry.* 1982 Oct;139(10):1297–1303.
72. Welch KA, Lawrie SM, Muir M, Johnstone E. Systematic review of the clinical presentation of schizophrenia in intellectual disability. *Journal of Psychopathology and Behavioral Assessment,* 2011, 33, 246–253.
73. Hatton C, Haddock G, Taylor JL, Coldwell J, Crossley R, Peckham N. The reliability and validity of general psychotic rating scales with people with mild and moderate intellectual disabilities: An empirical investigation. *J Intellect Disabil Res JIDR.* 2005;49, 490–500.
74 Mental health problems in people with learning disabilities: Prevention, assessment and management | Guidance and guidelines | NICE [Internet]. [cited 2016 Nov 1]. Available from: https://www.nice.org.uk/guidance/ng54.
75. Watson JE, Aman MG, Singh NN. The psychopathology instrument for mentally retarded adults: Psychometric characteristics, factor structure, and relationship to subject characteristics. *Res Dev Disabil.* 1988 Jan 1;9(3):277–90.
76. Bamburg JW, Cherry KE, Matson JL, Penn D. Assessment of schizophrenia in persons with severe and profound mental retardation using the diagnostic sssessment for the severely handicapped-II (DASH-II). *J Dev Phys Disabil.* 13(4):319–331.
77. Differential diagnosis of psychotic symptoms: Medical 'mimics' | *Psychiatric Times* [Internet]. 2012 [cited 2016 Nov 1]. Available from: http://www.psychiatrictimes.com/forensic-psychiatry/differential-diagnosis-psychotic-symptoms-medical-%E2%80%9Cmimics%E2%80%9D.
78. Ring H, Zia A, Lindeman S, Himlok K. Interactions between seizure frequency, psychopathology, and severity of intellectual disability in a population with epilepsy and a learning disability. *Epilepsy Behav EB.* 2007 Aug;11(1):92–97.
79. Larson FV, Wagner AP, Jones PB, Tantam D,Lai M-C, Baron-Cohen S, Holland AJ (2017). Psychosis in autism: Comparison of the features of both conditions in a dually affected cohort. *BJP* 2017 Apr;210(4):269–275.
80. Mental Health Act 1983. http://www.legislation.gov.uk/ukpga/1983/20/contents
81. Wiley: The Frith prescribing guidelines for people with intellectual disability, 3rd Edition—Sabyasachi Bhaumik, Satheesh Kumar Gangadharan, David Branford, et al [Internet]. [cited 2016 Nov 1]. Available from: http://www.wiley.com/WileyCDA/WileyTitle/productCd-111889720X.html.
82. Connor DF, Posever TA. A brief review of atypical antipsychotics in individuals with developmental disability. *Ment Health Asp Dev Disabil.* 1998;1:93–101.
83. Cohen S, Khan A, Zheng Y, Chiles J. Tardive dyskinesia in the mentally retarded: Comparison of prevalence, risk factors and topography with a schizophrenic population. *Acta Psychiatr Scand.* 1991 Mar;83(3):234–237.
84. Boyd RD. Recurrence of neuroleptic malignant syndrome via an inadvertent rechallenge in a woman with mental retardation. *ResearchGate.* 1992 May 1;30(2):77–79.
85. Fodstad JC, Bamburg JW, Matson JL, Mahan S, Hess JA, Neal D, et al. Tardive dyskinesia and intellectual disability: An examination of demographics and topography in adults with dual diagnosis and atypical antipsychotic use. *Res Dev Disabil.* 2010 May;31(3):750–759.
86. Newcomer JW. Metabolic considerations in the use of antipsychotic medications: a review of recent evidence. *J Clin Psychiatry.* 2007;68 Suppl 1:20–27.
87. Matson JL, Mahan S. Antipsychotic drug side effects for persons with intellectual disability. *Res Dev Disabil.* 2010 Dec;31(6):1570–1576.
88. Matson JL, Mayville EA, Bielecki J, Barnes WH, Bamburg JW, Baglio CS. Reliability of the Matson evaluation of drug side effects scale (MEDS). *Res Dev Disabil.* 1998;19(6):501–506.
89. Kane JM. Clinical efficacy of clozapine in treatment-refractory schizophrenia: An overview. *Br J Psychiatry Suppl.* 1992 May;(17):41–45.
90. Thalayasingam S, Alexander RT, Singh I. The use of clozapine in adults with intellectual disability. *J Intellect Disabil Res JIDR.* 2004 Sep;48(Pt 6):572–579.
91. Tharyan P, Adams CE. Electroconvulsive therapy for schizophrenia. *Cochrane Database Syst Rev.* 2002;(2):CD000076.
92. Chanpattana W. Maintenance ECT in mentally retarded, treatment-resistant schizophrenic patients. *J ECT.* 1999 Jun;15(2):150–153.
93. Devapriam J, Anand A, Raju LB, Bhaumik S. Monitoring for metabolic syndrome in adults with intellectual disability on atypical antipsychotic drugs. *Br J Dev Disabil.* 2009 Jan;55(108):3–13.
94. Teeluckdharry S, Sharma S, O'Rourke E, Tharian P, Gondalekar A, Nainar F, et al. Monitoring metabolic side effects of atypical antipsychotics in people with an intellectual disability. *J Intellect Disabil JOID.* 2013 Sep;17(3):223–235.
95. British Psychological Association. Psychological_therapies_and_people_who_have_id_pdf_for_review.pdf [Internet]. [cited 2016 Nov 1]. Available from: http://www.bps.org.uk/system/files/Public per cent20files/Policy/psychological_therapies_and_people_who_have_id_pdf_for_review.pdf.
96. Haddock G, Lobban F, Hatton C, Carson R. Cognitive–behaviour therapy for people with psychosis and mild intellectual disabilities: A case series. *Clin Psychol Psychother.* 2004 Jul;11(4): 282–298.
97. Crowley V, Rose J, Smith J, Hobster K, Ansell E. Psycho-educational groups for people with a dual diagnosis of psychosis and mild intellectual disability: a preliminary study. *J Intellect Disabil JOID.* 2008 Mar;12(1):25–39.

98. Hatton C. Psychosocial interventions for adults with intellectual disabilities and mental health problems: A review. *J Ment Health*. 2002 Jan;11(4):357–374.
99. Valuing people—A new strategy for learning disability for the 21st century—Publications—GOV.UK [Internet]. [cited 2016 Oct 31]. Available from: https://www.gov.uk/government/publications/valuing-people-a-new-strategy-for-learning-disability-for-the-21st-century.
100. Spiller MJ, Costello H, Bramley A, Bouras N, Martin G, Tsakanikos E, et al. Consumption of mental health services by people with intellectual disabilities. *J Appl Res Intellect Disabil*. 2007 Sep;20(5):430–438.
101. Balogh R, Brownell M, Ouellette-Kuntz H, Colantonio A. Hospitalisation rates for ambulatory care sensitive conditions for persons with and without an intellectual disability—a population perspective. *J Intellect Disabil Res JIDR*. 2010 Sep; 54(9):820–832.
102. Lai C-I, Hung W-J, Lin L-P, Chien W-C, Lin J-D. A retrospective population-based data analyses of inpatient care use and medical expenditure in people with intellectual disability co-occurring schizophrenia. *Res Dev Disabil*. 2011 Jun;32(3):1226–1231.
103. Balogh R, Ouellette-Kuntz H, Bourne L, Lunsky Y, Colantonio A. Organising health care services for persons with an intellectual disability. *Cochrane Database Syst Rev*. 2008 Oct 8;(4):CD007492.
104. Hemmings CP. Community services for people with intellectual disabilities and mental health problems: *Curr Opin Psychiatry*. 2008 Sep;21(5):459–462.
105. Chaplin E, O'Hara J, Holt G, Bouras N. Mental health services for people with intellectual disability: Challenges to care delivery. *Br J Learn Disabil*. 2009 Jun 1;37(2):157–164.
106. Raitasuo S, Taiminen T, Salokangas RK. Inpatient care and its outcome in a specialist psychiatric unit for people with intellectual disability: A prospective study. *J Intellect Disabil Res JIDR*. 1999 Apr;43 (Pt 2):119–1227.
107. Friedlander RI, Donnelly T. Early-onset psychosis in youth with intellectual disability. *J Intellect Disabil Res JIDR*. 2004 Sep;48(Pt 6):540–547.
108. Morgan VA, Leonard H, Bourke J, Jablensky A. Intellectual disability co-occurring with schizophrenia and other psychiatric illness: Population-based study. *Br J Psychiatry J Ment Sci*. 2008 Nov;193(5):364–372.
109. WHO | Mental health action plan 2013–2020 [Internet]. WHO. [cited 2016 Nov 5]. Available from: http://www.who.int/entity/mental_health/publications/action_plan/en/index.html.
110. WHO | WHO Mental Health Gap Action Programme (mhGAP) [Internet]. WHO. [cited 2016 Nov 5]. Available from: http://www.who.int/mental_health/mhgap/en/.

11

Depressive Disorders in People with Intellectual Disability

Samuel Tromans, Atiq Umar, Jennifer Torr, Regi Alexander, and Sabyasachi Bhaumik†

Introduction

Depressive disorders encompass a spectrum of low mood, loss of interest in and/or enjoyment of daily life, associated with cognitive, somatic, and psychomotor symptoms. Severity ranges from 'subthreshold' depression, dysthymia, to severe depression with self-neglect, psychotic symptoms, catatonia, and/or suicide risk (1). Depressive disorders are common in people with intellectual disability (ID), causing individual suffering, additional impairments in adaptive behaviour and functioning, disruption of interpersonal relationships, social exclusion, poor physical health outcomes and sometimes death. Improvements in detection, diagnosis, and treatment of depression have the potential to improve the well-being and quality of life of people with ID, as well as reducing carer stress (2).

Epidemiology

Prevalence

The reported prevalence of depression in people with ID varies considerably (3–5), depending upon the characteristics of the study sample, method of case ascertainment—using one of the many rating scales or by semi-structured clinical assessment (6), and the diagnostic criteria used (5). The point prevalence of affective disorder in a large population study (5) (n = 1023), was 6.6 per cent based upon expert clinical assessment, compared with 5.7 per cent, 4.8 per cent, 3.6 per cent for diagnoses made according to DC-LD (7), ICD-10 DCR (8) and DSM-IV-TR (9) criteria respectively, and is similar to the point prevalence of depression of ~5 per cent in the general population (10). Similarly, the prevalence of depression in population studies of older adults with ID is ~5-7 per cent, but subthreshold symptoms occur in ~15 per cent (3,11). In a major study of young people, the point prevalence of depression in children and adolescents with ID (n = 641) was 1.4 per cent, compared with 0.9 per cent in those who did not have ID (n = 17,774) (12). However, other studies have found the prevalence of depression is significantly higher in people with ID, up to four-fold in adults with ID (13). The consensus is that depressive disorder is at least as common in people with ID, and is likely to be more prevalent.

† It is with great regret that we report the death of Sabyasachi Bhaumik during the production of this textbook.

Correlates and risk factors for depression

Depression is the outcome of complex interactions between multiple biopsychosocial factors.

Many factors associated with depression have been identified, but the aetiological significance, if any, and pathophysiological mechanisms are yet to be determined.

Biological

Physical characteristics and comorbid conditions

People with ID have very high rates of comorbid conditions which may increase the risk for, modify the presentation of, and complicate the treatment of depression. Depression in adults with ID is associated with the number of prior primary care appointments (3), which might be a proxy measure for comorbidity, as well as female gender, and increasing age, but not with severity of ID, obesity, or sensory impairments (3, 5, 14, 15). Smoking is associated with higher point prevalence of depression (5), and there is a link between substance misuse and anxiety and depressive symptoms, especially in those with mild to borderline ID, who also have other personality, emotional, and behavioural problems (16, 17).

Depression in older adults with mild to borderline in ID is associated with anxiety, heart failure, stroke, chronic obstructive pulmonary disease, coronary artery disease, diabetes mellitus, and those with depression have lower scores on activities of daily living. Depressive symptoms are very common in dementia, especially in the early stages (3, 11, 18).

Genetics

A review of the genetics of psychiatric disorders concluded the heritability of major depressive disorder and bipolar disorder to be 0.37 and 0.75 respectively (1). The genetic disorders of ID are often associated with other neurodevelopment disorders such as autism spectrum disorder (ASD), epilepsy, and mood and psychotic disorders.

Box 11.1 DC-LD criteria for diagnosis of a depressive episode

A The symptoms/signs must be present nearly every day for at least two weeks
B They must not be a direct consequence of drugs or other physical disorders
C The criteria for mixed affective episode of schizoaffective episode are not met
D The symptoms/signs must represent a change from the individual's premorbid state
E Item a or b must be present and prominent
 a Depressed mood
  Or Irritable mood
 b Loss of interest of pleasure in activities
  Or Social withdrawal
  Or Reduction in self-care
  Or Reduction in the quantity of speech/communication
F Some of the following symptoms must be present, so that at least four symptoms from E and F are present in total:
 a Loss of energy/ increased lethargy
 b Loss of confidence
  Or Increase in reassurance-seeking behaviour
  Or Increase in anxiety or fearfulness
 c Increased tearfulness
 d Onset of or increase in somatic symptoms/physical health concerns
 e Reduced ability to concentrate/ distractibility
  Or Increased indecisiveness
 f Increase in a specific problem behaviour
 g Increased motor agitation
  Or Increased motor retardation
 h Onset of or increase in appetite disturbance
  Or Significant weight change
 i Onset of or increase in sleep disturbance

People with ID and co-existing ASD have higher rates of depression than those without ASD (19, 20). A meta-analysis of epilepsy in people with ID yielded an overall prevalence of ~20 per cent, increasing from ~7 per cent for less severe to ~40 per cent for more severe ID (21) and there is a link between epilepsy and symptoms of low mood (22). A prospective case control study found that adults with ID and epilepsy had significantly higher incidence of psychiatric disorder, including depression, than those without epilepsy (15).

Specific genetic syndromes confer an increased risk for depression, as illustrated by the following examples. People with Down syndrome (DS) have lower overall rates of mental ill-health but the prevalence of depression ranges from 5–13 per cent (1). This relative risk for depression is postulated to be due to deficits in monoamine neurotransmission, especially noradrenaline and serotonin (23–26), which increase with age and the development of the neuropathology of Alzheimer's disease (27). The prevalence of depression is twice as common in adults with DS, who have early onset dementia Alzheimer's disease (38 per cent vs. 18 per cent), being much more common in mid-stage than late stage dementia (48% vs. 18%) (28). The prevalence of depression is around 20 per cent in people with Prader-Willi syndrome and this is more common in those with uniparental disomy. These individuals also have a very high risk of bipolar and psychotic disorders (29–32). The prevalence of depression in adolescents with 22q.11 deletion syndrome peaks at 40 per cent, preceding the onset of psychosis in young adults (33, 34).

Psychosocial correlates and risk factors

Depression in people with ID is associated with adverse social circumstances, disruptive life events (5, 35), low levels of social support, social exclusion, perceived stigma, bullying (36, 37), poor social and coping skills (38, 39), and high levels of interpersonal difficulties and social strain (40). Cognitive factors such as hopelessness, low self-esteem, reassurance seeking, negative self-appraisal, downward social comparison, and automatic negative thoughts are highly correlated with depression (36, 41–43). The number of negative life events, quality, and frequency of social support, self-esteem and automatic negative thoughts are predictive of depression in people with mild/moderate ID, accounting for 58 per cent of the variance (36, 44–46). But negative self-appraisal, poor self-esteem, and hopelessness are not predictive of the future development of depression (46) and there is no interaction between experiencing life stressors and negative attributional style or hopelessness (45), suggesting that cognitive variables are symptoms of, more so, than causes of depression. While depression is correlated with negative self-appraisal, this is not so for negative appraisals of the world or the future, which are common in people ID who are not depressed and reflect adverse life circumstances, rather than being cognitive distortions to be corrected (46, 47). People with ID do experience more adverse social circumstances, including higher rates of physical, sexual, and emotional abuse (48, 49), hate crimes (50), social exclusion and less social support, including both formal and informal social networks, loss of significant relationships due to circumstances beyond their control, and few employment opportunities and financial insecurity, as well as financial and emotional support (51, 52). Supportive person-focused environments are essential for physical and mental well-being (52–54) but in reality people with ID have limited real control over their life circumstances and the environments in which they live (2).

Assessment and diagnosis

Expert psychiatric assessment remains the gold standard diagnosing depression in people with ID and has good inter-rater reliability (55). Using standard diagnostic criteria results in the under-diagnosis of depression in people with ID, less so in people with mild ID (56–59). The Diagnostic Criteria for Psychiatric Disorders for Use With Adults With Learning Disabilities/Mental Retardation (DC-LD) (7) (see Box 11.1) and Diagnostic Manual: Intellectual Disability (DM-ID) (60) have modified diagnostic criteria informed by the evidence base and expert consensus, to account for differences in presentation due to cognitive, communication, and functional impairments. Using DC-LD increases the diagnostic yield (5, 57). DM-ID criteria for depression are not been modified, although the number of required associated symptoms has been reduced, and is less effective in detecting depression (61). However, the manual provides detailed guidance on the interpretation and application of standard diagnostic criteria for people with ID.

Sadness, crying, tearfulness and sobbing, self-criticism, reassurance seeking, social withdrawal, decreased communication, loss of energy and tiredness, self-neglect, self-injury, screaming, irritability, verbal abuse, temper tantrums, and aggressive behaviour are observed in depressive disorder in people with ID (36, 62–65)—but which of these symptoms are core features versus associated features of depression? Factor analysis of a carer completed depression checklist of observable aspects of core and associated phenomena of depression identified a depression factor with high loadings for depressed mood, loss of interest and loss of enjoyment, and social interaction and communication. Anxiety, irritability, and aggressive behaviours did not load onto the depression factor but onto a second factor (66). In another study of observed symptoms, depression was characterized by depressed affect, as well as sleep disturbance, and other features were stratified according to the level of ID. Symptoms in mild ID included tearfulness, diurnal mood variation, loss of energy, loss of interest, loss of confidence, and weight loss. Social isolation, self-injurious behaviour, reduced communication, and weight loss characterized depression in moderate ID. Depression in people with severe-profound ID can present with screaming, aggression, self-injurious behaviour, and reduced communication (see Table 11.1) (67). Low mood in adults with severe-profound ID is associated with more frequent and severe challenging behaviour, compared with those who are euthymic, even when confounders such as ASD, health, and sensory impairments were controlled for (68). Aggression and challenging behaviours are frequent presenting symptoms in depression (69, 70), though subside with treatment (63, 64), allowing for the weaning of antipsychotics (71). However, aggression is more likely to occur in mania, psychosis, and anxiety.

Table 11.1 Depressive symptoms typically found in patients with different levels of ID

Level of ID	Symptoms
Mild	• Depressed affect • Anhedonia • Withdrawal • Agitation • Sleep disturbance • Tearfulness • Diurnal mood variation • Loss of energy • Loss of interest • Loss of confidence • Weight loss
Moderate	• Depressed affect • Anhedonia • Withdrawal • Agitation • Sleep disturbance • Social isolation • Self-injurious behaviour • Reduced communication • Weight loss
Severe/profound	• Depressed affect • Anhedonia • Withdrawal • Agitation • Sleep disturbance • Screaming • Self-injurious behaviour • Reduced communication

Adapted from *Journal of Intellectual Disability Research*, 4(1), 6, Marston G, Perry D, Roy A, Manifestations of depression in people with intellectual disability, pp. 476–480. Copyright (1997) John Wiley & Sons Ltd. DOI: https://doi.org/10.1111/j.1365-2788.1997.tb00739.x.

Aggression and other challenging behaviours are non-specific associated features of depression and are not 'equivalent' to the core features of depression (59, 66, 72–75).

For comprehensive guidance on conducting a psychiatric interview with a person with ID, please refer to Chapter 2. Clinical diagnosis is based upon history and mental state examination. The symptoms of depression can be determined from talking with the person with ID or from informants and careful clinical observation. People with ID can report or endorse symptoms of depression. When interviewed using the Glasgow Depression Scale (76) patients report or endorse more cognitive and affective symptoms of depression than do their carers (63, 77–79), although carer reports tend to be more consistent (39). Self-report and information rating scales can be used to screen for depression, identify depressive symptoms—especially for inexperienced clinicians—and to monitor response to treatment, but are no substitute for a thorough clinical assessment. Reviews of instruments for the assessment of depression in people with ID (6, 80) are primarily focused on the utility for research rather than on the availability, cost, and ease of use in accommodation and clinical settings. The Glasgow Depression Scale is brief, readily available, has good psychometrics, and self-report and informant versions (76). The mood, pleasure and interest questionnaire elicits observations pertaining to the core features of depression in people with severe and profound ID and has clinical potential when combined with clinical assessment (81). For further details pertaining to use of clinical rating scales in people with ID, please refer to Chapter 5.

Few people with ID are diagnosed and treated for depression by their general practitioner or receive other mental health services (36). Along the pathway to care a person must recognize a problem and present for assessment. Many people with ID are reliant upon others to recognize and or facilitate access to health services. Care staff, who are often responsible for facilitating access to health care, frequently fail to recognize sadness and other behaviours associated with depressed mood. Clinical care is sought for aggressive and challenging behaviours, while sadness and tearfulness are often overlooked (63, 77–79). When people with ID and depression present to specialist services, many have been prescribed sedating and antipsychotic medications, to contain associated challenging behaviour (69, 71, 82). Enabling caregivers, whether family or paid carers, to screen for and identify symptoms of depression, and defining pathways to care including providing clinical guidance for general practitioners might improve detection, diagnosis, and treatment of depression (36, 66, 83). The depression in adults with intellectual disability checklist, with good concurrent validity with other instruments, is a freely available tool to assist carers in identifying and documenting observed features of depression, with a section on the assessment and management of depression which is given to the person's general practitioner to assist in their clinical assessment (66, 84).

Assessment should encompass the person's circumstances and risk as well as diagnosis and management options. Suicide is not common in people with ID. A population study of people with ID (n = 2369), over 35 years, identified only 10 suicides, and eight unclassified deaths. All but one person had mild ID (85). However, we need to acknowledge that there are some individuals with mild/borderline ID who access generic mental health services may not have been included in such studies. Risk factors for suicide in people with

ID mirror those of the general population including major depression, a history of previous attempts, chronic mental illness, loneliness, bereavement, social exclusion and lack of interpersonal and social supports, and many were not receiving psychiatric care (85, 86). In one study a quarter of people with mild-borderline ID endorsed suicidal ideation with one-third having thought of potentially fatal methods and one-tenth reported suicide attempts of which a quarter of informants were unaware (87). Inpatient care might be required to manage suicide risk, severe self-neglect and poor oral intake, catatonia, or complex medical and medication issues, or if carers are not able to provide the level of support required.

Compounding the challenges of clinical assessment are the complexity of each person's neurodevelopment disorder and disability, comorbid conditions, polypharmacy, and their social circumstances. Physical illness and medication effects can mimic depression, or depression can be mistaken for dementia. Inadequate social support and lack of a good informant can make it difficult to establish baseline functioning, changes from baseline and timelines.

Management

Optimal management of depressive disorders in people with ID requires a biopsychosocial multidisciplinary collaborative approach, based on the best available evidence tailored to the needs and preferences of the individual. The management plan should be made collaboratively with the person and their carers, in liaison with other professionals.

Pharmacotherapy

The current evidence for the effectiveness of antidepressant medications in people with ID includes small prospective open-label studies (71), case series, and retrospective file reviews of all specified treatment episodes in specialist ID psychiatric services that provide an overview of naturalistic practice treatment in the context of polypharmacy and high rates of comorbid conditions, including epilepsy and cardiac conditions (82, 88–92). In the absence of population specific randomized controlled trials (RCT) the National Institute of Health and Care Excellence (NICE) recommends evidence-based treatments for the general adult population be used for people with ID (83). Selective serotonin reuptake inhibitors (SSRIs) are recommended as first line treatment, and appear to have similar efficacy to the general population and are better tolerated than the tricyclic/tetracyclic antidepressants they have superseded (71, 82, 88–92). Figure 11.1 provides an algorithm for the treatment for depression in people with ID. People with ID have high rates of comorbid physical and psychiatric comorbidity and the Frith prescribing guidelines have published recommended antidepressants of choice for specific patient groups (92) (Table 11.2).

Although treatment of depression in people with ID with antidepressants is generally effective and safe, there are significant levels of adverse effects including seizures, sedation, weight gain, cardiac, anticholinergic, and autonomic side effects, hyponatraemia, serotonin syndrome, delirium, and discontinuation syndromes (71, 82, 88–92). The risk for seizures is higher with tricyclic antidepressants (TCAs), compared to SSRIs and monoamine oxidase inhibitors (MAOIs) (92). Prescribing the lowest effective dose of antidepressant and careful monitoring of treatment effects is recommended (83).

People with ID have very high rates or polypharmacy. Central nervous system prescriptions include anticonvulsants (around 30%) and antipsychotics (30–50%), often in combination (69, 71, 82, 90). Drug-drug interactions need to be considered. For example, paroxetine, fluvoxamine and fluoxetine, and less so sertraline, inhibit cytochrome P450 enzymes involved in the metabolism of medications, including anticonvulsant and antipsychotic medications, and environmental toxins. The addition of paroxetine, fluvoxamine, or fluoxetine can cause clinically significant, sometimes dangerous, increases in the serum levels of some antipsychotic medications, causing sedation, akathisia, extrapyramidal side effects which could be attributed to the antidepressants (93). Many antidepressants and antipsychotic medications can increase the QTc interval and increase the risk of sudden death. ECG monitoring of the QTc interval is recommended (89).

The potential for treatment-emergent behavioural effects is significant and evident up to six months after commencing treating, and include agitation, increase in maladaptive behaviours and aggression, and precipitation of hypomania/mania (71, 82, 88–92). Assessment should include enquiry about a family history of bipolar disorder and careful history taking to identify possible prior episodes of mania.

- Note 1: Drug treatment is indicated for patients with moderate to severe depression. The choice of drug depends on the presence of any comorbid psychiatric diagnoses and whether the person falls into any special group (Table 11.2).
- Note 2: There are fewer dietary restrictions with moclobemide that the other MAOIs, but restrictions still apply.
- Note 3: The Maudsley guidelines provide a number of alternative treatments for treatment resistant depression (94).

Electroconvulsive therapy

Electroconvulsive therapy (ECT) is an established treatment for severe depression, mania, psychosis, and catatonia (95). Treatment of severe depression with ECT, when indicated, may be delayed or denied because of diagnostic overshadowing, uncertain diagnosis, limited guidance about efficacy and safety, and consent and legal issues, and multiple trials of medications often precede ECT (96). There are no RCTs or prospective studies of ECT in people with ID. Reviews of collected case reports conclude that ECT is effective (response rates ~80%) and safe in people with ID for the treatment of severe depression, including depression with psychotic or catatonic features. One-third of patients require maintenance treatment. Pharmacotherapy continues post treatment. Side effects occurred in 10–15 per cent, including delirium, transient cognitive impairment, respiratory conditions, seizures, and mania (97–99). Comorbid medical and physical conditions, including alterations in head and neck anatomy, poor dental health, and cardiopulmonary disease are common, hence anaesthetic consultation is recommended before commencing treatment (99).

Psychological

People with ID value warm, validating, empathic, supportive relationships with family, friends, carers, and clinicians, being able to talk about their feelings and problems, and learning how to cope (100, 101). Systematic reviews of small-scale studies of CBT for depression for people with ID, using pre-test, post-test design with non-equivalent

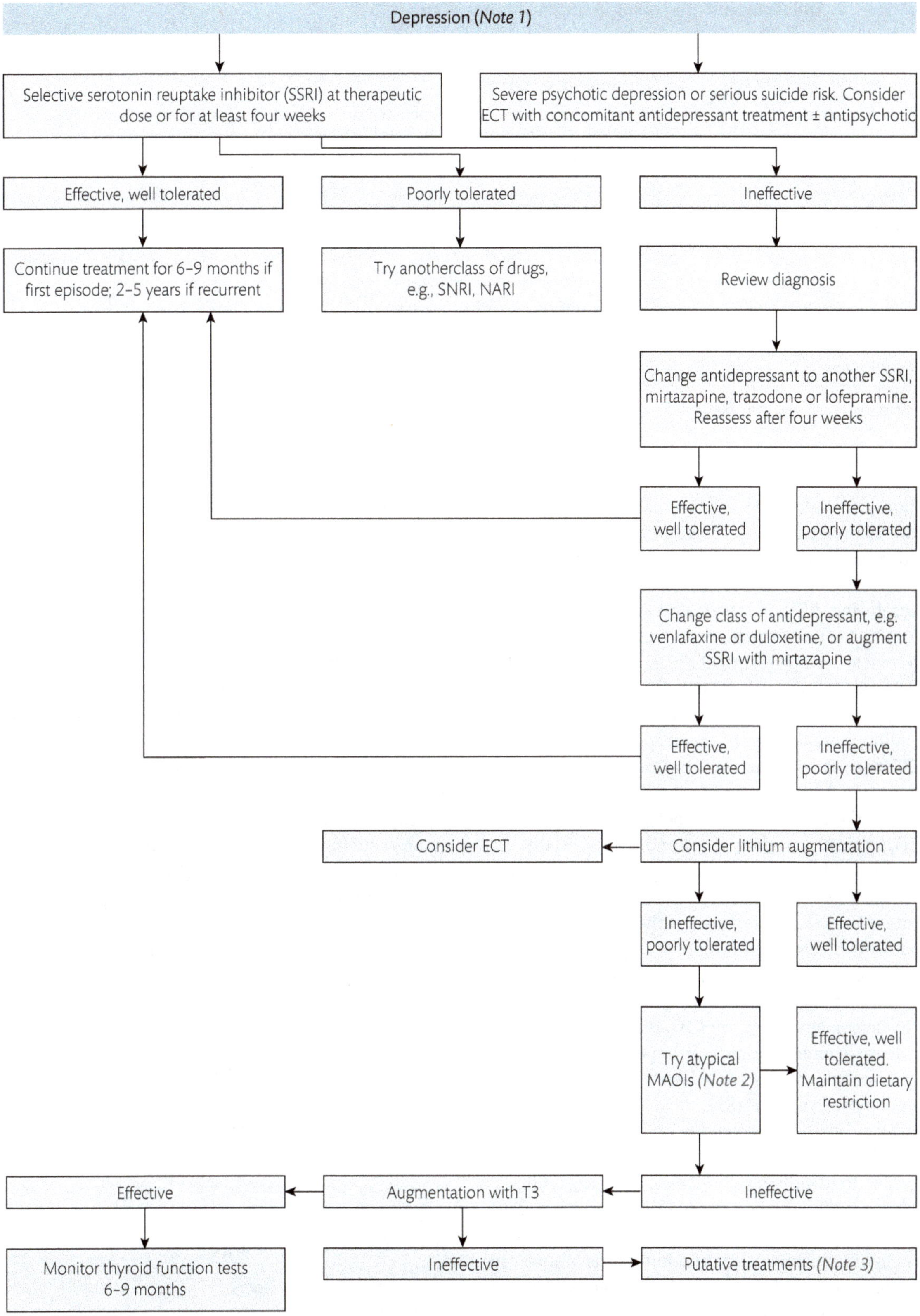

Figure 11.1 Treatment of depression in adults with ID

Reproduced from Hiremath A, Gangavati S, Gumber R, Barrett M. *Depression*. In: Bhaumik S, Gangadharan SK, Branford D, Barrett M (eds). *The Frith Prescribing Guidelines for People with Intellectual Disability*, 3rd edition. Copyright © 2015, John Wiley and Sons.

Table 11.2 Antidepressant prescribing in specific patient groups

Patient group	Recommended antidepressants
Women of childbearing age	SSRIs, especially fluoxetine
Pregnant women	Adequate experience with imipramine and amitriptyline. Also consider SSRIs, especially fluoxetine (risk with fluoxetine is reduced birthweight and preterm birth).
Breastfeeding women	Sertraline, paroxetine, nortriptyline, imipramine
Older persons	SSRIs, especially paroxetine, citalopram, sertraline, and venlafaxine. Avoid TCAs and reboxetine.
Down syndrome	SSRIs
Epilepsy	SSRIs. Consider moclobemide, other MAOIs, reboxetine, tryptophan, agomelatine. Adjust dose of antiepileptic drug if necessary. Avoid TCAs.
Cardiovascular problems	SSRIs. Avoid TCAs, especially dothiepin.
Renal impairment	Sertraline and citalopram. Avoid lithium.
Hepatic impairment	Imipramine, paroxetine, or citalopram.

control conditions, have identified seven studies with high heterogeneity and various methodological shortcomings, concluding that the current evidence is insufficient to confirm effectiveness, although some studies have moderate to large effect sizes (102–111). However, these reviews capturing different sets of studies, include studies of CBT for anger (103, 112), or for anxiety and depression (104, 111), or studies with control conditions with likely therapeutic effects (109, 113). A detailed review of six trials found effect sizes ranging from negligible to large (102). Of the two trials with negligible effect size the control conditions are likely to be therapeutic. One study compared group CBT against behaviour strategies, or cognitive strategies (109). The other study delivered individualized CBT for depression and/or anxiety and the control condition being treatment as usual by specialist ID services providing social and mental health care (111). Four studies of CBT specifically for depression, with waitlist or treatment as usual (with no expected benefit) as control conditions, showed moderate to large effect sizes, with improvement maintained for months following completion of therapy (105, 106, 108, 110). These studies explored innovative modes of delivering group CBT such as including caregivers in therapy sessions or training paid carers to identify depression and deliver CBT. It could be argued that the current evidence demonstrates that CBT specifically for depression is effective for people with ID. NICE has recommended CBT be considered for people with mild ID (83).

There is increasing interest in adaptations to and the components of CBT, such as the assessment of receptive language and ability to participate, training in identifying emotions and linking emotions, thoughts, and behaviours, and the use of Likert-type rating scales, modification of language, use of visual aids, and manualized therapy, behavioural vs cognitive components, mindfulness techniques, individual vs group, inclusion of carers, therapy by carers and more sessions (104–110, 114). The Self-Assessment and Intervention (SAINT) is a guided self-help tool for people with ID and depression and anxiety designed to help a person to recognize and report emotional states and develop coping strategies (115).

Social

The lack of social supports, resources, and opportunities can impact upon the potential for psychosocial interventions for depression (52, 116–118). It is important to consider environmental factors enhancing and discouraging social participation such as summarized in Table 11.3 (52).

Social interventions need to be tailored to the person's preferences and abilities. The importance of engagement in, or re-engagement in previously enjoyed activities is demonstrated by a pilot study for people with ID and depressive symptoms with a paid carer or family member. They received a manualized course of behaviour activation, focusing on meaningful activities and addressing avoidance, and found a strong effect size maintained at follow up. The programme was well received and is less reliant upon verbal communication (119). It is important to involve family and carers who can support the person and foster engagement is social and community activities, especially in the early stages of recovery from depression when motivation might be low and avoidance high (83). Other interventions might include training in social skills and social problem solving, and action to address adverse social environments and circumstances (120). The well-being and support of family and carers is integral to the care of the person with ID.

Table 11.3 Environmental factors affecting community participation in persons with ID

Factors encouraging participation	Factors detrimental to participation
• Opportunities to make choices • Variety and stimulation of the environment and facilities • Opportunities for residential involvement in policy making • Small residential facilities • Opportunities for autonomy • Vocational services • Social support • Family involvement • Assistive technology • Positive staff attitudes	• Lack of transport • Not feeling accepted

Summary

People with ID have significant biopsychosocial risks for depression, and depression is more common in this patient group than in the general population. Standard diagnostic criteria might be used in people with mild ID but modified diagnostic criteria that account for impairments in cognition and communication but including observational criteria and atypical presentation have been developed for use in people with more severe disability. Assessment and management is complicated by comorbidity conditions and polypharmacy There is a dearth of randomized controlled trials of all treatment modalities, however, the available evidence indicates that same range of treatment options for the general population are effective for people with ID and depression, albeit with modifications and careful monitoring.

Case study 1

Jill is a 40-year-old female with mild intellectual disability and epilepsy. Her grandmother, with whom Jill was especially close, passed away four months ago after a short illness. Jill attended the funeral with her family, and had been receiving some bereavement support from Sue, her community intellectual disability nurse. Jill has no previous history of depressive illness. Both Sue and Jill's family have noticed a consistent change in her since her grandmother's passing, manifesting as pervasive low mood and frequent tearfulness, especially in the morning. Jill had become reluctant to attend day centre and had stopped enjoying activities that she previously enjoyed, including listening to music, going to the cinema and going out for meals. She had been irritable with family members, which was out of keeping with her usual personality. Jill also had lost weight as well as having poor sleep, including early morning wakening. In the past week she had disclosed to Sue that she had experienced thoughts about ending her life, though had no imminent plans to act on such thoughts.

1. What antidepressant agents might you consider?

Selective Serotonin Reuptake Inhibitors (SSRI's) are the recommended first line antidepressant agents in patients with intellectual disability and comorbid epilepsy.

2. What are the issues related to prescribing antidepressant medication in individual's with comorbid epilepsy?

Hyponatraemia is a potential issue secondary to antidepressant therapy, which can cause fatigue and potentially further seizures secondary to this electrolyte imbalance. Additionally, some antidepressants can lower the seizure threshold, or interact with Jill's antiepileptic drug regime. It is also possible that the antidepressant medication could inhibit cytochrome P450 enzymes, impacting on Jill's ability to metabolize her antiepileptic medication.

3. Given that Jill has no prior history of depressive illness, how long would she require antidepressant therapy for?

As this is Jill's first episode of depression, she would require antidepressant treatment for at least six months at the dose required to achieve full remission (for episodes of recurrent depression, the duration would be 24 months).

Case study 2

David is a 32-year-old male with moderate intellectual disability and autism spectrum disorder, with associated social anxiety. He is prescribed low dose risperidone for long-standing challenging behaviours (mainly physical aggression to others and self-injury), as well as sodium valproate for epilepsy. David also benefits significantly from a strict adherence to his weekly routine; departure from this has historically caused significant anxiety. David also has a communication passport, to help inform others on how best to support him. Over the past three months, David has experienced increasingly frequent and intense episodes of significant irritability and aggression, manifesting as physical aggression toward others, damage to property and increased frequency of self-injury, predominantly taking the form of head-banging. This has happened with a background of a planned closure of his care home in three years' time; this has never been directly discussed with David. Due to this, there have been high rates of staff turnover, including staff whom David had positive relationships with, leading to difficulties in maintaining a structured routine pertaining to David's care.

A thorough behavioural analysis assessment was conducted by the community nursing team, to identify antecedents, behaviours, and consequences pertaining to David's episodes of aggression. On analysing this, the need for a steady group of staff, structure, and communication strategy was identified. However, despite these measures being implemented, David's symptoms got worse. The clinical psychologist then provided further support regarding behavioural issues, but this approach failed. Physical health comorbidities were also ruled out.

The lack of improvement in David's symptoms led to his risperidone dose being increased, which did not help at all. On the surface, there was no evidence of David demonstrating a depressive mood state, with no sleep disturbance and no change in his appetite from baseline (David has always been fussy with his eating). He was also attending his regular daily activities. Additionally, David's facial expression did not appear to demonstrate evidence of underlying depression, and whilst his eye contact was poor, this was consistent with his baseline functioning.

However, on further probing it was found that there was a qualitative difference in David's participation with daily activities; he was now only participating passively, rather than enjoying them as he would usually do. This, along with the evidence of significant agitation, led to the consideration of David possibly experiencing depressive illness and a therapeutic trial of sertraline. This was successful in treating David's depressive symptoms, and his risperidone dose was soon reduced to the previous dosage.

1. What factors related to David's medication regime could have masked his underlying depressive illness?

David's sleep could have remained undisturbed due to his sodium valproate medication. Additionally, whilst David's appetite has always been fussy with his eating, both his sodium valproate and risperidone medications may have prevented it being further compromised upon the development of his depressive illness.

2. What features related to David's diagnosis of autism could have masked his underlying depressive illness?

David's continued adherence to his routine, despite his depressive illness, is likely in part attributable to his autism diagnosis. Additionally, his facial expression failing to reveal his underlying emotions is also consistent with autism. Finally, as his baseline level of eye contact was also poor, a change in this was not seen upon the development of his depressive illness.

MULTIPLE CHOICE QUESTIONS

Questions

Please select the single most appropriate answer.

1. How does the presence of comorbid autism affect the risk of depression in individuals with ID?

A. Has no effect on depression risk
B. Increased risk of depression
C. Reduced risk of depression

2. How is the risk of completed suicide affected by level of ID in people with depression?

A. Increased risk of completed suicide with increasing severity of ID
B. Risk of completed suicide is greatest in individuals with mild ID
C. There does not appear to be a relationship between severity of ID and risk of completed suicide
D. Risk of completed suicide is greatest in individuals with moderate ID
E. People with ID do not undertake suicidal acts

3. Which of the following clinical features would you be least likely to identify in a patient with severe ID and depression?

A. Agitation
B. Sleep disturbance
C. Screaming
D. Loss of confidence
E. Self-injurious behaviours

4. Which of the following antidepressants should be generally avoided in patients with depression, ID, and epilepsy?

A. Citalopram
B. Sertraline
C. Reboxetine
D. Agomelatine
E. Lofepramine

5. Which of the following have not been found to encourage community participation in individuals with ID?

A. Opportunities for autonomy
B. Variety and stimulation of the environment and facilities
C. Large residential facilities
D. Positive staff attitudes
E. Family involvement

Answers

1. B. Autism has been found to be associated with an increased risk of depression in individuals with ID.
2. B. The risk of completed suicide is greatest in individuals with mild ID.
3. D. You would be least likely to identify loss of confidence in individuals with severe ID and depression.
4. E. You would generally avoid Lofepramine (a tricylic antidepressant) in patients with depression, ID, and epilepsy.
5. C. Large residential facilities have not been found to encourage community participation in individuals with ID (increased community participation is associated with small residential facilities).

REFERENCES

1. Sullivan PF, Daly MJ, O'Donovan M. Genetic architectures of psychiatric disorders: The emerging picture and its implications. *Nat Rev Genet.* 2012 Jul 10;13(8):537–551.
2. Dawson F, Shanahan S, Fitzsimons E, O'Malley G, Mac Giollabhui N, Bramham J. The impact of caring for an adult with intellectual disability and psychiatric comorbidity on carer stress and psychological distress. *Journal of Intellectual Disability Research.* 2016;60(6):553–563.
3. Cooper SA. Epidemiology of psychiatric disorders in elderly compared with younger adults with learning disabilities. *Br J Psychiatry.* 1997 Apr;170:375–380.
4. Deb S, Thomas M, Bright C. Mental disorder in adults with intellectual disability. 1: Prevalence of functional psychiatric illness among a community-based population aged between 16 and 64 years. *Journal of Intellectual Disability Research.* 2001;45(6): 495–505.
5. Cooper S, Smiley E, Morrison J, Williamson A, Allan L. An epidemiological investigation of affective disorders with a population-based cohort of 1023 adults with intellectual disabilities. *Psychol Med.* 2007;37(6):873–882.
6. Perez-Achiaga N, Nelson S, Hassiotis A. Instruments for the detection of depressive symptoms in people with intellectual disabilities: A systematic review. *J Intellect Disabil.* 2009 Mar;13(1): 55–76.
7. Royal College of Psychiatrists. *DC-LD: Diagnostic Criteria for Psychiatric Disorders for Use with Adults with Learning Disabilities/Mental Retardation.* London: Gaskell; 2001.
8. World Health Organization. *The ICD-10 Classification of Mental and Behavioural Disorders: Diagnostic Criteria for Research.* Geneva: World Health Organization; 1993.
9. American Psychiatric Association. *Diagnostic and Statistical Manual of Mental Disorders: DSM-IV-TR.* Washington, DC: American Psychiatric Association; 2000.
10. Johansson R, Carlbring P, Heedman Å, Paxling B, Andersson G. Depression, anxiety and their comorbidity in the Swedish general population: Point prevalence and the effect on health-related quality of life. *PeerJ* 2013;1:e98.
11. Hermans H, Beekman AT, Evenhuis HM. Prevalence of depression and anxiety in older users of formal Dutch intellectual disability services. *J Affect Disord.* 2013;144(1):94–100.
12. Emerson E, Hatton C. Mental health of children and adolescents with intellectual disabilities in Britain. *Br J Psychiatry.* 2007 Dec;191:493–499.
13. Richards M, Maughan B, Hardy R, Hall I, Strydom A, Wadsworth M. Long-term affective disorder in people with mild learning disability. *Br J Psychiatry.* 2001 Dec;179:523–527.

14. Maughan B, Collishaw S, Pickles A. Mild mental retardation: Psychosocial functioning in adulthood. *Psychol Med.* 1999;29(2):351–366.
15. Turky A, Felce D, Jones G, Kerr M. A prospective case control study of psychiatric disorders in adults with epilepsy and intellectual disability. *Epilepsia.* 2011;52(7):1223–1230.
16. Slayter EM. Demographic and clinical characteristics of people with intellectual disabilities with and without substance abuse disorders in a Medicaid population. Intellectual and developmental disabilities. 2010;48(6):417–431.
17. Didden R, Embregts P, van der Toorn M, Laarhoven N. Substance abuse, coping strategies, adaptive skills and behavioral and emotional problems in clients with mild to borderline intellectual disability admitted to a treatment facility: A pilot study. *Res Dev Disabil.* 2009;30(5):927–932.
18. Hermans H, Evenhuis HM. Factors associated with depression and anxiety in older adults with intellectual disabilities: results of the healthy ageing and intellectual disabilities study. *Int J Geriatr Psychiatry.* 2013;28(7):691–699.
19. Smith KR, Matson JL. Psychopathology: Differences among adults with intellectually disabled, comorbid autism spectrum disorders and epilepsy. *Res Dev Disabil.* 2010;31(3):743–749.
20. Fortuna RJ, Robinson L, Smith TH, Meccarello J, Bullen B, Nobis K, et al. Health conditions and functional status in adults with autism: A cross-sectional evaluation. *Journal of General Internal Medicine.* 2016;31(1):77–84.
21. Robertson J, Hatton C, Emerson E, Baines S. Prevalence of epilepsy among people with intellectual disabilities: A systematic review. *Seizure.* 2015;29:46–62.
22. van Ool JS, Snoeijen-Schouwenaars FM, Schelhaas HJ, Tan IY, Aldenkamp AP, Hendriksen JG. A systematic review of neuropsychiatric comorbidities in patients with both epilepsy and intellectual disability. *Epilepsy and Behavior.* 2016;60:130–137.
23. Walker J, Dosen A, Buitelaar J, Janzing J. Depression in Down syndrome: A review of the literature. *Res Dev Disabil.* 2011;32(5):1432–1440.
24. Seidl R, Kaehler S, Prast H, Singewald N, Cairns N, Gratzer M, et al. Serotonin (5-HT) in brains of adult patients with Down syndrome. The molecular biology of Down syndrome: Springer; 1999. pp. 221–232.
25. Phillips C, Fahimi A, Das D, S Mojabi F, Ponnusamy R, Salehi A. Noradrenergic system in Down syndrome and Alzheimer's disease a target for therapy. *Current Alzheimer Research.* 2016;13(1): 68–83.
26. Risser D, Lubec G, Cairns N, Herrera-Marschitz M. Excitatory amino acids and monoamines in parahippocampal gyrus and frontal cortical pole of adults with Down syndrome. *Life Sci.* 1997;60(15):1231–1237.
27. Mann D, Yates P, Marcyniuk B, Ravindra C. Pathological evidence for neurotransmitter deficits in Down's syndrome of middle age. *Journal of Intellectual Disability Research.* 1985;29(2):125–135.
28. McCarron M, Gill M, McCallion P, Begley C. Health co-morbidities in ageing persons with Down syndrome and Alzheimer's dementia. *Journal of Intellectual Disability Research.* 2005;49(7):560–566.
29. Hergüner S, Mukaddes NM. Psychosis associated with fluoxetine in Prader-Willi syndrome. *Journal of the American Academy of Child and Adolescent Psychiatry.* 2007;46(8):944–945.
30. Sinnema M, Boer H, Collin P, Maaskant MA, van Roozendaal KE, Schrander-Stumpel CT, et al. Psychiatric illness in a cohort of adults with Prader-Willi syndrome. *Res Dev Disabil.* 2011;32(5):1729–1735.
31. Soni S, Whittington J, Holland A, Webb T, Maina E, Boer H, et al. The course and outcome of psychiatric illness in people with Prader-Willi syndrome: Implications for management and treatment. *Journal of Intellectual Disability Research.* 2007;51(1):32–42.
32. Walton C, Kerr M. Prader Willi syndrome: Systematic review of the prevalence and nature of presentation of unipolar depression. *Advances in Mental Health and Intellectual Disabilities.* 2016;10(3):172–184.
33. Green T, Gothelf D, Glaser B, Debbane M, Frisch A, Kotler M, et al. Psychiatric disorders and intellectual functioning throughout development in velocardiofacial (22q11. 2 deletion) syndrome. *Journal of the American Academy of Child and Adolescent Psychiatry.* 2009;48(11):1060–1068.
34. da Silva Alves F, Schmitz N, Bloemen O, van der Meer J, Meijer J, Boot E, et al. White matter abnormalities in adults with 22q11 deletion syndrome with and without schizophrenia. *Schizophr Res.* 2011;132(1):75–83.
35. Hulbert-Williams L, Hastings RP. Life events as a risk factor for psychological problems in individuals with intellectual disabilities: A critical review. *Journal of Intellectual Disability Research.* 2008;52(11):883–895.
36. McGillivray JA, McCabe MP. Early detection of depression and associated risk factors in adults with mild/moderate intellectual disability. *Res Dev Disabil.* 2007;28(1):59–70.
37. Reiss S, Benson BA. Psychosocial correlates of depression in mentally retarded adults: I. Minimal social support and stigmatization. *Am J Ment Defic.* 1985;89(4):331–337.
38. Benson BA, Reiss S, Smith DC, Laman DS. Psychosocial correlates of depression in mentally retarded adults: II. Poor social skills. *Am J Ment Defic* 1985;89(6):657–659.
39. Laman DS, Reiss S. Social skill deficiencies associated with depressed mood of mentally retarded adults. Am J Ment Defic 1987 Sep;92(2):224–229.
40. Lunsky Y, Benson B. Association between perceived social support and strain, and positive and negative outcome for adults with mild intellectual disability. *Journal of Intellectual Disability Research.* 2001;45(2):106–114.
41. Esbensen AJ, Benson BA. Cognitive variables and depressed mood in adults with intellectual disability. *Journal of Intellectual Disability Research.* 2005;49(7):481–489.
42. Glenn E, Bihm EM, Lammers WJ. Depression, anxiety, and relevant cognitions in persons with mental retardation. *J Autism Dev Disord.* 2003;33(1):69–76.
43. Dagnan D, Sandhu S. Social comparison, self-esteem and depression in people with intellectual disability. *Journal of Intellectual Disability Research.* 1999;43(5):372–379.
44. Esbensen A, Benson B. A prospective analysis of life events, problem behaviours and depression in adults with intellectual disability. *Journal of Intellectual Disability Research.* 2006;50(4):248–258.
45. Esbensen AJ, Benson BA. Diathesis-stress and depressed mood among adults with mental retardation. *American Journal on Mental Retardation.* 2006;111(2):100–112.
46. Esbensen A, Benson B. An evaluation of Beck's cognitive theory of depression in adults with intellectual disability. *Journal of Intellectual Disability Research.* 2007;51(1):14–24.
47. Jahoda A, Dagnan D, Stenfert Kroese B, Pert C, Trower P. Cognitive behavioural therapy: from face to face interaction

to a broader contextual understanding of change. *Journal of Intellectual Disability Research*. 2009;53(9):759–771.
48. Horner-Johnson W, Drum CE. Prevalence of maltreatment of people with intellectual disabilities: A review of recently published research. *Developmental Disabilities Research Reviews*. 2006;12(1):57–69.
49. Jones L, Bellis MA, Wood S, Hughes K, McCoy E, Eckley L, et al. Prevalence and risk of violence against children with disabilities: a systematic review and meta-analysis of observational studies. *The Lancet*. 2012;380(9845):899–907.
50. Emerson E, Roulstone A. Developing an evidence base for violent and disablist hate crime in Britain: Findings from the life opportunities survey. *J Interpers Violence*. 2014;29(17):3086–3104.
51. Mithen J, Aitken Z, Ziersch A, Kavanagh AM. Inequalities in social capital and health between people with and without disabilities. *Soc Sci Med*. 2015;126:26–35.
52. Verdonschot MM, De Witte LP, Reichrath E, Buntinx W, Curfs LM. Community participation of people with an intellectual disability: A review of empirical findings. *Journal of Intellectual Disability Research*. 2009;53(4):303–318.
53. Kozma A, Mansell J, Beadle-Brown J, Emerson E. Outcomes in different residential settings for people with intellectual disability: A systematic review. *American Journal on Intellectual and Developmental Disabilities*. 2009;114(3):193–222.
54. Thompson JR, Bradley VJ, Buntinx WH, Schalock RL, Shogren KA, Snell ME, et al. Conceptualizing supports and the support needs of people with intellectual disability. *Intellectual and Developmental Disabilities*. 2009;47(2):135–146.
55. Einfeld S, Tonge B, Chapman L, Mohr C, Taffe J, Horstead S. Inter-rater reliability of the diagnoses of psychosis and depression in individuals with intellectual disabilities. *Journal of Applied Research in Intellectual Disabilities*. 2007;20(5):384–390.
56. Cooper SA, Collacott RA. Clinical features and diagnostic criteria of depression in Down's syndrome. *Br J Psychiatry*. 1994 Sep;165(3):399–403.
57. Smiley E, Cooper S. Intellectual disabilities, depressive episode, diagnostic criteria and Diagnostic Criteria for Psychiatric Disorders for Use with Adults with Learning Disabilities/Mental Retardation (DC-LD). *Journal of Intellectual Disability Research*. 2003;47(s1):62–71.
58. Davis JP, Judd FK, Herrman H. Depression in adults with intellectual disability. Part 1: A review. *Aust N Z J Psychiatry*. 1997 Apr;31(2):232–242.
59. Tsiouris J, Kim S, Brown W, Cohen I. Association of aggressive behaviours with psychiatric disorders, age, sex and degree of intellectual disability: A large-scale survey. *Journal of Intellectual Disability Research*. 2011;55(7):636–649.
60. Fletcher RJ, Loschen E, Stavrakaki C. *Diagnostic Manual: Intellectual Disability (DM-ID), a Textbook of Diagnosis of Mental Disorders in Persons with Intellectual Disability*. Kingston, NY: National Association for the Dually Diagnosed; 2007.
61. Hurley AD. Depression in adults with intellectual disability: Symptoms and challenging behaviour. *Journal of Intellectual Disability Research*. 2008;52(11):905–916.
62. Clarke D, Gomez G. Utility of modified DCR-10 criteria in the diagnosis of depression associated with intellectual disability. *Journal of Intellectual Disability Research*. 1999;43(5):413–420.
63. Davis JP, Judd FK, Herrman H. Depression in adults with intellectual disability. Part 2: A pilot study. *Australian and New Zealand Journal of Psychiatry*. 1997;31(2):243–251.
64. Koritsas S, Torr J, Carling-Jenkins R. *Depression, Behaviours of Concern, and Restrictive Interventions. Final Report*. Centre for Developmental Disability Health, Victoria, Monash University. 2011.
65. Hartley S, Lickel AH, MacLean W Jr. Reassurance seeking and depression in adults with mild intellectual disability. *Journal of Intellectual Disability Research*. 2008;52(11):917–929.
66. Torr J, Iacono T, Graham MJ, Galea J. Checklists for general practitioner diagnosis of depression in adults with intellectual disability. *Journal of Intellectual Disability Research*. 2008;52(11):930–941.
67. Marston G, Perry D, Roy A. Manifestations of depression in people with intellectual disability. *Journal of Intellectual Disability Research*. 1997;41(6):476–480.
68. Hayes S, McGuire B, O'Neill M, Oliver C, Morrison T. Low mood and challenging behaviour in people with severe and profound intellectual disabilities. *Journal of Intellectual Disability Research*. 2011;55(2):182–189.
69. Jennifer Torr. *The Psychiatry of Intellectual Disability: A Review of the Literature and Review of a Psychiatric Clinic for Intellectually Disabled Adults*. Melbourne: University of Melbourne; 2000.
70. Langlois L, Martin L. Relationship between diagnostic criteria, depressive equivalents and diagnosis of depression among older adults with intellectual disability. *Journal of Intellectual Disability Research* 2008;52(11):896–904.
71. Verhoeven W, Veendrik-Meekes M, Jacobs G, Van Den Berg Y, Tuinier S. Citalopram in mentally retarded patients with depression: A long-term clinical investigation. *European Psychiatry* 2001;16(2):104–108.
72. Tsiouris J, Mann R, Patti P, Sturmey P. Challenging behaviours should not be considered as depressive equivalents in individuals with intellectual disability. *Journal of Intellectual Disability Research*. 2003;47(1):14–21.
73. Tsiouris JA, Mann R, Patti PJ, Sturmey P. Symptoms of depression and challenging behaviours in people with intellectual disability: A Bayesian analysis. *Journal of Intellectual and Developmental Disability*. 2004;29(1):65–69.
74. Davies LE, Oliver C. The purported association between depression, aggression, and self-injury in people with intellectual disability: A critical review of the literature. *American Journal on Intellectual and Developmental Disabilities*. 2014;119(5): 452–471.
75. Sturmey P, Laud RB, Cooper CL, Matson JL, Fodstad JC. Challenging behaviors should not be considered depressive equivalents in individuals with intellectual disabilities. II. A replication study. *Res Dev Disabil*. 2010;31(5):1002–1007.
76. Cuthill FM, Espie CA, Cooper SA. Development and psychometric properties of the Glasgow Depression Scale for people with a learning disability. Individual and carer supplement versions. *Br J Psychiatry*. 2003 Apr;182:347–353.
77. Mileviciute I, Hartley S. Self-reported versus informant-reported depressive symptoms in adults with mild intellectual disability. *Journal of Intellectual Disability Research*. 2015;59(2):158–169.
78. Clark A, Reed J, Sturmey P. Staff perceptions of sadness among people with mental handicaps. *Journal of Intellectual Disability Research*. 1991;35(2):147–153.
79. Patel P, Goldberg D, Moss S. Psychiatric morbidity in older people with moderate and severe learning disability. II: The prevalence study. *Br J Psychiatry*. 1993 Oct;163:481–491.
80. Hermans H, Evenhuis HM. Characteristics of instruments screening for depression in adults with intellectual disabilities: Systematic review. *Res Dev Disabil*. 2010;31(6):1109–1120.
81. Ross E, Oliver C. Preliminary analysis of the psychometric properties of the Mood, Interest and Pleasure Questionnaire (MIPQ)

for adults with severe and profound learning disabilities. *British Journal of Clinical Psychology*. 2003;42(1):81–93.
82. Bhaumik S, Collacott R, Gandhi D, Duggirala C, Wildgust H. A naturalistic study in the use of antidepressants in adults with learning disabilities and affective disorders. *Hum Psychopharmacol Clin Exp*. 1995;10(4):283–288.
83. National Institute for Health and Care Excellence. Mental health problems in people with learning disabilities: Prevention, assessment and management (NG 54). 2016.
84. Torr J, Iacono T, Graham MJ, Galea J. Depression in adults with intellectual disability checklist. 2008; Available at: http://www.cddh.monashhealth.org/index.php/depression-in-adults-with-intellectual-disability-checklist/.
85. Patja K, Iivanainen M, Vesala H, Oksanen H, Ruoppila I. Life expectancy of people with intellectual disability: A 35-year follow-up study. *Journal of Intellectual Disability Research*. 2000;44(5):591–599.
86. Mollison E, Chaplin E, Underwood L, McCarthy J. A review of risk factors associated with suicide in adults with intellectual disability. *Advances in Mental Health and Intellectual Disabilities*. 2014;8(5):302–308.
87. Lunsky Y. Suicidality in a clinical and community sample of adults with mental retardation. *Res Dev Disabil*. 2004;25(3):231–243.
88. Bhaumik S, Wildgust HJ. Treatment outcomes including withdrawal phenomena with fluoxetine and paroxetine in patients with learning disabilities suffering from affective disorders. *Human Psychopharmacology: Clinical and Experimental*. 1996;11(4):337–338.
89. Santosh PJ, Baird G. Psychopharmacotherapy in children and adults with intellectual disability. *The Lancet*. 1999;354 (9174):233–242.
90. Bhaumik S, Branford D, Naik B, Biswas A. A retrospective audit of selective serotonin re-uptake inhibitors (fluoxetine and paroxetine) for the treatment of depressive episodes in adults with learning disabilities. *The British Journal of Development Disabilities*. 2000;46(91):131–138.
91. Rai PR, Kerr M. Antidepressant use in adults with intellectual disability. *The Psychiatrist*. 2010;34(4):123–126.
92. Hiremath A, Gangavati S, Gumber R, Barrett M. *Depression*. In: Bhaumik S, Gangadharan SK, Branford D, Barrett M, eds. *The Frith prescribing guidelines for people with intellectual disability*. 3rd ed.: John Wiley & Sons; 2015. p. 169–178.
93. Spina E, Scordo MG, D'arrigo C. Metabolic drug interactions with new psychotropic agents. *Fundam Clin Pharmacol*. 2003;17(5):517–538.
94. *Depression and Anxiety*. In: Taylor D, Paton C, Kapur S, eds. *The Maudsley prescribing guidelines in psychiatry*. 12th ed. West Sussex, UK: John Wiley & Sons; 2015. pp. 255–257.
95. Greenhalgh GH, Knight C, Hind D, Beverley C, Walters S. *Electro-Convulsive Therapy (ECT) for Depressive Illness, Schizophrenia Catatonia and Mania*. National Institute for Clinical Excellence 2002.
96. Little JD, McFarlane J, Ducharme H. ECT use delayed in the presence of comorbid mental retardation: A review of clinical and ethical issues. J ECT 2002;18(4):218–222.
97. van Waarde JA, Stolker JJ, van der Mast, Rose C. ECT in mental retardation: A review. *J ECT*. 2001;17(4):236–243.
98. Collins J, Halder N, Chaudhry N. Use of ECT in patients with an intellectual disability: Review. *The Psychiatrist Online* 2012;36(2):55–60.
99. Torr J, D'Abrera JC. Maintenance electroconvulsive therapy for depression with catatonia in a young woman with Down syndrome. *J ECT*. 2014 Dec;30(4):332–336.
100. McGillivray JA, McCabe MP. Detecting and treating depression in people with mild intellectual disability: The views of key stakeholders. *British Journal of Learning Disabilities*. 2010; 38(1):68–76.
101. Pert C, Jahoda A, Stenfert Kroese B, Trower P, Dagnan D, Selkirk M. Cognitive behavioural therapy from the perspective of clients with mild intellectual disabilities: A qualitative investigation of process issues. *Journal of Intellectual Disability Research*. 2013;57(4):359–369.
102. Jennings C, Hewitt O. The use of cognitive behaviour therapy to treat depression in people with learning disabilities: A systematic review. *Tizard Learning Disability Review*. 2015;20(2):54–64.
103. Koslowski N, Klein K, Arnold K, Kosters M, Schutzwohl M, Salize HJ, et al. Effectiveness of interventions for adults with mild to moderate intellectual disabilities and mental health problems: Systematic review and meta-analysis. *Br J Psychiatry*. 2016 Dec;209(6):469–474.
104. James JS. Cognitive-behavioral therapy for depression in individuals with intellectual disabilities: A review. *Journal of Mental Health Research in Intellectual Disabilities*. 2017;10(1):17–29.
105. McCabe M, McGillivray J, Newton DC. Effectiveness of treatment programmes for depression among adults with mild/moderate intellectual disability. *Journal of Intellectual Disability Research*. 2006;50(4):239–247.
106. McGillivray JA, McCabe MP, Kershaw MM. Depression in people with intellectual disability: An evaluation of a staff-administered treatment program. *Res Dev Disabil*. 2008;29(6):524–536.
107. Hassiotis A, Serfaty M, Azam K, Strydom A, Martin S, Parkes C, et al. Cognitive behaviour therapy (CBT) for anxiety and depression in adults with mild intellectual disabilities (ID): a pilot randomised controlled trial. *Trials*. 2011;12(1):95.
108. McGillivray JA, Kershaw MM. The impact of staff initiated referral and intervention protocols on symptoms of depression in people with mild intellectual disability. *Res Dev Disabil*. 2013;34(2):730–738.
109. McGillivray J, Kershaw M. Do we need both cognitive and behavioural components in interventions for depressed mood in people with mild intellectual disability? *Journal of Intellectual Disability Research*. 2015;59(2):105–115.
110. Hartley SL, Esbensen AJ, Shalev R, Vincent LB, Mihaila I, Bussanich P. Cognitive behavioral therapy for depressed adults with mild intellectual disability: A pilot study. *Journal of Mental Health Research in Intellectual Disabilities*. 2015;8(2):72–97.
111. Hassiotis A, Serfaty M, Azam K, Strydom A, Blizard R, Romeo R, et al. Manualised individual cognitive behavioural therapy for mood disorders in people with mild to moderate intellectual disability: A feasibility randomised controlled trial. *J Affect Disord*. 2013;151(1):186–195.
112. Willner P, Rose J, Jahoda A, Kroese BS, Felce D, Cohen D, et al. Group-based cognitive-behavioural anger management for people with mild to moderate intellectual disabilities: Cluster randomised controlled trial. *Br J Psychiatry*. 2013 Sep;203(3):288–296.
113. Hassiotis A, Robotham D, Canagasabey A, Romeo R, Langridge D, Blizard R, et al. Randomized, single-blind, controlled trial of a specialist behavior therapy team for challenging behavior in adults with intellectual disabilities. *Am J Psychiatry*. 2009;166(11):1278–1285.
114. Idusohan-Moizer H, Sawicka A, Dendle J, Albany M. Mindfulness-based cognitive therapy for adults with intellectual disabilities: An evaluation of the effectiveness of mindfulness in reducing symptoms of depression and anxiety. *Journal of Intellectual Disability Research*. 2015;59(2):93–104.

115. Chaplin E, Chester R, Tsakanikos E, McCarthy J, Craig T, Bouras N. Reliability and validity of the SAINT: A guided self-help tool for people with intellectual disabilities. *Journal of Mental Health Research in Intellectual Disabilities*. 2013;6(3):245–253.
116. Dodd P, Dowling S, Hollins S. A review of the emotional, psychiatric and behavioural responses to bereavement in people with intellectual disabilities. *Journal of Intellectual Disability Research*. 2005;49(7):537–543.
117. Stoddart KP, Burke L, Temple V. Outcome evaluation of bereavement groups for adults with intellectual disabilities. *Journal of Applied Research in Intellectual Disabilities*. 2002;15(1):28–35.
118. Ali A, King M, Strydom A, Hassiotis A. Self-reported stigma and symptoms of anxiety and depression in people with intellectual disabilities: Findings from a cross sectional study in England. *J Affect Disord*. 2015;187:224–231.
119. Jahoda A, Melville C, Pert C, Cooper S, Lynn H, Williams C, et al. A feasibility study of behavioural activation for depressive symptoms in adults with intellectual disabilities. *Journal of Intellectual Disability Research*. 2015;59(11):1010–1021.
120. Anderson G, Kazantzis N. Social problem-solving skills training for adults with mild intellectual disability: A multiple case study. *Behaviour Change*. 2008;25(2):97–108.

12

Bipolar Affective Disorder in Intellectual Disability

Samuel Tromans, Ian Jones, Ignatius Gunaratna, Natalie Orr, and Sabyasachi Bhaumik†

Introduction

Bipolar Affective Disorder (BPAD) encompasses a category of mood disturbances characterized by both episodes of depression (with low mood, anhedonia, and reduced energy and activity) and manic or hypomanic episodes (with elevated mood and increased energy and activity). Psychotic symptoms may also be present, and these are typically mood congruent in nature, with a persecutory and/or nihilistic quality during depressive episodes, and a grandiose quality during manic episodes. However, repeated episodes of hypomania or mania (without depressive episodes) also fall under the classification of bipolar disorder (1). Some of the key terms required in understanding BPAD are summarized in Box 12.1.

The World Health Organization (WHO) classified BPAD as the sixth leading cause of disability worldwide (2), associated with a considerable burden of both psychiatric impairment and socioeconomic deprivation (3–5).

Historically, BPAD has often gone unrecognized in people with Intellectual Disability (ID). This is likely in part due to communication deficits in this population. Additionally, the clinical presentation of BPAD can be somewhat different within this patient group, particularly in those with more severe ID, raising questions about the clinical utility of general (rather than ID-specific) diagnostic classification systems (6).

Epidemiology

General

Data from large-scale general population surveys confirm the significance of BPAD as a major public health issue. For example, in the 2014 UK-based Adult Psychiatry Morbidity Survey, 2.0 per cent per cent of the population screened positive for BPAD, based on self-completion of the Mood Disorder Questionnaire (11), a 15-item scale based on DSM-IV criteria. No significant gender differences were found, though BPAD was more prevalent among younger age groups. In contrast, a replication of the US National Comorbidity Survey of the general population found a 12-month prevalence of BPAD of around 1.4 per cent, with a lifetime prevalence of 2.1 per cent, though an estimated further 2.4 per cent experience subthreshold BPAD symptoms during their lifetime (12). Finally, the World Health Organization World Mental Health Survey Initiative, conducting surveys on 61,392 adults across 11 countries, found 12-month prevalences of 0.4 per cent for Bipolar I disorder, 0.3 per cent for Bipolar II disorder, 0.8 per cent for subthreshold BPAD and 1.5 per cent for Bipolar Spectrum Disorders (10).

The prevalence of BPAD in people with ID has been estimated in multiple community-based population studies. In administering the mini PAS-ADD to 90 persons with ID, Deb et al (13) found a prevalence of 2.2 per cent for BPAD. In another study, involving 1023 persons with ID, Cooper et al (2007) (14) reported a point prevalence of 2.3 per cent for BPAD, of which 0.5 per cent were bipolar depressive episodes, 0.6 per cent were manic episodes and 1.2 per cent were bipolar disorder where the individual was euthymic at the time of the assessment (in contrast, 4.1% of the participants were found to have unipolar depression). In a much larger scale study, Morgan et al. (2008) (15) found a prevalence of BPAD in persons with ID of around 1.0 per cent among younger and 1.2 per cent among older persons, representing a similar rate to that seen in the general population (16).

With regard to Rapid Cycling Bipolar Disorder (RCBPAD), a lack of related population survey evidence means that it is difficult to reliably estimate its prevalence (17), but cases have been reported in the literature (18, 19), suggesting that this disorder is also evident in individuals with ID.

Specific conditions

Prior to the late 1980s, individuals with Down Syndrome (DS) were previously thought to be protected from developing mania or hypomania (18). Though this theory is outdated, as multiple cases of BPAD in DS have since been reported in the literature (18, 20–23), the prevalence is not currently well established (24). However, a more recent study involving 49 patients with DS and 70

It is with great regret that we report the death of Sabyasachi Bhaumik during the production of this textbook.

Box 12.1 Key terminology relating to BPAD. Please note that bipolar type I and II are DSM-IV[1] subtypes and are not recognized in ICD-10[2]

- *Hypomania* is a disorder associated with persistent mild mood elevation, which is not of sufficient severity to cause marked impairment of social or occupation functioning. The patient may have heightened energy and activity levels, as well as feelings of heightened physical and mental efficiency. There is an absence of psychotic symptoms (1).
- *Mania* demonstrates a more significant level of mood elevation than hypomania, with significant impairment of the individual's social and/or occupational functioning. In addition to elation, overactivity, pressured speech, inattention, elevated self-esteem, disinhibition, and a lack of need for sleep may be present. Psychotic symptoms (delusions and hallucinations) may be present (1).
- *Mixed affective episodes* represent the coexistence or rapid alteration of manic and depressive symptoms (1, 8).
- *Rapid Cycling Bipolar Disorder (RCBPAD)* describes patients who experience ≥4 episodes of mania or depression per year; this BPAD subtype can be particularly treatment resistant (9).
- *Cyclothymia* is described by ICD-10 as a persistent instability of mood involving numerous periods of depression and mild elation, none of which is sufficiently severe or prolonged to justify a diagnosis of BPAD (1).
- *Bipolar I disorder* describes patients who have had at least one manic episode in the course of their illness (9).
- *Bipolar II disorder* describes patients who have had a mixture of one or more major depressive episodes and at least one hypomanic episode, with no episodes of full-blown mania (9).
- *Bipolar spectrum disorders* encompass Bipolar I, Bipolar II and subthreshold bipolar affective disorder, including cyclothymia (10).

Reprinted from *The Lancet*, 381, Phillips ML, Kupfer DJ, Bipolar disorder diagnosis: challenges and future directions, pp. 1663–1671. DOI:https://doi.org/10.1016/S0140-6736(13)60989-7.

[1] Diagnostic and Statistical Manual of Mental Disorders, fourth edition
[2] International Statistical Classification of Diseases and Related Health Problems, tenth edition

with other IDs, found a significantly reduced prevalence of BPAD among DS patients relative to their non-DS peers (4% vs. 29%) (25). Furthermore, a population study of psychiatric comorbidity in Western Australia appeared to suggest that psychiatric illness in general was underrepresented in DS compared persons with non-DS ID, with the notable exception of Alzheimer's dementia (15). Indeed, there is some evidence from post-mortem brain tissue examinations that people with DS have reduced levels of noradrenaline, serotonin, and cortisol at all ages (26–28), which could possibly explain both a predisposition to unipolar depression and a relative, albeit not absolute, protection from mania (18).

Though historically associated with an increased risk of schizophrenia, there is some evidence to suggest that individuals with velocardiofacial (DiGeorge) syndrome are also predisposed to developing BPAD. A small cohort study of 25 patients with velocardiofacial syndrome found that 64 per cent of them satisfied DSM III-R diagnostic criteria for a spectrum of BPAD (29).

Aetiology

The aetiology of BPAD is multifactorial, involving a complex interaction of genetic, psychosocial and medical factors (30).

Genetic

Epidemiological research involving a combination of family, twin, and adoption studies has provided substantial evidence to confirm a genetic component to BPAD (31). As would perhaps be expected, the risk of BPAD reduces with diminishing genetic relatedness to the affected individual, ranging from a risk of 40–70 per cent for a monozygotic twin, to about 5–10 per cent for a first degree relative, to around 0.5–1.5 per cent for an unrelated individual (31, 32). Familial studies have similarly found a relationship between polarities at the onset of BPAD among family members (33), which is clinically important as polarity at disease onset is predictive of the polarity of subsequent episodes. Additionally, ongoing genome-wide association studies are identifying risk loci associated with BPAD (34, 35), thereby progressively enhancing our understanding of the molecular basis of the disorder.

In conducting a systematic review on published literature pertaining to RCBPAD, Vanstraelen and Tyrer (17) found that the vast majority of patients had a positive family history of affective disorder, particularly among those with more severe ID, suggesting a genetic component to its aetiology. For 48 per cent of patients, the onset of the first episode of affective disturbance was before 18 years of age, potentially suggestive of genetic anticipation.

Environmental

Studies in the general population have found a relationship between BPAD episodes and stressful life events, though it is difficult to discern whether such life events are the cause or consequence of such relapse (36). The kindling hypothesis (37) suggests that psychosocial stressors likely play a greater role in the onset or early relapses of BPAD, whereas later relapse episodes are more autonomous in nature (i.e. less dependent on environmental influence), though clinical findings are only partially (rather than convincingly) supportive of this theory (38).

Medical

Though rare, manic episodes can occur as a consequence of physical illness, so-called 'secondary mania'. Conditions more frequently reported to precipitate this include stroke (39), traumatic brain injury (40) multiple sclerosis (41), epilepsy (42) and HIV (43). Though there is a lack of research in this area, it is reasonable to consider the possibility that people with ID may be at greater risk of secondary mania, in light of the greater prevalence of neurological disease among this group (44).

Iatrogenic

As in the general population, people with ID can potentially develop mania secondary to prescribed drugs, most notably levodopa (prescribed for Parkinsonism) and steroids, though other agents such as thyroxine and other dopaminergic anti-Parkinsonian drugs are more rarely reported causes (45).

Illicit substances

Illicit substances, including amphetamines (46), cocaine (47), and cannabis (48) may potentially precipitate manic symptoms.

Comorbidities

BPAD is associated with high rates of psychiatric (49, 50) and physical comorbidities (51), which can complicate its presentation, assessment, and treatment (52).

A meta-analysis, including worldwide data from 40 studies involving 14,914 patients within the general population (50), found a lifetime prevalence of anxiety disorder of 45 per cent among individuals with BPAD. Another study, based on DSM-IV diagnostic interviews of patients with BPAD, found a similarly high rate of 42 per cent, as well as increased prevalence of substance misuse (42 per cent), and, to a lesser extent, eating disorders (5 per cent), relative to the general population (49). There is currently no available research data on psychiatric comorbidity in individuals with both BPAD and ID, though one would suspect that similar trends would be observed.

Additionally, it is increasingly recognized that people with Autism Spectrum Disorders (ASD) are at increased risk of psychiatric comorbidities, including BPAD. In a retrospective review of 42 patients with ASD within an inpatient forensic ID service, 4 (9.5 per cent) were found to have comorbid BPAD (53).

With regard to medical comorbidity in BPAD, a study comparing 1,720 individuals with BPAD with 1,340 control subjects with no history of affective disorder (51) found that they were statistically significantly ($P<0.05$) more likely to have a wide range of conditions, including asthma, type 2 diabetes, elevated lipids, epilepsy, gastric ulcers, hypertension, renal disease, memory loss/dementia, migraine headaches, rheumatoid arthritis, osteoarthritis, stroke, and thyroid disease. Indeed, many of these conditions were still significantly more prevalent when also compared with a cohort of 1,737 individuals with unipolar depression.

Clinical features

As there are no known biological markers for BPAD, the diagnosis is currently based entirely on clinical history (including reports from both patient and carers) and mental state examination. The relevant NICE guidelines (54) state that staff and carers should consider the possibility of a mental health problem if a person with ID exhibits changes in their behaviour, including a loss in skills, irritability, agitation, avoidance, social withdrawal, or a loss of interest in activities that they previously enjoyed.

Even among the non-ID population, BPAD is notoriously difficult to diagnose accurately. This is partly due to the diagnostic requirements for depressive episodes in BPAD being the same as for unipolar depression, leading to BPAD often being mistaken for this. Thus it is clinically important to enquire regarding previously possible hypomanic or manic episodes in a patient presenting with depressive symptoms. Additionally, even where both depressive and possible hypomanic episodes have occurred, the absence of clear manic episodes can lead to diagnostic ambiguity (7).

Further challenges are present in making a BPAD diagnosis in someone with ID, as they typically have greater difficulties in communication, including readily expressing their thoughts and emotions (6). Additionally, there is a risk of diagnostic overshadowing, whereby symptoms in keeping with BPAD are misattributed to the patients pre-existing ID, thus effectively denying them of timely and appropriate treatment (55). Indeed, similar biases may be present in some caregivers, leading to underreporting of symptoms to clinicians or institution of inappropriate and/or ineffective forms of treatment by the carers themselves (56). Other reasons may include atypical presentation (57) and a lack of clarity regarding diagnostic criteria, though attempts have been made to address this through the development of diagnostic manuals designed specifically for persons with ID (58), as well as rating scales (59) and identifying behavioural equivalents for mania (60) in those with more severe ID.

Behavioural equivalents of mania in individuals with ID include excessive smiling, enthusiastic greeting of everyone, being easily provoked to scream or swear, reduced sleep, rapid and pressured speech, episodes of singing, pacing, and overly sexualized behaviours (61). Some of these features could undoubtedly manifest as challenging behaviour, but it is important to distinguish from challenging behaviour secondary to a mental disorder such as BPAD from those attributable to environmental factors. When clinically making a diagnosis of BPAD, one needs to bear in mind that all of these symptoms should represent a shift from the patient's normative behaviours.

There have also been some efforts to identify behavioural equivalents manifesting in persons with severe or profound ID. In a study involving 45 such individuals (60), 15 of whom were also diagnosed with BPAD, several symptoms were found to be statistically significantly associated with a diagnosis of mania, including psychomotor agitation (e.g. restlessness, agitation, motor activity), reduced sleep (e.g. difficulties with sleep initiation, waking frequently through the night, decreased need for sleep), mood disturbance (e.g. irritability and elevated mood) and disruptive/aggressive behaviours. Such findings demonstrate the importance of observation, and the patient explicitly communicating their symptoms is not essential in order to make an informed clinical diagnosis of BPAD. Table 12.1 summarizes the clinical features of mania according to level of ID.

Despite BPAD's classical association with mania, it should be noted that depressive symptoms are more prevalent in BPAD than either mania or hypomania. Major depressive episodes in BPAD present similarly to those seen in unipolar depression, though certain features are more likely to be present, including psychomotor retardation, feelings of worthlessness and atypical features, including hypersomnia and weight gain (7). For a more comprehensive overview of the presentation of depression in people with ID, please refer to Chapter 11.

Assessment and diagnosis

Individuals with ID and possible BPAD should be assessed by a psychiatrist with specialist expertise in the assessment and treatment of mental health problems in people with ID, as is the case in all other forms of severe mental illness (54).

Table 12.1 Clinical features of mania in patients with ID, according to level of ID.

Clinical feature	Severity of ID		
	Mild	Moderate	Severe-profound
Elevated mood	✓	✓	✓[1]
Pressured speech	✓	✓	
Excessive energy/psychomotor restlessness	✓	✓	✓
Elevated self-esteem/grandiosity	✓	✓	
Irritability/agitation	✓	✓	✓
Inappropriate social behaviours	✓	✓	
Increased libido/sexual disinhibition	✓	✓	✓
Inattention/ distractibility	✓	✓	✓
Reduced need for sleep	✓	✓	✓
Psychotic symptoms (reported)	✓		
Psychotic symptoms (apparent on observation)	✓	✓	
Reckless behaviour	✓	✓	

[1] May be evident on observation, though unlikely to be explicitly reported by the patient.

As mentioned before, the diagnosis of BPAD is made clinically; however, the criteria to make a diagnosis may be used, depending on clinician's choice. The diagnostic criteria for psychiatric disorders for the use with adults with ID (DC-LD) (58) was produced by the Royal College of Psychiatrists in 2001 to improve upon existing general population psychiatric classification systems for the use with adults with ID. Its utility may be somewhat contingent upon the severity of ID in the individual being assessed; DC-LD may be seen as complimentary to standard classification systems (ICD-10 and DSM-IV) in persons with mild ID, whereas it can be considered as more of a stand-alone text in those with more moderate-severe ID, whom present less similarly to the general population. The DC-LD diagnostic criteria for a manic episode are outlined in Box 12.2. For the DC-LD diagnostic criteria for a depressive episode, please refer to Chapter 11.

Box 12.2 DC-LD criteria for diagnosis of a manic episode

A The symptoms/signs must be present for at least one week
B They must not be a direct consequence of drugs or other physical disorders
C The criteria for mixed affective episode of schizoaffective episode are not met
D The symptoms/signs must represent a change from the individual's premorbid state
E An abnormally elevated, expansive or irritable mood must be present
F Three of the following symptoms must additionally be present:
- a Onset of or increase in overactivity; excessive energy
- b Increased talkativeness/pressure of speech
- c Flight of ideas
- d Loss of usual social inhibitions (excluding sexual inhibitions) and inappropriate social behaviour
- e Reduced sleep
- f Increase in self-esteem such that it is over-inflated; or grandiosity
- g Reduced concentration/distractibility
- h Reckless behaviour
- i Increased libido/sexual energy, or sexual indiscretions that are out of keeping with the person's usual behaviour

However, despite the development of specific criteria for persons with ID, diagnostic criteria used in the general population may still have some clinical utility. A retrospective chart review over a 3-year period of 166 adults with ID and comorbid psychiatric illness demonstrated that DSM-IV criteria can be useful in both the diagnosis of BPAD in ID, but also distinguishing it from other common psychiatric disorders, including schizophrenia and unipolar depression (6).

Matson and colleagues (60) investigated the use of two different rating scales for the evaluation of mania symptoms in people with ID. These were the Diagnostic Assessment for the Severely Handicapped-Revised (DASH-II), widely used in assessment of psychopathology in individuals with ID, and the parents' version of the Young Mania Rating Scale (P-YMRS), the most frequently used scale for assessment of children with mania in the non-ID population. They found that both measures produced similar results, converging on several symptom items as predictive of mania, particularly those related to psychomotor agitation and decreased sleep.

As for any patient with ID and mental health problems, risk assessment represents an essential component of the clinical assessment process. This encompasses the patient's risk to self and others, and these can manifest in a myriad of ways dependent upon the individual. Some of the commonly observed risks in mania are that of verbal aggression and physical aggression towards others, which in turn put the patient at risk of retaliation, as well as sexual disinhibition. It is important that strategies are implemented to mitigate such risks, as well as any risk plan being communicated thoroughly to both fellow professionals within the multidisciplinary team, as well as formal and informal carers (54).

Differential diagnosis

It is important to also consider other conditions that could manifest as over activity in someone with ID, such as Attention Deficit Hyperactivity Disorder (ADHD) and brain damage. Collateral history from informants who have known the patient for a long period can help distinguish between such these causes, which would be long-standing in nature (or, in the case of brain injury, likely present since the insult occurred), and thus not represent a shift from the patient's normative functioning, as opposed to in BPAD.

Another differential diagnosis is that of Emotionally Unstable Personality Disorder (EUPD). The episodes of elation and low mood in EUPD would be of shorter duration than would be expected in BPAD (though equally, this renders the patient vulnerable to being instead misdiagnosed as RCBPAD). Nevertheless, it can often be difficult to distinguish EUPD from BPAD, particularly the Bipolar II subtype (62).

Clinical course/prognosis

Within the general population, BPAD is a chronic and enduring mental illness, with a typical age of onset of 15–24 years, though there is often a delay of several years before a diagnosis is made and treatment is commenced (63). The risk of recurrence is high; a longitudinal study of 82 patients following a first BPAD episode found that 73 per cent of patients had a manic or depressive relapse within five years, with two thirds of these patients having multiple relapses (64). A similar subsequent study involving 162 patients found 40 per cent to have a recurrent manic or depressive episode within only a two-year period of follow-up (65). Over the course of a lifetime, around 10–15 per cent of patients will have >10 episodes of recurrence (66).

There is a relative scarcity of research data on the course of BPAD specifically within the ID population. However, a study by Wu and colleagues (2013) (57), analysing the courses of hospitalization of 17,899 patients with BPAD (including 544 with ID), observed significantly different outcomes in patients with ID relative to their non-ID counterparts, including a longer length of stay, lower daily dose of psychotropic medication, and a greater propensity for unsuccessful discharge into the community.

As the published evidence on RCBPAD in ID focuses on short-term aspects of the condition, there is a dearth of data on the clinical course of these patients, although a systematic review found severe ID to be statistically significantly associated with a greater number of episodes per year relative to those with borderline-moderate ID (17). However, based on the long-term follow-up findings of Coryell et al (66) within the general population, patients with RCBPAD have on average an earlier age of onset, as well as both a greater level of depressive morbidity and risk of suicide attempts than those with non-rapid cycling BPAD. Nevertheless, the rapid cycling resolved within two years of onset in over 80 per cent of the 89 patients observed in this study.

Management

There is a lack of research evidence on the treatment of BPAD specific to the ID population, but the NICE guidelines on mental health problems in people with learning disabilities (54) emphasizes the importance of referring to evidence and guidance from the general population under such circumstances. Additionally, it is essential that patients and carers are as actively involved in treatment decisions as possible, and that the management plan emerges from a process of collaboration.

Pharmacotherapy

General principles

In commencing pharmacological treatment for BPAD, the basic principles for prescribing any psychotropic medication in an individual with ID should be followed. This includes taking account of potential medication interactions and effects on comorbid conditions, assessing the risk of non-adherence, establishing a review schedule and monitoring both the therapeutic response as well as emergence of any side effects (54).

One should also consider the impact of any mood stabilizing medications on the patient's physical health, such as the possible effects of antipsychotic-induced weight gain and diabetes. As such, the clinician may wish to avoid antipsychotics such as Olanzapine, particularly in a patient who is already overweight and/or diabetic. Additionally, some mood stabilizers have anti-epileptic properties (e.g. sodium valproate, lamotrigine), whereas others can conversely lower seizure threshold (e.g. lithium); thus, it is essential to consider these factors in any patient with a history of epilepsy. However, due to its teratogenic effects, sodium valproate should generally be avoided in females of childbearing age.

The patient's other medications should also be taken into account to minimize the risk of drug interactions. For example, angiotensin converting enzyme (ACE) inhibitors, thiazide diuretics (67) and non-steroidal anti-inflammatory drugs (68) are all associated with an increased risk of lithium toxicity.

There has been a gradual movement away from lithium therapy in BPAD, in part due to patients living longer, and thus more likely to experience chronic kidney disease as a consequence of such treatment. Additionally, patients with ID may struggle to communicate the associated side effects of polydipsia and polyuria, rendering them vulnerable to hyponatraemia and seizures.

In commencing any medications for BPAD, one should always consider the monitoring requirements (Table 12.2) (69), particularly pertaining to blood testing, as needle phobia is prevalent among persons with ID, particularly those with Autism Spectrum Disorder (ASD) (70). Though desensitization interventions can be effective in some individuals with needle phobia (71), one must balance the potential therapeutic benefits against the distress for the patient caused by regular blood testing. In the case of Lithium therapy, it is important not to commence this unless the patient is able to adhere to the serum monitoring regime (69). The monitoring requirements for medications commonly used in the treatment of BPAD are summarized in Table 12.1.

In terms of the length of treatment course, the Frith prescribing guidelines (69) recommend at least two years routinely following an episode of BPAD, but up to five years if there are risk factors for a higher likelihood of relapse. Such risk factors include a history of recurrent relapses, associated psychotic symptoms, comorbid substance abuse, persistent significantly stressful life events and a lack of social support.

First episode mania or hypomania

- Note 1: For acute treatment of a first episode of mania or hypomania, antipsychotic medication (with possible use of a benzodiazepine as an adjunctive agent) has demonstrated therapeutic efficacy. The treatment course should be of 6–12 months' duration (Figure 12.1).

Table 12.2 Recommended list of monitoring requirements for medications frequently used in the treatment of BPAD

Test or measurement	Monitoring for all patients		Monitoring for specific drugs			
	Initial health check-up	Annual check-up	Antipsychotics	Lithium	Valproate	Carbamazepine
Thyroid function	✓	✓		At start and every 6 months, more often if evidence of deterioration		
Liver function	✓				At start and at 6 months	At start and at 6 months
Renal function	✓			At start and every 6 months, more often if there is evidence of deterioration or the patient starts taking drugs such as ACE inhibitors, diuretics or NSAIDs		
Full blood count	✓		Only if clinically indicated	At start and once during first 6 months		At start and at 6 months
Blood glucose	✓	✓	At start and at 3 months (and at 1 month if taking olanzapine); more often if there is evidence of elevated levels			
Lipid profile	✓	Over 40s only	At start and 3 months; more often if evidence of elevated levels			
Blood pressure	✓	✓				
Prolactin	Children and adolescents only		Risperidone only at start and if symptoms of raised prolactin develop			
ECG	If indicated by history or clinical picture		At start if there are risk factors for or existing cardiovascular disease	At start if there are risk factors for or existing cardiovascular disease		

Reproduced from Hiremath A, Gangavati S, Gumber R, Barrett M, Depression. In: Bhaumik S, Gangadharan SK, Branford D, Barrett M (eds), *The Frith Prescribing Guidelines For People With Intellectual Disability*, 3rd edition. Copyright © 2015, John Wiley and Sons.

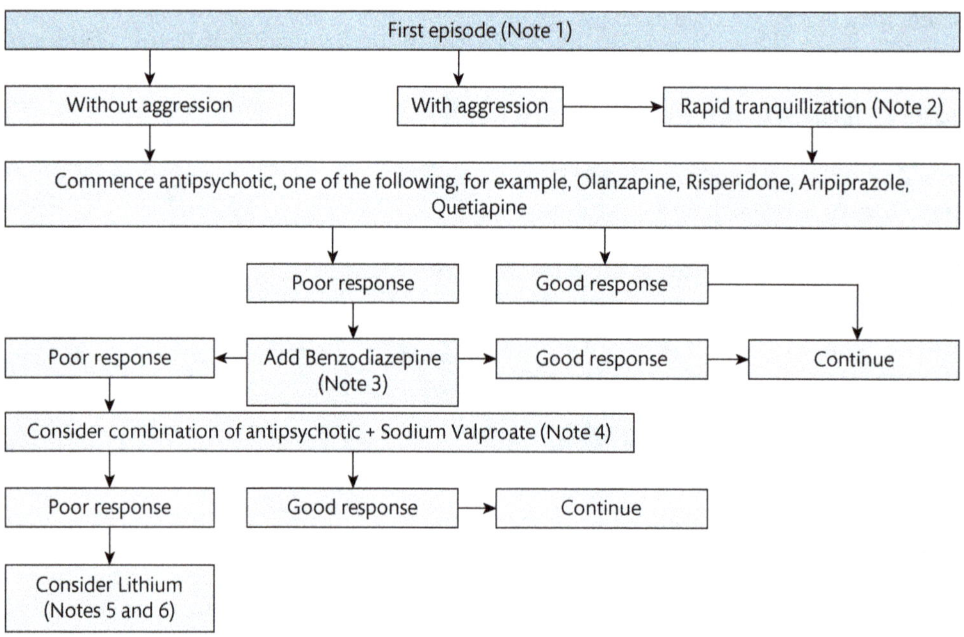

Figure 12.1 Treatment of first episode mania and hypomania in adults with ID

Reproduced from Hiremath A, Gangavati S, Gumber R, Barrett M. *Depression*. In: Bhaumik S, Gangadharan SK, Branford D, Barrett M (eds). *The Frith Prescribing Guidelines for People with Intellectual Disability*, 3rd edition. Copyright © 2015, John Wiley and Sons.

- Note 2: Rapid tranquillization may be indicated during the acute phase.
- Note 3: The use of benzodiazepines should not exceed four weeks, in order to reduce the risks of physical dependency and tolerance to the sedative effects (tolerance to the anxiolytic effects develop much more slowly, over several months) (72).
- Note 4: Commence valproate at a dose of 200mg twice daily, with gradual increases in dose according to therapeutic response.

Recurrent bipolar affective disorder

Figure 12.2 provides guidance on the treatment of adults with ID who have recurrent episodes of BPAD.

In a study involving 10 patients with BPAD and ID, Carta and colleagues (73) demonstrated a widespread positive response to Gabapentin when used as an adjunctive agent, particularly with regard to depressive and anxiety symptoms. However, further larger scale and more scientifically robust trials are required to build on these promising early findings.

- Note 1: Lithium treatment may take ten or more days before exerting its antimanic effects. As such, adjunctive treatment with either an antipsychotic or benzodiazepine medication is necessary.
- Note 2: If the patient is taking an antidepressant medication, abruptly or gradually reduce this, depending on the associated risk of discontinuation symptoms of the agent in question.
- Note 3: Before commencing treatment with a mood stabilizing medication, baseline investigations should be performed, including a Full Blood Count (FBC), Urea and Electrolytes (U+E), Liver Function Tests (LFTs), Thyroid Function Tests (TFTs) and an Electrocardiogram (ECG).
- Note 4: The serum lithium concentration for prophylaxis is 0.4-0.8mM, with dose adjustments often required to achieve this.
- Note 5: Other mood stabilizing medications:
  - Sodium valproate: Commence at 200mg twice daily, increasing the dose according to therapeutic response.
  - Carbamazepine: Commence at 100–200mg daily, again increasing the dose according to therapeutic response.
  - Antipsychotic medications, such as olanzapine, risperidone and quetiapine
  - Lamotrigine: May be useful for patients with BPAD presenting with primarily depressive episodes
- Note 6: Lithium has several contraindications. Firstly, it is a known teratogen, and is thus contraindicated in pregnancy, where it is

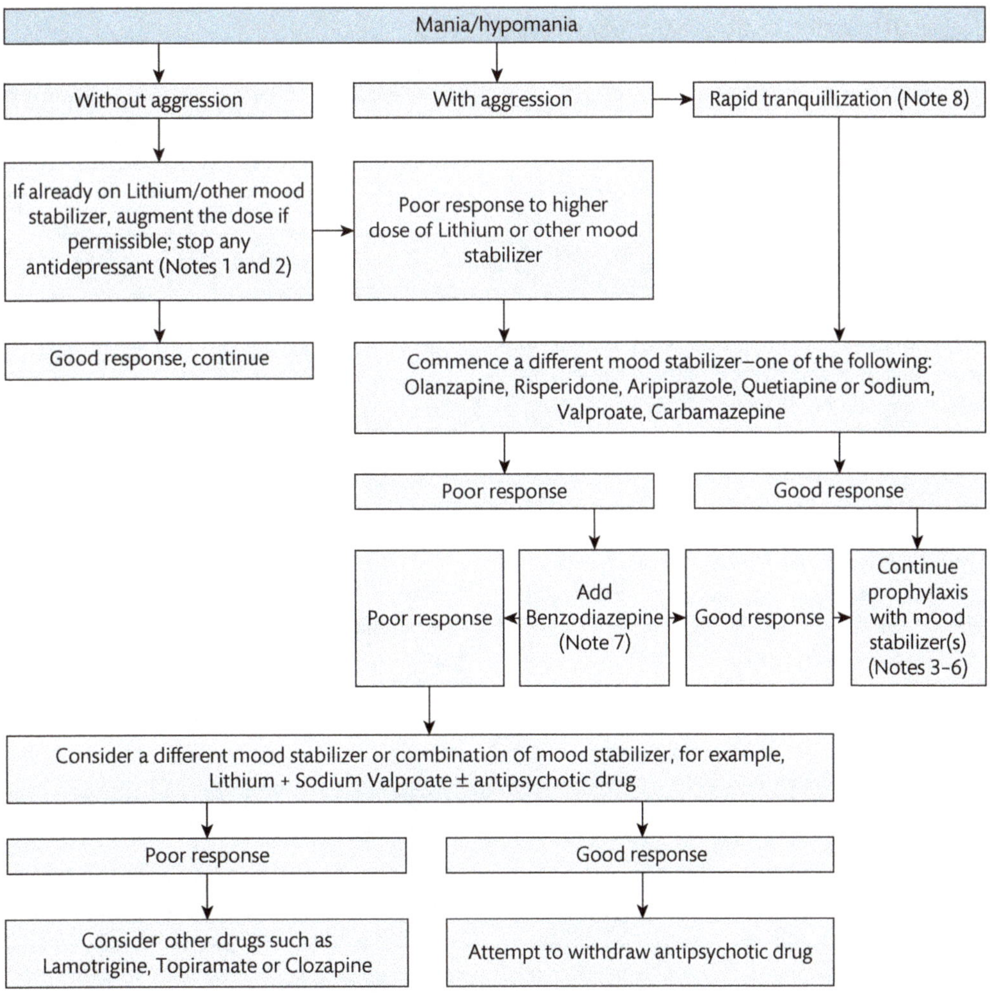

Figure 12.2 Treatment of mania and hypomania associated with BPAD in adults with ID

Reproduced from Hiremath A, Gangavati S, Gumber R, Barrett M. *Depression*. In: Bhaumik S, Gangadharan SK, Branford D, Barrett M (eds). *The Frith Prescribing Guidelines for People with Intellectual Disability*, 3rd edition. Copyright © 2015, John Wiley and Sons.

associated with a 1 in 1,000 risk of Ebstein's anomaly. However, there may be situations where, after weighing the associated risks of relapse against those of foetal abnormality, a decision to prescribe lithium is made, though this should be done through using the minimum effective dose, particularly during the first trimester. In patients with epilepsy, lithium may induce electroencephalogram (EEG) changes, as well as lowering the seizure threshold. Lithium is also contraindicated in Addison's disease, renal disease, and cardiac disease.

Depressive episodes

In treating a depressive episode in BPAD, one should recognize the risks of antidepressant-induced manic switch, and consider treatment with an adjunctive manic agent (69). However, meta-analyses conducted in the non-ID population have found that, contrary to popular belief, antidepressant agents are not significantly associated with a switch to mania, though they also demonstrate a lack of clinical efficacy in the treatment of bipolar depression (69).

If a patient experiences a depressive episode whilst already being prescribed mood stabilizing medication, one should first check compliance, then consider increasing the dose where appropriate (69).

Mixed affective episodes

In the Frith prescribing guidelines (3rd edition), Michael et al (69) recommend pharmacological treatment of mixed affective episodes to be the same as that for an acute manic episode, recommending against commencement of an antidepressant agent.

Rapid cycling BPAD

A systematic review of reported cases of RCBPAD in persons with ID found that lithium, carbamazepine and sodium valproate were the most commonly used medications, all of which had achieved mixed results for the patients concerned (17). Michael and colleagues (69), designed a treatment algorithm (Figure 12.3), as well as making several general recommendations, including adopting a long-term approach, with medication trials of at least six months' duration, reviewing previous medications and considering further trials of any agents that were incompletely adhered to in the initial trial.

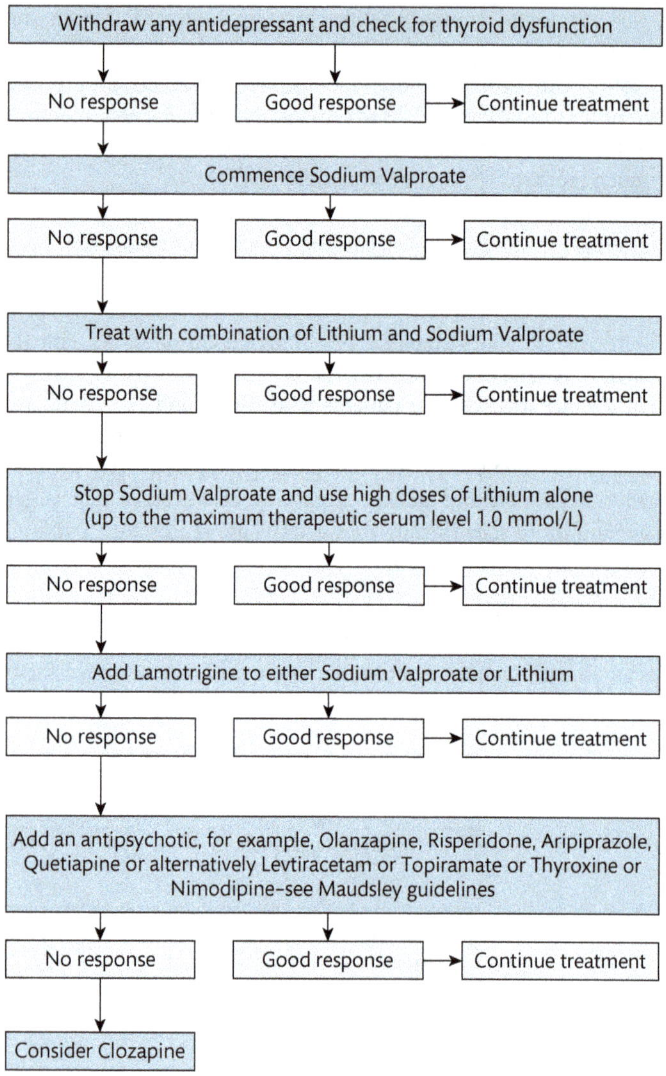

Figure 12.3 Algorithm for pharmacological treatment of RCBPAD in persons with ID

Reproduced from Hiremath A, Gangavati S, Gumber R, Barrett M. *Depression*. In: Bhaumik S, Gangadharan SK, Branford D, Barrett M (eds), *The Frith Prescribing Guidelines for People with Intellectual Disability*, 3rd edition.

Electroconvulsive Therapy (ECT)

Very little published research evidence exists on the use of ECT in patients with BPAD and ID, though the small number of cases reported (74, 75) suggest that it may have similarly positive effects to those seen with treatment-resistant BPAD in the non-ID population, where a study of 522 BPAD patients demonstrated response rates of 75 per cent for mania and 68 per cent for bipolar depression (76). Indications for ECT in patients with ID would be the same as those for the non-ID population, including severe depression, catatonia, or a prolonged, severe manic episode (77).

Psychological

The NICE guidelines for mental health problems in people with learning disabilities (54) make no mention to psychological treatments for hypomania or mania, though do recommend consideration of cognitive behavioural therapy (CBT) for depression or subthreshold depressive symptoms (such as those observed in cyclothymia) in those with mild ID, provided they have been appropriately adapted for the patient's level of functioning.

Social

Occupational interventions play an important role in treatment, particularly during the recovery phase of BPAD, where patients should be supported to engage in community activities and voluntary or paid work, wherever possible (54).

Summary

BPAD is likely prevalent in persons with ID at a similar rate as the general population, though its diagnosis is often delayed or missed. The evidence base specific to ID populations is scarce, and there is a real need for larger high quality research, particularly pertaining to epidemiology and management. One must recognize that BPAD may present atypically in persons with ID, and consider their symptomatology against the background of their communication skills and level of ID. It is essential to avoid diagnostic overshadowing, whereby new symptoms are attributed to the person's ID, and consider BPAD as a diagnostic possibility. The pharmacological treatment approach for BPAD in ID follows the principles of those used for the general population, though due consideration of the monitoring requirements of any medication, as well as any comorbid psychiatric or physical illness, is of paramount importance in this group. Treatment in general should be a collaborative, multidisciplinary process, with patients and their carers as active participants in decision-making processes wherever possible.

Case study

James is a 32-year-old gentleman with moderate intellectual disability (idiopathic in aetiology and present since birth) and a ten-year history of treatment-resistant Bipolar Affective Disorder (BPAD), for which he takes lithium 1200mg once nightly, carbamazepine 400mg twice daily (mornings and evenings) and risperidone 2mg twice daily (mornings and evenings). He takes no other medications and has no physical health comorbidities. He lives in a bungalow as the only resident, though receives 24-hour support from care staff, many of whom have worked with him for several years. When in remission, he accesses community-based activities on a regular basis, including visiting cafes, farms, and going bowling.

The majority of his multiple historical relapses are manic in nature, characterized by elation, pressured speech, motor restlessness, irritability, and poor sleep. He is also physically aggressive to other persons at such times, as well as sexually disinhibited, manifesting as exposing his genitalia and trying to kiss others, particularly care staff. His less frequent depressive episodes involve low mood, withdrawal from activities he usually enjoys, frequent tearfulness, and psychotic symptoms, including persecutory delusions (pertaining to staff and members of the public trying to harm him) and derogatory auditory hallucinations.

In the midst of James's most recent manic relapse, he demonstrated additional symptoms that had not been historically present, including polydipsia and polyuria. He also appeared unsteady on his feet, possibly suggesting dizziness, as well as demonstrating increased slurring of his speech. His psychiatrist was concerned about the possibility of lithium toxicity in addition to his manic relapse. James had historically been needle phobic, but when tested, he demonstrated a lack of capacity to make a decision pertaining to serum lithium testing, so the views of James's multidisciplinary team, carers, and family was sought with a view to making a decision in his best interests. A decision was made to take James's serum lithium levels, which, despite a concerted effort from the clinical team, was significantly distressing for him. His levels were subsequently found to be 1.52mmol/L (i.e. consistent with lithium toxicity).

James's lithium dose was subsequently reduced from 1200mg once nightly to 800mg once nightly. In the weeks following this reduction, James' manic symptoms persisted, though his polyuria and polydipsia reduced somewhat. Additionally, further more frequent blood testing (to ensure that James's lithium levels were returning to normal therapeutic range) continued to be distressing for him.

Following consultation with James's multidisciplinary team, carers, and family, a decision was made to gradually discontinue his lithium. This decision was made because of his more frequent relapses recently, suggesting that his current drug regime was diminishing in effectiveness as well as the risk of side effects and future toxicity associated with lithium. Additionally, the process of taking James's bloods caused significant distress for him, as well as being detrimental to both his well-being and relationship with his care team.

As the lithium dose was tapered off, James's carbamazepine dose was gradually increased from 400mg to 800mg twice daily. This gradually brought about a stabilization of his mood, without the need for concomitant lithium therapy. James's BPAD has remained in remission following these changes being made, and has started to access and gain enjoyment from his community-based activities, in keeping with his baseline functioning.

1. Why has there been a movement away from Lithium therapy in persons with ID and BPAD?

Patients are living longer, and are thus more likely to experience chronic kidney disease secondary to lithium therapy. Additionally, patients with ID may struggle to communicate the associated side effects of polydipsia and polyuria, rendering them vulnerable to hyponatraemia and seizures.

2. Though James's BPAD has stabilized, for how long would you recommend him continuing his remaining pharmacological treatment?

The Frith prescribing guidelines (69) would recommend James continuing his medication regime for up to five years following his recent relapse. This would be due to the presence of several risk factors, including a history of multiple relapses and associated psychotic symptoms.

MULTIPLE CHOICE QUESTIONS

Questions

Please select the single most appropriate answer.

1. What is the typical age of onset of Bipolar Affective Disorder (BPAD)?

A. 10–15 years
B. 15–24 years
C. 25–34 years
D. 35–44 years
E. ≥45 years

2. Which term best describes patients whom experience ≥4 episodes of mania or depression per year?

A. Mixed affective episodes
B. Cyclothymia
C. Bipolar I disorder
D. Rapid Cycling Bipolar Disorder
E. Bipolar II disorder

3. Which of the following physical illnesses is not associated with development of 'secondary mania'?

A. Diabetes
B. Multiple sclerosis
C. HIV

D. Stroke
E. Epilepsy

4. Which of the following symptoms are most prevalent in individuals with BPAD?
A. Manic symptoms
B. Hypomanic symptoms
C. Depressive symptoms

5. Which medication is recommended by the Frith prescribing guidelines as a first line agent for first episode mania in adults with ID?
A. Olanzapine
B. Lithium
C. Sodium valproate
D. Carbamazepine
E. Gabapentin

Answers

1. B. The typical age of onset of BPAD is between 15–24 years of age.
2. D. The description given is in line with that for Rapid Cycling Bipolar Disorder.
3. A. Diabetes is not associated with the development of secondary mania.
4. C. Despite BPAD being perhaps classically associated with mania, depressive symptoms are more prevalent in BPAD than either manic or hypomanic symptoms.
5. A. The Frith prescribing guidelines recommend the use of an antipsychotic agent such as olanzapine as a first line agent, possibly accompanied by a benzodiazepine as an adjunct).

REFERENCES

1. World Health Organization. *The ICD-10 Classification of Mental and Behavioural Disorders: Clinical Descriptions and Diagnostic Guidelines*. Geneva: World Health Organization; 1992.
2. Murray CJ, Lopez AD, World Health Organization. *The Global Burden of Disease: A Comprehensive Assessment of Mortality and Disability from Diseases, Injuries, and Risk Factors in 1990 and Projected to 2020: Summary*. 1996.
3. Marwaha S, Sal N, Bebbington P. Chapter 9: Bipolar disorder. Mental health and wellbeing in England: *Adult Psychiatric Morbidity Survey* 2014.
4. Coryell W, Scheftner W, Keller M, Endicott J, Maser J, Klerman GL. The enduring psychosocial consequences of mania and depression. *Am J Psychiatry* 1993.
5. Judd LL, Akiskal HS, Schettler PJ, Endicott J, Leon AC, Solomon DA, et al. Psychosocial disability in the course of bipolar I and II disorders: a prospective, comparative, longitudinal study. *Arch Gen Psychiatry* 2005;62(12):1322–1330.
6. Cain N, Davidson P, Burhan A, Andolsek M, Baxter J, Sullivan L, et al. Identifying bipolar disorders in individuals with intellectual disability. *Journal of Intellectual Disability Research* 2003;47(1):31–38.
7. Phillips ML, Kupfer DJ. Bipolar disorder diagnosis: Challenges and future directions. *The Lancet* 2013;381(9878):1663–1671.
8. Swann AC, Lafer B, Perugi G, Frye MA, Bauer M, Bahk W, et al. Bipolar mixed states: An international society for bipolar disorders task force report of symptom structure, course of illness, and diagnosis. *Am J Psychiatry* 2013;170(1):31–42.
9. Belmaker R. Bipolar disorder. *N Engl J Med* 2004;351(5):476–486.
10. Merikangas KR, Jin R, He J, Kessler RC, Lee S, Sampson NA, et al. Prevalence and correlates of bipolar spectrum disorder in the world mental health survey initiative. *Arch Gen Psychiatry* 2011;68(3):241–251.
11. Hirschfeld RM, Williams JB, Spitzer RL, Calabrese JR, Flynn L, Keck PE Jr, et al. Development and validation of a screening instrument for bipolar spectrum disorder: the Mood Disorder Questionnaire. *Am J Psychiatry* 2000;157(11):1873–1875.
12. Merikangas KR, Akiskal HS, Angst J, Greenberg PE, Hirschfeld RM, Petukhova M, et al. Lifetime and 12-month prevalence of bipolar spectrum disorder in the National Comorbidity Survey replication. *Arch Gen Psychiatry* 2007;64(5):543–552.
13. Deb S, Thomas M, Bright C. Mental disorder in adults with intellectual disability. 1: Prevalence of functional psychiatric illness among a community-based population aged between 16 and 64 years. *Journal of Intellectual Disability Research* 2001;45(6):495–505.
14. Cooper SA, Smiley E, Morrison J, Williamson A, Allan L. Mental ill-health in adults with intellectual disabilities: prevalence and associated factors. *Br J Psychiatry* 2007 Jan;190:27–35.
15. Morgan VA, Leonard H, Bourke J, Jablensky A. Intellectual disability co-occurring with schizophrenia and other psychiatric illness: population-based study. *Br J Psychiatry* 2008 Nov;193(5):364–372.
16. Judd LL, Akiskal HS. The prevalence and disability of bipolar spectrum disorders in the US population: Re-analysis of the ECA database taking into account subthreshold cases. *J Affect Disord* 2003;73(1):123–131.
17. Vanstraelen M, Tyrer S. Rapid cycling bipolar affective disorder in people with intellectual disability: A systematic review. *Journal of Intellectual Disability Research* 1999;43(5):349–359.
18. Cooper SA, Collacott RA. Mania and Down's syndrome. *Br J Psychiatry* 1993 Jun;162:739–743.
19. Glue P. Rapid cycling affective disorders in the mentally retarded. *Biol Psychiatry* 1989;26(3):250–256.
20. Cooper S, Collacott RA. Manic episodes in Down's syndrome: two case reports. *J Nerv Ment Dis* 1991;179(10):635–636.
21. Sovner R. Divalproex-responsive rapid cycling bipolar disorder in a patient with Down's syndrome: Implications for the Down's syndrome-mania hypothesis. *Journal of Intellectual Disability Research* 1991;35(2):171–173.
22. Cook EH, Leventhal BL. Down's syndrome with mania. *The British Journal of Psychiatry* 1987.
23. Singh I, Zolese G. Is mania really incompatible with Down's syndrome? *Br J Psychiatry* 1986 May;148:613–614.
24. McLaughlin M. Bipolar affective disorder in Down's syndrome. *Br J Psychiatry* 1987 Jul;151:116–117.
25. Dykens EM, Shah B, Davis B, Baker C, Fife T, Fitzpatrick J. Psychiatric disorders in adolescents and young adults with Down syndrome and other intellectual disabilities. *Journal of Neurodevelopmental Disorders* 2015;7(1):9.
26. Mann D, Yates P, Marcyniuk B, Ravindra C. Pathological evidence for neurotransmitter deficits in Down's syndrome of middle age. *Journal of Intellectual Disability Research* 1985;29(2):125–135.
27. Mann D, Lincoln J, Yates P, Brennan C. Monoamine metabolism in Down syndrome. *The Lancet* 1980;316 (8208–8209):1366–1367.

28. Reynolds G, Godridge H. Alzheimer-like brain monoamine deficits in adults with Down's syndrome. *The Lancet* 1985;326(8468):1368–1369.
29. Papolos DF, Faedda GL, Veit S, Goldberg R. Bipolar spectrum disorders in patients diagnosed with velo-cardio-facial syndrome: Does a hemizygous deletion of chromosome 22q11 result in bipolar affective disorder? *Am J Psychiatry* 1996;153(12):1541.
30. Kerner B. Genetics of bipolar disorder. *Appl Clin Genet* 2014 Feb 12;7:33–42.
31. Craddock N, Sklar P. Genetics of bipolar disorder. *The Lancet* 2013;381(9878):1654–1662.
32. Craddock N, Jones I. Genetics of bipolar disorder. *J Med Genet* 1999 Aug;36(8):585–594.
33. Kassem L, Lopez V, Hedeker D, Steele J, Zandi P, Bipolar Disorder Consortium, NIMH Genetics Initiative, et al. Familiality of polarity at illness onset in bipolar affective disorder. *Am J Psychiatry* 2006;163(10):1754–1759.
34. Barnett JH, Smoller JW. The genetics of bipolar disorder. *Neuroscience* 2009;164(1):331–343.
35. Mühleisen TW, Leber M, Schulze TG, Strohmaier J, Degenhardt F, Treutlein J, et al. Genome-wide association study reveals two new risk loci for bipolar disorder. *Nature Communications* 2014;5:3339.
36. Koenders M, Giltay E, Spijker A, Hoencamp E, Spinhoven P, Elzinga B. Stressful life events in bipolar I and II disorder: cause or consequence of mood symptoms? *J Affect Disord* 2014;161:55–64.
37. Post RM. Transduction of psychosocial stress into the neurobiology. *Am J Psychiatry* 1992;149:999–1010.
38. Weiss RB, Stange JP, Boland EM, Black SK, LaBelle DR, Abramson LY, et al. Kindling of life stress in bipolar disorder: comparison of sensitization and autonomy models. *J Abnorm Psychol* 2015 Feb;124(1):4–16.
39. Santos CO, Caeiro L, Ferro JM, Figueira ML. Mania and stroke: a systematic review. *Cerebrovasc Dis* 2011;32(1):11–21.
40. Jorge RE, Robinson RG, Starkstein SE, Arndt SV, Forrester AW, Geisler FH. Secondary mania following traumatic brain injury. *Am J Psychiatry* 1993;150:916–921.
41. Heila H, Turpeinen P, Erkinjuntti T. Case study: Mania associated with multiple sclerosis. *Journal of the American Academy of Child and Adolescent Psychiatry* 1995;34(12):1591–1595.
42. Schmitz B. Depression and mania in patients with epilepsy. *Epilepsia* 2005;46(s4):45–49.
43. Nakimuli-Mpungu E, Musisi S, Mpungu SK, Katabira E. Primary mania versus HIV-related secondary mania in Uganda. *Am J Psychiatry* 2006;163(8):1349–1354.
44. Emerson E, Baines S. Health inequalities and people with learning disabilities in the UK. *Tizard Learning Disability Review* 2011;16(1):42–48.
45. Peet M, Peters S. Drug-induced mania. *Drug Safety* 1995;12(2): 146–153.
46. Vergne DE, Whitham EA, Barroilhet S, Fradkin Y, Ghaemi SN. Adult ADHD and amphetamines: a new paradigm. *Neuropsychiatry* 2011;1(6):591–598.
47. Post RM, Weiss SR. Sensitization, kindling and anticonvulsants in mania. *J Clin Psychiatry* 1989;50:23–30.
48. Gibbs M, Winsper C, Marwaha S, Gilbert E, Broome M, Singh SP. Cannabis use and mania symptoms: a systematic review and meta-analysis. *J Affective Disord* 2015;171:39–47.
49. McElroy SL, Altshuler LL, Suppes T, Keck Jr PE, Frye MA, Denicoff KD, et al. Axis I psychiatric comorbidity and its relationship to historical illness variables in 288 patients with bipolar disorder. *Am J Psychiatry* 2001;158(3):420–426.
50. Pavlova B, Perlis RH, Alda M, Uher R. Lifetime prevalence of anxiety disorders in people with bipolar disorder: A systematic review and meta-analysis. *The Lancet Psychiatry* 2015;2(8):710–717.
51. Forty L, Ulanova A, Jones L, Jones I, Gordon-Smith K, Fraser C, et al. Comorbid medical illness in bipolar disorder. *Br J Psychiatry* 2014 Dec;205(6):465–472.
52. Krishnan KRR. Psychiatric and medical comorbidities of bipolar disorder. *Psychosom Med* 2005;67(1):1–8.
53. Esan F, Chester V, Gunaratna IJ, Hoare S, Alexander RT. The clinical, forensic and treatment outcome factors of patients with autism spectrum disorder treated in a forensic intellectual disability service. *Journal of Applied Research in Intellectual Disabilities* 2015;28(3):193–200.
54. National Institute for Health and Care Excellence. *Mental Health Problems in People with Learning Disabilities: Prevention, Assessment and Management* (NG 54). 2016.
55. Mason J, Scior K. 'Diagnostic overshadowing'amongst clinicians working with people with intellectual disabilities in the UK. *Journal of Applied Research in Intellectual Disabilities* 2004;17(2):85–90.
56. Arumainayagam M, Kumar A. Manic-depressive psychosis in a mentally handicapped person. Seasonality: a clue to a diagnostic problem. *Br J Psychiatry* 1990 Jun;156:886–889.
57. Wu C, Desarkar P, Palucka A, Lunsky Y, Liu S. Acute inpatient treatment, hospitalization course and direct costs in bipolar patients with intellectual disability. *Res Dev Disabil* 2013;34(11):4062–4072.
58. Royal College of Psychiatrists. *DC-LD: Diagnostic Criteria for Psychiatric Disorders for Use with Adults with Learning Disabilities/Mental Retardation* (Occasional Paper OP 48). Devon, England: Edward Gaskell Publishers; 2001.
59. Matson JL, Smiroldo BB. Validity of the mania subscale of the Diagnostic Assessment for the Severely Handicapped-II (DASH-II). *Res Dev Disabil* 1997;18(3):221–225.
60. Matson J, González M, Terlonge C, Thorson R, Laud R. What symptoms predict the diagnosis of mania in persons with severe/profound intellectual disability in clinical practice? *Journal of Intellectual Disability Research* 2007;51(1):25–31.
61. Lowry M. A clear link between problem behaviors and mood disorders. *Habilitative Mental Healthcare Newsletter* 1993;12:105–110.
62. Benazzi F. Borderline personality-bipolar spectrum relationship. *Prog Neuropsychopharmacol Biol Psychiatry* 2006;30(1):68–74.
63. Müller-Oerlinghausen B, Berghöfer A, Bauer M. Bipolar disorder. *The Lancet* 2002;359(9302):241–247.
64. Gitlin MJ, Swendsen J, Heller TL, Hammen C. Relapse and impairment in bipolar disorder. *Am J Psychiatry* 1995;152(11):1635.
65. Tohen M, Zarate Jr CA, Hennen J, Khalsa HK, Strakowski SM, Gebre-Medhin P, et al. The McLean-Harvard first-episode mania study: prediction of recovery and first recurrence. *Am J Psychiatry* 2003;160(12):2099–2107.
66. Coryell W, Solomon D, Turvey C, Keller M, Leon AC, Endicott J, et al. The long-term course of rapid-cycling bipolar disorder. *Arch Gen Psychiatry* 2003;60(9):914–920.
67. Juurlink DN, Mamdani MM, Kopp A, Rochon PA, Shulman KI, Redelmeier DA. Drug-Induced Lithium Toxicity in the Elderly: A Population-Based Study. *J Am Geriatr Soc* 2004;52(5): 794–798.
68. Ragheb M. The Clinical Significance of Lithium-Nonsteroidal: Anti-inflammatory Drug Interactions. *J Clin Psychopharmacol* 1990;10(5):350–354.
69. Michael DM, Brandford D, Barrett M. Bipolar Affective Disorder. In: Bhaumik S, Gangadharan SK, Branford D, Barrett M, editors. *The Frith Prescribing Guidelines for People with Intellectual Disability*. 3rd ed.: John Wiley & Sons; 2015. pp. 179–191.

70. Sukhodolsky DG, Scahill L, Gadow KD, Arnold LE, Aman MG, McDougle CJ, et al. Parent-rated anxiety symptoms in children with pervasive developmental disorders: Frequency and association with core autism symptoms and cognitive functioning. *J Abnorm Child Psychol* 2008;36(1):117–128.
71. Wolff JJ, Symons FJ. An evaluation of multi-component exposure treatment of needle phobia in an adult with autism and intellectual disability. *Journal of Applied Research in Intellectual Disabilities* 2013;26(4):344–348.
72. Ashton H. The diagnosis and management of benzodiazepine dependence. *Curr Opin Psychiatry* 2005 May;18(3):249–255.
73. Carta M, Hardoy M, Dessì I, Hardoy M, Carpiniello B. Adjunctive gabapentin in patients with intellectual disability and bipolar spectrum disorders. *Journal of Intellectual Disability Research* 2001;45(2):139–145.
74. Cutajar P, Wilson D. The use of ECT in intellectual disability. *Journal of Intellectual Disability Research* 1999;43(5):421–427.
75. Reinblatt SP, Rifkin A, Freeman J. The efficacy of ECT in adults with mental retardation experiencing psychiatric disorders. *J ECT* 2004;20(4):208–212.
76. Perugi G, Medda P, Toni C, Mariani MG, Socci C, Mauri M. The role of electroconvulsive therapy (ECT) in bipolar disorder: effectiveness in 522 patients with bipolar depression, mixed-state, mania and catatonic features. *Current Neuropharmacology* 2017;15(3):359–371.
77. National Institute for Clinical Excellence. Guidance on the use of electroconvulsive therapy [TA59]. 2003.

13

Anxiety and Related Disorders in People with Intellectual Disability

Sherva Cooray and Avinash Hiremath

Introduction

Anxiety disorders are a category of mental disorders characterized by excessive fear, anxiety, and related behavioural disturbances (DSM 5 2013) (3), with symptoms severe enough to result in severe distress or cause significant impairment in personal, family, social, educational, occupational, or other important areas of functioning. These conditions are highly prevalent, with significant morbidity and disability leading to substantial economic costs, but many who might benefit from treatment remain unrecognized or untreated. Anxiety disorders include generalized anxiety disorder (GAD), panic disorder, agoraphobia, social phobia, specific, simple or isolated phobia, somatic symptom related disorder, hypochondriasis, separation anxiety disorder, and selective mutism.

To understand anxiety disorders, it is useful to define the terms or phenomena associated with these disorders. Fear is defined as 'the emotional response to real or perceived danger' whereas anxiety is the 'anticipation of future threat' and worry is 'apprehensive expectation'. It involves 'unpleasant or uncomfortable thoughts that cannot be consciously controlled by trying to turn the attention to other subjects. The thoughts are often persistent, repetitive and out of proportion to the topic worried about.'(3). While many of these features underlie most anxiety disorders, a key differentiating feature is the stimulus, situation or the focus of apprehension. These could highly specific as in specific phobias or much broader as in generalized anxiety, or social anxiety disorder (2).

Some disorders have a significant component of 'worry' in addition to fear and anxiety. OCD involves recurrent thoughts, ruminations, images, or impulses (obsessions) and/or physical or mental rituals (compulsions) that cause interference with social and occupational functioning. While the source of anxiety can be difficult to establish in most of the anxiety disorders, PTSD is characterized by a history of exposure to identifiable trauma (actual or threatened death, serious injury, or threats to the physical integrity of the self or others).

Apart from cognitive limitations, People with Intellectual Disabilities (PWID) have a range of physical and psychological impairments that affect their ability to interact with their environment. The range and complexity of these impairments are covered in other chapters in this book, but one of the main impairments is the ability to comprehend and communicate. As clinical approaches and diagnostic criteria are based on the ability of the patients to describe their subjective experiences, it becomes difficult to reliably apply these approaches to this population. Therefore, mental disorders are often thought of as problem behaviours, consequently they are poorly recognized (88). This issue has been described by Sovner (83), who highlighted four factors reflecting the profound bio/psycho/social effects of Intellectual Disabilities (ID) that may influence the diagnostic process which include:

- Intellectual distortion (diminished ability for abstract thinking and effective communication),
- Psycho-social masking effect on content of psychiatric symptoms due to limitations in social skills and real-world experiences)
- Cognitive disintegration (becomes easily disorganized under stress)
- Baseline exaggeration (an increase in the frequency and intensity of pre-existing maladaptive behaviours during the course of a mental illness

There is also the phenomenon of diagnostic overshadowing, where a tendency in the clinician to overlook symptoms of mental illness by attributing them to ID may contribute to difficulties experienced by clinicians (76). In addition, the population of PWID is significantly heterogeneous, and without appropriate adaptations that take note of the different levels of ID, formulating a diagnosis may be difficult (16).

People with intellectual disabilities experience anxiety disorders, but the prevalence and issues associated with anxiety disorders are different to that of the mainstream population (16). Matson et al. (61) concluded that people with more severe degrees of ID experience difficulties in articulating key diagnostic concepts of anxiety particularly with relation to more complex subjective cognitive phenomena. In these people, anxiety may manifest as behavioural disorders. However, behaviours may also be a reflection of other triggers in the environment, and it is therefore important to distinguish behaviours due to anxiety disorders from behaviours due to other causes. In diagnosing anxiety, Khreim and Mikkelson (49) emphasized the relevance of phenomena such as agitation, screaming, crying, withdrawal, regressive/clingy behavior, or freezing, which could be interpreted as manifestations of fear in PWID.

To support the reliability of clinical diagnoses, a number of guidelines and diagnostic tools have been developed (81, 21). These include informant and self-report assessment instruments of psychopathology, for example, Psychopathology Instrument for Mentally Retarded Adults (PIMRA), based on DSM-III-R (59), Diagnostic Assessment for the Severely Handicapped (DASH) scale, based on DSM-III-R (60) and ICD-10 based Psychiatric Assessment Scale for Adults with Developmental Disability (PAS-ADD) (63). The concurrent validity of different informant and self-report assessment instruments of psychopathology, both general and specific for anxiety and/or depression, in adolescents with ID, according to DSM IV criteria positively correlated with anxiety measures and with PIMRA and Child Behaviour Check List (CBCL) total scores, as well as with the internalizing score of the CBCL. However, the reliability of these instruments is variable and the greatest unreliability when applying the PAS-ADD, is related to symptoms of anxiety.

The Diagnostic Criteria for Psychiatric Disorders for Use with Adults with Learning Disabilities/Mental Retardation (DC-LD) (79), (Royal College of Psychiatrists, 2001, a consensus-based system reflecting expert opinion), provides operationalized diagnostic criteria for psychiatric disorders for use with adults with moderate, severe or profound ID. This also complements the ICD-10 or DSM-IV-TR in adults with mild ID. The Diagnostic Manual—Intellectual Disability (DM-ID 2) was developed by the National Association for the Dually Diagnosed (NADD), in association with the American Psychiatric Association (APA) and outlines evidence-based guidelines for anxiety disorders in PWID aimed at facilitating the diagnosis of mental disorders in PWID from the perspective of clinical utility (17).

Clinical features of anxiety-related disorders

Generalized anxiety disorder

Generalized anxiety disorder (GAD) is characterized by excessive and inappropriate persistent worrying (lasting in excess of a few months) and not restricted to particular circumstances. Patients exhibit physical anxiety symptoms and key psychological symptoms (restlessness, fatigue, difficulty concentrating, irritability, muscle tension, and disturbed sleep).

Panic disorder

Panic disorder involves recurrent unexpected surges of severe anxiety ('panic attacks'), with varying degrees of anticipatory anxiety between attacks. Panic attacks involve discrete periods of intense fear or discomfort, accompanied by multiple physical or psychological anxiety symptoms. Panic attacks typically reach their peak within 10 minutes and last around 30–45 minutes. Most patients experience a fear of having further attacks.

Agoraphobia

Agoraphobia is defined as fear in places or situations from which escape might be difficult or in which help might not be available, in the event of having a panic attack. These include being in a crowd, being outside the home, or using public transport. Consequently, they are either avoided or endured with significant personal distress.

Social phobia

Social phobia consists of a marked, persistent, and unreasonable fear of being observed or evaluated negatively by other people, in social or performance situations, which is associated with physical and psychological anxiety symptoms. Feared situations (e.g. speaking to unfamiliar people or eating in public) are either avoided or are endured with significant distress.

Specific phobia

Specific/simple/isolated phobias involve excessive or unreasonable fear of (and restricted to) single people, animals, objects, or situations (e.g. dentists, spiders, seeing blood) which are either avoided or endured with significant personal distress

Separation anxiety disorder

Separation anxiety disorder is characterized by fear or anxiety concerning separation from those to whom an individual is attached: common features include excessive distress when experiencing or anticipating separation from home, and persistent and excessive worries about potential harms to attachment figures or untoward events that might result in separation.

Hypochondriasis

Hypochondriasis (somatic symptom related disorder) is characterized by excessive or disproportionate preoccupations with having or acquiring a serious illness, often leading to excessive health-seeking behaviours and high levels of reassurance seeking.

Obsessive compulsive disorder

The main features of OCD can be described in terms of thoughts, images, or ruminations that are repetitive, intrusive, distressing, and ego-dystonic (obsessions), often associated with rituals or actions (compulsions). Mostly, the compulsive behaviours are related to obsessions (e.g. repeated washing of hands in response to fears of contamination) and are devised as a mitigating behaviour, but in time become disabling in their own right. Commonly occurring obsessions include fear of contamination, need for order or symmetry, obsessive doubts, excessive conscientiousness (need to do the right thing, fear of committing a transgression, often religious), and unwanted, intrusive sexual/aggressive thoughts. Commonly occurring compulsions consist of hoarding, arranging and rearranging objects, reassurance seeking, list making, cleaning/washing rituals, counting/repeating actions a certain number of times or until it 'feels right', and checking (e.g. locks, cooker, safety of family members).

OCD is a heterogeneous condition (91), and generally follows a chronic course, waxing and waning in severity, having significant comorbidity with major depression, anxiety (91), as well as tic disorder (24). The differential diagnosis of OCD includes obsessive-compulsive personality disorder (OCPD). OCPD typically emerges in early adulthood and refers to individuals who are preoccupied with orderliness, perfectionism, and mental and interpersonal control, at the expense of flexibility, openness, and efficiency.

Post-traumatic stress disorder

PTSD involves a history of exposure to a traumatic event that that results in symptoms from each of four symptom clusters namely, intrusion, avoidance, negative alterations in cognitions and mood, and alterations in arousal and reactivity (3). Other requisites for a diagnosis concern symptom duration; and non-attribution of symptoms to a substance or comorbid medical condition. The individual initially responds with intense fear, helplessness, or horror to the traumatic exposure, later developing a response characterized by persistently re-experiencing the event, with resultant symptoms of numbness, avoidance, and hyperarousal causing clinically significant distress or functional impairment (70).

Clinical presentations of anxiety disorders in PWID

Matson et al. (61), investigating anxiety symptoms in individuals with severe and profound ID concluded that worry, fear of particular stimulus, and avoidance could not be reliably assessed in this group. Forte et al. (25) examined the content and salience of worries experienced by young people with mild ID during transition to adulthood, and found that this group ruminated significantly more about their worries and being more distressed by them. Hurley (38), investigating the presentation of depression, reported that PWID with anxiety disorders displayed significantly more fearfulness compared with people with depression, whereas people with depression were reported to have significantly more withdrawal, sadness, crying, anhedonia, aggression, and impulsivity than individuals with anxiety.

The manifestation of fear can be observed in individuals who are unable to self-report, through facial expression and or other physiological or psychological (table 13.1) manifestations (85, 61, 68). The DSM5 allows fear and anxiety in children to be expressed via crying, tantrums, freezing or clinging, shrinking, or failing to speak. Extrapolation of similar approaches using such modifiers to diagnostic criteria in adults with intellectual disability functioning at a similar developmental level could facilitate diagnosis.

Avoidance or requiring the presence of a companion may be problematic in people with severe and profound ID since they may not have opportunities to express choice and are invariably accompanied whenever in the community by due their adaptive functioning such as poor road skills, thereby making their phobic symptoms difficult to elicit. With agoraphobia, individuals with severe/profound ID are unlikely to express complex cognitions that drive their avoidance such as escape being difficult, or help might not be available. Similar problems arise in the criteria for panic disorder regarding concepts of derealization, depersonalization, fear of losing control, 'going crazy', or fear of dying. In GAD, symptoms such as poor concentration or mind going blank, or muscle tension are unlikely to be described by people with profound ID. However, restlessness, being easily fatigued, irritability, and sleep disturbance can possibly be observed by others particularly if more marked. There is an association of anxiety symptoms with self-injurious behaviours in people with intellectual disabilities (74).

The features of generalized anxiety in adoloscents and young adults with mild intellectual disabilities grossly parallel symptoms experienced by people with a normal IQ (57). Anxiety disorders typically first diagnosed in childhood include behavioural manifestations in their criteria. For example in separation anxiety disorder behavioural elements constitute half of the features of excessive fear concerning separation while selective mutism is entirely behaviourally defined. Facial expressions of children with severe and profound ID may be more subtle and have been shown to be recognized more frequently by parents compared with adults inexperienced in the care of children with ID. Behaviours associated with anxiety such as arguing, performing repetitive acts, and avoiding difficult tasks have also been described in children with fragile X syndrome and mild to moderate ID. Helverschou and Martinsen (33) explored the recognition of anxiety symptoms in people with ID and Autism from a small sample and demonstrated informants' ability to describe behavioural symptoms of anxiety in people with ID and autism, although they seem to recognize the severity of physiological signs less well.

OCD

Detection of OCD can be difficult in PWID. Vitiello (89) reported that OCD can be considered in PWID despite the absence of recognizable ego dystonic characteristics and that emphasis should be on the behavioural, externally observable components of the disorder, rather than on inner conflicts and anxiety. The assessment of observable behaviour is demonstrated to have good reliability in diagnosing OCD in such patients in diagnostic approach.

PTSD

Most of the current knowledge on PTSD has been extrapolated from the general population and from case studies. PTSD is characterized as age and developmental level specific (55). In the non-ID adult population, the most common symptoms reported include nightmares, trouble sleeping, and jumpiness (55). Misdiagnosis in PWID may arise when symptoms of extreme stress reactions may be interpreted as problem behaviour and flashbacks may be perceived as hallucinations. Emotional numbing, as commonly seen in response to trauma, may be confused with depression, lack of motivation, or confused with the negative symptoms of psychosis.

Mevissen et al. (62) concluded from a literature review on the prevalence, assessment, and treatment of PTSD in PWID, that individuals may be misdiagnosed when symptoms of extreme stress reaction are mistaken for behavioural problems or flashbacks misconceived as hallucinations. Rosenberg and colleagues (77) indicated that the most frequent diagnoses preceding PTSD were either no diagnosis or schizophrenia. Other candidates for misdiagnosis include autism and Intermittent Explosive Disorder (IED). Co-occurring diagnoses are likely to include depression, generalized anxiety, and pathological grief (55).

Prevalence

Anxiety disorders are common with a lifetime morbidity risk of 41.7 per cent (47, 48). Eighty per cent of consultations for mental health problems in primary care are for anxiety and depression (14). It is well known that PWID suffer from anxiety disorders (56), at

Table 13.1 Correlates of physiological and psychological symptoms of anxiety in PWID

Anxiety	Self-injurious behaviour
	Avoidance behaviour
	Physiological symptoms (sweating, increased pulse rate etc.) Hyperactivity
	Agitation
Dry mouth	Drinking excessive fluids
Shortness of breath	Hyperventilation

rates similar to the general population (20, 51, 82). The point prevalence of anxiety disorders in PWID is 3.8 per cent with GAD most common (1.7%), and agoraphobia (0.7%) (69). There is evidence to suggest that older adults with ID are likely to have higher rates of GAD compared to younger adults (14).

Due to limitations in language ability, it appears that a failure to understand the full physiological and cognitive manifestations of anxiety could lead to an under-reporting of anxiety disorders in PWID (Table 13.1) (41). A literature review by Charlot et al. (13) derived behavioural descriptors of DSM-IV symptoms of anxiety with good correlation with clinically made diagnoses. Anxiety disorders were identified as more prevalent in individuals with self-injurious behaviour than in those without such behaviour (66). A study cohort comparing PWID with the general population revealed significantly higher rates of phobic disorder in the former (20).

Comorbidity

Anxiety disorders exhibit high levels of co-morbidity with each other (30). Panic disorder with agoraphobia and AWOPD are frequently comorbid with social phobia, simple phobia, and GAD.

Comorbid conditions commonly occurring in OCD include anxiety and mood disorders, attention deficit hyperactivity disorder (ADHD), impulse control disorders, (especially kleptomania and trichotillomania), tic disorder, OCPD, somatoform disorders, (hypochondriasis and body dysmorphic disorder), and eating disorders. The symptoms of OCD, such as excessive hand washing may be associated with eczematous eruptions.

PTSD is highly comorbid with other psychiatric disorders, with the highest being personality disorders, followed by mood, and anxiety disorders (67).

They are also significantly co-morbid with physical illnesses, and influence their risks and outcomes (88). There are high comorbid rates between AD and major depression (47), bipolar disorder (29), schizophrenia(11) and substance abuse (19). Comorbidity was virtually ubiquitous especially in cases of GAD and social phobia (31).

The national comorbid study found that the presence of mood disorders with GAD correlates with significant increases in associated disability and dysfunction. This relationship has important implications for clinical course and prognosis. From a public health perspective, GAD emerges as a strong predictor of functional impairment, over and above than what can be explained by major depression (72).

It is possible that the experience of anxiety due to any syndromal cause may decrease the threshold for an individual to experience other anxiety symptoms or disorders. Clinicians should be aware of these patterns of comorbidity in order to formulate accurate differential diagnoses and prescribe treatments rationally (30).

Aetiology

While the definitive aetiology of anxiety and related disorders remains unclear, emerging evidence supports complex interactions of psycho/bio/social factors that include genetic, neurobiological, and environmental components. From a genetic perspective, no specific genes have been identified. However, research evidence demonstrates that panic disorder, GAD, phobias, and OCD all have significant familial aggregation and genes largely explain this phenomenon. In anxiety disorders, genes predispose to two broad groups of disorders dichotomized as panic-generalized-agoraphobic anxiety vs. the specific phobias (34).

Anxiety disorders appear to involve a variety of neuroendocrine, neurotransmitter, and neuroanatomical disruptions in the limbic, brain stem, and higher cortical brain areas. The identification of the most functionally relevant differences is complex because of the high degree of interconnectivity between neurotransmitter- and neuropeptide-containing circuits. Primary alteration in brain structure or function or in neurotransmitter signalling may result from environmental experiences and underlying genetic predisposition; such alterations can increase the risk for psychopathology (58).

The major mediators implicated in the symptoms of anxiety disorders within the central nervous system are noradrenaline, serotonin, dopamine, and gamma-aminobutyric acid (GABA). Other neurotransmitters and peptides possibly involved include corticotropin-releasing factor. Peripherally, the autonomic nervous system, especially the sympathetic nervous system, mediates many of the symptoms (28).

Positron emission tomography (PET) scanning demonstrated an increased flow in the right parahippocampal region and reduced serotonin type 1A receptor binding in the anterior and posterior cingulate and raphe of patients with panic disorder (43). Magnetic Resonance Imaging (MRI), demonstrated smaller temporal lobe volume in patients when compared with healthy subjects with normal hippocampal volumes in both patients and controls (90). The CSF in studies in humans show elevated levels of hypocretin, thought to play an important role in the pathogenesis of panic in rat models (43).

OCD

Research and treatment trials suggest that abnormalities in serotonin (5-HT and in some cases, dopamine) neurotransmission in the brain are meaningfully involved in OCD. This is strongly supported by the efficacy of serotonin reuptake inhibitors (SSRIs) in the treatment. From a genetic perspective, emerging evidence support the view that OCD co-varies in conditions such as Tourettes syndrome and multiple chronic tics in an autosomal dominant pattern. Bloch (9) reported that symptoms of OCD in such individuals respond preferentially to a combination therapy of SSRIs and antipsychotics.

Attention has also been focused on glutamatergic abnormalities and possible glutamatergic treatments for OCD. Although modulated by serotonin and other neurotransmitters, the synapses in the cortico-striato-thalamo-cortical circuits thought to be centrally involved in the pathology of OCD principally employ the neurotransmitters glutamate and gamma-aminobutyric acid (GABA).

The functional imaging studies in OCD such as magnetic resonance imaging (MRI) and PET scanning have demonstrated increases in blood flow and metabolic activity in the orbitofrontal cortex, limbic structures, caudate, and thalamus, with a trend towards right-sided predominance in OCD. Some studies report that these areas of overactivity have been shown to normalize following successful treatment with either SSRIs or cognitive-behavioural therapy (CBT) (8). This supports the hypothesis that symptoms of OCD are a consequence of impaired intracortical inhibition of specific orbitofrontal-subcortical circuitry that mediates strong emotions and the autonomic responses to those emotions It is noteworthy that a cingulotomy, sometimes used for severe and treatment-resistant OCD, interrupts this circuit.

Genetic influence in OCD

Evidence particularly from twin studies suggest that OCD is strongly heritable. Twin studies suggest that in children, obsessive-compulsive (OC) symptoms are heritable, with genetic influences in the range of 45 per cent to 65 per cent. In adults, studies are suggestive for a genetic influence on OC symptoms, ranging from 27 per cent to 47 per cent (92).

The role of infectious diseases have been implicated in case reports of OCD with and without tics arising in children and young adults following acute group A streptococcal infections. The Herpes simplex virus has also been cited as the apparent precipitating infectious event in a few case reports. It is posited that these infections trigger a CNS autoimmune response, resulting in neuropsychiatric symptoms (paediatric autoimmune neuropsychiatric disorders associated with streptococcal infections [PANDAS]).

PTSD

PTSD is a neurophysiological phenomenon, linked to disruptions in the neuroendocrine system that controls reactions to acute stress. Heightened arousal, one of the hallmarks of PTSD, has been linked to disruption in the hypothalamic-pituitary-adrenal (HPA) axis. It is also posited that the amygdala, a structure involved in emotional and fear response and the hippocampus involved in the consolidation of memory also has a role. PTSD has been associated with dysregulation of cortisol and linked to atrophy of hippocampus which is particularly evident in people with chronic PTSD (67).

Risk factors

All anxiety-related disorders share genetic and environmental risk factors (87). Current models of anxiety incorporate the role of the individual's vulnerability, which includes both genetic (82, 44) and acquired predispositions (18). Some genetic causes of ID have associations with anxiety, for example Fragile-X syndrome is associated with social anxiety disorder; Rubinstein-Taybi and Prader-Willi syndromes with obsessive-compulsive disorder (52); Williams syndrome with anxiety (23), and phobias (22) and Cornelia de Lange syndrome with significantly high compulsive behaviour (36).

Risk factors which may trigger anxiety and related disorders as a consequence of their effect on increasing vulnerability to stressful life events include adversity, inadequate social support, and poor coping skills commonly encountered in PWID. Women are reported to have elevated rates of anxiety disorders and it appears that all types of mental disorder, including anxiety, decline with increasing educational level (10, 48).

Studies on types of fear reported in PWID reflect similarities between children and adults of equivalent mental age, highlighting the developmental perspective (86). For example, individuals with moderate ID experience fears of: animals, thunder, and ghosts (preoperational thinking), and physical injuries (concrete operational), mirroring normal Piagetian transition in non-learning disabled children. However, in childhood, anxieties and phobias might also occur as transient phenomena, integral to normal early development.

OCD symptoms can worsen with stress; however, stress does not appear to be an etiologic factor.

PWID may be at a greater risk for exposure to traumatic events and consequently develop PTSD. There is growing evidence that individuals with disabilities constitute a particularly vulnerable group, with regard to likelihood of abusive experiences during childhood as well as later in life. Two recent meta-analyses have reported alarming prevalence rates of violence against disabled adults (37).

Treatment

Almost all of the evidence based practice in the field of intellectual disabilities has been drawn from adult mental services, due to several difficulties in establishing an evidence base in learning disabilities (66). The approach to the treatment of depression and anxiety includes psychotherapeutic and pharmacological approaches, with the evidence base leaning towards cognitive-behavioural and interpersonal therapies. The treatment of anxiety-related disorders broadly parallels that in the general population with evidence-based psychological interventions being first line (65) followed by pharmacological therapy. The need for treatment is influenced by the intensity and duration of illness and the impact of symptoms on everyday life (5).

In PWID, a range of effective psychological interventions (85), including reassurance, counselling, anxiety management (such as relaxation training), anger management, and self-help have been found to be useful. Desensitization and exposure therapy are effective management strategies in OCD and social phobia. Some studies suggest that optimum results are achieved by combining psychological and pharmacological interventions (27), such as the combination of CBT with SSRIs (71). Behavioural therapy and cognitive therapy alone or in combination have demonstrated clear evidence of efficacy in the treatment of anxiety disorders (73). It is important to involve patients in their treatment using comprehensible and clear communication, and this is known to improve outcomes.

Psychotherapy, such as exposure therapy, cognitive therapy and cognitive behavioural therapy (CBT), has largely consistent evidence of efficacy in the treatment of anxiety disorders (35). The efficacy of psychological and pharmacological approaches is broadly similar in the acute treatment of anxiety disorders.

In people with mild or borderline ID and anxiety disorders, evidence based on case studies demonstrate the effectiveness of CBT (53, 54). The core principles of CBT may require modification to meet the abilities of the individual. Overall the evidence base currently available for the efficacy of CBT for treatment of anxiety disorders in PWID is weak.

Pharmacological treatment of anxiety and related disorders is targeted at achieving maximum gains from the lowest effective dose and with minimum adverse effects. PWID need careful monitoring since they may not be able to report adverse effects. The possibility of drug interactions, lower doses, and the risk of worsening any pre-existing cognitive impairment particularly from medications with sedative effects should also be borne in mind.

Despite widespread belief that antidepressant drugs can lower the seizure threshold, systematic review of data from placebo-controlled trials indicates that that the frequency of seizures is significantly lower with psychotropic drugs than with placebo (1).

In GAD, OCD, panic disorder, PTSD, and social phobia, SSRIs may be used as first line treatment. The SNRIs duloxetine and venlafaxine have proven efficacy in short-term and long-term treatment of GAD (5). Placebo-controlled trials indicate that venlafaxine is also efficacious in the acute treatment and prevention of relapse in panic disorder (7). Tricyclics may be used as second-line intervention for all of these conditions with the exception of social phobia. Other pharmacological treatments with a weaker evidence base or which are less well tolerated include buspirone (GAD, OCD) and antipsychotics (quetiapine or risperidone as antidepressant augmentation for OCD). Treatment choice should ultimately be a consequence of the assessment process and shared decision-making, with emphasis on safety, tolerability, and the patient's preferences within the context of best available evidence.

In view of potentially adverse effects, benzodiazepines should be considered only for short-term (up to four weeks) treatment of acute, disabling anxiety which is causing significant distress, while longer-term strategies are instituted. A minority with intractable anxiety may benefit from long-term treatment, which should not be denied (86), (6).

It is probable that the combination of pharmacological and psychological treatment is superior to psychological approaches or medication, when either is given alone (5).

OCD

Spontaneous remission is rare without treatment. Most improve significantly with treatment but around 15 per cent have symptoms which worsen with functional impairment over time. A minority of approximately 5 per cent reportedly have complete remission of symptoms between episodes of exacerbation.

PTSD

There is robust evidence supporting the efficacy of SSRIs and SNRIs in the acute treatment of PTSD continuing for at least 12 months after response (5). All PTSD sufferers should be offered a course of trauma-focused psychological treatment (CBT) or eye movement desensitization and reprocessing (EMDR) which is safe and effective (42) preferably on an individual outpatient basis (Table 13.2). When evidence based psychological or pharmacological treatments fail, combination therapy may be considered. There is limited evidence in support of combination therapy with paroxetine and exposure therapy.

Prognosis

Continued pharmacological treatment is recommended where effective in anxiety and related disorders since discontinuation frequently precipitates relapse. Successful completion of CBT may bring about enduring relief following treatment. Evidence also suggests that extending top up CBT may further improve the outcome. Some patients may have treatment resistant CBT requiring multiple trials of medication. An even smaller proportion with intractable and disabling symptoms may benefit from neurosurgical interventions. OCD sufferers improve significantly with appropriate treatment including CBT and, often, medication.

Summary

Anxiety and fear-related disorders are a category of mental disorders characterized by excessive fear and anxiety and related behavioural disturbances, with symptoms that are severe enough to result in significant distress or significant impairment in personal, family, social, educational, occupational, or other important areas of functioning. Despite difficulties in diagnosis of anxiety and related disorders with increasing degrees of DID, there is substantial evidence that their prevalence is similar if not higher than in people with average intellectual functioning. The diagnosis of these

Table 13.2 Treatment algorithms

	First line	Second line	Third line
OCD	CBT	SSRI (Consider atypical antipsychotic if associated with Autism)	Combination of SSRI and atypical antipsychotics
Panic disorder	CBT	SSRI	SNRI's Imipramine or other tricyclic antidepressants
Generalized anxiety disorder	CBT	SSRI Consider propranolol if significant physiological symptoms	Imipramine or other tricyclic antidepressants

disorders in PWDID can be facilitated by using developmentally appropriate means of communication and placing greater reliance on observable/reported signs as well as behavioural equivalents of diagnostic criteria.

The treatment of anxiety-related disorders broadly parallels that in the general population with evidence-based psychological interventions being first line and pharmacological therapy second line as well as combination therapy where relevant.

Case study 1

Jill is a 27-year-old lady with a mild intellectual disability. She was referred by the GP to the intellectual disability team for support to obtain a blood sample required for an investigation into her physical health. The primary care team had experienced difficulties as Jill refused to co-operate. The intellectual disability team established that Jill had the mental capacity to make an informed decision, and had made the decision that offering the blood sample was in her best interests. She, however, would be overcome with significant anxiety at the time a venepuncture was attempted. This was tried a few times by the primary care team, and Jill had developed a degree of avoidance to contact by health teams. The extreme anxiety associated with needles, and development of avoidance behaviours, correlated to a diagnosis of specific phobia related to needles.

The intellectual disability team developed a rapport by working around the avoidance behaviour related to venepuncture, and agreed with Jill to attempt desensitization. A manualized desensitization approach based on carefully planned gradual exposure to needles was planned and agreed. After about eight weeks of gradual exposure, Jill was able to tolerate the needle on her skin, and then allowed the team to collect a blood sample.

1. Is the consideration of specific phobia important in people with intellectual disabilities?

Specific phobia is known to occur at a higher prevalence in people with intellectual disabilities. The consideration of specific phobia is as important in people with intellectual disabilities as in the mainstream population, but it is complicated by the need to consider the issue of mental capacity. Where a lack of mental capacity is suspected, the approach to intervening in cases of specific phobia must take into account the principles set out in the code of practice of the mental capacity act.

2. Does the treatment of specific phobia vary in people with intellectual disabilities?

The treatment of specific phobia, and anxiety disorders in general is not very different in people with intellectual disabilities. However, the psychological approach has to be adapted to the cognitive profile of the service user and take into account challenges with modifying the cognitive approach. The population of people with intellectual disability is heterogeneous in their cognitive profile, and therefore, the adaptations to the treatment need to be heterogeneous too. It is known anecdotally, particularly with needle phobia, a single use of benzodiazepines at the time of venepuncture can add to the benefit of the desensitization.

Case study 2

Jack is a 22-year-old man with mild intellectual disabilities and childhood autism. He lives with his parents, and volunteers at a local charity shop where he is responsible for cleaning and arranging items on display shelves. He prefers his own company and generally avoids social situations. He does not like change, and keeps to time and schedules. He has a need for ritualistic order, and prefers to keep items in his room in a certain pattern that he does not like other people to tamper with. His parents have noticed that in the last few months, he has seemed more anxious than usual. He takes a little longer with his morning routine, and is spending more time in the bathroom. This results in his routine schedule falling apart which adds to his anxiety. They have noticed that he is running out of soap earlier than usual and his hands appear very dry. He has also seemed anxious to check that the lights are switched off, and that the doors and windows are locked. He started doing it once or twice a day, and over the last few months, has been doing it more often. On some days, he tends to call home and ask his mother if she has turned the gas hobs off. His parents think this behaviour has possibly started after news of a fire-related event which was on the news a year ago.

He was assessed by the intellectual disability team who confirmed the diagnosis of childhood autism, and identified the behavioural needs associated with autism. Jack then shared that he needed to make sure he was always clean so that the germs don't get him, and he had to clean himself several times to achieve that level of cleanliness. He also felt it was important to check lights, locks, and gas hobs as a security measure. He was unable to explain why he did it several times, and whether he thought it was rational. The pattern of thoughts and behaviours indicated obsessive doubts of cleanliness with compulsive washing and fears of the house being broken into/catching fire with compulsive checking.

1. What are the issues related to diagnosing OCD in people with autism spectrum disorder?

Both Autism and OCD are known to present with a pattern of repetitive behaviours associated with anxiety. In people with intellectual disabilities and autism, there is a high likelihood that OCD may not be associated with insight, and therefore it may be difficult to establish the ego-dystonicity classically associated with OCD. However, it is possible to differentiate the two patterns of behaviour, in that, the behavioural patterns associated with autism are usually developmental in origin whereas the behaviours associated with OCD are usually new in onset. The behaviours associated with OCD are usually related to the themes of contamination and checking, both in people with and without intellectual disability and autism.

2. Is the treatment approach for OCD different in people with intellectual disability and autism spectrum disorder?

The pharmacological approach to treatment is the same as in mainstream populations, that is, SSRIs as the first-line treatment. A note of caution is advised about the initial surge of anxiety observed with initiation of SSRI's, which may need to be managed with short courses of benzodiazepines. The use of CBT needs to be modified to the level of intellectual functioning, and also take into account the needs related to language and communication, parental support, and the tolerability to increasing anxiety associated with CBT treatments for OCD.

MULTIPLE CHOICE QUESTIONS

Questions

Please select the single most appropriate answer.

1. In people with intellectual disability suffering from anxiety disorders, the psychological treatment with the most evidence base is

A. Interpersonal therapy
B. Intensive interaction
C. Cognitive behaviour therapy
D. Family therapy

2. The prevalence of anxiety disorders in intellectual disability is

A. Less than the mainstream population
B. More than the mainstream population
C. Same as the mainstream population
D. Not known

3. The ritualistic behaviours associated with OCD in people with intellectual disability are phenotypically similar to

A. Rituals associated with autism
B. Motor stereotypies
C. Magical thinking
D. Complex partial seizures

4. Anxiety in people with intellectual disability can present in the form of

A. Aggression
B. Self-injurious behaviour
C. Discrete physiological symptoms
D. All of the above

Answers

1. C. The overall evidence for psychological interventions for anxiety disorders leans towards CBT-based approaches. Intensive interaction is an intervention focused on enhancing communication abilities in people with intellectual disability and autism, rather than treatment for anxiety. There is no evidence for interpersonal or family therapy in the treatment of anxiety in people with intellectual disability.
2. B. Most of the literature published suggests a higher prevalence of mental illness, including anxiety disorders in people with intellectual disability. Various studies indicate that point prevalence of anxiety disorders are at least similar to the mainstream population, but the prevalence seems to increase if phobic disorders are taken into account; therefore it would be reasonable to state that the prevalence is higher than the mainstream population, in line with prevalence figures of other mental illnesses.
3. A. All the four phenomena are observed in people with intellectual disability, but the behaviours associated with OCD in people with intellectual disability closely resemble behaviours with autism. The similarity is marked with compulsive rituals such as checking, need for order, and counting compulsions. There is not much similarity with magical thinking as cognitive compulsions are difficult to establish in people with intellectual disability. Motor stereotypies are usually simple repetitive movements, unlike the sequential behavioural rituals of compulsive behaviour. Complex partial seizures are usually episodic in nature and are associated with impairment or loss of consciousness, while consciousness is retained in obsessive-compulsive behaviours.
4. D. Depending on the level of cognitive ability, all the described behaviours are known to be correlates of anxiety. As such behaviours are associated with other causes, such as various genetic conditions and distress associated with pain or physical health conditions, it is important to consider a detailed developmental, physical health, and psychiatric history to develop a behavioural formulation.

REFERENCES

1. Alper K, Schwartz KA, Kolts RL, Khan A. Seizure incidence in psychopharmacological clinical trials: An analysis of food and drug administration (FDA) summary basis of approval reports. *Biological Psychiatry*. 2007;62(4):345–354.
2. Expert Consensus Guideline Series: Treatment of psychiatric and behavioral problems in mental retardation. *American Journal of Mental Retardation*. 2000;105(3):159–226.
3. American Psychiatric Association. (2013). Diagnostic and statistical manual of mental disorders: DSM-5. Arlington, VA: American Psychiatric Association.
4. Bailey NM, Andrews TM. Diagnostic criteria for psychiatric disorders for use with adults with learning disabilities/mental retardation (DC-LD) and the diagnosis of anxiety disorders: A review. *Journal of Intellectual Disability Research*. 2003;47 suppl. 1:50–61.
5. Baldwin DS, Anderson IM, Nutt DJ, Allgulander C, Bandelow B, den Boer JA, Christmas DM, Davies S, Fineberg N, Lidbetter N, Malizia A, McCrone, P Nabarro D, O'Neill C, Scott, J van der Wee N, Wittchen, H-U. Evidence-based pharmacological treatment of anxiety disorders, post-traumatic stress disorder and obsessive-compulsive disorder: A revision of the 2005 guidelines from the British Association for Psychopharmacology. *Journal of Psychopharmacology*. 2014;28(5):403–439.
6. Baldwin DS, Talat B. Should benzodiazepines still have a role in treating patients with anxiety disorders? *Human Psychopharmacology*. 2012;27(3):237–238.
7. Batelaan NM, Van Balkom AJLM, Stein DJ. 'Evidence-based pharmacotherapy of panic disorder: an update'. *The International Journal of Neuropsychopharmacology*. 2011;15(3):403–415.
8. Baxter LR, Schwartz JM, Bergman KS, Szuba MP, Guze BH, Mazziotta JC, Alazraki A, Selin CE, Ferng H-K, Munford P, Phelps ME. Caudate glucose metabolic rate changes with both drug and behavior therapy for obsessive-compulsive disorder. *Arch Gen Psychiatry*. 1992;49(9):681–689.
9. Bloch MH, Landeros-Weisenberger A, Kelmendi B, Coric V, Bracken MB, Leckman JF. A systematic review: Antipsychotic augmentation with treatment refractory obsessive-compulsive disorder. *Molecular Psychiatry*. 2006;11(7):622–632.
10. Bradley E, Summers A, Wood HL, Bryson SE. Comparing rates of psychiatric and behaviour disorders in adolescents and young adults with severe intellectual disability with and

without autism. *Journal of Autism and Developmental Disorders.* 2004;34(2):151–161.

11. Buckley PF, Miller BJ, Lehrer DS, Castle DJ. Psychiatric comorbidities and schizophrenia. *Schizophrenia Bulletin* 2009;35(2):383–402.
12. Catani C, Sossalla IM. Child abuse predicts adult PTSD symptoms among individuals diagnosed with intellectual disabilities. *Frontiers in Psychology.* 2015;6:1600. http://doi.org/10.3389/fpsyg.2015.01600.
13. Charlot L, Deutsch C, Hunt A, Fletcher K, McLlvane W. Validation of the mood and anxiety semi-structured (MASS) interview for patients with intellectual disabilities. *Journal of Intellectual Disability Research.* 2007;51(Pt 10):821–834.
14. Cooper B. Clinical and social aspects of chronic neurosis. *Proceedings of the Royal Society of Medicine.* 1972;65(6):509–512.
15. Cooper S-A. Psychiatry of elderly compared to younger adults with intellectual disability. *Journal of Applied Research in Intellectual Disability.* 1997;10:303–311.
16. Cooray SE, Bakala A. Anxiety disorders in people with learning disabilities. *Advances in Psychiatric Treatment.* 2005;11(5):355–361.
17. Cooray SE, Cooper S-A, Gabriel S, et al. (2005) Anxiety disorders. In NADD Diagnostic Manual (DSM–IV–ID) (eds R. Fletcher, E. Loschen, C. Stavrakaki, et al.). Kingston, NY: NADD Press.
18. Coplan JD, Pine DS, Papp LA, Gorman JM. A view on noradrenergic, hypothalamic–pituitary–adrenal axis and extrahypothalamic corticotropin-releasing factor function in anxiety and affective disorders: The reduced growth hormone response to clonidine. *Psychopharmacology Bulletin.* 1997;33 (2):193–204.
19. Crippa, JA, Zuardi AW, Martin-Santos R, Bhattacharyya S, Atakan Z, McGuire P, Fusar-Poli P. Cannabis and anxiety: a critical review of the evidence. *Human Psychopharmacology.* 2009;24(7):515–523.
20. Deb S, Thomas M, Bright C. Mental disorder in adults with intellectual disability. Prevalence of functional psychiatric illness among a community-based population aged between 16 and 64 years. *Journal of Intellectual Disability Research.* 2001;45(Pt 6):495–505.
21. Deb S, Matthews T, Holt G, Bouras N. *Practice Guidelines for the Assessment and Diagnosis of Mental Health Problems in Adults with Intellectual Disability.* 2001. Brighton: Pavilion.
22. Dykens EM. Anxiety, fears, and phobias in persons with Williams syndrome. *Developmental Neuropsychology.* 2003;23(1-2):291–316.
23. Einfeld SL, Tonge BJ, Rees VW. Longitudinal course of behavioural and emotional problems in Williams syndrome. *American Journal on Mental Retardation.* 2001;106(1):73–81.
24. Fibbe LA, Cath DC, Van den Heuvel OA, Veltman DJ, Tijssen MA, Van Balkom AJ. The relationship of movement disorders with OCD: beyond the OCD-tic phenotype. A systematic review. *Journal of Neurology, Neurosurgery, and Psychiatry.* 2012;83(6):646–654.
25. Forte M, Jahoda A, Dagnan D. An anxious time? Exploring the nature of worries experienced by young people with a mild to moderate intellectual disability as they make the transition to adulthood. *The British Journal of Clinical Psychology/the British Psychological Society.* 2011;50(4):398–411.
26. Fineberg N, Drummond, LM. Anxiety disorders: Drug treatment or behavioural cognitive psychotherapy. *CNS Drugs.* 1995;3:448–466.
27. Fineberg NA, Brown A, Reghunandanan S, Pampaloni I. Evidence-based pharmacotherapy of obsessive-compulsive disorder. *The International Journal of Neuropsychopharmacology.* 2012;15(8):1173–1191.
28. Freitas-Ferrari MC, Hallak JE, Trzesniak C, Filho AS, Machado-de-Sousa JP, Chagas MH, Nardi AE, Cripa JA. Neuroimaging in social anxiety disorder: a systematic review of the literature. *Progress in Neuropsychopharmacology and Biological Psychiatry.* 2010;34(4):565–580.
29. Gaudiano BA, Miller IW. Anxiety disorder comorbidity in bipolar 1 disorder: Relationship to depression severity and treatment outcome. *Depression and Anxiety.* 2005;21(2):71–77.
30. Goisman RM, Goldenberg IM, Vasile RG, Keller MB. Comorbidity of anxiety disorder in a multicentre anxiety disorder study. *Comprehensive Psychiatry.* 1995;36:303–311.
31. Goldenberg IM, White K, Yonkers K, Reich J, Warshaw MG, Goisman RM, Keller MB. *The Infrequency of 'Pure Culture' Diagnoses Among the Anxiety Disorders. Journal of Clinical Psychiatry.* 1996;57:528–533.
32. Haynes RB, Devereaux PJ, Guyatt GH. Physicians' and patients' choices in evidence based practice : Evidence does not make decisions, people do. *BMJ: British Medical Journal.* 2002;324(7350):1350–1350.
33. Helverschou SB, Martinsen H. Anxiety in people diagnosed with autism and intellectual disability: Recognition and phenomenology. *Research in Autism Spectrum Disorders.* 2010. doi:10.1016/j.rasd.2010.05.003.
34. Hettema JM, Prescott CA, Myers JM, Neale MC, Kendler KS. The structure of genetic and environmental risk factors for anxiety disorders in men and women. *Archives of General Psychiatry.* 2005;62(2):182–189.
35. Hofmann SG, Smits JA. Cognitive-behavioral therapy for adult anxiety disorders: A meta-analysis of randomized placebo-controlled trials. *The Journal of Clinical Psychiatry.* 2008;69(4):621–632.
36. Hyman P, Oliver C, Hall S. Self-injurious behavior, self-restraint, and compulsive behaviors in Cornelia de Lange syndrome. *American Journal on Mental Retardation.* 2002;107:146–154.
37. Hughes K, Bellis MA, Jones L, Wood S, Bates G, Eckley L, McCoy E, Mikton C, Shakespeare T, Officer A. Prevalence and risk of violence against adults with disabilities: a systematic review and meta-analysis of observational studies. *Lancet.* 2012;6736(11):61851–61855.
38. Hurley AD. Depression in adults with intellectual disability: Symptoms and challenging behaviour. *Journal of Intellectual Disability Research.* 2008;52(11):905–916.
39. ICD-11-Beta Draft-2016) http://id.who.int/icd/entity/1336943699 accessed 09/08/2016.
40. Jones L, Bellis MA, Wood S, Hughes K, McCoy E, Eckley L, Bates G, Mikton C, Shakespeare T, Officer A. Prevalence and risk of violence against children with disabilities: A systematic review and meta-analysis of observational studies. *Lancet.* 2012;380(9845):899–907.
41. Judd LL, Kessler RC, Paulus MP, Zeller PV, Wittchen HU, Kunovac JL. Comorbidity as a fundamental feature of generalized anxiety disorders: Results from the National Comorbidity Study (NCS). *Acta Psychiatrica Scandinavica, Supplementum.* 1998; 393:6–11.
42. Jowatt S, Karatzias T, Brown M, Grieve A, Paterson D, Walley R. Psychological Trauma, Theory, Research and PracticeTrauma. 2016 1 Apr. [Epub ahead of print].
43. Katerndahl DA, Talamantes M. A comparison of persons with early-versus late-onset panic attacks. *The Journal of Clinical Psychiatry.* 2000;61(6):422–427.
44. Kendler KS, Eaves LJ, Loken EK, Pedersen NL, Middeldorp CM, Reynolds C, Boomsma D, Lichtenstein P, Silberg J, Gardner CO. The impact of environmental experiences on symptoms of anxiety and depression across the life span. *Psychological Science.* 2011;22(10):1343–1352.

45. Kogan CS, Stein DJ, Maj M, First MB, Emmelkamp PM, Reed GM. The Classification of Anxiety and Fear Related Disorders in the ICD-11. *Depression and Anxiety*. 2016. doi:10.1002/da.22530 [Epub ahead of print].
46. Kendler KS, Neale MC, Kessler RC, Heath AC, Eaves LJ. Major depression and generalized anxiety disorder. Same genes, (partly) different environments? *Archives of General Psychiatry*. 1992;49(9):716–722.
47. Kessler RC, Chiu WT, Demler O, Walters EE. Prevalence, severity, and comorbidity of twelve-month DSM-IV disorders in the National Comorbidity Survey Replication (NCS-R). *Archives of General Psychiatry*. 2005;62(6):617–627.
48. Kessler RC, Petukhova M, Sampson NA, Zaslavsky AM, Wittchen HU. Twelve-month and lifetime prevalence and lifetime morbid risk of anxiety and mood disorders in the United States. *International Journal of Methods in Psychiatric Research*. 2012;21(3):169–184.
49. Khreim I, Mikkelson E. Anxiety disorders in adults with mental retardation. *Psychiatric Annals*. 1997;27:271–281.
50. King BH, DeAntonio C, McCracken JT, Forness SR, Ackerland V. Psychiatric consultation in severe and profound mental retardation. *American Journal of Psychiatry*. 1994;151:1802–1808.
51. King R, Nixon J, Beatty K, Szalajko J, Marwick L, Prescott H. Post-traumatic stress disorder and phenotype behavior in an individual with Smith-Magenis Syndrome: A multimodal approach. *Mental Health Aspects of Developmental Disabilities*. 2004;7:131–141.
52. Levitas AS, Reid CS. Rubinstein-Taybi syndrome and psychiatric disorders. *Journal of Intellectual Disability Research*. 1998;42:284–292.
53. Lindsay WR. Cognitive therapy. *The Psychologist*. 1999;12:238–241.
54. Lindsay WR, Neilson C, Lawrenson H. In: Cognitive behaviour therapy for people with learning disabilities. Kroese BS, Dagnan D, Loumidis K, editor. London: Routledge. 1997. Cognitive behaviour therapy for anxiety in people with learning disabilities, pp. 124–140.
55. McCarthy J. Post-traumatic stress disorder in people with learning disability. *Advances in Psychiatric Treatment*. 2001;7:163–169.
56. McNally RJ, Ascher LM. Anxiety disorders in mentally retarded people. In Anxiety and Stress Disorders: Cognitive/Behavioural Assessment and Treatment (eds L. Michelson & M. L. Ascher). 1987, pp. 379–394. New York: Guildford Press.
57. Masi G, Favilla L, Mucci M. Generalised anxiety disorder in adolescents and young adults with mild mental retardation. *Psychiatry*. 2000;63:54–64.
58. Martin EI, Ressler KJ, BinderE, Nemeroff CB. The neurobiology of anxiety disorders: Brain imaging, genetics, and psychoneuroendocrinology. *The Psychiatric Clinics of North America*. 2009;32(3):549–575.
59. Matson JL, Kazdin AE, Senatore V. Psychometric properties of the Psychopathology Inventory for Mentally Retarded Adults. *Applied Research in Mental Retardation*. 1984;5:881–889.
60. Matson JL, Gardner WI, Coe DA, Sovner R. A scale for evaluating emotional disorders in severely and profoundly mentally retarded persons. Development of the Diagnostic Assessment for the Severely Handicapped (DASH) scale. *British Journal of Psychiatry*. 1991;159:404–409.
61. Matson JL, Smiroldo BB, Hamilton M, Baglio CS. Do anxiety disorders exist in persons with severe and profound retardation? *Research in Developmental Disabilities*. 1997;18:39–44.
62. Mevissen L, de Jongh A. PTSD and its treatment in people with intellectual disabilities: A review of the literature. *Clinical Psychology Review*. 2010;30(3):308–316.
63. Moss S, Emerson E, Kiernan C,Turner S, Hatton C, Alborz A. Psychiatric symptoms in adults with learning disability and challenging behaviour. *British Journal of Psychiatry*. 2000;177:452–456.
64. Michels R. Psychotherapeutic approaches to treatment of anxiety and depressive disorders. *Journal of Clinical Psychiatry*. 1997; 58(suppl. 13):30–32.
65. Anxiety Disorders NICE quality standard [QS53] Published date: February 2014.
66. Oliver PC, Piachaud J, Done J, Regan A, Cooray SE, Tyrer PJ. Difficulties developing evidence-based approaches in learning disabilities. *Evidence-Based Mental Health*. 2003;6:37–39.
67. Ozer EJ, Weiss DS. Who develops posttraumatic stress disorder? *Current Directions in Psychological Science*. 2004;13(4):169–172.
68. Pruijssers AC, van Meijel B, Maaskant M, Nijssen W, van Achterberg T. The relationship between challenging behaviour and anxiety in adults with intellectual disabilities: A literature review. *Journal of Intellectual Disability Research*. 2014;58(2):162–171.
69. Reid KA, Smiley E, Cooper SA. Prevalence and associations of anxiety disorders in adults with intellectual disabilities. *Journal of Intellectual Disability Research*. 2011;55(2):172–181.
70. Risser HJ, Hetzel-Riggin MD, Thomsen CJ, McCanne TR. PTSD as a mediator of sexual revictimization: The role of reexperiencing, avoidance, and arousal symptoms. *Journal of Traumatic Stress*. 2006;19(5):687–698.
71. Simpson HB, Foa EB, Liebowitz MR, Huppert JD, Cahill S, Maher MJ, McLean CP, Bender J Jr, Marcus SM, Williams MT, Weaver J, Vermes D, Van Meter PE, Rodriguez CI, Powers M, Pinto A, Imms P, Hahn CG, Campeas R. Cognitive-behavioral therapy vs risperidone for augmenting serotonin reuptake inhibitors in obsessive-compulsive disorder: A randomized clinical trial. *JAMA Psychiatry*. 2013;70(11):1190–1199.
72. Stein MB. Public health perspectives on generalized anxiety disorder. *The Journal of Clinical Psychiatry*. 2004;65(suppl 13):3–7.
73. Tyrer P, Cooper S, Salkovskis P, Tyrer H, Crawford M, Byford S, Dupont S, Finnis S, Green J, McLaren E, Murphy D, Reid S, Smith G, Wang D, Warwick H, Petkova H, Barrett B. Clinical and cost-effectiveness of cognitive behaviour therapy for health anxiety in medical patients: A multicentre randomised controlled trial. *Lancet*. 2014;383(9913):219–225.
74. Moss S, Emerson E, Kiernan C, et al. Psychiatric symptoms in adults with learning disability and challenging behaviour. *British Journal of Psychiatry*. 2000;17:452–456.
75. Raghavan R. Anxiety disorders in people with learning disabilities: A review of the literature. *Journal of Learning Disabilities for Nursing, Health and Social Care*. 1997;2:3–9.
76. Reiss S, Levitan GW, Szyszko J. Emotional disturbance and mental retardation: Diagnostic overshadowing. *American Journal of Mental Deficiency*. 1982;86:567–574.
77. Rosenberg SD, Mueser KT, Friedman MJ, Gorman PG, Drake RE, Vidaver RM, Torrey WC, Jankowski MK. Developing effective treatments for post traumatic disorders among people with severe mental illness. *Psychiatric Services* (Washington. D.C.), 2001;52(11):1453–1461.
78. Royal College of Psychiatrists. Benzodiazepine: Risks,Benefits and Dependence. A Re-evaluation (Council Report CR59). London: Royal College of Psychiatrists, 1997.
79. Royal College of Psychiatrists. DC-LD [Diagnostic Criteria for Psychiatric Disorders for Use with Adults with Learning Disabilities/Mental Retardation] (Occasional Paper OP48). London: Gaskell, 2001.

80. Roy-Byrne PP, Davidson KW, Kessler RC, Asmundson GJ, Goodwin RD, Kubzansky L, Lydiard RB, Massie MJ, Katon W, Laden SK, Stein MB. Anxiety disorders and comorbid medical illness. *General Hospital Psychiatry*. 2008;30(3):208–225.
81. Rush AJ, Frances A (eds). Expert consensus guideline series: Treatment of psychiatric and behavioural problems in mental retardation. *American Journal on Mental Retardation*. 2000;105(3) (special issue):159–226.
82. Smoller JW, Tsuang MT. Panic and phobic anxiety: Defining phenotypes for genetic studies. *American Journal of Psychiatry*. 1998;155:1152–1162.
83. Sovner R. Limiting factors in the use of DSM–III criteria with mentally ill/mentally retarded persons. *Psychopharmacology Bulletin* 1986;22:1055–1059.
84. Smith SM, Goldstein RB, Grant BF. The association between post-traumatic stress disorder and lifetime DSM-5 psychiatric disorders among veterans: Data from the National Epidemiologic Survey on Alcohol and Related Conditions-III (NESARC-III). *Journal of Psychiatric Research*. 2016;82:16–22. [Epub ahead of print].
85. Stavrakaki C, Mintsioulis G. Anxiety disorders in persons with mental retardation: Diagnostic, clinical and treatment issues. *Psychiatric Annals*. 1997;27:182–189.
86. Sternlicht M. Fears of institutionalised mentally retarded adults. *Journal of Psychology*. 1979;101:57–71.
87. Tambs K, Czajkowsky N, Røysamb E, Neale MC, Reichborn-Kjennerud T, Aggen SH, Harris JR, Ørstavik RE, Kendler KS. Structure of genetic and environmental risk factors for dimensional representations of DSM-IV anxiety disorders. *The British Journal of Psychiatry*. 2009;195(4):301–307.
88. Veerhoven WMA, Tuinier S. Neuropsychiatric consultation in mentally retarded patients. *European Psychiatry*. 2009;12: 242–248.
89. Vitiello B, Spreat S, Behar D. Obsessive-compulsive disorder in mentally retarded patients. *The Journal of Nervous and Mental Disease*. 1989;177(4):232–236.
90. Vythilingam M, Anderson ER, Goddard A, Woods SW, Staib LH, Charney DS, Bremner JD. Temporal lobe volume in panic disorder—A quantitative magnetic resonance imaging study. *Psychiatry Research*. 2000;99(2):75–82.
91. Zaudig M. Obsessive-compulsive disorder—Clinical picture, diagnosis, and therapy. *Psychosom Med Psychother*. 2011; 57(1):3–50.
92. Van Grootheest D, Cath D, Beekman A, & Boomsma D. Twin Studies on Obsessive–Compulsive Disorder: A Review. *Twin Research and Human Genetics*, 2005;8(5), 450–458.

14

The Assessment and Treatment of Personality Disorders in People with Intellectual and Developmental Disabilities

William R. Lindsay†, Verity Chester, and Regi Alexander

Introduction

The publications of DSM III and DSM IV (1, 2) stimulated an expansion of clinical and research interest in the field of Personality Disorder (PD) in general. The research was wide ranging and included work on prevalence (3), the longitudinal course for PDs (4), and the reliability, validity, and internal consistency of PD diagnoses (5). This interest spread to the field of Intellectual and Developmental Disabilities (IDD), albeit with much reduced activity, and studies found widely disparate prevalence for PD in populations of IDD. Khan, Cowan, and Roy (6) reported that 50 per cent of their sample had personality abnormalities and 31 per cent had a degree of impairment sufficient to warrant a diagnosis of PD. Goldberg, Gitta, and Puddephatt (7) reported very high levels of PD in samples of people with IDD. They used DSM III diagnostic criteria and two other screening measures for mental health symptomatology. They found abnormal personality traits in 57 per cent of individuals in an institutional sample and 91 per cent of individuals in a community sample. Flynn, Matthews, and Hollins (8) studied a hospital in patient sample of 36 cases and reported that 92 per cent were diagnosed with personality disorder using ICD-10 criteria. On the other hand, working with the same ICD-10 criteria, Naik, Gangadharan, and Alexander (9) found PD in 7 per cent of a community sample, while Alexander, Piachaud, Odebiyi, and Gangadharan (10) reported a 58 per cent prevalence among a sample of patients referred to a forensic hospital.

A turning point in research on PD and IDD came with Alexander and Cooray's (2003) review of studies (11). They noted that there was a lack of reliable diagnostic instruments, the use of different diagnostic systems (ICD-10 and DSM-IV), a confusion of definition and personality theory and difficulty in distinguishing PD from other problems integral to IDD such as communication problems, sensory disorders, and developmental delay. They concluded that 'the variation in the co-occurrence of personality disorder in learning disability, with prevalence ranging from less than 1 per cent to 91 per cent in a community setting and 22 per cent to 92 per cent in hospital settings, is very great and too large to be explained by real differences'. They recommended tighter diagnostic criteria and greater use of behavioural observation and informant information. Most studies published since have been more careful in their methodology and have employed their recommendations.

While the variation in rates means there can be little confidence as to the exact prevalence, PD is certainly common in clinical populations of people with IDD. A possible explanation for this is that people with IDD are much more vulnerable to early adversity and psychological, physical, and sexual abuse (12). This is due to their inherent dependence on other people for personal care; an 'imbalance of power' between the carer and the person being cared for, difficulties in communicating, lack of sexual knowledge and assertiveness, and guilt and shame at being disabled (13).

Lindsay et al (19) employed the recommendations made by Alexander and Cooray (11) in a study of 164 males with IDD in three forensic settings—high secure, medium/low secure, and community forensic services. They employed four independently rated measures of PD, a DSM-IV criteria checklist completed firstly from file review, secondly by a clinician and thirdly from nurse observations, and finally the Standardised Assessment of Personality (SAP) (20) completed by care staff. A consensus rating was derived from the four assessments and a total prevalence of PD in this forensic sample was 39.5 per cent. They reported that the ratings had high levels of reliability. As would be expected in a forensic population, antisocial PD was the largest category at 22 per cent of cases and rates of PD across the other categories were between 1 and 3 per cent. It should be noted that care was taken in these guidelines to avoid confusing developmental delay with immature or dependent PD and there were no cases with dependent PD in the entire sample. It is also

† It is with great regret that we report the death of William R. Lindsay during the production of this textbook.

interesting that a previous more general file review of mental disorder in this sample (21) had found PD recorded at 22.6 per cent in the case files. Lindsay et al. (22) compared the two systems (psychiatric review and systematic assessment) using the same population and they found that by far the highest level of under recording was in the community forensic sample, which was 1.4 per cent in the case files, compared to 33 per cent in the carefully organized assessment study. These authors noted that even the highest figures found in this forensic IDD sample were lower than the figures of over 90 per cent in studies on community samples reviewed by Alexander and Cooray (11).

Lindsay et al. (23) then reported a factor analysis of the PD categories. In mainstream PD research, Blackburn et al. (24) had previously investigated higher order dimensions with 168 male forensic psychiatric patients and found two higher order factors that appeared to underlie personality structure. They labelled these two factors as 'acting out' and 'anxious-inhibited' which was similar to higher order structures identified by Morey (25). In a similar confirmatory factor analysis on offenders with IDD Lindsay et al. (23) produced a two factor solution similar to that found previously with an 'avoidant/inhibition' factor with high loadings from schizotypal PD, avoidant PD, obsessive compulsive PD, and a lower loading from schizoid PD; and an 'acting out' factor with high loadings from borderline, narcissistic, and paranoid PD with a smaller loading from antisocial PD. Therefore the higher order dimensions of PD in this study (23) on forensic participants with IDD were similar to those found on populations with mental disorder found in other studies (24–26). These studies suggest that it is eminently feasible to assess PD in people with IDD and that the nature of PD in this population broadly conforms to that seen in the general population. In addition, these studies suggest that when clinicians follow the recommendations from Alexander and Cooray (11), they are likely to produce more accurate evaluations of PD in this client group.

Alexander, Crouch, Halstead, and Piachaud (27) reported on the outcome of 65 patients with ID treated in medium secure forensic hospital settings. They found that the main associations with reconviction were a previous offence of theft or burglary, being younger than 27 years of age and a presence of a PD. This relationship between PD and crime has been shown repeatedly with mainstream offending populations (28). Indeed, one of the main reasons promoting the study of PD has been on the one hand, the predictive relationship between antisocial PD and crime, while on the other, the predictive relationship between borderline PD and psychiatric patient status (29). Morrissey et al (30) found that the Psychopathy Checklist-Revised (PCL-R) was significantly associated with negative treatment progress in terms of a move to more restricted treatment conditions. The PCL-R is strongly associated with antisocial PD. These authors have consistently made the caution that the construct of PD is a highly devaluing label and should be used very carefully with the population of people with IDD who are already highly devalued.

Most of the more recent work on PD and IDD has focused on forensic populations. To give an estimation of the differences in rates of diagnosis, Lunsky et al. (28) compared 74 forensic patients and 282 non forensic mental health patients, all with IDD, referred to mental health in-patient services across Ontario. They found that 32.9 per cent of the forensic cohort and 10.3 per cent of the mental health cohort had been diagnosed with PD. Alexander et al. (49) compared the progress of 138 patients with IDD in a secure setting over a six-year period, 77 with a dissocial or emotionally unstable PD (ICD-10) and 61 without. They found that previous histories of aggression and violence were no different in the two groups, but convictions for violent offences and compulsory detentions were significantly more common in the group with PD. However, there were no clinically significant differences in terms of outcome for the groups and the authors concluded that patients with PD and ID could be successfully treated in a general service for people with ID and a range of mental disorders. Alexander, Chester, Gray, and Snowden (33) contrasted the progress of three groups following treatment in a secure hospital system, one with ID, a second with both ID and PD, and a third with PD only. The two groups with ID appeared to follow similar treatment and management trajectories while the group with PD followed a very different trajectory. Both ID groups had lower rates of post release conviction and lower rates of violent re-offences at two year follow up.

Lindsay et al. (34) studied the relationships between emotional problems and PD using a forensic sample of 212 male participants with IDD. The findings suggested an orderly convergence of emotional problems, personality, and risk. Externalizing emotional problems had a significant relationship with antisocial PD and narcissistic PD, while internalizing emotional problems correlated significantly with avoidant PD. There were similar strong relationships between externalizing emotional problems and dominant personality characteristics and significant negative correlations between externalizing emotional problems and nurturant personality dimensions. There was a strong relationship between narcissistic PD and dominant personality characteristics and further negative statistical relationships between avoidant PD and dominant personality characteristics and negative correlations between antisocial PD and nurturant personality characteristics. Therefore the existing research suggests that PD is a relevant and useful concept in the field of IDD.

Diagnosis: DSM and ICD classifications

This chapter will concentrate on DSM definitions with some reference to ICD. Both systems have been undergoing revisions and the result, especially in the case of the DSM-5 (14), has been a move in the direction of a major shift in the framework for the diagnosis of PD. While the DSM-5 retains the diagnostic system in the DSM-4, it also proposes an alternative system where the assessor uses a four-stage process that is based on both a sound theoretical model of personality development and diagnostic indicators. This system has strengths and weaknesses. Paris (15) has pointed out that it is a more complex process with unfamiliar terminology for busy clinicians who would find it time consuming to follow the precise instructions in the alternative DSM-5 system. However, it has considerable strengths as we shall discuss later.

The main system for the DSM-5 retains detailed trait descriptions for the 10 principal PD diagnoses. These remain paranoid, schizoid, schizotypal, antisocial, borderline, histrionic, narcissistic, avoidant, dependant, and obsessive compulsive PDs. PD Not Otherwise Specified is a final category, in which there may be a number of features of more than one PD, but not enough to meet the full criteria for any specific disorder. In fact this is one of the main criticisms of the system in that around half of the patients with PD are given this latter diagnosis rather than any specific category which is problematic for a classification system (5). The alternate system is a staged process that involves firstly making an assessment of the person's severity of personality functioning; secondly an appraisal of which maladaptive personality traits are present; thirdly, if personality functioning is maladaptive, making a decision on whether the patient conforms to any of six retained PD diagnoses, and finally deciding on the dysfunctional traits that comprise a possible diagnosis of PD trait specified when the person does not fit any of the six categories of PD. The traits specified conform to the five-factor model of personality (explained later) that has emerged from the extensive research on personality (16).

It should be noted that there has been a review of ICD-10 classifications, which takes account of an IDD perspective, the Diagnostic Criteria for Psychiatric Disorders for Use with Adults with Learning Disabilities/Mental Retardation (DC:LD) (17). From the viewpoint of PD there are interesting basic differences in DC-LD. Firstly it recommends that, because of developmental delay in these individuals, diagnosis should not be made until at least 21 years of age. In addition, DC-LD requires the initial confirmation of PD unspecified before progressing to more general diagnoses of PD. PD unspecified requires that the characteristics must not be a direct consequence of the person's IDD and also states specifically that there must be associated significant problems in occupational and/or social functioning. There have also been reviews of DSM-IV and DSM-5 diagnoses of PD with respect to people with IDD (15) resulting in the Diagnostic Manual-Intellectual Disability (DM-ID). The DC-LD and DM-ID have unique considerations for the diagnosis of PD that are designed to accommodate the intellectual and developmental delays that might produce characteristics that could be mistaken for PD. Both suggest that diagnosis should not be made until the age of 21 and both recommend that a provisional diagnosis should be made first and revisited in 12 months to ensure that the features are stable over time. The third major recommendation is that information should be gathered from three sources; self, staff, and observation so that a convergent diagnosis can be made. Other considerations include specific characteristics of IDD and are contained in DM-ID-2 (18). People with IDD may have been encouraged to develop a dependency on others either through institutionalization or through protective family environments. It is not unusual that those with IDD are necessarily dependent on others for several statutory functions especially if they are subject to legal status such as guardianship. These features are difficult to separate out from dependent PD but certainly thought should be given to them in any assessment for dependent PD. Lack of empathy for others is a feature of several PDs and it is also the case that empathy is a perspective taking ability predicated on intellectual development. The intellectual limitations of IDD mean that difficulties with empathy may well be a feature of the developmental delay rather than PD and assessors should be aware of this distinction. Behavioural disturbance is a common feature of IDD and while it might be an enduring personality trait it could also be a symptom of behavioural phenotypes or a consequence of mental illnesses which are more prevalent in people with IDD than in the general population (38). There is also the problem of whether it is even possible to diagnose PD in adults with severe and profound IDD. Both DC-LD and DM-ID-2 suggest that for individuals with severe or profound IDD, personality is not sufficiently developed or mature to allow for reliable diagnosis.

Diagnosis: Alternative system in DSM-5 and the five factor model

The criticism of the DSM-IV's 10 PD categories has been consistent, making the point that the categories have little reference to the predominant model for understanding personality. This is the Five Factor Model (FFM), which has been developed through a considerable body of empirical research. It is based on a trait theory perspective, in that individual differences characterize a person and these, in turn, will influence thoughts, feelings, and behaviours (16). The five factors are thought to be fully comprehensive and generally agreed to be the basic dimensions of 'normal' personality (39). Neuroticism (N) is the most consistent domain and runs on a continuum from neurotic to stable. A tendency to feel negative affect, for example, fear, guilt, or anger, is at the core of N. Extraversion (E) runs on a continuum from extraversion to introversion. E is sometimes known as the 'sociable' domain; however, it also includes factors such as sensation-seeking and assertiveness, which do not necessarily have a sociable component. Openness (O) refers to the individual's openness to experience and covers a wide range of attributes including intellect, imagination, and values. The Agreeableness (A) domain focuses most strongly on interpersonal abilities and needs, and runs on a continuum from agreeable to disagreeable. Conscientiousness (C) reflects determination, strong will, and a sense of duty and is also related to some aspects of N such as impulse control and self-regulation factors (16). Such is its ubiquity, it has been said that the FFM 'is the Christmas tree on which findings of stability, heritability, consensual validation, cross cultural invariance, and predictive utility are hung like ornaments' (40, p. 302).

Despite the extensive work in mainstream populations, at present, there are very few studies on the use of the FFM with people with IDD. Lindsay, Rzepecka, and Law (41) adapted and simplified the language of the measure based on the FFM, the NEO-PI, to be suitable for people with mild IDD. They first tested that the adapted assessment produced results with general population participants very similar to the full questionnaire. They then used the self and respondent versions to assess its applicability for the client group with 40 participants with IDD and carers who knew the person well. They found that there were consistent differences between self and respondent ratings with people with IDD rating themselves as significantly more agreeable, more extraverted, and more conscientious than observers. The difference was an average of 10 percentile points for E where the self-ratings were 5 percentiles above the mean and the respondent mean 5 percentiles below the mean. There was an average difference of 10 percentile points for the A factor and 19 percentile points for the C factor and in both factors respondents rated the participant lower in agreeableness and conscientiousness than the people with IDD did themselves. While this is interesting, it requires replication.

In stark contrast to mainstream research, the predominant models of understanding personality in people with IDD have been motivational. In short, these models assume that people are motivated to a greater or lesser extent by variables such as experience of failure, expectancy of success, creativity, rejection, and so on. For example, Zigler and colleagues have conducted extensive research into personality and IDD (42). They hypothesized that repeated experience of failure on academic and other tasks changed problem-solving style, leading to the avoidance of novel challenging tasks, expecting to fail, and the tendency to look to others for cues as to how to solve these tasks. Factor analytic studies on children and young adults with IDD led Zigler et al. (42) to hypothesize seven personality dimensions, based on motivation to interact with the environment, along which people with IDD varied as follows: Positive reaction tendency (a heightened motivation to both interact with, and be dependent upon, a supportive adult), negative reaction tendency (initial wariness shown when interacting with strange adults), expectancy of success (the degree to which one expects to succeed or fail when presented with a new task), outer directedness (tendency to look to others for the cues to solutions of difficult or ambiguous tasks), efficacy motivation (the pleasure derived from tackling and solving difficult problems), obedience (individual follows directions), and curiosity/creativity. It is immediately noticeable that these personality traits bear little resemblance to the FFM. It would appear that none of Zigler's factors are related to mood or emotion, which is one of the most enduring factors in personality research.

Lindsay, Finlay, Mulholland, Ansari, and Steptoe (43) studied the relationship between the FFM and the Zigler motivational model and found that both were valid in assessing the personality features they addressed in people with IDD and that there was an orderly relationship between the models. They hypothesized that negative reaction tendency would correlate negatively with A, E, O, and C while correlating positively with N and that other factors (apart from negative reaction tendency and N) in both assessments would relate positively together, or not at all. This was generally supported although not all correlations were significant. Using another motivational model for people with IDD, the FFM (44) concluded that 'domains (in the FFM) tended to relate in a rational manner to the Reiss Motives' (p. 214). Therefore, as far as the authors are aware, there are only three studies investigating the use of FFM with people with IDD but all three have validated the FFM for this client group.

As a result of these positive studies it seems appropriate to investigate the extension of the alternative model for assessment of PD to people with IDD. The model is based on empirical research into the relationship between the FFM and PD and employs a staged diagnostic process.

The first stage is recognizing a new general definition of PD that reviews deficits and core components of self and interpersonal personality functioning. Hopwood et al. (45) conducted a prospective study on 605 patients with PD, and found that those personality traits loading most highly on a severity dimension of PD were preoccupation with social rejection, fear of social ineptness, feelings of inadequacy, anger, identity disturbance, and paranoid ideation. They interpreted these items as being consistent with disturbances in the views of ones' self and of other people. These two dimensions—self and interpersonal—have been investigated extensively (46) and have been incorporated as the main dimensions for the initial conception of PD in the alternative DSM-5.

The second stage is based on an assessment of global personality functioning which is represented by five levels of severity in self and interpersonal functioning ranging from normal functioning to extreme deficits. The elements for rating level of personality functioning can be seen in Lindsay et al. (46) and, when they are rated 0–4 on increasing maladaptive personality functioning, constitute the Level of Personality Functioning Scale (LPFS). They are Self 1. Identity: Experience of oneself as unique; stability of self-esteem and accuracy of self-appraisal; capacity to regulate emotional experience; Self 2: Self direction: The pursuit of meaningful short term and life goals; ability to self-reflect productively; Interpersonal 1: Empathy—Comprehension and appreciation of others' experiences and motivations; tolerance of differing perspectives; understanding the effects of one's own behaviour on others; Interpersonal 2: Intimacy—connection with others; capacity for closeness; mutuality of regard. Generalized severity of personality functioning has been found to be the best single predictor of personality pathology. Hopwood et al. (45) found that 'generalised severity (of personality dysfunction) is the most important single predictor of concurrent and prospective dysfunction'. Therefore, there is a considerable amount of evidence supporting the conceptualization of PD in this way and for the clinical utility of evaluating severity. The degrees of disturbance in self and interpersonal dimensions are then continuously distributed from normal/no impairment through mild impairment, moderate impairment, serious impairment, and extreme impairment. DSM 5 contains good descriptions of personality functioning at each point in the scale. In general, a rating of 0 (no impairment) or 1 (some impairment) would indicate that the individual is below the threshold for any consideration of PD. A rating of 2, 3, or 4 (moderate, severe, and extreme impairment respectively) indicate increasing degrees of personality dysfunction when diagnosis of PD should be considered.

Once deficits in personality functioning have been established, the third stage consists of identifying whether or not the person conforms to any particular PD. Six PD types have been retained from the original ten in DSM-IV (and retained in the primary diagnostic system in DSM-V). The six retained PD types are antisocial PD, borderline PD, narcissistic PD, schizotypal PD, avoidant PD, and obsessive compulsive PD. Thus far, the system seems relatively straightforward and has parallels with the ICD-10 system where the assessor is required first to consider whether the person has sufficient dysfunction to be considered for a general diagnosis of PD and then to allocate one or more specific types of dysfunction such as dissocial PD, anankastic PD, impulsive PD, emotional type, and impulsive type.

The final stage in classification pertains to the category of 'personality disorder trait specified' and conforms to the five factor model of personality describing dysfunctional traits in terms of the facets that are associated to each factor. The description for the alternative DSM-5 is the pathological correlate of each FFM dimension as follows: negative affectivity versus emotional stability (neuroticism), detachment v extraversion, antagonism v agreeableness, disinhibition v conscientiousness, and psychoticism v lucidity. It can be seen that the only one that does not conform to the five factors is psychoticism, although it does have some aspects of lack of openness to experience.

In a recent evaluation of the system, Lindsey et al. (47) described the process with four clients with IDD. They used the Assessment of Global Personality Functioning from DSM-5, the International Personality Disorder Examination (IPDE) and the adapted NEO-PI by (20) assesses personality based on the FFM. Three sources of information (recommended by Alexander and Cooray (11)) combined for composite PD assessment: participant interview; interview with key nurse; observations of participant. PD ratings (self, staff, and observer) tended to converge for borderline, antisocial, and narcissistic PDs. NEO-PI ratings converged on Neuroticism,

Extraversion, Openness with discrepancies on agreeableness and conscientiousness (staff rating lower). They concluded that the structured DSM-5 system was easily usable but takes more time than diagnostic interview. Interestingly, the lower staff ratings on agreeableness and conscientiousness supported the findings of Lindsay et al. (23).

Treatment and treatment outcomes

Drawing on her experience in treating people with PD and IDD in an in-patient forensic hospital setting, Johnstone (48) described a four-stage treatment process consisting of:

(i) assessment and motivational work, (ii) interventions including foundation treatments, offence-specific treatments, and personality disorder symptom reduction treatments, (iii) consolidation or relapse prevention and (iv) discharge. This was further developed into the framework of a ten-point treatment programme (32, 49) that could be used both within hospital and community settings. The key elements of this include:

1. A multi-axial diagnostic assessment that covers the degree of intellectual disability, cause of intellectual disability, pervasive developmental disorders, other developmental disabilities, mental illnesses, substance misuse or dependence, personality disorders, physical disorders, psychosocial disadvantage, and types of behavioural problems (for personality disorders, the alternative diagnostic model that combines the FFM, motivational, and a DSM or ICD clinical diagnosis may be used)
2. A collaboratively developed psychological formulation
3. Risk assessments
4. A behaviour support plan
5. Pharmacotherapy, targeting co-morbid mental illnesses, and if clinically indicated predominant symptom complexes
6. Individual and group psychotherapy, guided by the psychological formulation (a range of approaches including dialectical behaviour therapy, cognitive behavioural, or cognitive analytical therapy can be used).
7. Offence-specific therapies, if relevant
8. Education, skills acquisition, and occupational/vocational rehabilitation
9. Increasing community participation
10. Preparation for transition

There is a dearth of treatment studies, be they psychological or pharmacological, reporting progress for people with IDD and PD. Three treatment studies have used an adapted version of Dialectical Behaviour Therapy (DBT) in small groups of people with IDD. Sakdalan, Shaw, and Collier (35) used a 13-week programme with six participants and although the sample size was very small, they found significant improvements on dynamic risk assessment scores. Morrissey and Ingamells (31) developed a longer sixty session DBT programme and reported anecdotal improvements in four out of six participants, maintained 12 months following treatment. Mason (32) reported a single case where assessment of personality and PD guided successful treatment. Regarding pharmacological treatment, the focus is on identifying and actively treating comorbid mental illnesses. If clinically indicated, short-term treatment to target four predominant symptom clusters: behaviour dyscontrol, affective dysregulation, anxiety symptoms, and psychotic symptoms has been suggested and found useful (50, 51). This however should be subject to strict monitoring of the following standards: (a) meticulously recording all the diagnoses, (b) initiating treatment only as part of a multidisciplinary treatment package, (c) clearly identifying the predominant symptom complexes being targeted, (d) identifying and recording in consultation with the patient the expected improvements and behavioural targets, (e) discussing and recording the rationale, effects and potential side-effects of the proposed treatment, (f) having regular follow-up appointments to monitor progress on the expected changes, and (g) specifying a length of time that the person will be tried on medication with the plan to stop if there is no improvement (50, 51).

In terms of longer term follow up, Alexander et al. (27) found that there were no clinically significant differences in terms of outcome between the groups with or without IDD treated in a forensic hospital service while Alexander, Chester, Gray, and Snowden (33) in contrasting the progress of three groups following treatment in the forensic hospital system, one with IDD, a second with both IDD and PD, and a third with PD only found that the two groups with IDD appeared to follow similar treatment and management trajectories with lower rates of violent re-offences while the group with PD alone followed a very different trajectory.

Conclusions and recommendations

The field of IDD and PD has seen huge advances in the last 10 to 15 years. These have produced a greater amount of research in the field and have changed practice towards this client group. The most important changes have been the recommendations to use three sources of information: interview with the person, with a significant other such as a key worker, and observations, in order to make a diagnosis. Using these guidelines the nature of research has altered and has become less conflicted, less contradictory, and more consistent with mainstream research. It would appear that we now have more valid methods to assess PD in this client group.

There is however, much to do in the field. The research that does exist suggests that personality functioning has the same underlying factors in people with IDD as in the general population. That being the case, the models that are currently being developed for assessment of PD are likely to be relevant for people with IDD as long as the relevant guidelines are followed. There are a number of important considerations for people with IDD. The assessor should bear in mind that perspective taking is a developmental skill and that deficits are likely to be features of the IDD itself. Therefore lack of empathy (clearly a perspective taking skill) should be considered in relation to the population of people with IDD in general. Other considerations are in relation to dependency, anger, and whether or not personality problems are stable or situationally specific giving rise to the recommendations that only provisional diagnoses should be made with a further assessment after a year and that diagnosis should not be made prior to the age of 21.

Case study

Mary is a 29-year-old lady with a mild intellectual disability and a long history of behaving aggressively towards people and seriously self-harming. Her mother had a history of alcohol abuse and her father subjected her to sexual abuse from a young age. As a teenager, Mary was involved in a series of abusive relationships with older men who groomed and abused her. Her mood swings became progressively worse in adulthood and she also had had at least three depressive episodes which lasted for about three months each. In between she would have periods of well-being and excessive cheerfulness interspersed with periods of extreme irritability and low mood—this could happen several times in the same week. Occasionally, she would talk about hearing voices in her head, particularly when stressed. She was very conscious of what professionals talked about her and would become very angry when people thought it was 'just behavioural'. A detailed diagnostic clarification suggested the presence of an emotionally unstable personality disorder. The affective symptoms did not always reach the threshold for the diagnosis of a major mood disorder nor was there evidence to support a diagnosis of a psychotic illness. However longitudinal history suggested the presence of a recurrent depressive disorder. Following a comprehensive psychological formulation, she was offered dialectical behaviour therapy and also treated with antidepressant and mood stabilizer prophylaxis. She was found a supported living placement in the community and had access to a community mental health team that could provide crisis care.

MULTIPLE CHOICE QUESTIONS

Questions

Please select the single most appropriate answer.

1. It is advised that the diagnosis of personality disorder in people with an intellectual disability should be made after the age of:

A. 16
B. 18
C. 21
D. 30
E. 65

2. Which of the following is most useful in making a clinical diagnosis of personality disorder in a person with an intellectual disability?

A. Interviewing the person
B. Interviewing an informant who knows the person well
C. Behavioural observations over a period of time
D. Use of structured instruments
E. All of the above

3. All of the following are true about making a diagnosis of personality disorder in a person with an intellectual disability except:

A. The DSM 5 offers a way of making a diagnosis based on criteria as well as an alternate method that draws on personality traits
B. The ICD 10 does not allow this diagnosis to be made
C. The DM-ID proposes that the diagnosis should be made only after the age of 21
D. The DC-LD proposes that the diagnosis should be made only after the age of 21
E. Diagnostic stability can be poor if made before the age of 21

4. The Five Factor Model (FFM) of personality includes all of the following except:

A. Efficacy motivation
B. Extroversion
C. Neuroticism
D. Openness
E. Agreeableness

5. All of the following are true about personality disorders in people with an intellectual disability except:

A. A full diagnostic evaluation and formulation is warranted as part of the treatment programme
B. Dialectical behaviour therapy has been conclusively shown to be the best therapeutic choice
C. An experience of past sexual abuse or childhood victimization is found in many people with the diagnosis
D. There is some evidence that long-term treatment outcomes of those with personality disorders and intellectual disability is different from those with a personality disorder alone
E. Education, skills acquisition, and vocational rehabilitation is part of the treatment process

Answers

1. C. The DC-LD and DM-ID classificatory systems are designed to accommodate the intellectual and developmental delays that might produce characteristics that could be mistaken for PD. Both suggest that diagnosis should not be made until the age of 21, that the provisional diagnosis should be made first and revisited in 12 months to ensure that the features are stable over time and that information should be gathered from multiple sources.
2. E. The use of multiple sources or informants and structured instruments help to make a reliable and valid diagnosis.
3. B. ICD10 does allow this diagnosis to be made.
4. A. The FFM of personality includes neuroticism, extroversion, openness, agreeableness, and conscientiousness. Efficacy motivation is one of seven personality dimensions, proposed by Zigler.
5. B. There are a limited number of treatment and outcome studies. There has been no conclusive evidence that any single mode of treatment is best.

REFERENCES

1. American Psychiatric Association. *Diagnostic and Statistical Manual of Mental Disorders* (3rd ed), DSM-III. Washington DC; 1980.
2. American Psychiatric Association. *Diagnostic and Statistical Manual of Mental Disorders* (4th ed), DSM-IV. 1994.

3. Weissman MM. The epidemiology of personality disorders: a 1990 update. *J Pers Disord* [Internet]. 1993 [cited 2017 Aug 7]; 7:44–62. Available from: http://cat.inist.fr/?aModele=afficheN&cpsidt=4694941.
4. Skodol AE, Gunderson JG, McGlashan TH, Dyck IR, Stout RL, Bender DS, et al. Functional impairment in patients with schizotypal, borderline, avoidant, or obsessive-compulsive personality disorder. *Am J Psychiatry* [Internet]. 2002 Feb [cited 2017 Aug 7];159(2):276–283. Available from: http://www.ncbi.nlm.nih.gov/pubmed/11823271.
5. Zimmerman M. Diagnosing personality disorders. A review of issues and research methods. [Internet]. Vol. 51, *Archives of General Psychiatry*. 1994 [cited 2017 Aug 7]. p. 225–45. Available from: http://www.ncbi.nlm.nih.gov/pubmed/8122959.
6. Khan A, Cowan C, Roy A. Personality disorders in people with learning disabilities: A community survey. *J Intellect Disabil Res* [Internet]. 1997 Aug [cited 2017 Aug 7];41(4):324–30. Available from: http://www.ncbi.nlm.nih.gov/pubmed/9297610.
7. Goldberg B, Gitta MZ, Puddephatt A. Personality and trait disturbances in an adult mental retardation population: Significance for psychiatric management. *J Intellect Disabil Res* [Internet]. 1995 Aug 1 [cited 2017 Aug 7];39(4):284–94. Available from: http://doi.wiley.com/10.1111/j.1365-2788.1995.tb00520.x.
8. Flynn A, Matthews H, Hollins S. Validity of the diagnosis of personality disorder in adults with learning disability and severe behavioural problems preliminary study. *Br J Psychiatry* [Internet]. 2002 [cited 2017 Aug 7];180(JUNE):543–6. Available from: http://bjp.rcpsych.org/content/180/6/543.
9. Naik BI, Gangadharan S, Alexander RT. Personality Disorders in Learning Disability—The Clinical Experience. *Br J Dev Disabil* [Internet]. 2002 Jul 18 [cited 2017 Aug 7];48(95):95–100. Available from: http://www.tandfonline.com/doi/full/10.1179/096979502799104210.
10. Alexander RT, Piachaud J, Odebiyi L, Gangadharan SK. Referrals to a forensic service in the psychiatry of learning disability. *Br J Forensic Pract* [Internet]. 2002 May 11 [cited 2017 Aug 7];4(2):29–33. Available from: http://www.emeraldinsight.com/doi/10.1108/14636646200200013.
11. Alexander R, Cooray S. Diagnosis of personality disorders in learning disability. In: *British Journal of Psychiatry* [Internet]. 2003 [cited 2017 Aug 7]. p. S28–31. Available from: http://www.ncbi.nlm.nih.gov/pubmed/12509306.
12. Brown H, Craft A. Thinking the Unthinkable. London: London; 1989.
13. Cooke LB, Sinason V. Abuse of People with Learning Disabilities and Other Vulnerable Adults. *Adv Psychiatr Treat* [Internet]. 1998 [cited 2017 Feb 23];4(2):119–125. Available from: http://apt.rcpsych.org/cgi/doi/10.1192/apt.4.2.119.
14. American Psychiatric Association. Diagnostic and Statistical Manual of Mental Disorders (5th ed), DSM-V. [Internet]. American Psychiatric Association; 2013 [cited 2017 Feb 20]. 991 pp. Available from: http://psychiatryonline.org/doi/book/10.1176/appi.books.9780890425596.
15. Paris J. The Intelligent Clinician's Guide to the DSM-5 [Internet]. 2013 [cited 2017 Aug 7]. pp. 40–54. Available from: https://books.google.ca/books?hl=en&lr=&id=xKOuBgAAQBAJ&oi=fnd&pg=PP1&dq=intelligent+clinician%27s+guide+dsm&ots=Ch7m9UOlI6&sig=wWydx0YbWveY0v5wG00XsVit0jA.
16. Costa PT, Mccrae RR. Domains and facets : Hierarchical personality assessment using the revised NEO personality inventory. 1995 Jan 1 [cited 2017 Aug 7];64(1):21–50. Available from: https://www.scienceopen.com/document?vid=4f108e6d-cd23-44f7-aa37-21667fa6afd4.
17. Royal College of Psychiatrists. Diagnostic Criteria for Psychiatric Disorders for Use with Adults with Learning Disabilities/Mental Retardation (DC:LD). London: Royal College of Psychiatrists; 2001.
18. Lindsay W, Dana L, Alexander RT, Griffiths D, Wilkinson S. Personality disorders. In: Fletcher R, Barnhill J, Cooper S-A, editors. *Diagnostic Manual—Intellectual Disability* (DM-ID-2). Kingston, NY.: National Association for the Dually Diagnosed; 2016. pp. 599–636.
19. Lindsay WR, Hogue T, Taylor JL, Mooney P, Steptoe L, Johnston S, et al. Two studies on the prevalence and validity of personality disorder in three forensic intellectual disability samples. *J Forensic Psychiatry Psychol* [Internet]. 2006 Sep [cited 2017 Aug 7];17(3):485–506. Available from: http://www.tandfonline.com/doi/abs/10.1080/14789940600821719.
20. Ballinger BR, Reid AH. A standardised assessment of personality disorder in mental handicap. *Br J Psychiatry* [Internet]. 1987 Apr [cited 2017 Aug 7];150:108–109. Available from: http://www.ncbi.nlm.nih.gov/pubmed/3167424.
21. Hogue T, Steptoe L, Taylor JL, Lindsay WR, Mooney P, Pinkney L, et al. A comparison of offenders with intellectual disability across three levels of security. *Crim Behav Ment Heal* [Internet]. 2006 Mar 1 [cited 2017 Aug 7];16(1):13–28. Available from: http://doi.wiley.com/10.1002/cbm.52.
22. Lindsay WR, van Logten A, Didden R, Steptoe L, Taylor JT, Hogue T. The validity of two diagnostic systems for personality disorder in people with intellectual disabilities: A short report. *J Intellect Disabil Offending Behav*. 8(3):104–110.
23. Lindsay WR, Steptoe L, Hogue TE, Taylor JL, Mooney P, Haut F, et al. Internal consistency and factor structure of personality disorders in a forensic intellectual disability sample. *J Intellect Dev Disabil* [Internet]. 2007 Jan [cited 2017 Aug 7];32(2):134–142. Available from: http://www.ncbi.nlm.nih.gov/pubmed/17613684.
24. Blackburn R, Logan C, Renwick SJD, Donnelly JP, Barrett P, Beadle MA, et al. Higher-order dimensions of personality disorder: Hierarchical structure and relationships with the five-factor model, the interpersonal circle, and psychopathy. *J Pers Disord* [Internet]. 2005 Dec [cited 2017 Aug 7];19(6):597–623. Available from: http://www.ncbi.nlm.nih.gov/pubmed/16553558.
25. Morey LC. The categorical representation of personality disorder: A cluster analysis of DSM-III-R personality features. *J Abnorm Psychol* [Internet]. 1988 Aug [cited 2017 Aug 7];97(3):314–321. Available from: http://www.ncbi.nlm.nih.gov/pubmed/3192824
26. Krueger RF, Skodol AE, Livesley WJ, Shrout PE, Huang Y. Synthesizing dimensional and categorical approaches to personality disorders: Refining the research agenda for DSM-V Axis II. *Int J Methods Psychiatr Res* [Internet]. 2007 Jun [cited 2017 Aug 7];16(S1):S65–73. Available from: http://www.ncbi.nlm.nih.gov/pubmed/17623397.
27. Alexander R, Crouch K, Halstead S, Piachaud J. Long-term outcome from a medium secure service for people with intellectual disability. J *Intellect Disabil Res* [Internet]. 2006 Apr [cited 2016 Jul 6];50(Pt 4):305–315. Available from: http://www.ncbi.nlm.nih.gov/pubmed/16507035.
28. Fazel S, Danesh J. Serious mental disorder in 23,000 prisoners: A systematic review of 62 surveys. *Lancet* [Internet]. 2002 Feb 16 [cited 2017 Aug 7];359(9306):545–550. Available from: http://www.ncbi.nlm.nih.gov/pubmed/11867106.
29. Widiger, TA, and Frances AJ. Epidemiology, diagnosis and comorbidity of borderline personality disorder. In: Tislan A, Hales RS, Frances AJ, editors. *Review of Psychiatry*, Volume 8. Washington DC: American Psychiatric Press; 1989. pp. 8–24.

30. Morrissey C, Mooney P, Hogue TE, Lindsay WR, Taylor JL. Predictive validity of the PCL-R for offenders with intellectual disability in a high security hospital: Treatment progress. *J Intellect Dev Disabil* [Internet]. 2007 Jun [cited 2016 Jul 12];32(2): 125–133. Available from: http://www.ncbi.nlm.nih.gov/pubmed/17613683.
31. Lunsky Y, Gracey C, Koegl C, Bradley E, Durbin J, Raina P. The clinical profile and service needs of psychiatric inpatients with intellectual disabilities and forensic involvement. *Psychol Crime Law* [Internet]. 2011 Jan [cited 2017 Feb 20];17(1):9–23. Available from: http://www.tandfonline.com/doi/abs/10.1080/10683160903392277.
32. Alexander RT, Green FN, O'Mahony B, Gunaratna IJ, Gangadharan SK, Hoare S. Personality disorders in offenders with intellectual disability: A comparison of clinical, forensic and outcome variables and implications for service provision. *J Intellect Disabil Res*. 2010;54(7):650–658.
33. Alexander RT, Chester V, Gray NS, Snowden RJ. Patients with personality disorders and intellectual disability—closer to personality disorders or intellectual disability? A three-way comparison. *J Forens Psychiatry Psychol* [Internet]. 2012;23(4):435–451. Available from: http://www.tandfonline.com/doi/abs/10.1080/14789949.2012.694462.
34. Lindsay WR, Taylor JL, Hogue TE, Mooney P, Steptoe L, Morrissey C. Relationship between assessed emotion, personality, disorder and risk in offenders with intellectual disability. *Psychiatry, Psychol Law* [Internet]. 2010 Aug [cited 2017 Aug 7];17(3):385–397. Available from: http://www.tandfonline.com/doi/abs/10.1080/13218710903443344.
35. Sakdalan JA, Shaw J, Collier V. Staying in the here-and-now: A pilot study on the use of dialectical behaviour therapy group skills training for forensic clients with intellectual disability. *J Intellect Disabil Res* [Internet]. 2010 Apr 28 [cited 2017 Aug 7];54(6):568–572. Available from: http://www.ncbi.nlm.nih.gov/pubmed/20456594.
36. Morrissey C, Ingamells B. Adapted dialectical behaviour therapy for male offenders with learning disabilities in a high secure environment: Six years on. *J Learn Disabil Offending Behav* [Internet]. 2011 Jan 24 [cited 2017 Aug 7];2(1):8–15. Available from: http://www.emeraldinsight.com/doi/10.5042/jldob.2011.0024.
37. Mason J. Personality assessment in offenders with mild and moderate intellectual disabilities. *Br J Forensic Pract* [Internet]. 2007 Apr 11 [cited 2017 Aug 7];9(1):31–39. Available from: http://www.emeraldinsight.com/doi/10.1108/14636646200700006.
38. Cooper S-A, Smiley E, Morrison J, Williamson A, Allan L. Mental ill-health in adults with intellectual disabilities: Prevalence and associated factors. *Br J Psychiatry* [Internet]. 2007 Jan 1 [cited 2017 Aug 4];190(1):27–35. Available from: http://www.ncbi.nlm.nih.gov/pubmed/17197653.
39. Emmons RA. Levels and domains in personality: An introduction. *J Pers* [Internet]. 1995 Sep [cited 2017 Aug 7];63(3):341–64. Available from: http://www.ncbi.nlm.nih.gov/pubmed/7562359.
40. Costa PT Jr. and McCrae RR. Bullish on personality psychology. *Psychologist*. 1993;6:302–303.
41. Lindsay WR, Rzepecka H, Law J. An exploratory study into the use of the five factor model of personality with individuals with intellectual disabilities. *Clin Psychol Psychother* [Internet]. 2007 Nov 1 [cited 2017 Aug 7];14(6):428–437. Available from: http://doi.wiley.com/10.1002/cpp.553.
42. Zigler E, Bennett-Gates D, Hodapp R, Henrich CC. Assessing personality traits of individuals with mental retardation. *Am J Ment Retard* [Internet]. 2002 May [cited 2017 Aug 7];107(3):181. Available from: http://www.ncbi.nlm.nih.gov/pubmed/11966331.
43. Lindsay WR, Finlay C, Mulholland P, Ansari D, Steptoe L. The relationship between intellectual disability specific personality assessment and the five factor personality model. *Personal Communication- Lindsay WR.*
44. Boyd S. Five factor model personality functioning in adults with intellectual disabilities. In: Widiger T, Costa P, editors. *Personality disorders and the five factor model of personality*, 3rd edition. Washington DC.: *American Psychological Association*; 2013.
45. Hopwood CJ, Malone JC, Ansell EB, Sanislow CA, Grilo CM, McGlashan TH, et al. Personality assessment in DSM-5: Empirical support for rating severity, style, and traits. *J Pers Disord* [Internet]. 2011 Jun [cited 2017 Aug 7];25(3):305–320. Available from: http://www.ncbi.nlm.nih.gov/pubmed/21699393.
46. Bender DS, Morey LC, Skodol AE. Toward a model for assessing level of personality functioning in DSM-5, part I: A review of theory and methods. *J Pers Assess* [Internet]. 2011 Jul [cited 2017 Aug 7];93(August):332–346. Available from: http://www.ncbi.nlm.nih.gov/pubmed/22804672.
47. Lindsay WR, Steptoe L, McVicker R, Haut F, Robertson C. DSM-IV, DSM-5, and the five-factor model: The diagnosis of personality disorder with intellectual and developmental disabilities. *J Ment Health Res Intellect Disabil* [Internet]. 2017 Aug 14 [cited 2017 Aug 15];1–15. Available from: https://www.tandfonline.com/doi/full/10.1080/19315864.2017.1350226.
48. Johnstone S (2005) 'Intellectually disabled offenders with personality disorder.' Presentation at the 4th International Conference on the Care and Treatment of Offenders with a Learning Disability. University of Central Lancashire, Preston.
49. Alexander RT, Hiremath A, Chester V, Green FN, Gunaratna IJ, Hoare S Evaluation of treatment outcomes from a medium secure unit for people with intellectual disability. *Advances in Mental Health and Intellectual Disabilities* 2011;5(1):22–32.
50. Alexander R, Bhaumik S. Psychotropic medication in the treatment of personality disorders in Intellectual Disability. In Bhaumik S., Branford D, Barrett M. (Eds). *The Frith Prescribing Guidelines for Adults with Learning Disability*, 2016, 3rd Edition.
51. Alexander RT, Tajuddin M, Gangadharan SK. Personality disorders in intellectual disability approaches to pharmacotherapy. *Mental Health Aspects of Developmental Disabilities* 2007;10(4): 129–136.

15

Alcohol and Substance Misuse and People with Intellectual and/or Developmental Disabilities

Tobias Buxton, Verity Chester, Bijil Arackal, Divya Devulapally, and Yona Lunsky

Introduction

Substance misuse is defined as intoxication; regular excessive consumption of and/or dependence on substances that leads to social, psychological, physical, or legal problems. This includes problematic use of both legal and illegal substances (1). Historically, people with intellectual and/or developmental disability (IDD) were considered to have lower rates of alcohol and substance misuse (2). However, since deinstitutionalization, increasing numbers of people with IDD are living within community settings, which correlates with an increase in the use of both illicit and legal intoxicants (3). Knowledge regarding addictions in this population is largely based on small-scale community samples (4, 5). These studies suggested rates of substance use or abuse ranging between 0.5 per cent and 2.6 per cent, but these are likely to be underestimates, due to methodological difficulties and under-recognition of substance misuse in this population (6). Public Health England (7) recently highlighted that many studies underestimate the problem, due to reliance on self-report measures, or including only people known to services, therefore not capturing the 'hidden majority' of people with IDD most likely to misuse alcohol or drugs.

More recent large-scale studies, using linked data, have found that rates of misuse can be as high as the general population, if not higher in those with IDD (8). In clinical samples, substance abuse has been reported as highly prevalent. Salavert and colleagues (9) found that 36.4 per cent (N = 32) of 88 people with ID (40 men and 48 women), met criteria for substance use disorder (SUD). The main SUD was cannabis use disorder (25 per cent), followed by alcohol use disorder (22.7 per cent) and cocaine use disorder (13.6 per cent). The use of more than one substance was the most frequent pattern. A study from a specialized treatment unit reported that nearly 46 per cent of 39 clients with mild to moderate IDD, and severe behavioural and emotional problems, also had histories of alcohol and substance misuse (10). Alcohol is most commonly misused, at rates matching those of the general population (5, 11, 12), followed by cannabis (13, 14). This may reflect the legal status and availability of these substances, and usage in the general population (15). Other drugs known to be misused by people with IDD include amphetamines, caffeine, cocaine, hallucinogens, inhalants, opioids, anxiolytics, hypnotics, and phencyclidine (16); however the exact rates are unknown.

Risk factors

Risk factors for alcohol and substance misuse among those with IDD appear very similar to the general population, and include being a younger age, lower socioeconomic status (17), living in the poorest neighbourhoods, and male gender (8). In one study, those with 'broken families' (i.e. divorce or no family contact) were more likely to use substances, whereas having an 'intact family' was a protective factor, alongside ethnic minority status, and being a younger adolescent (18). Further risk factors include living independently, having comorbid mental disorder, and a disability in the mild rather than moderate to profound range (19,20).

Several psychological and psychosocial risk factors have also been identified. Taggart, McLaughlin, Quinn, and McFarlane (20) interviewed people with IDD who misused substances. These interviews revealed a theme of 'self-medicating against life's negative experiences', with sub-themes of 'psychological trauma' and 'social distance from community'. Furthermore, Hammink, VanDerNagel, and van de Mheen (21) suggested that substance use/misuse in an IDD population may be facilitated by inadequate coping abilities, feelings of loneliness, stigmatization and limited social skills. Taggart, Huxley, and Baker (19) also highlight low self-esteem, disempowerment, inadequate self-control/regulatory behaviour, unemployment, and peer group pressure as further reasons for engaging in substance misuse among those with IDD. Taggart, McLaughlin, Quinn, and McFarlane (20) report past psychological trauma as a further risk factor, such as physical and sexual abuse, which disproportionally affects people with IDD (23). Therefore, individuals with an IDD may use/misuse substances as a way to fit in with others and to feel socially included (24), as a method of coping, stress relief, and soothing during difficult life experiences (25), and in response to loneliness and isolation from the wider community (21), past bullying, separation, and exploitation by others (26).

Poelen, Schijven, Otten, and Didden (27) assessed the role of four personality dimensions (anxiety sensitivity, negative thinking, impulsivity, and sensation seeking) in substance use in individuals with mild to borderline intellectual disabilities (MBID) using the revised version of the Substance Use Risk Profile Scale (SURPS). Findings showed that individuals with higher levels of negative thinking and sensation seeking had more severe drug and alcohol use, while anxiety, sensitivity, and impulsivity were associated with severe alcohol use. The authors concluded these were important targets within therapy for this group. These psychological risk factors make those with IDD uniquely vulnerable with regard to how they use substances and how they interact with other substance users.

Consequences and sequelae

People with IDD experience the same sequelae of drug misuse as the general population, such as mood changes, physical health complications, negative impact on daily living activities and social interactions/relationships, increased risk of physical and/or sexual assault, robbery, accidental injury, criminal prosecution, and damage to reputation and/or employment prospects (28, 29). However, people with IDD also experience additional sequelae, and appear to be particularly vulnerable to developing mental health issues as a result of alcohol/substance misuse (30), with lower amounts of substances precipitating a deterioration in the mental state, and higher rates of psychiatric crisis (31). This deterioration impacts on the functioning of those individuals within society (24, 29).

Further ID-specific consequences include increased social isolation, victimization whilst under the influence, increased cognitive disability, physical impairment, poor impulse control, substance abuse-related medical conditions, and the potential for life-threatening cross-reactions with commonly prescribed psychotropic medications (32). A case study highlighted that an individual with ID, autism, and alcohol use disorder regularly vandalized property, was hospitalized, became doubly incontinent, neglected to eat or take anti-hypertensive medication and unable to attend to his self-care (33). Huxley, Copello, and Day (34) described loss of housing placements and increased likelihood of inpatient admissions as negative social risk factors faced by individuals with IDD who use substances. This opens up a paradox that substances may be used as a form of relief or respite from negative experiences, yet increase isolation and negative experiences (35). Although there is generally a focus on psychological effects of drinking for patients with IDD, there are also physical effects due to vulnerabilities associated with specific genetic syndromes (36). For example, those with physical vulnerabilities associated with Down syndrome are likely to be impacted more by side effects of substance and alcohol misuse.

A recent study compared substance-related and addictive disorders (SRAD) in adults with IDD and examined the sociodemographic and clinical characteristics of adults with both IDD and SRAD, to those with IDD or SRAD only (8). Individuals with both IDD and SRAD had the highest rates of overall morbidity (78.8%, psychiatric comorbidity; 59.5%, high or very high morbidity) and of specific illnesses. The most common psychiatric comorbidities were anxiety disorders (67.6%), followed by affective (44.6%), psychotic (35.8%) and personality disorders (23.5%), while the most common chronic diseases were asthma (27.3%), hypertension (15.3%), chronic obstructive pulmonary disease (13.6%) and diabetes (12.6%). It is currently unclear whether substance misuse precedes mental disorders, or vice versa (8).

There is a well-documented association between mild IDD, substance use, personality factors, and offending behaviour. Rates of substance or alcohol use in those with an IDD in contact with forensic or criminal justice agencies are considerably higher than in those without such contact (4). Studies examining rates of substance or alcohol use in the IDD forensic community vary greatly from 11 per cent (37) to 40–50 per cent (14) (38). This is likely due to differences in definitions of substance misuse (14) Hassiotis et al. (13) found similar rates of lifetime exposure to drugs and drug dependence among a sample of prisoners in England and Wales with IDD and the general prison population. There were few differences in the rates of alcohol dependence, but more prisoners with IDD were dependent on cannabis than peers without IDD (51.2% v. 42.1%, P = 0.01). However, prisoners with IDD and co-morbid substance dependence were less likely to receive help with their dependence or drug education than the general prison population (11.5% v. 22.1%, P = 0.01).

McGillivray and Moore (2001) described a correlation between the 'amount' and frequency of substances used, and the frequency of offences perpetrated by the individual. Plant, McDermott, Chester, and Alexander (14) reported that 47 per cent of inpatients in a forensic unit for people with IDD had a history of harmful use of alcohol or other illicit drugs, with similar rates of prevalence among both genders. Approximately a third of the individuals (35 per cent) had used illicit drugs or alcohol almost immediately prior to being admitted to the hospital or during their index offence. Cannabis and alcohol were most frequently consumed but other illicit substances, such as opiates, cocaine, and stimulants were also used by a significant minority. Previous convictions for violent offences were significantly higher in those with a history of substance misuse, while convictions for sexual offences were less likely.

In a 20-year cohort study including people treated in a community forensic intellectual disability service cohort, Lindsay et al. (39) found that patients with alcohol and substance abuse had a significantly higher rate of previous offending in all offence categories except verbal aggression and non-contact sexual offences. In the general forensic psychiatric population, patients with substance misuse histories were significantly more likely to be reconvicted following admission than those without substance misuse difficulties (40). Though long term follow up is lacking, it is likely these findings will extrapolate to those with IDD. This suggests a need for violence reduction programmes to include substance misuse work, in order to improve treatment outcomes among people with IDD and forensic needs (41).

Alcohol

Historically, studies have suggested people with IDD have lower rates of alcohol misuse than in the general population (42). However, more recent studies suggest rates are closer to those of the general population (5). Secondary analysis of child self-report data collected at age eleven years in the UK's Millennium Cohort indicated that children with IDD are more likely to experiment at an early age with potentially harmful levels of alcohol (43). Public health work aimed at reducing harmful drinking in children must recognize that those with IDD are a high-risk group, and interventions should be targeted appropriately (7).

It has been suggested that when people with IDD drink alcohol, they are more likely to develop alcohol problems than people without IDD (44), for example, drinking to problematic levels (45). It has been highlighted that people with IDD may have difficulties moderating their drinking, due to struggling to understand concepts of quantity, strength of alcoholic beverages and units of alcohol (21). Furthermore, they may be less attuned to effects of alcohol in their body, and experience challenges with behaviours to limit use. Alcohol misuse can have greater ramifications for people with IDD (24, 29). Kerr, Lawrence, Darbyshire, Middleton, and Fitzsimmons (46) stated that excessive alcohol consumption in people with mild/moderate ID presents risks to personal safety via accidental injury, unintended unprotected sex, impaired judgement and risk taking affecting interpersonal relationships, and physical and mental health. The authors also highlighted the physical effects of long-term health problems associated with persistent heavy drinking, including skin and hair damage, circulatory disorders, anaemia, cancer, gastric irritation, cardiac and cerebrovascular disease, neurological disorders, and liver disease, as well as mental effects, including stress, anxiety, and depression.

The ICD-10 (47) defines alcohol dependence syndrome as a cluster of phenomena, that together indicate a diagnosis of dependence. This can include craving for the drug, difficulties in restricting use, primacy, tolerance, withdrawal and persistent use despite associated harmful consequences. Primacy (from ICD-10) is firstly about reduced attention towards family/school/work besides an increase in efforts to obtain alcohol. DSM-V (1) gives a time frame of twelve months, for the following features to occur, for a diagnosis of substance dependence. Criteria include tolerance, craving, withdrawal and perseverance of use despite harm. These criteria are in the context of increased use of the substance, and inability to reduce use of the substance. The DSM includes two other criteria, reduction in social/occupational engagements and use of alcohol in settings that are dangerous to do so (i.e. driving). Assessing the effect of alcohol on social and occupational engagement requires careful consideration in people with ID, as this group have limited social and occupational opportunities generally (48, 49), which should be taken into account before concluding there is no impact on engagement.

Psycho-social treatment of alcohol misuse/dependence

A systematic review of the literature reported that only five studies met inclusion criteria for inclusion as an alcohol intervention for people with IDD (46). Included studies largely aimed to increase knowledge and motivation to change behaviour. These authors highlighted that most of the published work in this area had methodological issues, including small sample sizes, lack of control groups, lack of long term follow up, and use of data collection instruments not tested for reliability and validity. These authors concluded that although a number of potential psychological therapies have been developed or adapted for the IDD population, there is still a dearth of evidence on their success in achieving long-term abstinence. A systematic review investigating autism found no specific intervention studies for alcohol (50).

One of the most popular alcohol programmes, the 12-step approach, used by Alcoholics Anonymous (AA), has been criticized as not accessible for those with IDD (51). The approach requires significant cognitive and social skills in order to comprehend the 12 steps, as well as the use of analogues and metaphors, and requires talking in front of the group. To better tailor these groups to the needs of those with IDD, Sinclair (52) proposed that information be provided more visually, repeating core themes, and checking for comprehension. A further change is to move away from the 'opportunistic' model, whereby educational experiences are stories brought by individuals to the meetings, which are then discussed by group participants. Sinclair felt that this approach requires highly complex social skills, including well-developed empathy and the ability to interpret complex language. Therefore, the learning experience changed to a dialectic one, where key themes are acted out by facilitators in role play. Although this approach showed potential, further research is required on its application and efficacy in people with IDD. Another component of the 12-step approach is the role of the sponsor. Sponsors are established members of AA, who have been sober for a substantial period and mentor other members, give advice and support, and assist them in completing the 12 steps (53). Sponsors are unlikely to have training in intellectual disability or autism, and expecting them to be able to adapt their approach to meet the needs of this client group may be unrealistic (33).

In the general population, motivational interviewing has been used effectively to guide individuals through the cycle of change (54). The efficacy of motivational interviewing has been compared to the 12-step approach and CBT in those with alcoholism and other psychiatric diagnoses but without IDD, and demonstrated comparable outcomes (55). Such approaches have been implemented with people with alcohol dependence without IDD, and have been demonstrably more effective than advice alone (56). Mendel and Hipkins (57) also used motivational interviewing techniques with people with IDD, within group sessions over a period of two weeks, in addition to visual aids and vignettes, reporting that their cohort had an 'improved readiness to change' their behaviours, after completing the course. However, as the participants (n = 7) had no access to alcohol (they were currently in secure accommodation and no details of their release dates were provided), the relevance of moving participants into the 'action' phase is difficult to judge (46).

A number of educational interventions have been described, aiming to support a greater understanding of the risks also associated with substance misuse (58). Lindsay, Smith, Tinsley, Macer, and Miller (59) noted that while alcohol knowledge and awareness do not often feature as necessary in standard programmes, they are included in IDD specific programmes, because for people with IDD, it cannot be assumed that there is equal knowledge across all participants as a starting point for therapeutic intervention. A number of such educational programmes have been described (60, 61). The most recent (62) was set in an inpatient forensic intellectual disability service, and included information on different types of drink and their images, alcohol content/strength, concept of units, and safe limits. The effects of alcohol on behaviour, emotions, and on the body, attitudes to drink, 'sensible', and 'heavy' drinkers were also covered. Topics were introduced by facilitators using multimodal methods including videos, quizzes, assignments, posters, large/small group discussion, and observation. The authors noted the concerns of some support staff, that teaching patients about alcohol might encourage the behaviour. These authors felt that conversely, teaching sensible drinking enabled attendees to make an informed choice and take responsibility for their drinking, with less trial and error. Furthermore, the authors discussed the ethics of imposing abstinence on people with IDD (42), through their living arrangements, lack of opportunity, or as a treatment goal, while simultaneously promoting values such as choice and autonomy in making decisions, to lead as ordinary a lifestyle as any other person in society. Furthermore, these authors noted that substance misuse literature recognizes that whatever external goals are imposed, people will choose their own goals.

A number of alcohol programmes have been described for people with IDD who misuse alcohol and are engaged with criminal justice services (62) (59). These programmes tended to combine alcohol and anger management therapies in order to address both issues concurrently. However, descriptions and evaluations of substance misuse therapies are scarce. Authors have criticized the availability, design, lack of standardization, and absent research evaluations of alcohol and substance misuse treatment programmes for this population, suggesting a large unmet need (40, 63–65).

While preventative, public health initiatives are not specifically targeted towards people with IDD, there are some promising approaches emerging. Kiewik, VanDerNagel, Engels, and de Jong (66) described and evaluated the feasibility and efficacy of an e-learning prevention programme 'prepared on time', for adolescents with intellectual disabilities attending secondary special-needs schools in the Netherlands. While the intervention had no significant impact on substance knowledge, participants in the study group were less influenced by negative modelling of drinking with classmates/friends and their direct environment, than the control group. The authors suggested that individuals with IDD can benefit from direct, in-vivo, role play skills development to practice assertiveness and refusal (62) (19).

Drake and colleagues (33) described a case which highlights some of the clinical and legal challenges faced when treating alcohol use disorder in a person with autism and intellectual disability. The patient (John) was initially offered weekly sessions focused on harm minimization using motivational interviewing and cognitive behavioural therapy (CBT) techniques. John struggled to apply the suggested coping strategies, and later went through three weeks of detoxification followed by a four-week admission to a step-down unit, after which he returned home. One of the main challenges was John's preference for controlled drinking, and to take holidays abroad where alcoholic drinks were included in his holiday package. During a holiday, hotel staff had tried to evict him, following incidents of being intoxicated, incoherent, doubly incontinent, and anti-social. John was arrested, hospitalized, and was eventually chaperoned home, where he continued to drink uncontrollably, and was evicted from his home. Following a second attempt at detoxification, his care team offered weekly psychology sessions, and found a landlord who offered John a tenancy stipulating that he abstain from alcohol, and who provided time-tabled sessions to teach daily living skills. This combination of approaches supported John to remain sober for at least five years.

Pharmacological treatment of alcohol misuse/dependence

The principles and administration of acute treatment of alcohol withdrawal does not differ greatly between the IDD and the general population. The main adaptations required relate to explaining the approach to the patient in an accessible manner, and the considerations of relevant comorbidity, particularly epilepsy. Rates of epilepsy increase relative to the level of intellectual impairment, from 6 per cent in those with mild IDD to 50 per cent in those with profound impairment, a rate between 10 and 100 times the general population (67). Hence, those with the diagnoses of IDD, epilepsy, and alcohol dependence will need closer monitoring than those without such diagnoses.

Looking at the evidence for detoxification, or the withdrawal process in the general population, benzodiazepines are the first line choice. The specific benzodiazepine used will vary geographically or with specific patient issues (68). Other preparations, such as beta blockers, clonidine, carbamazepine, and neuroleptics (phenothiazines and haloperidol) can be used as an adjunct to benzodiazepine. Beta-blockers and clonidine reduce the symptoms of withdrawal but have no effect on seizures. Carbamazepine could be used in those with high risk or past withdrawal seizures and neuroleptics would be used to treat agitation and delirium (68). Neuroleptics are considered to reduce the seizure threshold but those recommended are those with lower effect on the seizure threshold (phenothiazines and haloperidol) and are expected to be used in those with severe delirium despite adequate benzodiazepine (69).

Following the withdrawal phase of treatment, two pharmacological treatments can be used to promote abstinence. These are disulfiram (antabuse) and naltrexone (70, 71). Disulfiram prompts unpleasant symptoms including dizziness and nausea if alcohol is consumed after taking the drug, and these side effects can become dangerous if drinking is continued. For this reason, it is important that this medication is prescribed to individuals with IDD with even more care, that is, they should have the ability to understand the ramifications of continued drinking. Due to this, naltrexone may be first choice for maintaining abstinence (16). Naltrexone affects the enjoyment or 'high' from the alcohol consumed, rather than affecting the craving for alcohol, or a deterrent response observed with disulfiram (72).

Smoking

The exact prevalence of smoking in people with IDD is unknown (73). However, it is expected that smoking is equally as prevalent, particularly among those with mild levels of IDD. A number of factors influence the likelihood of smoking among people with IDD. Rimmer, Braddock, and Marks (42) reported that people with IDD living in the least restrictive settings were more likely to smoke. It has also been suggested that people with IDD are particularly influenced if their care staff/role models are smokers (5, 74). It would be expected that this influence would be somewhat reduced today, as policies surrounding smoking have changed in many jurisdictions, and it is no longer acceptable for care workers to smoke when they are with their clients, or conversely, for staff to be at risk of second hand smoke when supporting clients.

The risks of smoking are equally high for people with IDD, with increased risk of developing a range of health problems including cancer, heart disease, chronic obstructive pulmonary disease, circulatory problems, stroke, and cognitive decline (46). Further considerations relate to the presence of common comorbid physical and mental disorders. A recent study highlighted that 49 per cent of people with IDD are prescribed psychotropic medication (75). As nicotine can alter the metabolism of many antipsychotic drugs, potentially altering their efficacy and contributing to resistance (76, 77), it is important that smoking is screened for when treating mental or behavioural health in this population. Unfortunately, it has been suggested those with IDD may be less likely to be screened, asked about their smoking status, or offered smoking-related advice by health professionals, most likely due to prevailing views that people with IDD do not smoke (78).

Few published studies have reported outcomes from smoking intervention programmes for those with IDD. Tracy and Hosken (79) described the adaptation of an existing smoking cessation programme, as it was felt that the existing course relied on levels of literacy and abstract thinking which would have excluded this population. The study had a small sample (N = 11) and was aimed specifically at those living independently in the community. The programme components were group discussions, short information-giving segments, videos, role playing, and a board game based on smoking education. The course consisted of a weekly two-hour session over seven weeks. The results were encouraging, with 55 per cent of the sample either quitting smoking altogether or significantly cutting down post-intervention. All patients who participated in the programme demonstrated increased knowledge and concern about the effects of smoking. Chester et al. (73) described a smoking cessation programme and its outcomes in a forensic IDD service. The programme included accessible health information provision, either via one-to-one sessions with their primary nurse, within group health promotion sessions, or through primary care. The service also implemented a smoking timetable which restricted the number of cigarettes which could be smoked daily. The findings of this evaluation were positive, with roughly a third of smokers giving up during their hospital stay. Though small-scale studies, both demonstrate that people with IDD are able to benefit from psychoeducational intervention programmes, when these interventions are adapted to ensure accessibility.

Along with the use of psychoeducational interventions, guidance supports nicotine replacement therapy (NRT) for all who smoke. There is a lack of research on the use of NRT and people with IDD, and additional education and information may be required for this group (The National Institute for Health and Care Excellence [NICE], 77). Further to NRT, NICE also suggest bupropion or varenicline, as long as risks are fully explained to the individual before starting the medication. There is some concern that varenicline could cause both a worsening of psychiatric disorders and increased risk of suicide (81), though recent evidence suggests these risks may be over reported (82). Despite this, a degree of caution should be used when prescribing, until this issue is clarified in further research.

The accessibility and impact of public health initiatives on the smoking behaviour of people with IDD is unclear. For example, one primary prevention strategy is to increase taxes and therefore the price of cigarettes (83). While this may support smoking cessation at the population level, people with IDD are known to experience difficulties in budgeting and may get into further difficulties due to continued smoking despite price increases. Burtner et al. (77) highlighted that many people with IDD have a reduced capacity to understand the complications and implications of smoking, and as a result, this group are more susceptible to the health risks, financial implications, and stigma associated with smoking (84). It is therefore necessary to tailor smoking awareness and cessation programmes (80) to the unique needs of those with IDD.

Barriers to effective treatment and interventions

When the substance use of an individual with IDD becomes problematic, they require equal access to treatments and interventions for this issue. However, people with IDD face additional difficulties accessing addiction services. Adults with IDD are underrepresented within specialist substance misuse services (5). Often, individuals may only be seen by a single team, which tends to be their IDD service (5, 85). Typically, there is lack of referral from IDD services to specialist drug misuse services, and a lack of recognition of need. McLaughlin, Taggart, Quinn, and Milligan (86) report that individuals referred to mainstream support services for substance use had negative experiences.

In America a large study indicated that young people with an IDD were less likely to engage in treatment for substance misuse following a referral into mainstream services (32, 87), while others have pointed out that apparent lack of co-operation may be due to a lack of understanding, rather than a lack of motivation to engage in treatment (7). This report also highlighted that people with IDD may be dependent upon carers and paid staff to make the positive life changes emphasized in mainstream drug and alcohol services. Drake and colleagues (33) noted that elements of standard treatment for alcohol dependence may not be appropriate for people with autism and learning disability, including psychoeducation, psychological therapy (e.g. CBT and motivational interviewing), outcome monitoring, support groups (e.g. AA), community and inpatient detoxification, and assisted withdrawal treatment. Forced involvement in group sessions may be anxiety and anger provoking for ASD patients and may precipitate drop out or rejection from the group (50).

This indicates barriers for this population in accessing generic support. While patients may prefer to be treated by a specialized IDD service, van Duijvenbode et al. (2015) note that those working in IDD services insufficiently incorporate scientific developments in addiction medicine and general psychiatry into the care of their patients, and therefore inaccurately view substance misuse as a relatively simple behavioural problem rather than a chronic brain disease, characterized by the persistent desire to use and the inability to cut down or control their intake. Furthermore, there is a lack of screening and formal assessment of substance use within IDD services, with staff members relying on their clinical judgement, which are unreliable, and prone to underestimation. Due to this, it has been suggested only more serious cases are picked up, missing chances to intervene earlier for those with less severe difficulties (88).

Staff in drug and alcohol services do not have appropriate training for working with people with IDD (7). Alcohol and drug professionals reported using the same assessments they use for the general population (7), yet commonly used screening and assessment measures are inappropriate for those with IDD, because of the requirement of substance-related knowledge that individuals with IDD often lack, use lengthy phrases, difficult wordings, and double negative phrases, and the tendency of individuals with IDD to acquiescence, as well as to 'naysay' (88). Training for both service professionals is required to ensure the needs of this group are not overlooked (32). Screening, referrals, and increased partnership working between mainstream addiction services and IDD teams, via the utilization of liaison professionals is recommended (7).

A further barrier to care is regarding the accessibility of population level preventative measures, such as generic government alcohol and substance misuse public health campaigns, and alcohol and substance education in schools (14). It has been suggested that people with IDD often struggle to access and interpret generic health campaigns, due to difficulties in reading, interpreting, and understanding written information (77). Children and young people with IDD are similarly excluded from alcohol and substance education and other preventative measures (28). People with IDD also experience considerable difficulties in voicing and asserting their health care needs.

Improving care for those with IDD and substance misuse

While research has established the current issues relative to the provision of services for those with IDD and substance misuse issues, few have focused on the implementation of practice improvements for this group. Therefore, the recent publication of a clinical resource by Public Health England (7) is both timely and welcomed. The resource describes a number of practical improvements and service examples which have been implemented in the UK, and how these could be rolled out elsewhere. Practice examples included joint working between substance misuse and IDD services, by:

- Raising awareness of IDD in the local drug and alcohol team through training delivered by IDD nurses and the health Expert by Experience, a young man with learning disabilities
- Identifying a IDD champion within substance misuse teams, and a substance misuse champion within the IDD team
- Introducing the IDD Screening Tool, to assist with identifying people who have intellectual disabilities
- Introducing a number of reasonable adjustments, including easy-read leaflets and information (for example, the service leaflet), harm minimization and making a complaint. Developing an easy-read section of the drug and alcohol website
- Recognition by the drug and alcohol team of how to support people with additional needs by using relevant and targeted approaches to recovery.
- Environmental improvements to building access, toilets and signage
- Developing flagging systems and audits—to track people with intellectual disabilities within substance misuse treatment and audit cases to monitor effective joint working.
- Joint working including developing a local referral pathway for people with intellectual disabilities with substance abuse problems between drug and alcohol, and the community IDD nurses
- Developing a discharge plan—many common issues can come up when someone needs to be discharged from services.

While these ideas were examples implemented in single teams (more examples in the full report), not yet adopted nationally, they provide inspiration for good practice. Furthermore, while costs of such adaptations were not described in the report, it is likely that any costs are offset by savings elsewhere in the care pathway and across the lifetime care of an individual with IDD. It will be important to carry out economic analyses alongside the development of new services.

Summary

As people with IDD are increasingly living within community settings, there is an associated rise in the contact with, use and misuse of, and addiction to, both illicit and legal intoxicants. While risk factors are largely similar to the general population, trauma and social factors disproportionately affect people with IDD. Consequences of substance misuse mirror, and also exceed those of the general population, with increased likelihood of mental, social, and physical health consequences. Many people with IDD and substance misuse histories come into contact with criminal justice agencies and forensic services, thus highlighting a need for improved access to substance misuse interventions in both community settings, and while within forensic services in order to reduce negative outcomes for this group. Any medical treatment for substance misuse has to consider the additional physical and mental comorbidities which commonly co-occur with IDD.

There is a developing evidence base of the application of psychological treatments to this population. Any application of therapies developed for the general population require significant adaption to ensure accessibility to those with IDD. Intervention development and evaluations are therefore urgently required for this group. Furthermore, focus on population level, public health, and preventative initiatives are required. It is recommended that health services review their current provision of services to those with both IDD and substance misuse at a national level, working towards joint working, sharing referrals, and coordinating care between both service types.

MULTIPLE CHOICE QUESTIONS

Questions

Please select the single most appropriate answer.

1. Reported risk factors for engaging in substance misuse among people with ID include all the following except:

A. Younger age
B. Lower socioeconomic status
C. Male gender
D. Moderate degree of learning disability
E. Living independently

2. Consequences and sequalae of substance misuse in people with ID include all the following except:

A. A paradoxical improvement in impulse control
B. Lower amounts of substance use producing adverse mental states
C. Increased occurrence of psychiatric crises
D. Increased risk of victimization while under the influence
E. Increased cognitive disability

3. Which of the following is true about alcohol use or abuse in people with ID?

A. When people with ID drink alcohol, they are less likely to develop alcohol problems than people without ID

B. The UK millennium cohort data suggest that children with ID are more likely to experiment at an early age with potentially harmful levels of alcohol
C. The 12-step approach can be used without any adaptation in people with ID and alcohol misuse or dependence.
D. Motivational interviewing techniques cannot be used in people with ID.
E. Individuals with ID do not benefit from direct, in-vivo, role-play skills development to practise assertiveness and refusal

4. All the following are true about pharmacological management of alcohol withdrawal and dependence except:
A. Benzodiazepines are the first line of managing acute withdrawal symptoms
B. The prescriber must consider commonly comorbid ID genetic syndromes
C. Naltrexone may be preferable to disulfuram as the drug of choice to maintain abstinence
D. The prescriber must consider diagnostic comorbidity such as epilepsy
E. Acute withdrawal symptoms rarely need treatment in people with ID and alcohol dependence.

5. Which of the following is true about smoking (tobacco) in people with ID?
A. People with ID are not particularly influenced if their care staff are smokers
B. In people with ID, nicotine does not alter the metabolism of antipsychotic drugs
C. Among those with mild ID, smoking is as prevalent as among those without an ID
D. People with ID living in the least restrictive settings are much less likely to smoke
E. NRT, varenicline and bupropion are contraindicated in people with ID and smoking

Answers

1. D. Risk factors appear very similar to the general population, and include younger age, lower socioeconomic status, living in the poorest neighbourhoods, male gender, living independently, and having a disability in the mild rather than moderate to profound range.
2. A. Impulse control tends to worsen.
3. B. People with ID are more likely to develop problems when abusing alcohol. Alcohol problems than people without ID. The 12-step approach and motivational interviewing techniques may need adaptations for people with ID. Therapy which includes direct, in-vivo, role-play skills development to practise assertiveness and refusal is of benefit to people with ID.
4. E. The broad principles of pharmacological management are the same as in the general population. Disulfiram prompts extremely unpleasant and potentially dangerous symptoms if alcohol is consumed after taking the drug. Understanding this fully may be problematic for many people with ID and hence naltrexone may be first choice for maintaining abstinence.
5. C. The prevalence of smoking in those with mild ID is similar to the general population. It is higher in those living in less restrictive settings. The pharmacological approach to treatment is similar to that in the general population.

REFERENCES

1. American Psychiatric Association. Diagnostic and statistical manual of mental disorders (5th ed.). Arlington, VA: *American Psychiatric Publishing*; 2013.
2. Edgerton RB. Alcohol and drug use by mentally retarded adults. *Am J Ment Defic.* 1986 May [cited 2017 Apr 3];90(6):602–609.
3. Slayter EM. Understanding and overcoming barriers to substance abuse treatment access for people with mental retardation. *J Soc Work Disabil Rehabil.* 2008 [cited 2017 Feb 20];7(2):63–80.
4. McGillivray JA, Moore MR. Substance use by offenders with mild intellectual disability. *J Intellect Dev Disabil.* 2001 Jan [cited 2017 Feb 20];26(4):297–310.
5. McGillicuddy NB. A review of substance use research among those with mental retardation. Vol. 12, *Mental Retardation and Developmental Disabilities Research Reviews.* 2006 [cited 2017 Feb 20]. pp. 41–47.
6. VanDerNagel JEL, Kiewik M, van Dijk M, Didden R, Korzilius HPLM, van der Palen J, et al. Substance use in individuals with mild to borderline intellectual disability: A comparison between self-report, collateral-report and biomarker analysis. *Research in Developmental Disabilities.* 2015 [cited 2017 Apr 3];151–159.
7. Public Health England. Substance Misuse and People with learning Disabilities: Making Reasonable Adjustments to Services. London; 2017.
8. Lin E, Balogh R, Mcgarry C, Selick A, Dobranowski K, Wilton AS, et al. Substance-related and addictive disorders among adults with intellectual and developmental disabilities (IDD): an Ontario population cohort study Conclusions: SRAD is a significant concern for adults. *BMJ Open.* 2016 Sep 2 [cited 2017 Mar 14];6(9):e011638.
9. Salavert J, Clarabuch A, Fernández-Gómez MJ, Barrau V, Giráldez MP, Borràs J. Substance use disorders in patients with intellectual disability admitted to psychiatric hospitalisation. *J Intellect Disabil Res.* 2018 Nov 1 [cited 2019 Mar 26];62(11):923–930.
10. Didden R, Embregts P, van der Toorn M, Laarhoven N. Substance abuse, coping strategies, adaptive skills and behavioral and emotional problems in clients with mild to borderline intellectual disability admitted to a treatment facility: A pilot study. *Res Dev Disabil.* 2009 Sep [cited 2017 Apr 3];30(5):927–932.
11. Burgard JF, Donohue B, Azrin NH, Teichner G. Prevalence and treatment of substance abuse in the mentally retarded population: An empirical review. *J Psychoactive Drugs.* 2000 Sep 6 [cited 2017 Feb 16];32(3):293–298.
12. Pacoricona Alfaro DL, Ehlinger V, Spilka S, Ross J, Sentenac M, Godeau E. Alcohol, tobacco and cannabis use: Do students with mild-intellectual disability mimic students in the general population? *Research in Developmental Disabilities.* 2015 [cited 2017 Apr 3];118–131.
13. Hassiotis A, Gazizova D, Akinlonu L, Bebbington P, Meltzer H, Strydom A. Psychiatric morbidity in prisoners with intellectual disabilities: Analysis of prison survey data for England and Wales. *Br J Psychiatry.* 2011 Aug 1 [cited 2017 Feb 20];199(2):156–157.

14. Plant A, McDermott E, Chester V, Alexander RT. Substance misuse among offenders in a forensic intellectual disability service. *J Learn Disabil Offending Behav*. 2011 Jul 15 [cited 2017 Feb 20];2(3):127.
15. Chaplin E, Gilvarry C, Tsakanikos E. Recreational substance use patterns and co-morbid psychopathology in adults with intellectual disability. *Res Dev Disabil*. 2011;32(6):2981–6.
16. Stavrakaki C. Substance related disorders in persons with developmental disabilities. In: *Mental Health Needs of Persons with Developmental Disabilities*. 2002. pp. 455–81.
17. Poulton R, Caspi A, Milne BJ, Thomson WM, Taylor A, Sears MR, et al. Association between children's experience of socioeconomic disadvantage and adult health: A life-course study. *Lancet*. 2002 Nov 23 [cited 2017 Feb 20];360(9346):1640–1645.
18. Kepper A, Monshouwer K, van Dorsselaer S, Vollebergh W. Substance use by adolescents in special education and residential youth care institutions. *Eur Child Adolesc Psychiatry*. 2011 Jun 14 [cited 2017 Apr 2];20(6):311–319.
19. Frielink N, Schuengel C, Kroon A, Embregts PJCM. Pretreatment for substance-abusing people with intellectual disabilities: Intervening on autonomous motivation for treatment entry. *J Intellect Disabil Res*. 2015 Dec [cited 2017 Feb 20];59(12):1168–1182.
20. Taggart L, Huxley A, Baker G. Alcohol and illicit drug misuse in people with learning disabilities: Implications for Research and Service Development. *Adv Ment Heal Learn Disabil*. 2008 Mar [cited 2017 Feb 20];2(1):11–21.
21. Taggart L, McLaughlin D, Quinn B, McFarlane C. Listening to people with intellectual disabilities who misuse alcohol and drugs. *Heal Soc Care Community*. 2007 Feb 7 [cited 2019 Mar 25];15(4):360–368.
22. Hammink AB, Vandernagel J, Van De Mheen D. Dual disorders: Mild intellectual disability and substance abuse. In: *Co-Occurring Addictive and Psychiatric Disorders: A Practice-Based Handbook from A European Perspective*. Berlin, Heidelberg: Springer Berlin Heidelberg; 2015 [cited 2017 Apr 2]. pp. 205–220.
23. Cooke LB, Sinason V. Abuse of people with learning disabilities and other vulnerable adults. *Adv Psychiatr Treat*. 1998 Mar 1 [cited 2017 Feb 23];4(2):119–125.
24. Chapman SL, Wu L-T. Substance abuse among individuals with intellectual disabilities. *Res Dev Disabil*. 2012 [cited 2017 Feb 20];33(4):1147–1156.
25. Kouimtsidis C, Fodor-Wynne L, Scior K, Hunter R, Baio G, Pezzoni V, et al. Extended brief intervention to address alcohol misuse in people with mild to moderate intellectual disabilities living in the community (EBI-ID): Study protocol for a randomised controlled trial. *Trials*. 2015 Mar 25 [cited 2017 Mar 23];16:114.
26. Thomas P. 'Mate crime': Ridicule, hostility and targeted attacks against disabled people. *Disabil Soc*. 2011 Jan [cited 2017 Mar 13];26(1):107–111.
27. Poelen EAP, Schijven EP, Otten R, Didden R. Personality dimensions and substance use in individuals with mild to borderline intellectual disabilities. *Res Dev Disabil*. 2016 [cited 2017 Apr 3];63:1–9.
28. Snow PC, Wallace SD, Munro GD. Drug education with special needs populations: Identifying and understanding the challenges. *Drugs Educ Prev Policy*. 2001 Jan 10 [cited 2017 Feb 20];8(3):261–273.
29. Neirynck S, Vanderplasschen W, Vanheule S, Vandevelde S. Substance use and misuse in persons with intellectual disabilities (ID): Results of a survey in ID and addiction services in Flanders. *Res Dev Disabil*. 2014 Jan [cited 2017 Feb 20];35(1):1–9.
30. Papachristou E, Anagnostopoulos D. Behavioral disorders and substance abuse in adolescents with mental retardation. *Psychiatriki*. 2014;25(2):139–150.
31. Westermeijer J, Kemp K, Nugent S. Substance disorders among persons with mild mental retardation. *Am J Addict*. 1996 Jan [cited 2017 Feb 20];5(1):23–31.
32. Slayter EM. Disparities in access substance abuse treatment among people with intellectual disabilities and serious mental illness. *Health Soc Work*. 2010 Feb 1 [cited 2017 Apr 2];35(1):49–59.
33. Drake ACLL, Hank D, Edwards R, Ensum I, Bateman L. The bounds of liberty: Lessons learnt from treating a man with alcohol use disorder, autism and learning disability. *Tizard Learn Disabil Rev*. 2018 Jan 2 [cited 2019 Mar 24];23(1):27–34.
34. Huxley A, Copello A, Day E. Substance misuse and the need for integrated services. *Learn Disabil Pract*. 2005 Jul [cited 2017 Apr 2];8(6):14–17.
35. Day C, Lampraki A, Ridings D, Currell K. Intellectual disability and substance use/misuse: A narrative review. *J Intellect Disabil Offending Behav*. 2016 Mar 14 [cited 2017 Apr 2];7(1):25–34.
36. Ryan R, Sunada K. Medical evaluation of persons with mental retardation referred for psychiatric assessment. *Gen Hosp Psychiatry*. 1997 Jul [cited 2017 Feb 20];19(4):274–280.
37. Lunsky Y, Gracey C, Koegl C, Bradley E, Durbin J, Raina P. The clinical profile and service needs of psychiatric inpatients with intellectual disabilities and forensic involvement. *Psychol Crime Law*. 2011 Jan [cited 2017 Feb 20];17(1):9–23.
38. Søndenaa E, Rasmussen K, Palmstierna T, Nøttestad J. The prevalence and nature of intellectual disability in Norwegian prisons. *J Intellect Disabil Res*. 2008 Dec [cited 2017 Feb 20];52(12):1129–1137.
39. Lindsay WR, Steptoe L, Wallace L, Haut F, Brewster E. An evaluation and 20-year follow-up of a community forensic intellectual disability service. *Crim Behav Ment Health*. 2013 Apr;23(2):138–149.
40. Scott F, Whyte S, Burnett R, Hawley C, Maden T. A national survey of substance misuse and treatment outcome in psychiatric patients in medium security. *J Forens Psychiatry Psychol*. 2004 Dec [cited 2017 Apr 3];15(4):595–605. Available from: http://www.tandfonline.com/doi/abs/10.1080/14789940412331305556.
41. Alexander RT, Hiremath A, Chester V, Green FN, Gunaratna IJ, Hoare S. Evaluation of treatment outcomes from a medium secure unit for people with intellectual disability. *Adv Ment Heal Intellect Disabil*. 2011 Jan 24 [cited 2019 Mar 11];5(1):22–32.
42. Rimmer JH, Braddock D, Marks B. Health characteristics and behaviors of adults with mental retardation residing in three living arrangements. *Res Dev Disabil*. 1995;16:489–499.
43. Emerson E, Robertson J, Baines S, Hatton C. Predictors of self-reported alcohol use and attitudes toward alcohol among 11-year-old British children with and without intellectual disability. *J Intellect Disabil Res*. 2016 Dec [cited 2017 Apr 14];60(12):1212–1226.
44. Reis O, Wetzel B, Häßler F. Mild or borderline intellectual disability as a risk for alcohol consumption in adolescents—A matched-pair study. *Research in Developmental Disabilities*. 2015 [cited 2017 Apr 3];132–141.
45. McGillicuddy NB, Blane HT. Substance use in individuals with mental retardation. *Addict Behav*. 1999 [cited 2017 Apr 14];24(6):869–878.
46. Kerr S, Lawrence M, Darbyshire C, Middleton AR, Fitzsimmons L. Tobacco and alcohol-related interventions for people with

mild/moderate intellectual disabilities: A systematic review of the literature. *J Intellect Disabil Res*. 2013 May [cited 2017 Feb 21];57(5):393–408.
47. World Health Organization. ICD-10 Classification of Mental and Behavioural Disorders; Diagnostic Criteria for Research. World Health Organization; 1992. 248 pp.
48. Forrester-Jones R, Carpenter J, Coolen-Schrijner P, Cambridge P, Tate A, Beecham J, et al. The social networks of people with intellectual disability living in the community 12 years after resettlement from long-stay hospitals. *J Appl Res Intellect Disabil*. 2006 Dec [cited 2017 Mar 7];19(4):285–295.
49. Cox A, Simmons H, Painter G, Philipson P, Hill R, Chester V. Real work opportunities: Establishing an accessible vocational rehabilitation programme within a forensic intellectual disability service. *J Intellect Disabil Offending Behav*. 2014;5(4):160–166.
50. Arnevik EA, Helverschou SB. Autism spectrum disorder and co-occurring substance use disorder—A systematic review. *Subst Abuse*. 2016;10:69–75.
51. Quintero M. Substance abuse in people with intellectual disabilities. *Soc Work Today*. 2011 [cited 2017 Feb 20];11(4):26.
52. Sinclair TJJ. Meeting the needs of persons with mental retardation within a twelve-step program of recovery. *NADD Bull*. 2004 [cited 2017 Feb 20];7(6).
53. Whelan PJP, Marshall EJ, Ball DM, Humphreys K. The role of AA sponsors: A pilot study. *Alcohol Alcohol*. 2009 Jul 1 [cited 2019 Mar 25];44(4):416–422.
54. Prochaska JO, DiClemente CC. Transtheoretical therapy: Toward a more integrative model of change. *Psychother Theory, Res Pract*. 1982 [cited 2017 Feb 20];19(3):276–288.
55. Project Match Research Group. Matching alcoholism treatments to client heterogeneity: Project MATCH posttreatment drinking outcomes. *J Stud Alcohol*. 1997 Jan [cited 2017 Feb 20];58(1): 7–29.
56. Rubak S, Sandbæk A, Lauritzen T, Christensen B. Motivational interviewing: A systematic review and meta-analysis. Vol. 55, *British Journal of General Practice*. Royal College of General Practitioners; 2005 [cited 2017 Feb 20]. pp. 305–312.
57. Mendel E, Hipkins J. Motivating learning disabled offenders with alcohol-related problems: A pilot study. *Br J Learn Disabil*. 2002;30(4):153–158.
58. Steel A, Ritchie G. Psycho-educational approach to addiction—a case study. *Drugs and Alcohol Today*. 2004 Dec [cited 2017 Feb 20];4(4):30–33.
59. Lindsay WR, Smith KJ, Tinsley S, Macer J, Miller S. A programme for alcohol related violence with offenders with intellectual disability. *J Intellect Disabil Offending Behav*. 2014 Jun 3 [cited 2017 Apr 3];5(2):107–119.
60. McCusker CG, Clare ICH, Cullen C, Reep J. Alcohol related knowledge and attitudes in people with a mild learning disability: The effects of a sensible drinking group. *J Community Appl Soc Psychol*. 1993 Apr [cited 2017 Apr 3];3(1):29–40.
61. Lindsay WR, Allen R, Walker P, Lawrenson H, Smith AHW. An alcohol education service for people with learning difficulties. *Ment Handicap*. 1991 Aug 26 [cited 2017 Apr 3];19(3):96–100.
62. Brown G, Coldwell B. Developing a controlled drinking programme for people with learning disabilities living in conditions of medium security. *Addict Res Theory*. 2006 Jan 11 [cited 2017 Apr 3];14(1):87–95.
63. Sandbrook J, Clark T, Cocksedge KA. Addressing substance misuse in medium secure settings in the UK and Ireland—a survey of current practice. *J Forensic Pract*. 2015 Aug 10 [cited 2017 Apr 3];17(3):192–203.
64. Weldon S, Ritchie G. Treatment of dual diagnosis in mentally disordered offenders: Application of evidence from the mainstream. *Adv Dual Diagn*. 2010 Jul 6 [cited 2017 Apr 3];3(2):18–23.
65. Whyte S, Harrison C. Substance misuse services in secure psychiatric units. *Med Sci Law*. 2004 Jan [cited 2017 Apr 3];44(1):71–74.
66. Kiewik M, VanDerNagel JEL, Engels RCME, de Jong CAJ. The efficacy of an e-learning prevention program for substance use among adolescents with intellectual disabilities: A pilot study. *Res Dev Disabil*. 2016 [cited 2017 Apr 3];60:191–200.
67. Lhatoo SD, Sander JWAS. The epidemiology of epilepsy and learning disability. *Epilepsia*. 2001 Mar [cited 2017 Feb 20];42(14):6–9.
68. Mayo-Smith MF. Pharmacological management of alcohol withdrawal. A meta-analysis and evidence-based practice guideline. American Society of Addiction Medicine Working Group on Pharmacological Management of Alcohol Withdrawal. *JAMA*. 1997 Jul 9 [cited 2017 Feb 20];278(2):144–151.
69. Taylor D, Paton C, Kapur S. The Maudsley Prescribing Guidelines in Psychiatry. Wiley-Blackwell; 2015.
70. Azrin NH, Sisson RW, Meyers R, Godley M. Alcoholism treatment by disulfiram and community reinforcement therapy. *J Behav Ther Exp Psychiatry*. 1982 Jun [cited 2017 Feb 20];13(2):105–112.
71. O'Malley SS, Jaffe AJ, Chang G, Schottenfeld RS, Meyer RE, Rounsaville B. Naltrexone and coping skills therapy for alcohol dependence. A controlled study. *Arch Gen Psychiatry*. 1992 Nov [cited 2017 Feb 20];49(11):881–887.
72. Volpicelli JR, Watson NT, King AC, Sherman CE, O'Brien CP. Effect of naltrexone on alcohol 'high' in alcoholics. *Am J Psychiatry*. 1995 Apr [cited 2017 Feb 20];152(4):613–615.
73. Chester V, Green F, Alexander R. An audit of a smoking cessation programme for people with an intellectual disability resident in a forensic unit. *Adv Ment Heal Intellect Disabil*. 2011 Jan 24 [cited 2017 Feb 20];5(1):33–41.
74. Minihan PM. Smoking policies and practices in a state-supported residential system for people with mental retardation. *Am J Ment Retard*. 1999 [cited 2017 Feb 20];104(2):131.
75. Sheehan R, Hassiotis A, Walters K, Osborn D, Strydom A, Horsfall L. Mental illness, challenging behaviour, and psychotropic drug prescribing in people with intellectual disability: UK population based cohort study. *BMJ*. 2015;351.
76. El-Guebaly N, Cathcart J, Currie S, Brown D, Gloster S. Public health and therapeutic aspects of smoking bans in mental health and addiction settings. *Psychiatr Serv*. 2002 Dec [cited 2017 Feb 20];53(12):1617–1622.
77. Burtner AP, Wakham MD, McNeal DR, Garvey TP. Tobacco and the institutionalized mentally retarded: Usage choices and ethical considerations. *Spec Care Dent*. 1995 Mar [cited 2017 Feb 20];15(2):56–60.
78. Kalyva E. Prevalence and influences on self-reported smoking among adolescents with mild learning disabilities, attention deficit hyperactivity disorder, and their typically developing peers. *J Intellect Disabil*. 2007 Sep 1 [cited 2017 Feb 20];11(3):267–279.
79. Tracy J, Hosken R. The importance of smoking education and preventative health strategies for people with intellectual disability. *J Intellect Disabil Res*. 1997 Oct [cited 2017 Feb 20];41(5):416–421.
80. The National Institute for Health and Care Excellence (NICE). Stop smoking services. 2008.
81. British Medical Association, Royal Pharmaceutical Society of Great Britain. BNF 72. London: *BMJ Group and Pharmaceutical Press*; 2016. 1447 pp.

82. Thomas KH, Martin RM, Knipe DW, Higgins JPT, Gunnell D. Risk of neuropsychiatric adverse events associated with varenicline: Systematic review and meta-analysis. *Br Med J.* 2015 Aug [cited 2017 Feb 20];350(mar12 8):h1109–h1109.
83. Townsend J, Roderick P, Cooper J. Cigarette smoking by socio-economic group, sex, and age: Effects of price, income, and health publicity. BMJ. 1994 Oct 8 [cited 2017 Feb 20];309(6959): 923–927.
84. Steinberg ML, Heimlich L, Williams JM. Tobacco use among individuals with intellectual or developmental disabilities: A brief review. *Intellectual and Developmental Disabilities NIH Public Access*; Jun, 2009 pp. 197–207.
85. Taggart L, McLaughlin D, Quinn B, Milligan V. An exploration of substance misuse in people with intellectual disabilities. *J Intellect Disabil Res.* 2006 Aug [cited 2017 Feb 20];50(8):588–597.
86. McLaughlin DF, Taggart L, Quinn B, Milligan V. The experiences of professionals who care for people with intellectual disability who have substance-related problems. *J Subst Use.* 2007 Jan 12 [cited 2017 Mar 14];12(2):133–143.
87. Slayter E. Not immune: Access to substance abuse treatment among Medicaid-covered youth with mental retardation. *J Disabil Policy Stud.* 2009 Mar 1 [cited 2017 Apr 2];20(4): 195–204.
88. van Duijvenbode N, VanDerNagel JEL, Didden R, Engels RCME, Buitelaar JK, Kiewik M, et al. Substance use disorders in individuals with mild to borderline intellectual disability: Current status and future directions. Vol. 38, *Research in Developmental Disabilities.* 2015 [cited 2017 Feb 21]. pp. 319–328.

16

Challenging Behaviours in People with Intellectual Disabilities

Glynis H. Murphy and Peter McGill

Introduction and definitions

It is widely recognized that people with an intellectual disability (ID) are at increased risk of various mental and physical health difficulties (see Chapters 1, 2 and 6). In addition, some people engage in unusual behaviours that historically were termed 'inappropriate', 'abnormal', 'disordered', 'dysfunctional', 'problem', or 'maladaptive' behaviour. These terms are now considered out-dated, for three reasons:

- They are generally pejorative terms
- They do not reflect reality (since some of the behaviours are functional, predictable, and not disordered, for the individual)
- They imply that the 'problem' is internal to the individual, whereas research has shown that the behaviours are generally heavily dependent on the physical and social environment.

Consequently, Emerson coined a new term, 'challenging behaviour' and he defined it as:

> Culturally abnormal behaviour(s) of such an intensity, frequency or duration that the physical safety of the person or others is likely to be placed in serious jeopardy, or behaviour which is likely to seriously limit use of, or result in the person being denied access to, ordinary community facilities (1).

The Royal College of Psychiatrists and British Psychological Society in their document 'A Unified Approach' (2), defined 'challenging behaviour' very similarly as:

> Behaviour of such an intensity, frequency or duration as to threaten the quality of life and/or the physical safety of the individual or others and is likely to lead to responses that are restrictive, aversive or result in exclusion.

This newer term, 'challenging behaviour', was expected to have some advantages over the earlier terms, in that it was less pejorative, made fewer assumptions about causality, and should have reminded professionals, staff, and policy makers that such behaviour was *a challenge to services*. The intention of the term was to prevent the phrase 'challenging behaviour' being used as a diagnosis. It was also hoped that the term would stop people feeling that they needed to 'fix' the person, so that they would instead concentrate on 'fixing' the physical and social environment. However, since the introduction of the term, many professionals and carers have felt that the change in terminology has been losing its effect: frequently people talk about 'his' challenging or about someone 'having' challenging behaviour, again implying that it belongs to them and is internal to them. New terms have been proposed: 'behaviour that challenges' and/or 'behaviours of concern'. But these terms may well turn out to have similar consequences.

The kinds of behaviour referred to include: aggressive behaviour (such as verbal abuse, threats, and physical violence), destructive or dangerous behaviours (such as breaking or destroying furniture and other objects, and setting fires), disruptive behaviours (such as repetitive screaming, smearing faeces, setting off fire alarms when there is no fire, calling the emergency services when there is no emergency), self-injurious behaviour (including self-biting, skin picking, head banging), and sexually harmful behaviour (including sexual assaults, rape, and stalking). Some of these behaviours may fall under the purview of the criminal justice system and these behaviours are dealt with further in Chapter 17. Generally speaking, behaviour that would be considered illegal in someone with mild/moderate ID may elicit intervention from the police, whereas for those with severe/profound ID the police are not typically involved, due to the *mens rea* requirement in law in many jurisdictions (see (3) for a review). Nevertheless, it should be recognized that for the more mildly disabled whose behaviour challenges, this is a grey area and some individuals may experience an inconsistent response in relation to the CJS (4).

When people with an ID engage in behaviour that challenges, they often experience a reduction in their quality of life (5). In practice this may include:

- Placement moves, often to more restrictive environments, that may be far from their home town and family (6, 7)
- Physical restraint by staff or carers, or seclusion in locked areas (8)
- Being prevented from entering parts of the building, such as their own kitchen, or being prevented from leaving the building (8)
- Sedation by rapid tranquillization or use of psychoactive medication, in the absence of psychiatric disorders (9, 10)

Families, carers, and staff also frequently experience a reduction in quality of life, often reporting frustration, fatigue, exhaustion, burnout, and feeling unable to continue in their caring role (11, 12). Meanwhile, when families, carers, or staff are unable to cope, service commissioners are often uncertain about what to do. At times, they fund the person's care in poor-quality services that are out of area, that may be very expensive, and that may increase the risk of behaviour that challenges even further (13–15). Such placements are often a very long distance from families, meaning that their quality of life, and that of their family member, may be even more compromised. From time to time the conditions in such services (which are often classified as hospitals or nursing homes) are called into question and in the UK, as in many other countries, there has been a series of enquiries into such settings. In the UK, the most recent such enquiry was that into Winterbourne View, and as a result of the enquiry, which had been triggered by undercover reporting in the service in question, NHS-England established the *Transforming Care* team to improve services (16). One of the related actions involved setting up a database of all those people with ID in hospital settings (see, http://content.digital.nhs.uk/catalogue/PUB16760/ld-census-initial-sep14-rep_version_2.pdf). It transpired that somewhat over 3000 people with ID were in hospital settings, in each of the 2013 and 2014 censuses. About 80 per cent of them were detained under the Mental Health Act and about 70 per cent were receiving psychotropic medication (Health and Social Care Information Centre, 2015). However, there was enormous variation in figures across regions of the country and this suggested that some areas were doing far better at commissioning care to suit people with challenging behaviour and/or forensic behaviours than others. A number of initiatives such as Care and Treatment Reviews are now under way to try to reduce numbers of people in hospital. In addition, community-based forensic teams are being set up to prevent and reduce criminal offending in the vulnerable population with ID.

Prevalence of challenging behaviour and risk factors

By no means everyone with ID engages in challenging behaviour (CB), but the prevalence is higher in those with ID than in those without. A few studies have compared the rates of behaviours such as conduct disorders, in children with and without developmental disabilities (17) and found that children with ID seem to show about three to five times as much of this kind of behaviour as typically developing children at any particular age (5). Most studies of prevalence though have been completed just amongst those with ID, and the generally accepted view of the overall prevalence of challenging behaviour in this population is that it lies between 10–15 per cent of those known to services, though this figure does vary with the exact definition of challenging behaviours that is used, the age and characteristics of the sample, the types of services being surveyed, and other methodological variables (see (5), for a review).

Studies of the rates of challenging behaviour across hospital settings, residential settings, schools, and family homes in children and adults with ID and in those with particular disorders, have led to an understanding of the variety of factors likely to affect the appearance and persistence of challenging behaviour. Early studies often focused on one particular behaviour (e.g. self-injurious behaviour (18) or aggressive behaviour (19)) but later researchers investigated a variety of types of challenging behaviour and found that they often occurred together (20, 21). Moreover, it has become clear that some children and adults with ID are far more vulnerable than others to developing challenging behaviour (9, 22–25) and often such behaviours are very persistent, even over decades of time (26–28). The long-term high risk factors for challenging behaviour are as follows:

- Autism spectrum conditions
- Degree of ID (more severe ID being associated with higher risk, apart from in verbal aggression)
- Age (there being an inverted U curve in prevalence of CB with age, with lower rates in young children, rising to the highest rates in the teens, twenties, and thirties, thereafter dropping again with increasing age)
- Settings (hospital settings and more restrictive settings being linked to higher prevalence rates for CB, though this may be partly the cause of admission and partly the effect of admission)
- Genetic disorders (the behavioural phenotypes of different genetic disorders varies considerably, with Down Syndrome being associated with low rates of challenging behaviour on the whole, whereas some other disorders are linked to high rates, sometimes of specific behaviours, such as over-eating in Prader-Willi syndrome and self-injury in Lesch-Nyhan syndrome)—see below for further discussion of this point
- Sensory impairments (blindness, for example, being a risk factor for self-injurious eye poking)

Interestingly, gender does not reliably predict a raised risk of challenging behaviours once autistic spectrum conditions are taken into account (23). There are also a number of very powerful short-term risk factors, which include physical health and mental health issues, and social factors. These are discussed in more detail below.

Assessment and intervention planning with individuals, families and care staff

Ideally, the best guide to effective interventions for challenging behaviour would be large-scale empirical studies, with a randomized controlled trial (RCT) design, and reliable, valid outcome measures, or alternatively systematic reviews with meta analyses combining study results (given that many studies involve only small numbers of participants). However, there are few RCT studies in existence in the field of ID and challenging behaviour, though there are rather more systematic reviews and meta-analyses. The RCTs have mainly reported on the effectiveness of parent training for young children with IDD (see below) but only one RCT so far has evaluated behavioural methods for adults with ID and challenging behaviour (29).[1] This chapter will briefly review the effectiveness of parent training for young children and will then concentrate on behavioural methods, which are likely to be the most widely effective method for reducing CB for people with severe or profound ID.

1. There are also a small number of RCTs that have tested cognitive behavioural interventions (e.g. for anger and aggression) in mildly disabled individuals and a few RCTs that have examined the effects of medication (30). Trials of CBT are reviewed in Chapter 18 and medication is reviewed in Chapter 19.

Parent training

According to NICE (30), there were 15 RCTs of parent training for young children with ID, in which various types of parent training were compared to a control condition. Typically, parent training included help to understand and intervene with the behaviour of children using a broadly behavioural approach. Of these 15 RCTs, 13 had sufficient data for a meta-analysis and many took place in Australia, using the Stepping Stones Triple P model (31–36). The meta-analysis showed that parent training did result in a significant reduction in challenging behaviour in the children, whether group or individual training was used. There were too few trials to recommend particular programmes but NICE did recommend that parents of young children with ID should be offered parent training and, since group training seemed as effective as individual training but was clearly more cost effective, the group parent training was the preferred model.

Behavioural approaches

There is considerable evidence that the most effective psychological approach to assessment and intervention for those with severe or profound intellectual disabilities seems to be the individualized behavioural approach, and recent systematic reviews and meta-analyses (37–42) have consistently shown that such approaches significantly reduce challenging behaviour, especially if preceded by a functional assessment.

Early on, behavioural approaches were criticized for lacking an ethical stance and concentrating too much on eliminating specific behaviours, rather than building up pro-social behaviours. More recently, the approach of positive behaviour(al) support (PBS) has emerged which has developed out of the behavioural approach (43), taking into account previous criticisms. PBS was defined by Ted Carr, one of the originators of the approach, as follows:

> PBS is an intervention technology based on social, behavioural, educational, and biomedical science that combines evidence-based practices with formal systems change strategies, focused on both improving the valued lifestyle options available for an individual and reducing problem behaviours (44).

Thus PBS is a framework, rather than a specific intervention (45), and it involves placing assessment and intervention within a broad framework that can draw on a range of specific, evidence-based interventions, based on an integrated formulation of the biological, psychological, social, and environmental factors contributing to the occurrence of a specific individual's challenging behaviour.

PBS: a practical guide

Confronted with the referral of an individual with challenging behaviour it is very important to remember the broad framework proposed by PBS and not jump to conclusions about the causes of the behaviour. It may help to draw on the sequence of steps outlined below and in Figure 16.1.

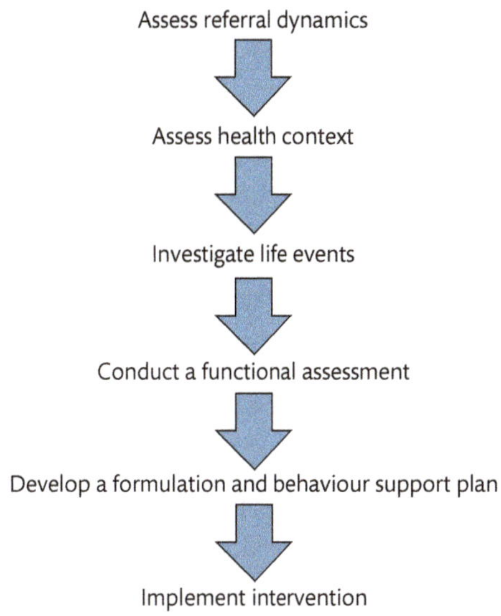

Figure 16.1 The assessment and intervention process with individuals

1. Assessing referral dynamics

Most individuals whose behaviour is described as challenging do not refer themselves to a psychologist, psychiatrist, or other mental health professional. Rather, the individual is likely to be referred by others who are affected by the person's behaviour in some way, for example, family or paid carers. In such circumstances it is very important to ask questions such as: Why is the behaviour considered challenging? Why has the referral been made now? For whom is changing the behaviour important? The importance of such questions is illustrated by Nunkoosing and Haydon-Laurelut (46) in their review of referrals from residential social care settings to a community learning disability team (CLDT). One referral included the following:

> Verbally aggressive toward other people. Unwilling to listen to reason. I can be very bossy, often involving myself in other people's affairs that do not concern me ... Provocation of others into losing their temper with me, striking out at me or shouting at me.'

There are many interesting things about this referral. For current purposes it is noteworthy that the person being referred (the 'I' in the referral, even though this is written by staff) is 'verbally aggressive' while others 'shout'. Others are 'provoked' while the person referred is 'unwilling to listen to reason'. In other words behaviours which may be very similar are constructed quite differently when it is the person being referred displaying them, than when it is others.

More generally, the definition and treatment of a behaviour as 'challenging' is a social process and, therefore, subject to a range of influences beyond the individual's actual behaviour. In a situation like this referral, it would be problematic to treat the individual's behaviour without addressing what would, in this case, seem to be problematic social processes amongst staff.

2. Assessing the health context

There is now considerable evidence of challenging behaviour being more likely when the person is suffering from a range of chronic or acute, physical, or mental health conditions (47). The conditions implicated are many and varied,[2] for example otitis media, allergies, constipation, infection, GORD, depression, schizophrenia etc. The

2. Note that ill-health may of course be related to an individual's genetic background. For example, GORD is part of the phenotype of Cornelia de Lange syndrome and seems to be related to the higher prevalence of self-injury of individuals with that syndrome (48).

impact of ill-health is often compounded by the difficulties experienced by the person with intellectual disabilities in identifying and communicating problems to others. The person may be in pain but not able to describe the location or type of pain. They may be having unusual experiences which they are unable to describe accurately and do not identify as requiring attention. It is vital, therefore, that consideration is given with all referrals to the possibility of ill-health and to its possible connection with the individual's behaviour, especially where the behaviour has recently developed or worsened. The identification of health problems should lead to their standard treatment. Of course, this is not necessarily simple. Diagnosis may be difficult, especially with respect to mental health problems in people with more severe disabilities. Treatment may be difficult to obtain because of continuing, underlying prejudice against people with intellectual disabilities (49). Treatment may be difficult to administer because of issues related to the person's disability, for example, the person may resist injections or it may be dangerous to administer a general anaesthetic. And all treatment, especially the more intrusive, will raise issues of capacity and consent that need to be tackled sensitively. Despite all of these problems, it is often vital to robustly identify and treat ill-health in order to resolve an individual's challenging behaviour and improve their quality of life.

Treatment of mental ill-health raises particular concerns. Because of a failure to make reasonable accommodations for the person's intellectual disability, and because of the inherent difficulties of doing so in respect of people with more severe disabilities, treatment will usually be pharmacological rather than a "talking therapy". Research suggests that 40 per cent of people with challenging behaviour are prescribed psychotropic medication in the absence of any reported mental health need (50). Because of these kinds of findings and the limited evidence of the effectiveness of psychotropic medication, NICE provided guidance that antipsychotic medication should only be used to manage challenging behaviour (as opposed to the treatment of psychotic disorder) alongside other interventions and with great care to ensure minimum doses, as well as monitoring impact and frequent review (51).

Given the high levels of use of psychotropic medications it is not surprising that side effects are frequently reported (52) and that in some cases, these side effects are implicated (possibly in interaction with other factors) in the occurrence of challenging behaviour. In a small sample (53), an average of 8.6 reported side effects were found, most commonly neurological, mood, health, gastrointestinal, and sleep effects. It is not hard to imagine how such effects, especially in a person with intellectual disabilities who may lack the ability to rationalize their pain/discomfort as a necessary evil to help them overcome another health problem, can contribute to challenging behaviour. Sleep deprivation, for example, has been implicated in previous research as a factor associated with daytime challenging behaviour (54). The implication here, of course, is that the treating clinician should always be aware of the range of medication an individual is taking (which may be extensive) and be considering the possible impact of this medication and its side effects on their behaviour.

3. Investigating life events

People with ID are at least as subject to adverse life events as others. Indeed, evidence about the high prevalence of abuse and hate crime against people with ID suggests that they are likely to experience such events at higher than average levels (55). It is important also to be aware of the possible impact of social network changes on an individual. People with ID generally have smaller social networks and they often consist largely of family members and/or care staff (56). As a result, the death of a significant member of their network or the kind of frequent staff turnover that is all too common in social care services may have a more disruptive effect on them than it would have for other members of the population. Adverse life events are recognized as contributing to the development of psychiatric, psychological (and also physical) disorders, which may be associated with challenging behaviour (57–59). Adverse life events may also be associated very directly with challenging behaviour as when a bereaved individual responds with aggression to the perhaps well-intentioned but insensitive encouragement of a naïve member of staff.

In assessment, it is therefore very important to investigate the extent to which an individual has recently experienced adverse life events. A number of measures designed for use with people with ID now exist, for example, the Bangor Life Events Schedule for Intellectual Disability (60). Identification of life events implicated in the person's behaviour should lead to attempts to reverse the event (where this is possible) or to provide culturally normative, evidence-based interventions (e.g. bereavement counselling, cognitive behaviour therapy) where feasible. Even if, because of the nature of the person's disabilities, it is not possible to provide such treatment, the likely role of life events should continue to be acknowledged as this will inform the wider formulation and may have an impact on the attributions made by others regarding the person's behaviour.

4. Conducting a functional assessment/analysis

Absolutely central to a PBS approach is the notion that challenging behaviour 'means' something. In particular, research suggests that challenging behaviour serves, in most cases, one of a relatively small number of common functions. For example, a report of the results of 981 published functional analyses (almost 90% of which were conducted with children or adults with developmental disabilities) (61), identified the following:

- In 32 per cent of analyses, the function was identified as 'escape'. That is, the challenging behaviour led to the individual getting away from demands or other 'aversive' stimulation
- In 22 per cent of analyses the function was identified as 'attention'. That is, the challenging behaviour increased the probability of the individual receiving attention from another person, usually a carer or member of staff
- In 16 per cent of analyses, the function was 'automatic'. That is, the challenging behaviour led to the individual receiving some kind of sensory stimulation without the intervention of a carer or member of staff
- In 11 per cent of analyses, the function was 'tangible'. That is, the challenging behaviour made it more likely that the individual received some kind of tangible reinforcement such as something to eat or drink, access to a preferred object, or activity
- In 19 per cent of analyses, the function was 'multiple'. That is, the challenging behaviour served more than one of the above functions.

Undoubtedly, the understanding of an individual's behaviour is more complex than the ascribing of a one-word function. Imagine, however, if we were not able to ascribe function or got it wrong. Supporting an individual under the assumption that the function of their behaviour is to gain attention when actually it is escape (perhaps from that very same attention) is likely not just to be ineffective but to actively make matters worse.

It is critical, therefore, to gather detailed information about the circumstances within which challenging behaviour occurs so as to reach an informed judgement about its function. The NICE guidance (30) suggests that this process may best be carried out in two steps with the second, more detailed analysis only being conducted where necessary. The first step would involve gathering a range of information about the behaviour through interviews with carers/staff (62), observations (63, 64) and questionnaires (65, 66). This information, coupled with the more general information already gained will often allow a conclusion, or at least a working hypothesis, about the function of the behaviour. In some individuals, however, where the behaviour is complex or it is particularly important to get the function right, more detailed and time-consuming assessments would be justified. In particular, these would be likely to involve structured direct observations in the natural environment (67) or carrying out an '"analogue"' assessment in which the person's behaviour is monitored in carefully designed conditions (68). In the former, the aim would be to identify a number of incidents of challenging behaviour and to detect relationships between the behaviour and environmental events. These relationships are likely to be behaviour analytic in nature with some events antecedent to the behaviour creating motivation for challenging behaviour (e.g. a lack of attention may act as a motivating operation for self-injury), or signalling the availability of reinforcement for challenging behaviour (e.g. the presence of a particular member of staff may act as a discriminative stimulus for aggressive behaviour that allows the person to escape), or events consequent upon the behaviour making it more likely the behaviour will occur again (e.g. the provision of attention may reinforce destructive behaviour). In analogue assessment, the aim would also be to detect such relationships between the behaviour and environmental events but, instead of just waiting for the behaviour to occur naturally, circumstances would be set up where the behaviour may be more likely. For example, the person may be asked to carry out difficult tasks which it is thought may trigger challenging behaviour. This kind of approach does raise ethical concerns but may be justified in circumstances where a more experimental approach is required to identify the true causes of (rather than simply those events correlated with) challenging behaviour.

5. Developing a formulation and behaviour support plan

Intervention strategies should directly follow from functional assessment. Such intervention may well be multi-component and is likely to involve the following elements:

Environmental modification

If the functional assessment identifies certain events as provoking challenging behaviour then intervention will often seek to remove or modify these events. If, for example, the behaviour seems to serve the function of escaping from demands that should not be being made on the person (e.g. to do tasks that are too difficult for them or to engage in activities which distress them) then, clearly, changes to these demands are required and are likely to have a major impact on the person's behaviour (69).

Developing new behaviours

Of course, sometimes the problem is not only, or not so much, the circumstances to which the person is exposed but, reflecting their intellectual disability, the lack of adaptive behaviours for controlling the situation. So a highly appropriate intervention may involve teaching the person new skills. Such skills often focus on communication. For example, in the case of the individual displaying challenging behaviour to escape from non-preferred activities, the teaching of a communication response (whether a word, sign, use of a motor response etc.) means that they can now control difficult situations to which they are exposed without needing to display challenging behaviour (63).

Changing the consequences of challenging behaviour

Challenging behaviour is difficult to ignore and, as a result, is often reinforced. Behaviour which serves the function of attention will often generate attention where none has previously been forthcoming. Likewise, behaviour serving the function of escape will often be responded to, where the person's increasing, preceding distress has not. So, sometimes it is important to ensure that challenging behaviour no longer gains reinforcing consequences. In doing this, however, it is vital that the person is given alternative ways to gain the same reinforcers and that punitive responses are avoided (70).

The causes of behaviour described as challenging are sometimes relatively straightforward to detect and address, but it is often the case, especially where the behaviour is well-established and of a serious nature, that it is a result of multiple, interacting causes. Such causes are much harder to detect and it is essential that findings are drawn from a holistic, often multidisciplinary approach to assessment. Intervention planning is then substantially aided by the development of an idiographic formulation which encapsulates the key influences (or, sometimes, the key, hypothesized influences) on the behaviour. An example case study follows.

Case study 1

Tom (not a real person but based on an amalgam of real individuals) is a young man with autism and severe ID who lives in a residential care home with four other young men. All the residents display challenging behaviour. Tom has recently been referred because his behaviour (hitting staff, other residents, and banging on walls) has recently got worse. Several staff and residents have been hurt, there have been a number of safeguarding alerts and there is visible damage to a number of the walls. The clinician interviews the acting manager of Tom's home. It quickly becomes apparent that Tom's placement is under threat and that urgent action is likely to be required. Further enquiry with the manager reveals that, while Tom's behaviour has been described as challenging since childhood, it is said to have worsened over the last three months. However, the manager has only been in place for two months and has limited knowledge of what happened before. Fortunately, Tom retains significant involvement with his family who live locally. The clinician is able to talk to Tom's mother and sister who tell her how well Tom was doing until a few months ago. They attribute this to the previous manager who Tom had known for three years and with whom he had an excellent relationship. 'Tom was always willing to do things for Jonathon (the previous manager)' said Tom's sister, 'they used to go out running together and to watch the football. Since he left it's not been the same.' 'And he's not been sleeping well', added Tom's mother, 'Jonathon had this routine for bedtime and he made the staff use it every night. Tom slept much better as a result. Now there's no routine and Tom's up and down all night.' The clinician spends some time with Tom and his current keyworker (also newly appointed). It's clear that Tom is using some signs but neither the clinician nor the keyworker know what they mean and they stop the session as Tom seems to be getting upset. The clinician later talks to Tom's sister who says that Tom makes up his own signs and the only person in the home who knew what they meant was Jonathon. The clinician decides to complete some informal observations of Tom and also to get the staff to keep some records of what happens during a number of incidents. While it proves challenging to collect any records, both sources suggest a similar pattern. Incidents are usually preceded by staff interacting with Tom, asking him to do things including self-care and household activities. Staff are polite but use rather complex language and the clinician thinks it likely that Tom doesn't understand what he's being asked to do. When Tom becomes aggressive, staff use their established plan of rounding up other residents and leaving Tom in whatever room of the house he is currently in until he has calmed down.

Accepting the limitations of the evidence gathered, the formulation in this case would likely include the following:

Referral dynamics: Substantial staff turnover means that most staff do not know Tom well. The referral may have the underlying intention of triggering a review of Tom's placement and possible move elsewhere.

Biological/health/personal context: Challenging behaviour is more likely in individuals with autism and those with restricted communication. The communication skills Tom has are limited and not well understood by staff. Tom also seems to be suffering from sleep deprivation/disruption, a known trigger for challenging behaviour.

Life events: It seems clear that the departure of the former manager three months previously was a highly significant event for Tom. He seems to have had good rapport with Jonathon as well as Jonathon being responsible for putting in place arrangements to support Tom's sleep which have since lapsed.

Functional assessment: Tom's behaviours happen when he is asked to do things (that he may not understand) and this results in his being left alone. It seems very likely that these behaviours serve as an escape function for Tom, being left alone acting as a reinforcer.

This formulation has very clear implications for the elements of an appropriate behaviour support plan for Tom:

- Building rapport between staff and Tom. Challenging behaviour is more likely when the person has a poor relationship with those who support him (71). Rapport can be built by sharing mutually pleasurable activities and by ensuring that Tom receives frequent reinforcement from staff
- Reinstating Tom's sleep routine
- Ensuring that Tom has frequent access to the kinds of preferred activities he previously shared with Jonathon
- Supporting the use of Tom's signing. This might be done with the assistance of family members to teach staff what Tom's signs mean
- Modification of the way in which demands are placed on Tom. This might include a temporary reduction in demands and/or the placing of demands in a more positive context, and/or simplifying demands.

6. Implementing intervention

Much intervention around the behaviour of people with ID depends upon 'mediators'—family members and care staff—for its implementation (72). It is vital, therefore, that intervention is developed in partnership with them, that it takes account of the situation in which they will carry out intervention and that adequate training is provided. Professional staff who are developing and overseeing interventions have a responsibility to ensure that intervention procedures are being followed (else failure may be attributed to the intervention rather than to its limited implementation) and to ensure the collection of data that allows informed judgements about the effectiveness of intervention. All too often such judgements are unreliable because they have been based upon informal, anecdotal reports. The specifics of data collection will depend on the circumstances.

The broader context—beyond the individual

Tom's situation, as described above, contains a number of elements that are relatively common correlates of challenging behaviour and that suggest the importance of considering the broader context within which challenging behaviour develops and is maintained. This broader context clearly includes biological/health elements (73) but here the focus has been mainly on environmental elements. In particular, it seems clear that attempts to assess and intervene with challenging behaviour should not treat the behaviour as being an entirely individual problem, requiring intervention only by clinicians such as psychiatrists, psychologists, and so on. Additionally, we should see challenging behaviour as being an indicator of how capable the health/social care environment is. In the example of Tom it was clear that his social care environment was not at all capable and had, effectively, produced challenging behaviour where none or little had been before. This carries an important implication. If we can improve the quality of care provided, especially in ways of most significance to challenging behaviour, we might hope to significantly reduce the need to refer individuals for assessment and intervention (74, 75).

MULTIPLE CHOICE QUESTIONS

Questions

Please select the single most appropriate answer.

1. Challenging behaviour in people with severe or profound ID is:

A. More likely in men
B. More likely in Down syndrome
C. More likely in those with poor communication skills
D. More likely in very young children

2. Challenging behaviour is not related to:
A. Life events
B. Mental health needs
C. Physical health
D. Social class

3. Functional analysis means:
A. Assessing someone's IQ
B. Assessing someone's self-care skills
C. Assessing the functions of staff and carers
D. Assessing the function of challenging behaviour

4. Parent training for families with children with challenging behaviour:
A. Is a waste of time
B. Has been recommended by NICE
C. Is very widespread
D. Has not been shown to be effective

5. PBS stands for:
A. Personal Behaviour Standards
B. Positive Behavioural Support
C. Positive Behaviour Services
D. Psychological and Behavioural Services

Answers

1. C. Challenging behaviour in severe/profound ID is not more likely in males, is relatively rare in people with Down syndrome, and peaks in the teens and early twenties. It is very commonly associated with communication deficits, hence C is correct.
2. D. Challenging behaviour tends to worsen after life events, and be more problematic when mental or physical health problems arise. It has no association with social class, hence D is correct.
3. D. Functional analysis refers to techniques used to assess what function a person's challenging behaviour may have for them (for example, gaining social attention, avoiding demands, etc). It can involve the use of direct observations, questionnaire data or interviews, and sometimes may include all three. D is therefore correct.
4. B. Parent training has been subject to rigorous RCTs and has been shown to provide considerable benefits. It has been recommended by NICE, so B is correct.
5. B. PBS is an abbreviation of Positive Behavioural Support. It is a broadly behavioural approach with a growing evidence base and a strong grounding in human rights and ethical standards.

REFERENCES

1. Emerson E. Challenging Behaviour: *Analysis and Intervention in People with Learning Disabilities*. Cambridge: Cambridge University Press; 1995.
2. Royal College of Psychiatrists, British Psychological Society, Royal College of Speech and Language Therapists. *Challenging Behaviour: A Unified Approach*. London: Royal College of Psychiatrists; 2007.
3. Murphy GH, Mason J. People with intellectual disabilities and offending behaviours. In: Tsakanikos E, McCarthy J, editors. *Handbook of Psychopathology in Intellectual Disability*. New York: Springer Science; 2014.
4. Wheeler JR, Holland AJ, Bambrick M, Lindsay WR, Carson D, Steptoe L, et al. Community services and people with intellectual disabilities who engage in anti-social or offending behaviour: Referral rates, characteristics, and care pathways. *Journal of Forensic Psychiatry and Psychology*. 2009;20(5):717–740.
5. Emerson E, Einfeld SL. *Challenging Behaviour*. Cambridge: Cambridge University Press; 2011.
6. Bonell S, Ali A, Hall I, Chinn D, Patkas I. People with intellectual disabilities in out-of-area specialist hospitals: What do families think? *Journal of Applied Research in Intellectual Disabilities*. 2011;24(5):389–397.
7. Chinn D, Hall I, Ali A, Hassell H, Patkas I. Psychiatric in-patients away from home: Accounts by people with intellectual disabilities in specialist hospitals outside their home localities. *Journal of Applied Research in Intellectual Disabilities*. 2011;24(1): 50–60.
8. McGill P, Murphy G, Kelly-Pike A. Frequency of use and characteristics of people with intellectual disabilities subject to physical interventions. *Journal of Applied Research in Intellectual Disabilities*. 2009;22:152–158.
9. Lundqvist L-O. Prevalence and risk markers of behavior problems among adults with intellectual disabilities: A total population study in Örebro County, Sweden. *Research in Developmental Disabilities*. 2013;34(4):1346–1356.
10. Robertson J, Emerson E, Gregory N, Hatton C, Kessissoglou S, Hallam A. Receipt of psychotropic medication by people with intellectual disability in residential settings. *Journal of Intellectual Disability Research*. 2000;44(6):666–676.
11. Hastings R. Parental stress and behaviour problems of children with developmental disability. *Journal of Intellectual and Developmental Disability*. 2002;27(3):149–160.
12. Lecavalier L, Leone S, Wiltz J. The impact of behaviour problems on caregiver stress in young people with autism spectrum disorders. *Journal of Intellectual Disability Research*. 2006;50(3):172–183.
13. Allen D, Lowe K, Moore K, Brophy S. Predictors, costs and characteristics of out of area placement for people with intellectual disability and challenging behaviour. *Journal of Intellectual Disability Research*. 2007;51(6):409–416.
14. Barron DA, Hassiotis A, Paschos D. Out-of-area provision for adults with intellectual disabilities and challenging behaviour in England: Policy perspectives and clinical reality. *Journal of Intellectual Disability Research*. 2011;55(9):832–843.
15. McGill P, Poynter J. High cost residential placements for adults with intellectual disabilities. *Journal of Applied Research in Intellectual Disabilities*. 2012;25(6):584–587.
16. Department of Health. *Transforming Care: A National Response to Winterbourne View Hospital*. London: Department of Health; 2012.
17. Emerson E, Hatton C. Mental health of children and adolescents with intellectual disabilities in Britain. *The British Journal of Psychiatry*. 2007;191(6):493–499.
18. Oliver C, Murphy G, Corbett J. Self-injurious behaviour in people with mental handicap: A total population study. *Journal of Mental Deficiency Research*. 1987;31:147–162.
19. Harris P. The nature and extent of aggressive behaviour amongst people with learning difficulties (mental handicap) in a single

health district. *Journal of Intellectual Disability Research.* 1993;37(3):221–242.

20. Emerson E, Kiernan C, Alborz A, Reeves D, Mason H, Swarbrick R, et al. The prevalence of challenging behaviors: A total population study. *Research in Developmental Disabilities.* 2001;22:77–93.
21. Kiernan C, Kiernan D. Challenging behaviour in schools for pupils with severe learning difficulties. *Mental Handicap Research.* 1994;7(3):177–201.
22. Davies L, Oliver C. The age related prevalence of aggression and self-injury in persons with an intellectual disability: A review. *Research in Developmental Disabilities.* 2013;34(2):764–775.
23. Felce D, Kerr M. Investigating low adaptive behaviour and presence of the triad of impairments characteristic of autistic spectrum disorder as indicators of risk for challenging behaviour among adults with intellectual disabilities. *Journal of Intellectual Disability Research.* 2013;57(2):128–138.
24. Holden B, Gitlesen JP. A total population study of challenging behaviour in the county of Hedmark, Norway: Prevalence, and risk markers. *Research in Developmental Disabilities.* 2006;27(4):456–465.
25. McLintock K, Hall S, Oliver C. Risk markers associated with challenging behaviours in people with intellectual disabilities: A meta-analytic study. *Journal of Intellectual Disability Research.* 2003;47(6):405–416.
26. Murphy GH, Beadle-Brown J, Wing L, Gould J, Shah A, Holmes N. Chronicity of challenging behaviours in people with severe intellectual disabilities and/or autism: A total population sample. *Journal of Autism and Developmental Disorders.* 2005;35(4): 405–418.
27. Murphy GH, Oliver C, Corbett J. Epidemiology of self-injury, characteristics of people with severe self-injury and initial treatment outcome. In: Kiernan C, editor. Research to Practice? Implications of Research on the Challenging Behaviour of People with Learning Disability. Clevedon, Avon: BILD Publications; 1993. p. 1–35.
28. Totsika V, Toogood S, Hastings RP, Lewis S. Persistence of challenging behaviours in adults with intellectual disability over a period of 11 years. *Journal of Intellectual Disability Research.* 2008;52(5):446–457.
29. Hassiotis A, Robotham D, Canagasabey A, Romeo R, Langridge D, Blizard R, et al. Randomised, single-blind, controlled trial of a specialist behaviour therapy team for challenging behaviour in adults with intellectual disabilities. *American Journal of Psychiatry.* 2009;166:1278–1285.
30. Challenging behaviour and learning disabilities: Prevention and interventions for people with learning disabilities whose behaviour challenges [Internet]. 2015. Available from: https://www.nice.org.uk/guidance/ng11.
31. Plant KM, Sanders MR. Reducing problem behavior during care-giving in families of preschool-aged children with developmental disabilities. *Research in Developmental Disabilities.* 2007;28(4):362–385.
32. Roberts C, Mazzucchelli T, Studman L, Sanders MR. Behavioral family intervention for children with developmental disabilities and behavioral problems. *Journal of Clinical Child and Adolescent Psychology.* 2006;35(2):180–193.
33. Roux G, Sofronoff K, Sanders M. A randomized controlled trial of group Stepping Stones Triple P: A mixed-disability trial. *Family Process.* 2013;52(3):411–424.
34. Sofronoff K, Jahnel D, Sanders M. Stepping Stones Triple P seminars for parents of a child with a disability: A randomized controlled trial. *Research in Developmental Disabilities.* 2011;32(6):2253–2262.
35. Tellegen CL, Sanders MR. A randomized controlled trial evaluating a brief parenting program with children with autism spectrum disorders. *Journal of Consulting and Clinical Psychology.* 2014;82(6):1193.
36. Whittingham K, Sofronoff K, Sheffield J, Sanders MR. Stepping Stones Triple P: An RCT of a parenting program with parents of a child diagnosed with an autism spectrum disorder. *Journal of Abnormal Child Psychology.* 2009;37(4):469–480.
37. Campbell JM. Efficicacy of behavioral interventions for reducing problem behavior in persons with autism: A quantitative synthesis of single-subject research. *Research in Developmental Disabilities.* 2003;24:120–138.
38. Didden R, Korzilius H, van Oorsouw W, Sturmey P. Behavioral treatment of challenging behaviors in individuals with mild mental retardation: Meta-analysis of single-subject research. *American Journal on Mental Retardation.* 2006;111(4):290–298.
39. Harvey ST, Boer D, Meyer LH, Evans IM. Updating a meta-analysis of intervention research with challenging behaviour: Treatment validity and standards of practice. *Journal of Intellectual and Developmental Disability.* 2009;34(1):67–80.
40. Heyvaert M, Maes B, van den Noortgate W, Kuppens S, Onghena P. A multilevel meta-analysis of single-case and small-n research on interventions for reducing challenging behaviour in persons with intellectual disabilities. *Research in Developmental Disabilities.* 2012;33:766–780.
41. Heyvaert M, Saenen L, Campbell JM, Maes B, Onghena P. Efficacy of behavioral interventions for reducing problem behavior in persons with autism: An updated quantitative synthesis of single-subject research. *Research in Developmental Disabilities.* 2014;35(10):2463–2476.
42. Walker VL, Snell ME. Effects of augmentative and alternative communication on challenging behavior: A meta-analysis. *Augmentative and Alternative Communication.* 2013;29(2):117–131.
43. Dunlap G, Carr EG, Horner RH, Zarcone JR, Schwartz I. Positive behavior support and applied behavior analysis: A familial alliance. *Behavior Modification.* 2008;32(5):682–698.
44. Carr EG, Dunlap G, Horner RH, Koegel RL, Turnbull AP, Sailor W, et al. Positive behavior support: Evolution of an applied science. *Journal of Positive Behavior Interventions.* 2002;4(1):4–16.
45. Gore NJ, McGill P, Toogood S, Allen D, Hughes JC, Baker PA, et al. Definition and scope for positive behavioural support. *International Journal of Positive Behavioural Support.* 2013;3(2):14–23.
46. Nunkoosing K, Haydon-Laurelut M. Intellectual disabilities, challenging behaviour and referral texts: A critical discourse analysis. *Disability and Society.* 2011;26(4):405–417.
47. May ME, Kennedy CH. Health and problem behavior among people with intellectual disabilities. *Behavior Analysis in Practice.* 2010;3(2):4.
48. Luzzani S, Macchini F, Valade A, Milani D, Selicorni A. Gastroesophageal reflux and Cornelia de Lange syndrome: Typical and atypical symptoms. *American Journal of Medical Genetics Part A.* 2003;119(3):283–287.
49. Michael J. Healthcare for All. London: Department of Health; 2008.
50. Sheehan R, Hassiotis A, Walters K, Osborn, D, Strydom A, Horsfall, L. Mental illness, challenging behaviour and psychotropic drug prescribing in people with intellectual disability: UK

population based cohort study. *British Medical Journal.* 2015;351:4326.
51. Murphy G. The NICE guidelines on learning disabilities and behaviour that challenges. *Tizard Learning Disability Review.* 2017;22(2):71–81.
52. Scheifes A, Walraven S, Stolker JJ, Nijman HLI, Egberts TCG, Heerdink ER. Adverse events and the relation with quality of life in adults with intellectual disability and challenging behaviour using psychotropic drugs. *Research in Developmental Disabilities.* 2016;49–50:13–21.
53. Valdovinos MG, Caruso M, Roberts C, Kim G, Kennedy CH. Medical and behavioral symptoms as potential medication side effects in adults with developmental disabilities. *American Journal on Mental Retardation.* 2005;110(3):164–170.
54. O'Reilly MF, Lancioni G. Response covariation of escape-maintained aberrant behavior correlated with sleep deprivation. *Research in Developmental Disabilities.* 2000;21(2):125–136.
55. Macdonald SJ. 'Community fear and harassment': Learning difficulties and hate crime incidents in the north-east of England. *Disability and Society.* 2015;30(3):353–367.
56. Forrester-Jones R, Carpenter J, Coolen-Schrijner P, Cambridge P, Tate A, Beecham J, et al. The social networks of people with intellectual disability living in the community 12 years after resettlement from long-stay hospitals. *Journal of Applied Research in Intellectual Disabilities.* 2006;19(4):285–295.
57. Murphy GH, O'Callaghan AC, Clare ICH. The impact of alleged abuse on behaviour in adults with severe intellectual disabilities. *Journal of Intellectual Disability Research.* 2007;51(10):741–749.
58. Rowsell A, Clare IC, Murphy GH. The psychological impact of abuse on men and women with severe intellectual disabilities. *Journal of Applied Research in Intellectual Disabilities.* 2013;26(4):257–270.
59. Sequeira H, Howlin P, Hollins S. Psychological disturbance associated with sexual abuse in people with learning disabilities. *The British Journal of Psychiatry.* 2003;183(5):451–456.
60. Hulbert-Williams L, Hastings RP, Crowe R, Pemberton J. Self-reported life events, social support and psychological problems in adults with intellectual disabilities. *Journal of Applied Research in Intellectual Disabilities.* 2011;24(5):427–436.
61. Beavers GA, Iwata BA, Lerman DC. Thirty years of research on the functional analysis of problem behavior. *Journal of Applied Behavior Analysis.* 2013;46(1):1–21.
62. O'Neill RE, Albin RW, Storey K, Horner RH, Sprague JR. *Functional Assessment and Program Development for Problem Behavior: A Practical Handbook.* Stamford, CT: Cengage Learning; 2014.
63. Carr EG. *Communication-based Intervention for Problem Behavior: A User's Guide for Producing Positive Change.* Baltimore: P.H. Brookes; 1994.
64. Touchette PE, MacDonald RF, Langer SN. A scatter plot for identifying stimulus control of problem behavior. *Journal of Applied Behavior Analysis.* 1985;18:343–351.
65. Durand VM, Crimmins DB. Identifying the variables maintaining self-injurious behavior. *Journal of Autism and Developmental Disorders.* 1988;18(1):99–117.
66. Matson JL, Bamburg JW, Cherry KE, Paclawskyj TR. A validity study on the Questions About Behavioral Function (QABF) scale: Predicting treatment success for self-injury, aggression, and stereotypies. *Research in Developmental Disabilities.* 1999;20(2):163–175.
67. Anderson CM, Long ES. Use of a structured descriptive assessment methodology to identify variables affecting problem behavior. *Journal of Applied Behavior Analysis.* 2002;35(2):137–154.
68. Hanley GP, Iwata BA, McCord BE. Functional analysis of problem behavior: A review. *Journal of Applied Behavior Analysis.* 2003;36(2):147–185.
69. Miltenberger RG. Antecedent interventions for challenging behaviors maintained by escape from instructional activities. In: Luiselli JK, editor. *Antecedent Assessment and Intervention: Supporting Children and Adults with Developmental Disabilities in Community Settings.* Baltimore, MD: Paul H. Brookes; 2006. pp. 101–124.
70. Ricciardi JN. Combining antecedent and consequence procedures in multicomponent behaviour support plans: A guide to writing plans with functional efficacy. In: Luiselli JK, editor. *Antecedent Assessment and Intervention: Supporting Children and Adults with Developmental Disabilities in Community Settings.* Baltimore, MD: Paul H. Brookes; 2006. pp. 227–245.
71. Magito-McLaughlin D, Carr EG. Quality of rapport as a setting event for problem behavior: Assessment and intervention. *Journal of Positive Behavior Interventions.* 2005;7(2):68–91.
72. Allen D. Mediator analysis: An overview of recent research on carers supporting people with intellectual disability and challenging behaviour. *Journal of Intellectual Disability Research.* 1999;43(4):325–339.
73. Langthorne P, McGill P, O'Reilly M. Incorporating 'motivation' into the functional analysis of challenging behaviour: On the interactive and integrative potential of the motivating operation. *Behavior Modification.* 2007;31(4):466–487.
74. Allen D, McGill P, Hastings RP, Toogood S, Baker P, Gore NJ, et al. Implementing positive behavioural support: Changing social and organisational contexts. *International Journal of Positive Behavioural Support.* 2013;3(2):32–41.
75. McGill P, Vanono L, Clover W, Smyth E, Cooper V, Hopkins L, et al. Reducing challenging behaviour of adults with intellectual disabilities in supported accommodation: A cluster randomized controlled trial of setting-wide positive behaviour support. *Research in Developmental Disabilities* 2018;81(October): 143–154.

17

Offending Behaviours in People with Intellectual Disabilities

John L. Taylor, William R. Lindsay†, and John Devapriam

Introduction

Public policy and clinical practice have long been susceptible to manipulation and distortion concerning offenders with intellectual disabilities (ID). Crime can be an inflammatory topic for the media, then the public, and consequently politicians. Fear of crime can lead to the easy manipulation of public perception concerning the culpability of one section of society or another. People with ID have a long history of being the target of such unwarranted scapegoating.

During the nineteenth century several potent influences came together. First came the development of the concept of institutions as a solution to educating people with ID. In 1844 John Conolly, chief physician at the Hanwell Asylum in London visited two institutions in Paris—the Salpetriere and the Bicertre, opened by Edouard Seguin, a French physician who pioneered educational approaches for children with ID (1). Conolly witnessed humane management of 'idiots', education of even the most disabled, and a large reduction in the use of restraint. His enthusiasm for Seguin's regime was reflected in his writings (2) which were circulated throughout Britain and North America. This resulted in widespread enthusiasm for institutional care. One early North American institution for people with ID was opened in South Boston in 1847 for people 'condemned in hopeless idiocy' (3). The originators of these establishments were influential and similar institutions opened in New York and Philadelphia. The early institute superintendents wrote of the educative potential of these places and created the concept of idiocy as a social construction while offering an ostensibly humane solution in the form of institutions.

By the mid-1850s, however, influential figures were already asserting a link between idiocy and delinquency. Isaac Newton Kerlin, an important figure in the field of ID, published a series of 22 case illustrations in 1858 in which he coined the term 'moral imbecile'(4). Subsequent institution superintendents were particularly successful in exploiting the supposed links between ID and criminality to make an argument for the expansion of their services, with medicine rather than education becoming the dominant ethos. Consequently, increasingly persuasive arguments were made for removing people with ID from society for their own, as well as for society's good. State funding followed, leading to the expansion of many such establishments and the increasing segregation of people with ID (5).

Up until the middle of the nineteenth century, people with ID were generally considered a burden on, rather than a menace to society. Scheerenberger (5) noted, however, that by the 1880s, people with ID were no longer viewed as unfortunates who with training could make a positive contribution to society. They had come to be seen as criminal, parasitic, and delinquent. In 1889, Kerlin (6) expounded on the association between ID and crime and argued that crime was the result of an individual's inability to understand moral sense and their physical infirmity, both of which were non-remediable and inherited.

The association between low intelligence and crime persisted well into the twentieth century and influenced policy on the management of people with ID. Terman (7), one of the pioneers of psychometric testing, wrote that: '[t]here is no investigator who denies the fearful role of mental deficiency in the production of vice, crime and delinquency … not all criminals are feeble minded but all feeble minded are at least potential criminals' (p. 11). In his book, *The Criminal Imbecile*, Goddard (8) concluded that 'probably from 25–50 per cent of the people in our prisons are mentally defective and incapable of managing their affairs with ordinary prudence' (p. 7). From 1910 to around 1925, with the influence of Mendelian theories of inheritance, advances in mental testing and concerns about increasing numbers, the association between ID and delinquency transformed into an acceptance that feeble mindedness caused crime.

Intellectual disability and offending behaviour

One might imagine that the historical association between crime and ID has no currency today. It is sobering to note then that official UK government census data show that a disproportionate number of people with ID, that is 7.7 per cent or one in 13 overall, are detained under Mental Health Act (MHA) 1983 in England (9). In NHS hospitals the number is more than double what would be expected in the general population (5.6% or 1 in 18); this rises to more than five times the expected number in independent hospitals (13.1% or 1 in

It is with great regret that we report the death of William R. Lindsay during the production of this textbook.

8). The median length of stay for male inpatients with ID in NHS hospitals in England and Wales was five times greater (at 31 months) than that (5.8 months) for non-ID male mental health inpatients (10). The situation was even worse for female inpatients with intellectual disabilities. Their median length of stay was 11 times longer than for non-ID women mental health inpatients (31 months and 2.5 months respectively).

The seeming bias concerning the extent to which ID is associated with crime extends also to the scientific literature. Consider the landmark study published by Hodgins (11) that found that 50 per cent of 'intellectually handicapped' men in the study sample had been convicted of an offence and men in this category were three times more likely to offend than men with no handicap or mental disorder. The study involved a Swedish administrative birth cohort sample that was analysed retrospectively. No clinical assessment or formal measurement of IQ was carried out. The 'intellectual handicap' group comprised just 1.3 per cent of the total cohort of 15,117, so the authors were missing around about 50 per cent of people with ID we would expect to see in a normal distribution. This is perhaps explained by the fact that those included in the 'intellectual handicap' group comprised 192 people who had been placed in special classes in 'high schools' in Stockholm. So, it would appear that the 'intellectual handicap' subjects were possibly low functioning but not necessarily ID in conventional terms. The frequency of offences by type seems to confirm this. Just under a quarter (23.7%) of offences committed by males in the 'intellectual handicap' group were labelled 'traffic' (mainly 'drunken driving and driving without a licence'). This is not the typical offence profile of people with ID referred to services in the UK due to offending or offending-type behaviour (12). Lindsay and Dernevik (13) considered this issue in detail and concluded that Hodgins' (11) 'intellectual handicapped' group probably included people who had experienced conduct disorder or similar behavioural problems as children or adolescents, but were not those with conventional ID.

Another, more recent study that appears to confirm the bias concerning the link between ID and offending is that by Nixon et al. (14), who used a data-linking approach to investigate the rates of commission and victimization of offending behaviour in people with ID. They used the register of people with ID in Victoria, Australia and linked this to the state-wide police database. Using these methods Nixon (14) compared 2,220 people with ID and a history of criminal charges with 4,830 non-ID offenders. It was reported that people with ID were found to be twice as likely to have a criminal charge against them when compared to the non-ID group. One in five people with ID had been charged while one in ten of the mainstream group had a conviction. However, they found no differences between the two groups in the number of previous charges. People with ID were 15 times more likely to be charged with a sexual offence and three times more likely to be charged with a violent offence.

On the face of it these findings appear to confirm the notion that ID is associated with higher rates of offending. However, there are some very significant methodological problems with this study. Most concerning is that the authors included people with ID who had been *charged* with an offence and compared these data to non-disabled people in the community who had been *convicted*. The reason given for this was the suggestion that those with ID are much more likely to be diverted from the criminal justice system than the general population. This reasoning doesn't, however, off-set the bias of applying a more inclusive offending criterion and lower standard of criminal behaviour to people with ID than was applied to the non-disabled sample.

So, given the apparent persistence of this historical association, what does the evidence tell us about the link between ID and offending behaviour?

Prevalence

The research evidence supporting the relationship between IQ and offending is robust (15, 16, 17), with those in lower IQ groups having greater rates of offending than those in higher functioning groups. Even when socio-economic status is controlled for, offending behaviour has been found to be significantly related to IQ (18, 19). However, most studies involve participants with IQs in the 80–120 range and there is some evidence that when participants with IQs between one and two standard deviations below the mean (<80) are included, the relationship with offending is less straightforward. For example, McCord and McCord (20) found that while the offending rate for those in the low average IQ group (81–90 IQ points) was higher than that for those with above average IQ, those in the lowest IQ group (less than 80 IQ points) had an offending rate lower than that for the low average group. More recently, Mears and Cochran (21) reported data from the National Longitudinal Survey of Youth project in the US that indicated that relationship between IQ and offending is curvilinear with lower IQs (<85) associated with lower levels of offending. Thus, while there would seem to be a clear relationship between offending rates and intellectual functioning, when studies are extended to include people with IQs below 80–85, the relationship does not appear to be simple or linear.

Further, it is not clear whether people with ID commit more crime than those without ID or, in fact, whether the nature and frequency of offending by people with ID differs from that committed by offenders in the general population. The ambiguity concerning these issues is due in large part to methodological problems in prevalence studies in this area (22). One source of variation of prevalence of offending reported across studies is the location of the study (community, prison-remand, prison-sentenced, hospital–high/medium/low secure) which can result in sampling bias and filtering effects. Frequently, the inclusion criteria used in prevalence studies vary or are not clear and this can affect the rates obtained—particularly if people with borderline intelligence are included. Also, the method used to identify ID (standardized vs. screening IQ tests, educational history, clinical assessment) can have a significant impact.

These methodological issues are well illustrated in the research literature concerning the prevalence of offenders with ID in prisons. MacEachron (23) reviewed the literature for prevalence of offenders with ID in prisons in the USA and found a range of 2.6–39.6 per cent. Fazel et al. (24) reviewed 10 well-conducted studies of prevalence of ID in prisons (remand and sentenced) conducted between 1988 and 1997 in five common law countries and reported rates between 0–2.9 per cent.

More recently, Crocker et al. (25) assessed 281 pre-trial prisoners in Montreal, Canada using three subscales of a standardized ability scale and reported that 18.9 per cent were in the ID range. Sondenaa et al. (26) used an IQ screening assessment with 143 prisoners in Norway and found that 10.8 per cent fell in the ID range. Contrast these findings with a study of prisoners in Victoria, Australia in which Holland and Persson (27) found a prevalence of less than 1.3 per cent using the Wechsler Adult Intelligence Scale; and the results of a study of 389 remand prisoners in Scotland that indicated that less than 0.5 per cent of those assessed had ID (28). It is difficult to reconcile these findings without concluding that the location, assessment, and sampling methods account for the variance in large part.

Recidivism

Studies of recidivism rates for offenders with ID are affected by similar methodological problems. Reported rates tend to be high but vary considerably depending on research setting, procedures, and definitions of re-offending used (29). For example, Lund (30) found a re-offending rate of 67–72 per cent in a follow-up study involving 155 Danish offenders with ID who had been detained on statutory orders—while Klimecki et al. (31) reported a re-offending rate of 41.3 per cent for 75 released prisoners with ID in Victoria, Australia. More recently, Linhorst et al. (29) reported that 25 per cent of 252 offenders with developmental disabilities who completed a case management community programme were re-arrested within a six-month period following case closure; 43 per cent of those who dropped out of the programme were re-arrested during the same period.

Due to the lack of controlled studies involving ID and non-ID offenders it is difficult to make direct comparisons of recidivism rates. It would appear, however, that recidivism rates for offenders with ID are no higher than those for populations of general offenders. Gray et al. (32) conducted a two year follow-up of 145 offenders with ID and 996 offenders without ID, all discharged from independent sector hospitals in the UK. The ID group had a lower rate of reconviction for violent offences after two years (4.8%) than the non-ID group (11.2%). This trend held true for general offences also (9.7% and 18.7% for the respective groups).

The Northgate, Cambridge, and Abertay Pathways (NCAP) project reported on the offence characteristics of 477 adults with ID referred to ID services in three regions of the UK during a 12-month period because of antisocial or offending behaviour (12). They found that aggression (physical and verbal) accounted for over 80 per cent of the antisocial and offending behaviour referred, with sex offences (contact and non-contact) making up almost 30 per cent. Just 4 per cent of referrals concerned fire-setting whilst 19 per cent were related to property damage.

Assessment and treatment of offenders with intellectual disabilities

Work has been underway in recent years to develop assessment and intervention approaches to address the main types of offending behaviour that causes people with ID to come to the attention of the criminal justice system and specialist health services. Broadly, the assessment and treatment framework in secure hospital-based services follows a ten-point treatment programme (33) and includes:

1. A multi-axial diagnostic assessment that covers the degree of ID, cause of ID, pervasive developmental disorders, other developmental disabilities, mental illnesses, substance misuse or dependence, personality disorders, physical disorders, psychosocial disadvantage, and types of behavioural problems
2. A collaboratively developed psychological formulation
3. Risk assessments
4. A behaviour support plan
5. Pharmacotherapy, targeting both comorbid mental illnesses and physical conditions
6. Individual and group psychotherapy, guided by the psychological formulation
7. Offence-specific therapies, particularly targeting violent and sexual offending
8. Education, skills acquisition, and occupational/vocational rehabilitation
9. Community participation through a system of graded leave periods
10. Preparation for transition

Risk assessment

Risk assessment is the foundation for therapeutic efforts aimed at reducing offending behaviour and is the basis for clinical formulations of treatment need. Advances in the development of measures designed to accurately predict future violence and sexual aggression has now been extended to include offenders with intellectual disabilities. For example, Quinsey et al. (34) demonstrated that the Violence Risk Appraisal Guide (VRAG), one of the best established actuarial risk measures in the general offender literature, has good predictive accuracy when used with ID offenders. Gray et al. (32) conducted a more extensive investigation into the VRAG. They compared 145 patients with ID and 996 mainstream patients all discharged from hospital having been admitted due to serious offending-type behaviour. They found that the VRAG predicted reconviction rates in the ID sample with an effect size as large as that for the non-ID sample. Similarly, the HCR-20 and the VRAG have been found to have excellent predictive efficacy in offenders with an ID with a structured clinical judgement based on the HCR-20 being especially predictive (35).

Important research on the assessment and management of risk in offenders with ID has continued in a study (the '212 Multi-Centre Risk Study') involving 212 clients across a range of security settings: hospital high, medium, and low security, and community forensic ID services (36). The most complex presentations, in particular co-morbid personality disorder, were found in the more secure samples. Lindsay et al. (37) combined the total cohort of offenders with intellectual disabilities from the 212 risk study to evaluate the predictive validity of a range of static and dynamic risk assessments. They found that the VRAG, the HCR-20 (38), the short dynamic risk scale (34), and the emotional problems scale (39) all showed significant 'areas-under-the-curve' (AUC using receiver operator characteristics, ROC analyses) in relation to the prediction of violent incidents. The static-99 (40) also showed a significant area-under-the-curve in relation to the prediction of sexual incidents.

Dynamic risk assessments (e.g. SDRS) contrast with static risk assessments such as the VRAG in that the variables are amenable to change through treatment and management of the individual. As there seemed to be strong relationships between dynamic risk factors and future incidents for this client group, Lofthouse et al. (41) re-analysed the risk assessment data published by Lindsay et al (37) which showed that both the actuarial VRAG and the SDRS (an easy and quick to complete dynamic risk assessment) had equivalent risk predictive values of AUC = 0.71 and 0.72 respectively. They investigated the functional relationships between VRAG and SDRS items to determine whether they were independent, mediating/moderating, or acting as a proxy and found that the dynamic variables on the SDRS acted as a proxy for the VRAG variables. They concluded that since these risk factors captured elements of the same underlying risk construct associated with violence, and as dynamic variables are more accessible and clinically meaningful, dynamic assessment, in the form of the SDRS, could provide more immediate and clinically relevant information to manage patients' risk needs.

This research has demonstrated that there are a number of actuarial, dynamic, and clinical instruments, some of which have been developed specifically for this client group, that have good reliability, discriminative validity, and predictive validity with offenders with ID. If we are able to confirm that proximal dynamic indicators of risk not only have more clinical utility, but are also as predictive as established static risk indicators, this could have a significant impact on developing practice to help offenders with ID to access better services in the least restrictive environments.

Fire setting behaviour

Although recent research found that fire setting accounted for only a small proportion (4%) of those referred to ID services due to offending and antisocial behaviour (12), the proportion of people in secure ID services with histories of fire setting is significant. Hogue et al. (36) found that just over 21 per cent of those detained in low/medium secure services in a UK study sample had an index offence of arson.

In North America, Rice and Chaplin (42) delivered a social skills training intervention to two groups of five fire-setters in a maximum security psychiatric facility. One of the groups was reported to be functioning in the mild-borderline ID range. Both treatment groups improved significantly on an observational rating scale of role-played assertive behaviour. Following treatment, ten of the treated patients were discharged from hospital and none had been convicted or suspected of setting fires at 12-month follow-up.

Clare et al. (43) reported on a single case study involving a man with mild ID who had been transferred from a maximum security hospital to a specialist inpatient unit in the UK. He had prior convictions for arson and a history of making hoax telephone calls to the fire services. He underwent a comprehensive treatment package that included assertiveness and social skills training, coping skills training, covert sensitization, and surgery for a severe facial disfigurement. Significant clinical improvements were observed following treatment, and 30 months post-discharge to a community placement there had been no reports of fire setting or associated offending behaviour. Hall et al. (44) described the delivery of a sixteen-session group cognitive-behavioural approach to six male patients with ID and histories of fire-setting detained in a UK specialist NHS medium secure unit. Unfortunately outcome data were not provided although most group participants were reported to have responded positively to the intervention in terms of their clinical presentations, and two patients were successfully transferred to less secure placements following completion of the programme.

Taylor et al. (45) reported on a case series of four men with intellectual disabilities and convictions for arson offences detained at Northgate Hospital in north-east England. They received a 40-session group-based intervention that involved work on offence cycles, education about the costs associated with setting fires, training of skills to enhance future coping with emotional problems associated with previous fire setting behaviour, and work on personalized plans to prevent relapse. Given the demonstrated importance of anger/revenge as an antecedent to fire setting in this population (46, 47) up to 10 sessions are dedicated to developing anger-coping strategies using an evidence-based intervention developed by Taylor and Novaco (48). The fire setter treatment is a cognitive behaviourally framed approach developed especially for this patient group. It is a multi-faceted programme based on the approach first outlined by Jackson (49) which is underpinned by the functional analysis paradigm (50). The intervention successfully engaged these patients, all of whom completed the programme delivered over a period of four months. Despite their intellectual and cognitive limitations, all participants showed high levels of motivation and commitment that was reflected in generally improved attitudes with regard to personal responsibility, victim issues, and awareness of risk factors associated with their fire setting behaviour.

In a further series of case studies on six women with mild-borderline ID and histories of fire setting, Taylor et al. (51) also employed the same group intervention to successfully engage participants in the therapy process. All participants completed the programme and scores on measures related to fire treatment targets generally improved following the intervention. All but one of the treatment group participants had been discharged to community placements at two-year follow-up and there had been no reports of participants setting any fires or engaging in fire risk related behaviour.

Using the same assessment and treatment approach as that used by Taylor and colleagues above, Taylor et al. (47) investigated the outcomes for 14 men and women with ID and arson convictions. Study participants were assessed pre- and post-treatment on a number of fire-specific, anger, self-esteem, and depression measures. Following treatment, significant improvements were found in all areas assessed, except for depression. Taylor (52) reported on a follow-up of 24 fire setters (16 men and eight women) with ID who had completed the Northgate group treatment programme. The follow-up period ranged between four and 13 years post-treatment. Seventeen participants were living in the community, four remained in hospital placements and two women were deceased. At follow-up there had been no further arrests or convictions for arson in this cohort. File data available for 17 study participants showed that prior to treatment that sub-group had been responsible for setting a total of 425 fires. This suggests that the group fire setters intervention used by Taylor et al. above is associated with a significant harm reduction effect.

The results of these small and methodologically weak pilot studies do provide some limited encouragement and guidance to practitioners concerning the utility of group-based interventions for fire setting behaviour by people with ID. These cognitive-behaviourally orientated approaches are associated with significant improvements on fire setter specific and clinically relevant measures and reductions in fire setter behaviour following treatment.

Sexual aggression

Psychological treatment interventions for sex offenders with ID were reviewed by Courtney and Rose (53). Nineteen studies published post-1990 were reviewed. These included drug treatment, problem-solving, psycho-educational, and cognitive-behavioural approaches. Eleven studies were single case or small case series designs—four involved drug therapy and seven psychological interventions. The reported outcomes in these studies were generally positive. Eight 'larger' studies including one drug therapy, three service/management interventions and five psychological treatments were also reviewed. In terms of outcomes, psychological interventions appeared to be marginally superior. Eight of the studies involved group therapy interventions which were found to yield mixed outcomes, with reported recidivism rates ranging between 0–40 per cent. Based on this review and that by Lindsay (54), it appears that most treatment approaches show some promise, but the studies were quite limited—involving small, heterogeneous samples, utilizing measures with limited reliability and validity, using poorly defined outcomes, and incorporating treatment interventions that were often described poorly. The main methodological shortcoming, however, is the absence of any controlled studies. This is due primarily to the ethical difficulty in withholding a potentially beneficial treatment given the social and legal issues involved.

More recently there has been some support for the use of cognitive and problem solving techniques in therapy for sex offenders with ID that have been shown to be effective in reducing re-offending rates in the mainstream sex offender field (55). Support for the centrality of cognitive distortions in the sex offending perpetrated by people with ID came from a qualitative study of nine male sex offenders by Courtney et al. (56). They concluded that all aspects of the offence process were linked to offender attitudes and beliefs such as denial of the offence, blaming others and seeing themselves as the victim.

To date there have been three fairly large-scale reports on the outcome of treatment and management programmes for sexually aggressive men with ID. Following a policy of total deinstitutionalization in Vermont, USA, McGrath et al. (57) reviewed the treatment and management regimes of 103 adult men with ID who had exhibited harmful sexual behaviour (HSB). All participants lived in staffed or private homes with paid caregivers. Social and daily living skills were taught to participants and they were encouraged to participate in community activities. There were also treatments to promote risk management skills. Therefore, the treatment was focused on skills development rather than on changing attitudes and beliefs. In an 11-year follow-up period, with an average of 5.8 years follow-up, the authors reported a 10.7 per cent rate for further HSB. As a comparison, the authors reported on 195 treated and untreated adult male sexual offenders without ID who had been followed up for an average period of 5.72 years. They found that 23.1 per cent of these individuals had been charged with a new sexual offence at some point during the follow-up period.

Murphy et al. (58) conducted a treatment study involving 46 male sex offenders with ID who were living in community and/or secure settings in the UK. Separately, Murphy and Sinclair (59) had reported that although this study was designed as a waiting list controlled treatment trial, it proved impossible to obtain control participants data at time 2. Control data were therefore not reported. Treatment groups ran over a one-year period and assessments included measures of sexual knowledge, victim empathy, and cognitive distortions as measured by the Questionnaire on Attitudes Consistent with Sexual Offences (QACSO; 60). Treatment was manualized and conducted across a number of settings with men attending from services such as community residential homes as well as secure services. The detailed manual described methods for addressing deficits in sexual knowledge, poor victim empathy, cognitive distortions, offending patterns and routines, and inadequate relationships, in addition to sections guiding therapists through disclosure exercises. Sexual knowledge, victim empathy, and cognitive distortions improved significantly following treatment, however, in Murphy et al (58) only treatment gains on sexual knowledge and cognitive distortion measures were maintained at six-month follow-up. It was reported also that 8.7 per cent of the sample (4/46) engaged in further sexually aggressive behaviour in the six months after completing the treatment programme. In an extension of this study, involving a long-term follow-up of 34 of the men who had completed SOTSEC-ID treatment, on average 3.5 years after the end of their treatment, Heaton and Murphy (61) reported that the improvements in sexual knowledge, empathy, and cognitive distortions that occurred during treatment were maintained at follow-up. However 32 per cent (11/34) of the men had shown further sexually abusive behaviour, albeit of lesser severity than their original behaviours. Only two (i.e. 6%) of these men had been convicted. These data illustrate the importance of being clear whether men have engaged in harmful sexual behaviour or have actually been convicted when comparing the outcomes for different interventions.

Lindsay et al. (62) reported a 20-year follow-up of 156 male sexual offenders, 126 male non-sexual offenders and 27 female offenders seen in community forensic ID services. All received at least four weeks assessment and treatment directed at their criminogenic need (deviant sexuality, anger, alcohol related treatment, etc.). All but 15 participants continued to have unrestricted access to the community throughout the follow-up period during which time 16 per cent of the sex offender cohort was reported to have carried out further HSBs (all could be classified as offending-like behaviours but not all were prosecuted). For non-sexual male offenders, 43 per cent committed another incident (mostly violent). This between-group difference in re-offending rates was significant.

Lindsay et al. (62) also recorded the number of incidents perpetrated by the recidivists over the follow-up period. This was possible because the study was conducted in a circumscribed region where incident records were gathered routinely via six-monthly case reviews that were held on each client for as long as any agency involved with the client wished them to continue. They found that, for recidivists only, there was a significant reduction in the number of incidents committed when comparing figures from two years prior to the referral and up to 20 years after referral. In conducting this exercise, they used a cut-off of 15 incidents for any one individual, in order not to increase the likelihood of finding a positive result for harm reduction. They argued that some individuals had committed dozens of incidents prior to referral and this would have significantly biased the analysis in favour of the harm reduction hypothesis. The highest number of HSB incidents committed by an individual following referral was 13 (below the cut-off of 15). The 16 per cent of recidivists in the sex offender cohort had committed 287 HSBs prior to referral and 76 after referral. This represents around a 70 per cent reduction in the number of HSBs and a significant amount of harm reduction amongst recidivists. If one takes into account that the majority of the sex offender cohort (84%) did not re-offend, then the reduction in HSB following referral is over 95 per cent.

Constructing a treatment effectiveness study for sex offenders is very difficult because referring agencies, such as the care services, courts, or the criminal justice system, are reluctant for public protection reasons to allow any delay of sex offender treatment. This means that having study waiting list control conditions is very difficult. It certainly means that randomized allocation of participants to experimental and no treatment conditions is, in reality, almost impossible. For these reasons there have been few RCTs in the non-ID literature on sexually aggressive behaviour, and none at all in the ID literature. Based on the limited evidence available however, it is possible to conclude, albeit tentatively, that psychologically informed and well-structured interventions appear to yield reasonable outcomes in the treatment of sex offenders with ID. Cognitive behavioural treatment appears to have a positive effect on offence-related attitudes and cognitions, sexual knowledge, and victim empathy. Longer periods of treatment may result in better outcomes that are maintained for longer periods. Comparison studies, although limited methodologically, indicate that psychological interventions may significantly reduce recidivism rates in sex offenders with ID—and where recidivism does occur, treatment may result in significant harm reduction effects.

Anger and aggression

Research on several continents has found high rates of aggression amongst people with ID—with much higher rates for those living in institutional and secure forensic facilities than for those residing in community settings (63). The impact of aggression is significant in a number of ways for people with ID and those who provide support and services to them. Aggression has been shown to be the main reason for individuals in this client group to be prescribed anti-psychotic and behavioural control drugs (64), despite there being little or no evidence for their efficacy (65, 66); and is the primary reason for people with ID to be admitted or re-admitted to institutional settings (67).

While it is neither necessary nor sufficient for aggression to occur, anger has been shown to be strongly associated with and predictive of violence in men with ID and offending histories (68). Thus anger has become a legitimate therapeutic target. The treatment of anger and aggression using cognitive-behavioural interventions has been extensively evaluated with a range of clinical populations (48). Further, there is evidence from studies in non-ID fields that for a range of psychological problems the effects of cognitive-behavioural treatments are maintained and increase over time compared to control conditions (48).

Willner (69) reviewed nine controlled studies involving people with ID that compared cognitive behavioural treatment for anger control problems with wait-list control conditions. Most of these interventions were based on the treatment approach developed by Novaco (70) that incorporates Meichenbaum's (71) stress inoculation paradigm. All of these studies reported significant improvements on outcome measures for those in treatment conditions that were maintained at three to 12-month follow-up. Nicoll et al. (72) systematically reviewed 12 studies of cognitive behavioural treatment for anger in adults with ID published between 1999 and 2011. Nine studies were included in a meta-analysis that yielded a large uncontrolled effect size (average ES = 0.84).

Taylor and colleagues have evaluated individual cognitive-behavioural anger treatment with detained male patients with ID and significant histories of violence in a linked series of studies (73, 74, 75). The 18-session treatment package included a six-session broadly psycho-educational and motivational preparatory phase; followed by a 12-session treatment phase based an individual formulation of each participant's anger problems and needs, following the classical cognitive-behavioural stages of cognitive preparation, skills acquisition, skills rehearsal, and then practice *in vivo*. These studies showed significant improvements on self-reported measures of anger disposition, reactivity, and imaginal provocation following intervention in the treatment groups compared with scores for the control groups, and these differences were maintained for up to four months following treatment.

The impact of these anger interventions on aggressive behaviour, including physical violence, has been investigated empirically on only a few occasions. Allan et al. (76) and Lindsay et al. (77) reported reductions in violence following a group intervention in case series of six women and six men respectively with violence convictions living in the community. In a larger study involving 47 people with ID and histories of aggression, Lindsay et al. (78) showed that following a community group anger intervention 14 per cent of participants had been aggressive during follow-up, compared with 45 per cent of people in a control condition.

Novaco and Taylor (79) described an evaluation of the impact of the cognitive behavioural anger treatment described earlier (73) on violent behaviour by offenders with ID living in secure forensic hospital settings. Violence incident data were collected retrospectively from hospital case notes over a 24-month period. The participants in this study were 44 men and six women referred by their clinical teams for anger treatment on the basis of their histories of aggression and/or current presentation. The total number of physical attacks against staff and patients fell from 319 in the 12-months before treatment to 153 in the 12-month period following treatment. This represents a reduction after treatment of 52 per cent. Importantly, the reduction in physical assaults was associated with measured reductions in anger over the course of treatment as indexed by several anger measures validated for use with this population.

In summary, there is an emerging research evidence base that cognitive behavioural anger interventions can be effective in the treatment of offenders with ID and histories of aggression and violence in terms of improvements on self-report and informant anger dependent measures that are associated with significant reductions in the number of violent incidents recorded following treatment.

Service level treatment outcome studies

There is limited empirical information on service-level outcome domains and indicators for people with ID being treated in secure hospitals. Based on a systematic review which identified 60 eligible

Table 17.1 Framework of outcome domains and sub-domains

Domain	Sub-domain
Effectiveness	1. Discharge outcome/direction of care pathway
	2. Delayed discharge/current placement appropriateness
	3. Readmission
	4. Length of hospital stay
	5. Adaptive functioning
	6. Clinical symptom severity/treatment needs (patient rated)
	7. Clinical symptom severity/treatment needs (clinician rated)
	8. Recovery/engagement/progress on treatment goals (patient rated)
	9. Recovery/engagement/progress on treatment goals (clinician rated)
	10. Re-offending (charges or convictions)
	11. Offending like behaviour (no charges or convictions)
	12. Incidents in care setting (violence or self-harm)
	13. Risk assessment measures
	14. Security need (physical, procedural, escort level/leave)
Patient safety	15. Premature death/suicide
	16. Physical health
	17. Medication use (exceeding BNF maximum doses, patient-rated side effects, PRN medication usage)
	18. Restrictive practices (restraint)
	19. Restrictive practices (seclusion or segregation)
	20. Victimization/safeguarding alerts
Patient (or carer) experience	21. Involvement in care
	22. Satisfaction/complaints
	23. Quality of life (patient rated)
	24. Therapeutic climate
	25. Access to meaningful activity or work
	26. Level of support/involvement in community (post discharge)
	27. Carer experience: communication with service/involvement in care

Adapted from *BJPsych Open*, 3,1 Morrissey C, Langdon PE, Geach N et al., A systematic review and synthesis of outcome domains for use within forensic services for people with intellectual disabilities, pp. 41–56.
DOI: https://doi.org/10.1192/bjpo.bp.116.003616.

studies, an outcomes framework that identified and developed three domains and 27 sub-domains that could be used to measure treatment outcomes for this population has been developed (80) (see Table 17.1).

A further systematic review of 52 studies to review treatment outcomes from hospitals that treat people with ID and mental health and/or behavioural problems found that in-patient forensic services offer a genuine alternative to prison. Well-resourced and appropriately staffed forensic community teams are needed to help support discharge from these services ((81), in press).

Conclusions

Recent political, health, and social care policies such as deinstitutionalization and Transforming Care in England (82) have had a significant impact on offenders with ID who are now more visible in the wider community than before. This in turn has meant that more people with ID who engage in antisocial or offending behaviour are being dealt with by the criminal justice system, and local generic ID services are managing more complex and forensically risky cases. This phenomenon is demonstrated by Lund (83) in a study of 123 offenders with ID on statutory care orders in Denmark which found 2–3 times increases in the incidence of sex, violence, and arson offences when comparing sentencing in 1973 and 1983. Lund suggested that these increases were less to do with an increase in offending per se in this population, but a result of deinstitutionalization policies during this period, whereby people with ID were no longer detained in hospital for indeterminate lengths of time, but living in the community where their offending behaviour was more likely to be subject to normal legal processes.

In England, approximately 191,000, or 20 per cent of people with ID are in contact with community services and 3035, or 0.3 per cent are treated within inpatient psychiatric, including forensic services (84). Another 6,000 are in prison settings (85), and there is wide geographical variation in care or criminal justice pathways depending on commissioning intent, availability specialist skills/services and system response to offences committed by people with ID (86, 87). Although more visible than in the past, it remains unclear whether people with ID are over- or under-represented in offender populations, or whether offending is more prevalent among people with ID than the general population. There is a need for controlled studies involving offenders with ID vs. non-ID offenders vs. non-offenders with ID in order to make direct comparisons of prevalence. This same requirement applies to recidivism studies.

To date, the treatment and management of offenders with ID have not been informed by good quality research. This is beginning to change. There have been some developments in the treatment of offenders with ID based on interventions using cognitive behavioural approaches. The most significant development has been in the field of anger treatment where programmes have been evaluated in a number of controlled studies. Although these studies have generally involved wait-list control rather than randomized designs, a host of positive outcomes indicate that anger treatment programmes can be incorporated into the general management of violent and aggressive offenders with ID with some confidence.

Another area of development has been in cognitive behavioural approaches for people with ID who display sexually aggressive behaviour. There have been a number of single-case reports producing encouraging results and, more importantly, employing lengthy follow-up periods. Comparisons of convenience samples have produced positive outcomes. Given the methodological weaknesses of these studies, the results should be treated cautiously but with optimism.

There have been a small number of studies concerning cognitive behaviourally framed interventions for fire setters with ID which have provided promising outcomes and guidance for practitioners. However, controlled evaluations of these interventions are certainly required. Similarly there are some early indications that interventions for alcohol misuse (88, 89) and cognitive skills training (90) adapted from mainstream offender practice may have value in work with offenders with ID.

For the future, larger, more powerful, and better-designed controlled trials are needed to show if the effects of treatment interventions obtained to date can be replicated, and longer-term follow-up would help to evaluate the impact of psychological treatment gains on reducing future offending behaviour. A range of process issues, including the active ingredients and optimum length of treatment and relative costs, also require further investigation.

MULTIPLE CHOICE QUESTIONS

Questions

Please select the single most appropriate answer.

1. Which of the following statements are true when comparing people with intellectual disabilities with general population?

A. There are disproportionately higher numbers of people with intellectual disabilities detained in hospitals in England
B. The length of stay for people with intellectual disabilities is unknown
C. People with intellectual disabilities commit more sexual offences
D. People with intellectual disabilities commit more fire setting offences
E. People with intellectual disabilities commit more driving offences

2. What factors influence the prevalence of offending in people with intellectual disabilities?

A. Definition of intellectual disability used to inform criteria for studies
B. Methods used to determine or diagnose intellectual disability
C. Setting that the study takes place in (prison, police cells, courts etc)
D. Availability of health, social care, and criminal justice liaison services where the study takes place.
E. All of the above

3. What is the most common (forensic) reason for contact with intellectual disability services?

A. Aggression (physical and verbal)
B. Property damage
C. Sexual inappropriate behavior (contact and non-contact)
D. Fire setting
E. Driving offences

4. What is the ten-point treatment programme in forensic learning disability services?

A. A protocol for medication optimization
B. A framework to deliver assessment and treatment in secure services
C. A framework to deliver assessment and treatment in primary care
D. Policy directive in England for people with intellectual disability
E. A framework for integrating healthcare with social care

5. All of the following are true except:

A. Anger has been shown to be strongly associated violence in men with intellectual disabilities and offending histories
B. Anger has been shown to be predictive of violence in men with intellectual disabilities and offending histories
C. Cognitive behavior therapy has little efficacy in the treatment of anger in this population
D. Cognitive behaviour therapy in the treatment of anger in this population incorporates the stress inoculation paradigm
E. Aggression is one of the commonest reasons for use of psychotropic medication prescribing in men with intellectual disabilities

Answers

1. A. True. Compared to the number of people with mental health problems in the general population being treated in in-patient settings, there is a comparatively higher proportion of people with LD receiving in-patient care at any point in time. In England, approximately 191,000, or 20 per cent of people with ID are in contact with community services and 3,035, or 0.3 per cent are treated within in-patient

psychiatric, including forensic services. Official UK government census data show that a disproportionate number of people with ID, that is 7.7 per cent or one in 13 overall, are detained under the Mental Health Act (MHA) 1983 in England. In NHS hospitals the number is more than double what would be expected in the general population (5.6% or 1 in 18); this rises to more than five times the expected number in independent hospitals (13.1% or 1 in 8).

B. False. The LoS in different categories of beds (standard and actual) are available in publications and guidance documents including benchmarking reports. The median length of stay for male in-patients with ID in NHS hospitals in England and Wales was five times greater (at 31 months) than that (5.8 months) for non-ID male mental health inpatients (10). The situation was even worse for female in-patients with intellectual disabilities. Their median length of stay was 11 times longer than for non-ID women mental health in-patients (31 months and 2.5 months respectively).

C. False. People with LD who sexually offend are overrepresented in offender study populations.

D. False. People with LD who set fire are overrepresented in offender study populations. Although recent research found that fire setting accounted for only a small proportion (4%) of those referred to ID services due to offending and antisocial behaviour (12), the proportion of people in secure ID services with histories of fire setting is significant.

E. False. There is no evidence for this.

2. E. All of the above are reasons for the variation seen reported prevalence of offending in people with LD. The ambiguity concerning these issues is due in large part to methodological problems in prevalence studies in this area. One source of variation of prevalence of offending reported across studies is the location of the study (community, prison-remand, prison-sentenced, hospital—high/medium/low secure) which can result in sampling bias and filtering effects. Frequently, the inclusion criteria used in prevalence studies vary or are not clear and this can affect the rates obtained—particularly if people with borderline intelligence are included. Also, the method used to identify ID (standardized vs. screening IQ tests, educational history, clinical assessment) can have a significant impact.

3. A. Aggression both outwards and towards self is the most common reason for contact with LD services.

4. B. This programme provides a systematic approach to multidisciplinary and multi-modal assessment and treatment in secure services.

5. C. There is an emerging research evidence base that cognitive behavioural anger interventions can be effective in the treatment of offenders with ID and histories of aggression and violence in terms of improvements on self-report and informant anger-dependent measures that are associated with significant reductions in the number of violent incidents recorded following treatment.

REFERENCES

1. Seguin E (1846). *Traitement moral, hygiène et éducation des idiots et des autres enfants arriérés*. Paris, France: J.B. Bailliere.
2. Conolly J (1847). *The construction and government of lunatic asylums and hospitals for the insane*. London: John Churchill, https://books.google.co.uk.
3. Trent JW (1994). *Inventing the feeble mind. A history of mental retardation in the United States*. Berkeley, CA: University of California Press.
4. Kerlin IN (1858). *A brief history of twenty-two imbecile children*. Philadelphia, PA: Hunt.
5. Scheerenberger RC (1983). *A history of mental retardation*. London: Brooks Publishing Company.
6. Kerlin IN (1890). *The moral imbecile*. Reprinted from the 17th annual report of the National Conference of Charities and Correction, held at Baltimore, 14–21 May, 1890.
7. Terman L (1911). *The measurement of intelligence*. Boston, MA: Houghton Mifflin.
8. Goddard H (1921). *The criminal imbecile*. New York, NY: Dodd, Mead and Co.
9. Health and Social Care Information Centre (2014). *Inpatients formally detained in hospitals under the Mental Health Act 1983, and patients subject to community treatment: Annual report, England, 2013/14*. London: Health and Social Care Information Centre.
10. Care Quality Commission (2011). *Count me in 2010: Results of the 2010 national census of inpatients and patients on supervised community treatment in mental health and learning disability services in England and Wales*. London: Care Quality Commission.
11. Hodgins S (1992). Mental disorder, intellectual deficiency, and crime. Evidence from a birth cohort. *Arch Gen Psychiatry*. Jun;49(6):476–483.
12. O'Brien, G., Taylor, J.L., Lindsay, W.R., Holland, A.J., Carson, D., Steptoe, L., et al. (2010). A multi-centre study of adults with learning disabilities referred to services for antisocial or offending behaviour: Demographic, individual, offending and service characteristics. *Journal of Learning Disabilities and Offending Behaviour*, 1(2), 5–15.
13. Lindsay and Dernevik (2013). Risk and offenders with intellectual disabilities. *Criminal Behaviour and Mental Health* 23: 151–157.
14. Nixon M, Thomas S, Daffern M, Ogloff J (2017). Estimating the risk of crime and victimisation in people with intellectual disability: A data-linkage study. *Social Psychiatry and Psychiatric Epidemiology*. 52. 10.1007/s00127-017-1371-3.
15. Hirschi T, Hindelang MJ (1977). Intelligence and delinquency: A revisionist view. *American Sociological Review*, 42, 571–587.
16. Goodman R, Simonoff E, Stevenson J (1995). The impact of child IQ, parent IQ and sibling IQ on child and behaviour deviance scores. *Journal of Child Psychology and Psychiatry*, 36, 409–425.
17. West DJ, Farrington DP (1973). *Who becomes delinquent?* London: Heinemann.
18. Moffit TE, Gabrielli WF, Mednick SA, Schulsinger F (1991). Socio-economic status, IQ and delinquency. *Journal of Abnormal Psychology*, 90, 152–157.
19. Farrington DP (1995). The development of offending and antisocial behaviour from childhood: Key findings from the Cambridge study in delinquent development. *Journal of Child Psychology and Psychiatry*, 36, 929–964.

20. McCord W, McCord J (1959). *Origins of crime: A new evaluation of the Cambridge-Somerville*. New York: Columbia Press.
21. Mears DP, Cochran JC (2013). What is the effect of IQ on offending? *Criminal Justice and Behavior*, 40, 1280–1300.
22. Lindsay WR, Taylor JL (2010). Mentally disordered offenders: Intellectual Disability. In GJ Towl and DA Crighton (Eds.), *Forensic Psychology* (pp. 285–308). Chichester: BPS Blackwell.
23. MacEachron AE (1979). Mentally retarded offenders prevalence and characteristics. *American Journal of Mental Deficiency*, 84, 165–176.
24. Fazel S, Xenitidis K, Powell J (2008). The prevalence of intellectual disabilities among 12,000 prisoners: A systematic review. *International Journal of Law and Psychiatry*, 31, 369–373.
25. Crocker AJ, Cote G, Toupin J, St-Onge B (2007). Rate and characteristics of men with an intellectual disability in pre-trial detention. *Journal of Intellectual and Developmental Disabilities*, 32, 143–152.
26. Søndenaa E, Rasmussen K, Palmstierna T, Nøttestad J (2008). The prevalence and nature of intellectual disability in Norwegian prisons. *Journal of Research in Intellectual Disabilities*, 53, 1129–1137.
27. Holland., S, Persson P (2011). Intellectual disability in the Victorian prison system: Characteristics of prisoners with an intellectual disability released from prison in 2003–2006. *Psychology, Crime and Law*, 17, 25–41.
28. Davidson M, Humphreys MS, Johnstone EC, Owens DG (1995). Prevalence of psychiatric morbidity among remand prisoners in Scotland. *British Journal of Psychiatry*, 167, 548–554.
29. Linhorst DM, McCutchen TA, Bennett L (2003). Recidivism among offenders with developmental disabilities participating in a case management programme. *Research in Developmental Disabilities*, 24, 210–230.
30. Lund J (1990). Mentally retarded criminal offenders in Denmark. *British Journal of Psychiatry*, 156, 726–731.
31. Klimecki MR, Jenkinson J, Wilson, L. (1994). A study of recidivism among offenders with intellectual disability. *Australia & New Zealand Journal of Developmental Disabilities (Journal of Intellectual & Developmental Disabilities)*, 19, 209–219.
32. Gray NS, Fitzgerald S, Taylor J, MacCulloch M, Snowden R (2007). Predicting future reconviction in offenders with intellectual disabilities: The predictive efficacy of the VRAG, PCL-SV and the HCR-20. *Psychological Assessment*, 19, 474–479.
33. Alexander RT, Hiremath A, Chester V, Green FN, Gunaratna IJ, Hoare S (2011). Evaluation of treatment outcomes from a medium secure unit for people with intellectual disability. *Advances in Mental Health and Intellectual Disabilities* 5(1), 22–32.
34. Quinsey, V.L. (2004). Risk assessment and management in community settings. In W.R. Lindsay, J.L. Taylor and P. Sturmey (Eds.), *Offenders with developmental disabilities* (pp. 131–142), Chichester: John Wiley & Sons.
35. Fitzgerald S., Gray NS, Alexander RT, Bagshaw R, Chesterman R, Huckle P, Jones,SK, Taylor J, Williams T, Snowden RJ (2013). Predicting institutional violence in offenders with intellectual disabilities: The predictive efficacy of the VRAG and the HCR-20. *Journal of Applied Research in Intellectual Disabilities*, 26, 384–393.
36. Hogue T, Steptoe L, Taylor JL, Lindsay WR, Mooney P, Pinkney L, Johnston S, Smith AHW, O'Brien G (2006). A comparison of offenders with intellectual disability across three levels of security. *Criminal Behaviour and Mental Health*, 16, 13–28.
37. Lindsay WR, Hogue TE, Taylor JL, Steptoe L, Mooney P, O'Brien G, Johnston,S, Smith AHW (2008). Risk assessment in offenders with intellectual disability: A comparison across three levels of security. *International Journal of Offender Therapy and Comparative Criminology*, 52, 90–111.
38. Webster CD, Eaves D, Douglas KS, Wintrup A (1997). *The HCR-20: The assessment of dangerousness and risk. Version 2*. Vancouver, Canada: Simon Fraser University and British Colombia Forensic Psychiatric Services Commission.
39. Prout HT, Strohmer DC, 1991. EPS, emotional problem scale. In: Professional Manual for the Behaviour Rating Sacles and the Self-Report Inventory, *Psychological Assessment Resources*, Inc. Odessa, FL, p. 31.
40. Hanson RK, Thornton D (1999). *Static-99: improving actuarial risk assessments for sex offenders.* (User report 1999-02). Ottowa: Department of the Solicitor General of Canada.
41. Lofthouse RE, Totsika V, Hastings RP, Lindsay WR, Hogue T, Taylor JL (2014). How do static and dynamic risk factors work together to predict violence amongst offenders with an intellectual disability? *Journal of Intellectual Disability Research*, 58, 125–133.
42. Rice ME, Chaplin TC (1979). Social skills training for hospitalised male arsonists. *Journal of Behaviour Therapy and Experimental Psychiatry*, 10, 105–108.
43. Clare ICH, Murphy GH, Cox D, Chaplin EH (1992). Assessment and treatment of firesetting: A single case investigation using a cognitive behavioural model. *Criminal Behaviour and Mental Health*, 2, 253–268.
44. Hall I, Clayton P, Johnson P (2005). In T. Riding, C. Swann, B. Swann (Eds.), *The Handbook of Forensic Learning Disabilities* (pp. 51–72). Oxford: Radcliffe Publishing.
45. Taylor JL, Thorne I, Slavkin., M. (2004). Treatment of firesetters. In W.R. Lindsay, J.L. Taylor and P. Sturmey (Eds.), *Offenders with Developmental Disabilities* (pp. 221–240). Chichester: Wiley.
46. Murphy GH, Clare ICH (1996). Analysis of motivation in people with mild learning disabilities (mental handicap) who set fires. *Psychology, Crime and Law*, 2(3), 153–164. doi:10.1080/10683169608409774.
47. Taylor JL, Thorne I, Robertson A, Avery G (2002). Evaluation of a group intervention for convicted arsonists with mild and borderline intellectual disabilities. *Criminal Behaviour and Mental Health*, 12, 282–293.
48. Taylor JL, Novaco RW (2005). *Anger treatment for people with developmental disabilities: A theory, evidence and manual based approach*. Chichester: Wiley.
49. Jackson HF (1994). Assessment of fire-setters. In M. McMurran and J. Hodge (Eds.), *The Assessment of Criminal Behaviours in Secure Settings* (pp. 94–126). London: Jessica Kingsley.
50. Jackson H, Glass C, Hope S (1987a). Why are arsonists not violent offenders? *International Journal of Offender Therapy and Comparative Criminology*, 31, 143–151.
51. Taylor JL, Robertson A, Thorne I, Belshaw T, Watson A.(2006). Responses of female firesetters with mild and borderline intellectual disabilities to a group-based intervention. *Journal of Applied Research in Intellectual Disabilities*, 19, 179–190.
52. Taylor JL (2014). Roots, referrals, risks and remedies for offenders with intellectual disabilities. Paper presented to 'A

Risky Business' BPS conference, October, 2014, University of Manchester, UK.

53. Courtney J, Rose, J. (2004). The effectiveness of treatment for male sex offenders with learning disabilities: A review of the literature. *Journal of Sexual Aggression*, 10, 215–236.
54. Lindsay WR (2002). Research and literature on sex offenders with intellectual and developmental disabilities. *Journal of Intellectual Disability Research*, 46 (Suppl. 1), 74–85.
55. Hanson RK, Gordon A, Harris AJR, Marques JK, Murphy W, Quinsey VL, Seto MC (2002). First report of the collaborative outcome data project on the effectiveness of psychological treatment for sex offenders. *Sexual Abuse: A Journal of Research and Treatment*, 14, 169–194.
56. Courtney J, Rose J, Mason O (2006). The offence process of sex offenders with intellectual disabilities: A qualitative study. *Sexual Abuse: A Journal of Research and Treatment*, 18, 169–191.
57. McGrath RJ, Livingston JA, Falk G. 2007. Community management of sex offenders with intellectual disabilities: Characteristics, services, and outcome of a state-wide program. *Intellect Dev Disability*, 45(6):391–398.
58. Murphy GH, Sinclair N, Hays S-J, Heaton K, Powell S, Langdon P et al. (2010). Effectiveness of group cognitive-behavioural treatment for men with intellectual disabilities at risk of sexual offending. *Journal of Applied Research in Intellectual Disabilities*, 23, 537–551.
59. Murphy G, Sinclair N. (2006). Group cognitive behaviour treatment for men with sexually abusive behaviour. Paper presented to 6th Seattle Club Conference on Research and People with Intellectual Disabilities.
60. Lindsay WR, Whitefield E, Carson D (2007). An assessment for attitudes consistent with sexual offending for use with offenders with intellectual disability. *Legal and Criminological Psychology*, 12, 55–68.
61. Heaton KM, Murphy GM (2013). Men with intellectual disabilities who have attended sex offender treatment groups: A follow-up. *Journal of Applied Research in Intellectual Disabilities*, 26, 489–500.
62. Lindsay WR, Steptoe L, Wallace L, Haut F, Brewster E (2013). An evaluation and 20 year follow up of recidivism in a community intellectual disability service. *Criminal Behaviour and Mental Health*, 23, 138–149.
63. Taylor JL, Novaco RW (2013). Anger control problems. In J.L. Taylor, W.R. Lindsay, R. Hastings, C. Hatton (Eds.). *Psychological therapies for adults with intellectual disabilities* (pp. 133–155). Chichester: Wiley.
64. Aman MG, Richmond G, Stewart AW, Bell JC, Kissell R (1987). The Aberrant Behavior Checklist: Factor structure and the effect of subject variables in American and New Zealand facilities. *American Journal on Mental Deficiency*, 91, 570–578.
65. Brylewski J, Duggan, L. (1999). Antipsychotic medication for challenging behaviour in people with learning disability. *Journal of Intellectual Disability Research*, 43, 360–371.
66. Tyrer P, Oliver-Africano P C, Ahmed Z, Bouras N, Cooray S, Deb S, et al. (2008). Risperidone, haloperidol, and placebo in the treatment of aggressive challenging behaviour in patients with intellectual disabilities: A randomised controlled trial. *The Lancet*, 371, 57–63.
67. Lakin KC, Hill BK, Hauber FA, Bruininks RH, Heal LW (1983). New admissions to a national sample of public residential facilities. *American Journal on Mental Retardation*, 88, 13–20.
68. Novaco RW, Taylor JL (2004). Assessment of anger and aggression in male offenders with developmental disabilities. *Psychological Assessment*, 16, 42–50.
69. Willner P (2007). Cognitive behaviour therapy for people with learning disabilities: Focus on anger. *Advances in Mental Health and Learning Disabilities*, 1(2), 14–21.
70. Novaco RW (1975). *Anger control: The development and evaluation of an experimental treatment*. Lexington, MA: Heath.
71. Meichenbaum D (1985). *Stress inoculation training*. Oxford: Pergamon Press.
72. Nicoll M, Beail N, Saxon D (2013). Cognitive behavioural treatment for anger in adults with intellectual disabilities: A systematic review and meta-analysis. *Journal of Applied Research in Intellectual Disabilities*, 26, 47–62.
73. Taylor JL, Novaco RW, Gillmer BT, Robertson A, Thorne I (2005). Individual cognitive-behavioural anger treatment for people with mild-borderline intellectual disabilities and histories of aggression: A controlled trial. *British Journal of Clinical Psychology*, 44, 367–382.
74. Taylor JL, Novaco RW, Gillmer B, Thorne I (2002). Cognitive-behavioural treatment of anger intensity among offenders with intellectual disabilities. *Journal of Applied Research in Intellectual Disabilities*, 15, 151–165.
75. Taylor JL, Novaco, RW, Guinan C, Street N (2004). Development of an imaginal provocation test to evaluate treatment for anger problems in people with intellectual disabilities. *Clinical Psychology and Psychotherapy*, 11, 233–246.
76. Allan R, Lindsay WR, Macleod F, Smith AHW (2001). Treatment of women with intellectual disabilities who have been involved with the criminal justice system for reasons of aggression. *Journal of Applied Research in Intellectual Disabilities*, 14, 340–347.
77. Lindsay WR, Allan R, Macleod F, Smart N, Smith AHW (2003). Long term treatment and management of violent tendencies of men with intellectual disabilities convicted of assault. *Mental Retardation*, 41, 47–56.
78. Lindsay WR, Allan R, Parry,C, Macleod F, Cottrell J, Overend H, Smith AHW (2004). Anger and aggression in people with intellectual disabilities: Treatment and follow-up of consecutive referrals and a waiting list comparison. *Clinical Psychology and Psychotherapy*, 11, 225–264.
79. Novaco RW, Taylor JL (2015). Reduction of assualtive behaviour following anger treatment of forensic hospital patients with intellectual disabilities. *Behaviour Research and Therapy*, 65, 52–59.
80. Morrissey C, Langdon P, Geach N, Chester V, Ferriter M, Lindsay W, McCarthy J, Devapriam J, Walker DM, Duggan C, Alexander R (2017). A systematic review and synthesis of outcome domains for use within forensic services for people with intellectual disabilities. *British Journal of Psychiatry Open*, 3, 1–16. *doi: 10.1192/bjpo.bp.116.003616*.
81. Langdon P, Melvin C, Barnoux M, Shepstone L, Chester V, Roy A, Devapriam J, Lovell M, Alexander R (2018, in press) *People with Intellectual Disabilities and Mental Health, Behavioural or Forensic Problems: National Data about Inpatient Bed Usage and Workforce*, HEE RCPsych Report.
82. NHS England (2015). *Building the right support: A national plan to develop community services and close inpatient facilities for people with a learning disability and/or autism who display behaviour that challenges, including those with a mental health condition*. https://www.england.nhs.uk/wp-content/uploads/2015/10/ld-nat-imp-plan-oct15.pdf.

83. Lund J (1990). Mentally retarded criminal offenders in Denmark. *British Journal of Psychiatry*, 156, 726–731.
84. Devapriam J, Rosenbach A, Alexander R (2015). In-patient services for people with intellectual disability and mental health or behavioural difficulties. *BJPsych Advances*, 21, 116–123.
85. Prison Reform Trust (2007) Indefinitely Maybe? How the Indeterminate Sentence for Public Protection is Unjust and Unsustainable. Prison Reform Trust.
86. Royal College of Psychiatrists (2013) Psychiatry of Intellectual Disability Faculty Report on People with Learning Disability and Mental Health, Behavioural or Forensic Problems: The Role of In-Patient Services. Royal College of Psychiatrists, London.
87. Royal College of Psychiatrists (2014) Psychiatry of Intellectual Disability Faculty Report on Forensic Care Pathways in People with Learning Disabilities. Royal College of Psychiatrists, London.
88. Gillmer BT (2013). *Intellectual and developmental disability, alcohol misuse and risk for violence*. Paper presented at the 8th European Conference on Violence in Clinical Psychiatry, Ghent, Belgium, 24 October 2013.
89. Lindsay WR, Smith JS, Tinsley S, Macer J, Miller S (2014). A programme for alcohol related violence with offenders with intellectual disability. *Journal of Intellectual Disabilities and Offending Behaviour*, 5, 107–119.
90. Lindsay WR, Hamilton C, Moulton S, Scott S, Doyle M, McMurran M (2011). Assessment and treatment of social problem solving in offenders with intellectual disability. *Psychology, Crime & Law*, 17, 181–197.

18

Psychological Therapies with People who have Intellectual Disabilities

Peter E. Langdon, Tawakalitu Kehinde, and Georgina Parkes

Introduction

There is substantial evidence that children, adolescents and adults with intellectual disabilities (ID) are at increased risk of developing mental health problems, with some estimating the prevalence of mental health problems amongst this population to be as high as 50 per cent (1–12). There are a variety of reasons why people with ID are more likely to develop enduring mental health problems that require treatment. These include an increased rate of disadvantageous social factors, including significant life events, family and developmental factors, as well as poor socioeconomic status, alongside an increased probability of having a predisposing genetic or biological vulnerability, often inherently associated with ID (5, 13--15). There is evidence to suggest a relationship between the severity of ID and some mental health problems (11, 16). Hove and Havik (16) demonstrated that severity of ID explained a proportion of the variance associated with mental health symptoms across a range of disorders, after controlling for age, gender, autism, genetic syndromes, neurological conditions, and psychosocial variables; some of these relationships were linear, while some were curvilinear.

Regardless of the relationship between ID and comorbid mental health problems, historically, many people were simply excluded from 'talking' psychological therapies, which has been described as an enduring 'therapeutic disdain' towards this population (17), not entirely dissimilar from the longstanding more generalized negative attitudes towards people with ID seen within wider society. This 'therapeutic disdain', while reflecting wider societal attitudes, was often portrayed as driven by an assumption that people with ID were unable to benefit from 'talking' psychological therapies because of difficulties associated with their general intellectual functioning, which would likely have a negative impact upon their ability to take part and benefit from the process of 'talking' therapy.

Many researchers have tried to tackle this assumption, and while there is no doubt that there is a remarkably high need for psychological therapies amongst this population, many have demonstrated that there is a relationship between verbal reasoning skills and ability to complete tasks thought to be integral to successfully completing some aspects of certain psychological therapies; for example, cognitive mediation skills are considered an important skillset for cognitive behavioural therapy, which may be difficult for some people with ID (18–23). Others have reported that people with ID may have difficulties discriminating between differing emotional states, and again, this is important, as some ability to understand, report, and discuss emotions are part of some psychological interventions (18, 21, 24, 25). However, there is also evidence that while there may be a relationship between improved psychotherapy outcomes and increasing verbal reasoning skills, there is also evidence that those with poorer verbal reasoning skills may actually make greater improvements following therapy (26).

Can people with ID take part in psychological therapies?

Considering that the evidence to support the use of cognitive-behavioural therapy (CBT) across a range of disorders is clearly the most robust (27), it is not unsurprising that many researchers have tended to focus on whether people with ID have the necessary skillset to allow them to successfully take part in CBT. Some authors have suggested that many of the interventions for people with ID making use of cognitive therapy actually tend to focus more heavily on the use of behavioural therapy (28, 29), at the expense of cognitive interventions, bearing in mind that CBT for many disorders does focus heavily on behavioural interventions (e.g. exposure and response prevention). Nevertheless, the underlying issue is whether people with ID can take part in the 'cognitive' interventions which are thought to require increasing verbal reasoning skills, an understanding of emotional states, and cognitive mediation skills.

Similar issues have been considered in relation to people without ID regarding whether they have the required skills needed to take part in CBT. Fennell and Teasdale (30) reported that people who tended to respond positively to some aspects of CBT (e.g. written homework tasks) tended to have more positive outcomes, and clearly written homework tasks are likely to be problematic for many people with ID. Over 40 years ago, Sifneos (31) argued that intelligence, having a history of meaningful relationships, an ability to relate to the therapist, an ability to describe the symptoms, and having motivation were all likely to predict good outcome from psychotherapy. Others have talked about 'psychological mindedness' as being both important for people with and without ID when taking part in therapy (25, 32).

Safran et al. (33) outlined a series of selection criteria which formed the Suitability for Short-Term Cognitive Therapy Scale (SSCT) administered as an interview in order to assess whether CBT was an appropriate intervention to use with an individual. These criteria were whether a person is able to: (a) access negative automatic thoughts about the difficulties they are experiencing, (b) distinguish between differing emotions, and identify those relevant to their difficulties, (c) identify that they are active as opposed to passive within the process of change, (d) consider and understand the tasks within CBT as relevant to them, such as cognitive mediation, and identify a goal, and (e) form an appropriate therapeutic alliance with the therapist. The criteria also included, (f) some consideration of how long-term and enduring the difficulties have been, (g) the nature and degree of strategies which are used to avoid dealing with difficult problems, which were referred to as 'security operations', which may inhibit appropriate exploration, and finally, (h) the ability of an individual to maintain a focus on their difficulties within therapy. There is evidence that scores on the SSCT predict treatment outcome (33–36), with more recent factor analytic work using the SSCT suggesting that capacity to take part in CBT is related to treatment outcome (36).

There are clear implications for people with ID, who may have difficulties with many of the aforementioned variables considered important for successfully taking part in, and benefiting from CBT. Others have highlighted that many people with ID encounter difficulties ensuring their mental health problems are successfully recognized, as they may be mistakenly considered inherent to having ID (37), or incorrectly seen as 'challenging behaviour' (38). Clinicians may not communicate collaboratively with people who have ID about the reason why they are being considered for psychological therapy (25), and there may be associated difficulties with establishing a therapeutic relationship, with a tendency for some to have difficulties avoiding overly dependent relationships (39). The most frequently considered issue is whether people with ID have the necessary cognitive skills to undertake some of the complex tasks within cognitive therapy, many of which draw on cognitive perspective-taking or mentalization, emotional recognition, verbal communication, and self-monitoring, along with the use of homework tasks, which may involve reading and writing skills. Focusing on more complex skills, such as cognitive mediation, there is evidence that people with ID can indeed complete tasks related to some of these abilities. For example in one study, approximately two-thirds were able to link basic emotions to a scenario, although such abilities are related to verbal reasoning skills (40). Others have reported similar findings, and while not all people with ID are able to complete aspects of these tasks, it is the case that many can (18–23).

There have been some successful experiments investigating whether people with ID can be taught some of the skills that are thought to be necessary to successfully take part in CBT. Within the first study to consider this, adults with mild ID were randomized to either an attention control arm, where they received relaxation training, or an intervention arm, where they were taught using a series of pictorial aids to identify thoughts, feeling and behaviours, and practice linking thoughts to feelings, or in other words, cognitive mediation. The intervention attempted to replicate aspects of what might happen in therapy for people with ID as a therapist may have to spend extra time teaching concepts. The intervention led to a significant improvement in cognitive mediation skills, while ability to discriminate between thoughts, feelings, and behaviours did not improve, suggesting that some of the skills needed in order to take part in CBT could be taught to some people with mild ID within a one-hour session (41).

Two further recent experiments have made use of technology to teach people with ID some of the skills needed to take part in CBT. The first involved randomizing adults with ID to an intervention arm where a training task in cognitive mediation, using comic strips with accompanying audio was presented on a computer, based upon those used in an earlier study (40). Participants randomized to an attention-control condition viewed the comic strips and listened to the audio, but the learning prompts and questions were not administered. Participants who received the training had a significantly improved ability to select an appropriate emotion within the context of a situation linked to a belief. Ability to select an appropriate mediating belief, within the context of a situation linked to an emotion, did not improve significantly following training, after controlling for intelligence and pre-test scores (42). In a second study, again using a training intervention delivered using a computer, participants with moderate to mild ID were randomized to a training intervention which aimed to teach cognitive mediation and ability to discriminate between thoughts, feelings, and behaviours (43). The intervention led to a significant improvement in the ability of participants to discriminate between thoughts, feelings, and behaviours, while there were no significant improvements in skills related to cognitive mediation. The average full-scale IQ of participants included in this study was 50, which is substantially lower than that found in related studies.

While the majority of studies examining whether people with ID can successfully take part in psychological therapies have tended to focus on CBT and related psychotherapies, there is evidence that while this is related to verbal reasoning skills, many can successfully complete some of the tasks thought to be important and related to a successful outcome. Further, there have been several experimental studies demonstrating that many people with ID can be taught some of the skills thought necessary to be able to successfully take part in CBT. While such interventions can be easily integrated into psychological therapies, there is still a lack of evidence to indicate that they are associated with improved outcomes for this population within the context of well-designed psychotherapy trials.

Several authors have suggested a variety of augmentations that can be made to psychological therapies to help improve accessibility. Over 50 years ago, Sternlicht (44) wrote about how Rogers's (45) view was that insight, verbal communication, and intelligence were needed in order to take part in psychotherapy, and as a consequence, people with ID were excluded. Sternlicht (44) challenged this view, and argued that having ID does not mean that a person does not have 'intelligent behaviour', as many people with ID have strengths, and while some people with ID will have difficulties with verbal communication, non-verbal communication provides a wealth of information which is helpful to the psychotherapeutic process. He went on to discuss how aids, such as drawings, painting, music, and dance can be helpful with encouraging communication, while building relationships was vitally important. Interestingly, he also suggested that more directive psychotherapies may have benefits for people with ID, contrasting them at the time to non-directive counselling and psychodynamic approaches, while he also suggested that play therapy, dramatherapy, and group therapy could be helpful in overcoming some of the perceived difficulties.

Hurley et al. (46) outlined a variety of techniques and modifications that can be made to psychological therapies when used with people who have ID, drawn from the literature at the time. These included: (a) simplification by breaking down interventions and making sessions shorter, (b) reducing the use of complex language, (c) including drawings and homework assignments which have been augmented to help understanding, (d) including developmental level within therapy by ensuring that sessions, content, and materials are appropriate, (e) increasing directedness by clearly outlining treatment goals, progress, and using visual guides, (f) ensuring flexibility and using change techniques related to cognitive level, (g) involving support staff and carers, (h) making use of strong boundaries to guard against increased risk of transference and countertransference, as there is a risk of attachments with a parental theme, and (i) discussing issues related to disability within therapy in order to work on the development of positive self-image.

More recent summaries of the techniques and modifications to psychological therapies for people with ID have been summarized for both CBT and psychodynamic approaches (47). In a similar vein to Hurley (46), simplification of techniques and language, using shorter sessions, incorporating drawings, pictures, videos and audiotapes, including adaptations and materials relating to developmental level, increasing use of directive methods, increasing flexibility, the inclusion of carers, paying further attention to transference and countertransference, and including issues relating to having ID within therapy were all included across the studies reviewed. However, as discussed by the authors, there has been little research into the effectiveness of many of the included components of therapy with people with ID, including many of the adaptations that have been used or developed. One of the difficulties that the authors found within the literature was that many had not sufficiently detailed the augmentations they made to therapies for people with ID, which of course made it difficult to describe the therapeutic content and process. Some of these issues were discussed by Vereenooghe and Langdon (48) who further recommended that the effectiveness of these augmentations need to be considered within the context of therapy for people with ID, while pointing out that people with ID are a heterogeneous population, and modern directive psychotherapies are formulation driven, and as such, interventions should be tailored, based upon the formulation, as should any adaptations to the techniques and therapeutic process.

Are psychological therapies effective?

Several groups have examined the effectiveness of psychological therapies for people with ID within meta-analyses. The majority of these have focused on structured and directive psychotherapies, such as CBT, while there is preponderance of case studies, and small single group designs investigating other psychological therapies, including psychodynamic approaches. Across all the therapeutic modalities, there are a lack of well-designed clinical trials, and of the studies that do exist, many have not employed adequate allocation concealment, appropriate randomization, or comparison groups. Further still, many have made use of insufficient sample sizes, while often sampling bias has not been thoroughly addressed, as people with ID may not be afforded opportunities to take part in psychological therapy research, as participation is often reliant upon having supportive carers.

Cognitive Behavioural Therapy. Bearing the difficulties mentioned above in mind, Vereenooghe and Langdon (48) completed a meta-analysis, which while not limited to studies involving CBT, included a majority of studies that examined the effectiveness of CBT with people who have ID. The majority of the included studies attempted to address anger problems, while other studies treated depression, or attempted to improve interpersonal functioning. They reported that studies where participants were randomized were associated with a moderate effective size, $g = 0.56$, while studies that did not employ randomization were associated with a higher and large effect size, $g = 0.85$, and combining both groups of studies was associated with a moderate effect size, $g = 0.68$. They also contrasted studies that delivered therapy within a group vs. an individual format, and reported that the effect size of group-based interventions, while moderate, $g = 0.56$, was lower than that associated with individual therapy, $g = 0.78$. Further still, examining treatment effectiveness according to the disorder or presenting problem being treated revealed that treatment effectiveness for anger was associated with a large effect size, $g = 0.83$, while for depression, treatment was associated with a moderate to large effect size, $g = 0.74$. Treatment for interpersonal problems was associated with a negative treatment effect, $g = -0.34$. The authors went on to consider their findings in relation to some of the previously completed reviews (49–51), where some had attempted to include treatments focused solely on teaching relaxation or social skills, or excluded interventions that were delivered by staff members working directly with people who have ID. They commented that their calculation of the effect size associated with interventions for the treatment of anger problems was similar across studies (50, 51). They considered that there were no trials of psychological interventions for children and adolescents, nor were there any trials of psychodynamic interventions, which met the inclusion criteria for their review. The authors made a series of recommendations for future clinical trials within this area which were that researchers need to: (a) measure and report the level of general intellectual functioning of participants, (b) describe methods and interventions clearly, (c) describe the adaptations that are made to therapy, and (e) conduct robust and well-designed clinical trials involving adults, as well as children and adolescents with ID.

More recently, Koslowski et al. (52) completed a meta-analysis where they excluded studies that failed to report the level of ID across participants, eventually including only 10 studies in their analysis. They noted an unclear risk of bias associated with masking of research staff, allocation concealment, and selective reporting. Symptoms or disorders treated within studies included behavioural problems, depression, anxiety, quality of life, and functioning. Only six of the 10 included studies made use of CBT as the intervention, while the remaining studies used medication or system-level interventions. They reported that CBT for the treatment of depression was associated with a nonsignificant moderate effect size, $d = 0.49$, while this was nonsignificant and small, $d = 0.15$, for the treatment of anxiety.

Unwin et al. (53) undertook a systematic review of CBT when used as a treatment for anxiety and depression with people with ID, including both the qualitative and quantitative literature. While they did not complete a meta-analysis, owing to the methodological difficulties with the literature, they did conclude that CBT appears feasible and well-tolerated by people with ID. Many of the qualitative studies tended to reflect positive attitudes towards treatment amongst patients and carers. The authors discussed whether it would be helpful to train carers in some of the techniques associated with CBT to help improve the generalizability of treatment effects, commenting further that this may lead to improved knowledge and attitudes, and an increased ability amongst carers to respond to distress.

Mindfulness. Often used in conjunction with CBT (54), mindfulness is a technique that probably originated from Buddhism and Yoga. It is a mental state of focusing on the present moment in a non-judgemental way (55), and has been reported to have a moderate effect size (56) in the general population. There is some emerging evidence to suggest that mindfulness may be helpful for people with ID who have anger problems (57), and Hwang and Kearney (58) reviewed 12 studies which involved teaching mindfulness to people with intellectual and developmental disabilities, some of whom were adolescents, concluding that there was emerging evidence to suggest that the intervention is efficacious. The majority of the studies made use of single case designs, and mindfulness had been used most frequently with aggressive behaviour, but there were studies using the technique as an intervention for deviant sexual arousal (59), anxiety, and obsessive compulsive disorder (60), smoking (61), and for weight loss with someone who had Prader-Willi syndrome (62). A variety of modifications to the techniques were described when used with people with ID, including longer self-practice periods of up to one year, often for those with increasing complexity, and a greater degree of ID. Role play, verbal instructions, pictorial aids, and the use of audio recordings to help with instruction was also employed. Mindfulness had also been used as a technique for supporting carers and staff working with people who have ID (63), parents caring for a child with ID (64), while a recent randomized controlled trial using 'mindfulness-based positive behavioural support' with staff members within an institution for people with severe and profound ID had been completed. The intervention involved training staff in positive behavioural support, while also training them to practice mindfulness. The intervention led to an improved ability of staff members to manage their stress, and reductions in the use of physical restraint and 'as required' medication for service users (65). The authors also reported a reduction in aggression displayed by service users, and staff turnover.

Dialectical Behavioural Therapy. Linehan's (66) dialectical behavioural therapy (DBT) was developed in an attempt to help individuals who were feeling suicidal, who have difficulties with emotional dysregulation, frequently seen in personality disorder. The therapy includes helping individuals to shift towards increasing control over their behaviour, while encouraging the development of new skills, increasing motivation, and with a focus on the generalization of skills within the context of everyday life. The therapy includes the use of group and individual therapy, coaching, which in many settings is delivered by telephone, and team consultation. Meta-analytic work has suggested that DBT is associated with a moderate effect size, but whether DBT is more efficacious than other interventions for similar difficulties remains unclear (67).

A recent systematic review examined the use of DBT with people who have ID, reviewing seven studies (68). DBT had been used within community and inpatient settings for people with ID, and many had made adaptations to the programme, including the use of visual aids, simplified language, more feedback and rehearsal of skills, and the inclusion of carers within the therapy to help with coaching. While many made use of telephone coaching, some did not because the therapy was delivered within an inpatient setting, and coaching was provided by staff members. While the included studies reported improvements in functioning for many of the participants, the designs used did not allow for conclusions regarding causality. It was unclear whether some of the interventions were complete DBT programmes, or instead were informed by DBT.

Behavioural Therapy. While often considered in relation to the treatment of challenging behaviour, behaviour therapy (BT) is often an integral and important part of many modern directive psychotherapies, including CBT. This includes interventions like behavioural activation (69), and exposure and response prevention (70), as well as other techniques, collaboratively informed by learning theory. There is evidence that applied behavioural analysis is associated with moderate to large effect sizes when used with children who have autism (71), and meta-analytic work analysing single-subject designs has demonstrated that behavioural interventions are effective in treating challenging behaviour, drawing on techniques such as differential reinforcement, extinction, and antecedent control procedures; effect sizes were larger for those studies where a functional assessment had been conducted before implementing the intervention, outlining the important role that high quality assessment and formulation has in informing clinical interventions (72), something which has been reinforced by others (73).

Positive behavioural support (PBS; 74, 75) is directly informed by applied behavioural analysis, and many have argued that the focus within PBS, in comparison to applied behavioural analysis, is more upon the social values and the rights of people with ID (76), which includes a focus on meaningful outcomes, normalization, and self-determination (77). It would be rather unethical, and exceptionally concerning, if any psychotherapy did not embrace such values when being used with any person, including people with ID. PBS is an organizational multicomponent framework for intervention, driven by a functional assessment; the goal is to implement evidence-based intervention to bring about an improvement in quality of life by reducing the probability of challenging behaviour. Techniques include the use of antecedent control strategies, which includes the manipulation of environmental conditions, along with reinforcement-based intervention strategies. These are organized into: (a) ecological strategies, (b) teaching functionally equivalent skills, (c) interventions drawn on our understanding of learning theory (e.g. differential reinforcement), and (d) reactive strategies. Meta-analytic studies of the effectiveness of PBS, while drawn primarily on single case designs, have indicated that it is associated with a large effect size, but this is when PBS incorporates both antecedent control strategies and interventions using reinforcement, based upon a functional assessment (78). It is relatively clear that PBS is most effective when based upon a good functional assessment.

Psychodynamic psychotherapy. This particular type of therapy focuses on the use of the relationship between the patient and therapist as the mechanism for change. Significant attention is paid to developing a trusting relationship, which makes use of attentive listening, noting body language. Some may incorporate education and advice, which may not be included as part of therapy for people without ID. Ensuring that the therapist has a warm affect, coupled with friendliness, and making use of modelling around labelling emotions is useful. There are additional challenges for therapists, who may experience guilt because they may not have a disability, associated with fears of not understanding individuals, coupled with powerful projections and countertransference which may become magnified because of communication difficulties. However, Jackson and Beail (79), while considering many of the aforementioned modifications, commented that the majority of the literature in this area is reliant on descriptive case reports, and outlined how the therapeutic process draws on information gathering, formulation, and understanding, along with communication of meaning within a circular process nested within the therapeutic frame. They also stated that within the literature there was a general absence of clear information about formulation with people who have ID (79).

Changes can be slow, subtle, and tend to occur after therapy has ended (80), or they can be sudden, which may be associated with the first stage of therapy. Some aspects of therapy, while beneficial for people with ID, may be judged by others as negative, as individuals increasingly develop a sense of self-efficacy. For example, in an early paper, Symington (81) reported how a person with ID announced that they were 'retired' and no longer wished to attend a day centre, resulting in a perception that symptoms were 'worsening'. However, Symington (81) further discussed how this individual presented as more 'disabled', retreating into his disability as a psychic defence; over time he began to use the bus independently to travel to sessions, and tended to use his disability as a mechanism for integrating more into his peer group. This illustrated how a 'secondary handicap', which is often an unconscious process, reduced early within therapy. This does involve acknowledging the pain of having a disability within a society inherently geared towards people who do not have disabilities.

The second stage of therapy is a 'depressive' stage, and some have considered that it can take up to 12 months (82), while it may be shorter for others. During this stage, there can be a dip in affect and presentation, and working effectively with carers to support an individual is important, often to guard against dropout from therapy. Some may present as acutely distressed, and additional support may have to be offered, which may include hospitalization for those who have experienced severe trauma. This is not commonly encountered within community settings, but it is important to be aware of this process during therapy. Once this stage has been reached, it is important for people to continue with therapy for two to three months to reach resolution. There is evidence that people with ID use the same defence mechanisms, although some have considered there may be more of a reliance on 'primitive' defence mechanisms, such as 'acting out' (83). However, people with ID have been shown to make use of psychodynamic psychotherapy in such a way as to effect change (84).

People with ID tend to face higher rates of loss and trauma (85–87), and many have considered that having an ID in itself can be inherently traumatizing (88). Emotional attachments may be fragile, and it may take longer for individuals to develop a sense of self, while dependency upon others can lead to greater psychological dependency and reduced autonomy. Some individuals may take much longer to address difficult issues, and many may have developed strategies to avoid upsetting or distressing others, in an attempt to supress negative emotions (89).

There are no clinical trials of psychodynamic psychotherapy involving people with ID. Recently, Shepherd and Beail (90) completed a systematic review of 13 studies in this area, concluding that this type of psychotherapy may be effective, but there were no controlled trials, and there were concerns about methodological quality. Box 18.1 summarizes the key points regarding the evidence base for psychological therapies for people with ID.

Box 18.1 Key points

- There is a relationship between cognitive development and the ability to successfully understand some of the skills taught within psychological therapies.
- There is evidence that people with ID can be successfully taught some of these skills.
- There is some evidence that people with ID can benefit from cognitive-behavioural therapy, but further robust studies are needed.
- There is also some emerging evidence that mindfulness may be helpful for people with ID, but larger randomized controlled trials are needed.
- There is some evidence to support the use of dialectal behaviour therapy with people with ID, but this evidence is weak.
- There is evidence that behavioural interventions are effective with people who have ID and challenging behaviour, but much of this evidence comes from single-case designs.
- There is some evidence to support the use of psychodynamic therapy with people who have ID, but this evidence is weak.
- Psychological interventions for mental health problems when used with people who have ID need to be based on a well-developed and theory-driven psychological formulation. Adaptations to therapy need to be tailored to meet the needs of the individual, but we still do not understand whether the adaptations made leads to improved outcomes.
- Psychological therapies need to be delivered by an expert with formal and recognized training in therapy who is also experienced in working with people who have ID.

Conclusions

The evidence base for the use of psychological interventions for people with mental health problems who do not have ID is well established, while a comparable evidence base for people with ID remains lacking. The most thorough evidence exists for the use of interventions drawn on cognitive-behavioural therapy, and while there has been a focus on modifications and adaptations to help with accessibility, the evidence is not markedly robust. There is emerging evidence to support the use of mindfulness. The evidence for behavioural therapy is drawn predominantly upon single case designs, while the evidence for DBT and psychodynamic therapy, although promising, remains sparse. This should not be used as a reason to not offer psychological therapies to people with ID.

MULTIPLE CHOICE QUESTIONS

Questions

Please select the single most appropriate answer.

1. All of the following are true about modifications to CBT and psychodynamic psychological therapies for people with intellectual disabilities except:

A. Simplification of techniques and language
B. Using longer sessions
C. Incorporating drawings, pictures, videos, and audiotapes
D. Including adaptations and materials relating to developmental level
E. Increasing use of directive methods

2. All of the following are true about studies on the effectiveness of therapy using mindfulness in people with intellectual disability except:

A. The majority of the studies made use of single case designs
B. It has been used most frequently with aggressive behaviour
C. Modifications to the techniques include longer self-practice periods
D. It may not be helpful for people with intellectual disabilities who have anger problems
E. When used to support carers, there can be an improved ability to manage their stress

3. All of the following are true about studies on the effectiveness of behaviour therapy in people with intellectual disability except:

A. It is associated with moderate to large effect sizes when used with children who have autism
B. Effect sizes were smaller for those studies where a functional assessment had been conducted before implementing the intervention
C. Meta-analytic work analysing single-subject designs has demonstrated that it is effective in treating challenging behaviour
D. Positive behavioural support (PBS) is informed by applied behavioural analysis and includes a focus on meaningful outcomes, normalization, and self-determination
E. A good functional assessment makes PBS effective

4. All of the following are true about studies on psychodynamic therapy in people with intellectual disability except:

A. Changes can be slow and tend to occur after therapy has ended
B. Changes may be associated with the first stage of therapy
C. It may take longer for individuals to develop a sense of self
D. There can be a depressive stage where there is a dip in affect and presentation
E. For those who reach a depressive stage, therapy should be stopped immediately

5. Dialectical Behaviour Therapy for people with intellectual disabilities:

A. Is effective only in in-patient settings
B. Has been shown to be effective through a meta-analysis of randomized controlled trials
C. Adaptations like the use of visual aids are not recommended
D. The inclusion of carers within the therapy to help with coaching is recommended
E. Telephone coaching is not recommended

Answers

1. B. Making sessions longer may make increasing demands upon information processing skills and interfere with learning.
2. D. There is no evidence that mindfulness is ineffective when used with those who have anger problems.
3. B. Effect sizes are larger when interventions are delivered having completed a functional assessment first.
4. E. Therapy should not be stopped when the client is experiencing the depressive stage as they need to continue to progress through to resolution.
5. D. Including carers within therapy can be a helpful adjunct as clients can continued to be supported with practising and using skills outside of the therapy session.

REFERENCES

1. Borthwick-Duffy SA. Prevalence of destructive behaviors. In: Thompson T, Gray DB, editors. Destructive Behavior in Developmental Disabilities: Diagnosis and Treatment. Thousand Oaks: Sage; 1994. pp. 3–23.
2. Deb S, Thomas M, Bright C. Mental disorder in adults with intellectual disability 1: Prevalence of functional psychiatric illness among a community-based population aged between 16 and 64 years. *Journal of Intellectual Disability Research*. 2001;45:495–505.
3. Deb S, Thomas M, Bright C. Mental disorder in adults with intellectual disability. 2: The rate of behaviour disorders among a community-based population aged between 16 and 64 years. *Journal of Intellectual Disability Research*. 2001;45:506–514.
4. Cooper SA, Smiley E, Jackson A, Finlayson J, Allan L, Mantry D, et al. Adults with intellectual disabilities: Prevalence, incidence and remission of aggressive behaviour and related factors. *Journal of Intellectual Disability Research*. 2009;53:217–232.
5. Cooper SA, Smiley E, Morrison J, Allan L, Williamson A. Prevalence of and association with mental ill health in adults with intellectual disabilities. *British Journal of Psychiatry*. 2007;190:27–35.
6. Emerson E, Hatton C. Mental health of children and adolescents with intellectual disabilities in Britain. *The British Journal of Psychiatry*. 2007;191(6):493–499.
7. Emerson E. Prevalence of psychiatric disorders in children and adolescents with and without intellectual disability. *Journal of Intellectual Disability Research*. 2003;47(1):51–58.
8. Morgan VA, Leonard H, Bourke J, Jablensky A. Intellectual disability co-occurring with schizophrenia and other psychiatric illness: Population-based study. *The British Journal of Psychiatry*. 2008;193(5):364–372.
9. Einfeld SL, Ellis LA, Emerson E. Comorbidity of intellectual disability and mental disorder in children and adolescents: A systematic review. *Journal of Intellectual and Developmental Disability*. 2011;36(2):137–143.

10. Smiley E. Epidemiology of mental health problems in adults with learning disability: An update. *Advances in psychiatric treatment*. 2005;11(3):214–222.
11. Smiley E, Cooper SA, Finlayson J, Jackson A, Allan L, Mantry D, et al. The incidence and predictors of mental ill health in adults with intellectual disabilities. *British Journal of Psychiatry*. 2007;191:313–319.
12. Whitaker S, Read S. The prevalence of psychiatric disorders among people with intellectual disabilities: An analysis of the literature. *Journal of Applied Research in Intellectual Disabilities*. 2006;19(4):330–345.
13. Clarke D. Diagnostic criteria for psychiatric disorders for use with adults with learning disabilities/mental retardation (DC-LD) and psychiatric phenotypes. *Journal of Intellectual Disability Research*. 2003;47:43–49.
14. Hulbert-Williams L, Hastings RP. Life events as a risk factor for psychological problems in individuals with intellectual disabilities: A critical review. *Journal of Intellectual Disability Research*. 2008;52(11):883–895.
15. Koskentausta T, Iivanainen M, Almqvist F. Risk factors for psychiatric disturbance in children with intellectual disability. *Journal of Intellectual Disability Research*. 2007;51(1):43–53.
16. Hove O, Havik OE. Developmental level and other factors associated with symptoms of mental disorders and problem behaviour in adults with intellectual disabilities living in the community. *Social Psychiatry and Psychiatric Epidemiology*. 2010;45:105–113.
17. Bender M. The unoffered chair: The history of therapeutic disdain toward people with a learning difficulty. *Clinical Psychology Forum*. 1993;54:7–12.
18. Joyce T, Globe A, Moody C. Assessment of component skills for cognitive therapy in adults with intellectual disability. *Journal of Applied Research in Intellectual Disabilities*. 2006;19:17–23.
19. Oathamshaw SC, Haddock G. Do people with intellectual disabilities and psychosis have the cognitive skills required to undertake cognitive behavioural therapy? *Journal of Applied Research in Intellectual Disabilities*. 2006;19(1):35–46.
20. Sams K, Collins S, Reynolds S. Can people with intellectual disabilities (ID) engage in cognitive components of cognitive behaviour therapy (CBT)? *Journal of Intellectual Disability Research*. 2006;19:25–33.
21. Dagnan D, Chadwick D. Cognitive-behaviour therapy for people with learning disabilities: Assessment and intervention. In: Stenfert-Kroese B, Dagnan D, Loumidis K, editors. *Cognitive-Behaviour Therapy for People with Learning Disabilities*. London: Routledge; 1997. pp. 110–123.
22. Dagnan D, Chadwick D, Proudlove J. Toward an assessment of suitability of people with mental retardation for cognitive therapy. *Cognitive Therapy and Research*. 2000;24:627–636.
23. Sams K, Collins S, Reynolds S. Cognitive therapy abilities in people with learning disabilities. *Journal of Applied Research in Intellectual Disabilities*. 2006;19(1):25–33.
24. McKenzie K, Matheson E, McKaskie K, Hamilton L, Murray GC. A picture of happiness: Emotion recognition in individuals with a learning disability. *Learning Disability Practice*. 2001;4:26–29.
25. Willner P. Readiness for cognitive therapy in people with intellectual disabilities. *Journal of Applied Research in Intellectual Disabilities*. 2006;19(1):5–16.
26. Taylor JL, Lindsay WR, Willner P. CBT for people with intellectual disabilities: Emerging evidence, cognitive ability and IQ effects. *Behavioural and Cognitive Psychotherapy*. 2008;36:723–734.
27. Butler AC, Chapman JE, Forman EM, Beck AT. The empirical status of cognitive-behavioral therapy: A review of meta-analyses. *Clinical Psychology Review*. 2006;26(1):17–31.
28. Sturmey P. Cognitive therapy with people with intellectual disabilities: A selective review and critique. *Clinical Psychology and Psychotherapy*. 2004;11(4):222–232.
29. Sturmey P. On some recent claims for the efficacy of cognitive therapy for people with intellectual disabilities. *Journal of Applied Research in Intellectual Disabilities*. 2006;19(1):109–17.
30. Fennell MJ, Teasdale JD. Cognitive therapy for depression: Individual differences and the process of change. *Cognitive Therapy and Research*. 1987;11(2):253–271.
31. Sifneos PE. Short-term psychotherapy and emotional crisis: Harvard University Press; 1972.
32. Davanloo H. Short-term dynamic psychotherapy: Jason Aronson; 1980.
33. Safran JD, Segal ZV, Vallis TM, Shaw BF, Samstag LW. Assessing patient suitability for short-term cognitive therapy with an interpersonal focus. *Cognitive Therapy and Research*. 1993;17(1): 23–38.
34. Myhr G, Talbot J, Annable L, Pinard G. Suitability for short-term cognitive-behavioral therapy. *Journal of Cognitive Psychotherapy*. 2007;21(4):334–345.
35. Renaud J, Russell JJ, Myhr G. The association between positive outcome expectancies and avoidance in predicting the outcome of cognitive behavioural therapy for major depressive disorder. *British Journal of Clinical Psychology*. 2013;52(1):42–52.
36. Renaud J, Russell JJ, Myhr G. Predicting who benefits most from cognitive-behavioral therapy for anxiety and depression. *Journal of Clinical Psychology*. 2014;70(10):924–932.
37. Reiss S, Levitan G, Szyszko J. Emotional disturbance and mental retardation: Diagnostic overshadowing. *American Journal of Mental Deficiency*. 1982;86:567–574.
38. Azam K, Sinai A, Hassiotis A. Mental ill-health in adults with learning disabilities. *Psychiatry*. 2009;8(10):376–381.
39. Jahoda A, Selkirk M, Trower P, Pert C, Kroese BS, Dagnan D, et al. The balance of power in therapeutic interactions with individuals who have intellectual disabilities. *British Journal of Clinical Psychology*. 2009;48(1):63–78.
40. Reed J, Clements J. Assessing the understanding of emotional states in a population of adolescents and young adults with mental handicaps. *Journal of Intellectual Disability Research*. 1989;33(3):229–233.
41. Bruce M, Collins S, Langdon P, Powlitch S, Reynolds S. Does training improve understanding of core concepts in cognitive behaviour therapy by people with intellectual disabilities? A randomized experiment. *British Journal of Clinical Psychology*. 2010;49:1–13.
42. Vereenooghe L, Reynolds S, Gega L, Langdon PE. Can a computerised training paradigm assist people with intellectual disabilities to learn cognitive mediation skills? A randomised experiment. *Behaviour Research and Therapy*. 2015;71:10–19.
43. Vereenooghe L, Gega L, Reynolds S, Langdon PE. Using computers to teach people with intellectual disabilities to perform some of the tasks used within cognitive behavioural therapy: A randomised experiment. *Behaviour Research and Therapy*. 2016;76:13–23.
44. Sternlicht M. Psychotherapeutic techniques useful with the mentally retarded: A review and critique. *Psychiatric Quarterly*. 1965;39(1):84–90.

45. Rogers CR. Client-centered therapy. 1951. Boston: Hoghton-Mifflin.
46. Hurley AD, Tomasulo DJ, Pfadt AG. Individual and group psychotherapy approaches for persons with mental retardation and developmental disabilities. *Journal of Developmental and Physical Disabilities*. 1998;10(4):365–386.
47. Whitehouse RM, Tudway JA, Look R, Kroese BS. Adapting individual psychotherapy for adults with intellectual disabilities: A comparative review of the cognitive-behavioural and psychodynamic literature. *Journal of Applied Research in Intellectual Disabilities*. 2006;19(1):55–65.
48. Vereenooghe L, Langdon PE. Psychological therapies for people with intellectual disabilities: A systematic review and meta-analysis. *Research in Developmental Disabilities*. 2013;34:4085–4102.
49. Prout HT, Nowak-Drabik KM. Psychotherapy with persons who have mental retardation: An evaluation of effectiveness. *American Journal on Mental Retardation*. 2003;108:82–93.
50. Nicoll M, Beail N, Saxon D. Cognitive behavioural treatment for anger in adults with intellectual disabilities: A systematic review and meta-analysis. *Journal of Applied Research in Intellectual Disabilities*. 2013;26(1):47–62.
51. Hamelin J, Travis R, Sturmey P. Anger management and intellectual disabilities: A systematic review. *Journal of Mental Health Research in Intellectual Disabilities*. 2013;6(1):60–70.
52. Koslowski N, Klein K, Arnold K, Kösters M, Schützwohl M, Salize HJ, et al. Effectiveness of interventions for adults with mild to moderate intellectual disabilities and mental health problems: Systematic review and meta-analysis. *The British Journal of Psychiatry*. 2016:bjp. bp. 114.162313.
53. Unwin G, Tsimopoulou I, Kroese BS, Azmi S. Effectiveness of cognitive behavioural therapy (CBT) programmes for anxiety or depression in adults with intellectual disabilities: A review of the literature. *Research in Developmental Disabilities*. 2016;51:60–75.
54. Kuyken W, Byford S, Taylor RS, Watkins E, Holden E, White K, et al. Mindfulness-based cognitive therapy to prevent relapse in recurrent depression. *Journal of Consulting and Clinical Psychology*. 2008;76(6):966.
55. Childs D. Mindfulness and clinical psychology. *Psychology and Psychotherapy: Theory, Research and Practice*. 2011;84(3):288–298.
56. Khoury B, Lecomte T, Fortin G, Masse M, Therien P, Bouchard V, et al. Mindfulness-based therapy: A comprehensive meta-analysis. *Clinical Psychology Review*. 2013;33(6):763–771.
57. Singh NN, Wahler RG, Adkins AD, Myers RE, Group MR. Soles of the feet: A mindfulness-based self-control intervention for aggression by an individual with mild mental retardation and mental illness. *Research in Developmental Disabilities*. 2003;24(3):158–169.
58. Hwang Y-S, Kearney P. A systematic review of mindfulness intervention for individuals with developmental disabilities: Long-term practice and long-lasting effects. *Research in Developmental Disabilities*. 2013;34(1):314–326.
59. Singh NN, Lancioni GE, Winton AS, Singh AN, Adkins AD, Singh J. Can adult offenders with intellectual disabilities use mindfulness-based procedures to control their deviant sexual arousal? *Psychology, Crime and Law*. 2011;17(2):165–179.
60. Brown FJ, Hooper S. Acceptance and Commitment Therapy (ACT) with a learning disabled young person experiencing anxious and obsessive thoughts. *Journal of Intellectual Disabilities*. 2009;13(3):195–201.
61. Singh NN, Lancioni GE, Winton AS, Singh AN, Singh J, Singh AD. Effects of a mindfulness-based smoking cessation program for an adult with mild intellectual disability. *Research in Developmental Disabilities*. 2011;32(3):1180–1185.
62. Singh NN, Lancioni GE, Singh AN, Winton AS, Singh J, McAleavey KM, et al. A mindfulness-based health wellness program for an adolescent with Prader-Willi syndrome. *Behavior Modification*. 2008;32(2):167–181.
63. McConachie DAJ, McKenzie K, Morris PG, Walley RM. Acceptance and mindfulness-based stress management for support staff caring for individuals with intellectual disabilities. *Research in Developmental Disabilities*. 2014;35(6):1216–1227.
64. Reid C, Gill F, Gore N, Brady S. New ways of seeing and being: Evaluating an acceptance and mindfulness group for parents of young people with intellectual disabilities who display challenging behaviour. *Journal of Intellectual Disabilities*. 2016;20(1):5–17.
65. Singh NN, Lancioni GE, Karazsia BT, Chan J, Winton AS. Effectiveness of caregiver training in Mindfulness-Based Positive Behavior Support (MBPBS) vs. Training-as-Usual (TAU): A randomized controlled trial. *Frontiers in Psychology*. 2016;7.
66. Linehan M. Dialectical behavioural therapy: A cognitive behavioural approach to parasuicide. *Journal of Personality Disorders*. 1987;1(4):328–333.
67. Kliem S, Kröger C, Kosfelder J. Dialectical behavior therapy for borderline personality disorder: A meta-analysis using mixed-effects modeling. *American Psychological Association*; 2010.
68. McNair L, Woodrow C, Hare D. Dialectical Behaviour Therapy [DBT] with people with intellectual disabilities: A systematic review and narrative analysis. *Journal of Applied Research in Intellectual Disabilities*. 2016.
69. Jahoda A, Melville C, Cooper S-A, Hastings R, Briggs A, Dagnan D, et al. BEAT-IT: Comparing a behavioural activation treatment for depression in adults with intellectual disabilities with an attention control: Study protocol for a randomised controlled trial. *Trials*. 2015;16(1):595.
70. Boyd BA, Woodard CR, Bodfish JW. Feasibility of exposure response prevention to treat repetitive behaviors of children with autism and an intellectual disability: A brief report. *Autism*. 2013;17(2):196–204.
71. Virués-Ortega J. Applied behavior analytic intervention for autism in early childhood: Meta-analysis, meta-regression and dose-response meta-analysis of multiple outcomes. *Clinical Psychology Review*. 2010;30(4):387–399.
72. Didden R, Duker PC, Korzilius H. Meta-analytic study on treatment effectiveness for problem behaviors with individuals who have mental retardation. *American Journal on Mental Retardation*. 1997;101(4):387–399.
73. Harvey ST, Boer D, Meyer LH, Evans IM. Updating a meta-analysis of intervention research with challenging behaviour: Treatment validity and standards of practice. *Journal of Intellectual and Developmental Disability*. 2009;34(1):67–80.
74. Carr EG. Invited commentary: The evolution of applied behavior analysis into positive behavior support. *Journal of the Association for Persons with Severe Handicaps*. 1997;22(4):208–209.
75. Horner RH, Carr EG. Behavioral support for students with severe disabilities: Functional assessment and comprehensive intervention. *The Journal of Special Education*. 1997;31(1):84–104.
76. Horner RH. Positive behavior supports. Focus on autism and other developmental disabilities. 2000;15(2):97–105.

77. Johnston J, Foxx RM, Jacobson JW, Green G, Mulick JA. Positive behavior support and applied behavior analysis. *Behavior Analyst*. 2006;29(1):51.
78. Marquis JG, Horner RH, Carr EG, Turnbull AP, Thompson M, Behrens GA, et al. A meta-analysis of positive behavior support. *Contemporary Special Education Research: Syntheses of the Knowledge Base on Critical Instructional Issues*. 2000: 137–178.
79. Jackson T, Beail N. The practice of individual psychodynamic psychotherapy with people who have intellectual disabilities. *Psychoanalytic Psychotherapy*. 2013;27(2):108–23.
80. Fonagy P, Rost F, Carlyle Ja, McPherson S, Thomas R, Pasco Fearon R, et al. Pragmatic randomized controlled trial of long-term psychoanalytic psychotherapy for treatment-resistant depression: The Tavistock Adult Depression Study (TADS). *World Psychiatry*. 2015;14(3):312–321.
81. Symington N. The psychotherapy of a subnormal patient. *British Journal of Medical Psychology*. 1981;54(2):187–199.
82. Carlsson B. Psychoanalytic psychotherapy with intellectually disabled adults—evaluation by using projective tests: A collaboration project between a psychiatric clinic and the services for mentally handicapped. *NADD Bulletin*. 2000;5.
83. Newman D, Beail N. An exploratory study of the defence mechanisms used in psychotherapy by adults who have intellectual disabilities. *Journal of Intellectual Disability Research*. 2010;54(7):579–583.
84. Newman DW, Beail N, MacLean J, William E. Analysis of assimilation during psychotherapy with people who have mental retardation. *American Journal on Mental Retardation*. 2005;110(5):359–365.
85. Beail N, Warden S. Sexual abuse of adults with learning disabilities. *Journal of Intellectual Disability Research*. 1995;39:382–387.
86. Sequeira H, Howlin P, Hollins S. Psychological disturbance associated with sexual abuse in people with intellectual disabilities (ID): A case-control study. *Journal of Intellectual Disability Research*. 2003;183:451–456.
87. Martorell A, Tsakanikos E. Traumatic experiences and life events in people with intellectual disability. *Current Opinion in Psychiatry*. 2008;21(5):445–448.
88. Hollins S, Sinason V. Psychotherapy, learning disabilities and trauma: New perspectives. *British Journal of Psychiatry*. 2000;176:32–36.
89. Sinason V. *Mental handicap and the human condition: New approaches from the Tavistock*: Free Association Books; 1992.
90. Shepherd C, Beail N. A systematic review of the effectiveness of psychoanalysis, psychoanalytic and psychodynamic psychotherapy with adults with intellectual and developmental disabilities: Progress and challenges. *Psychoanalytic Psychotherapy*. 2017:1–24

19

Pharmacotherapy for Mental Illness and Behaviours that Challenge in People with Intellectual Disabilities

David Branford, Reena Tharian, Regi Alexander, and Sabyasachi Bhaumik[†]

Background

Although there are many surveys of the use of psychotropic medication in intellectual disability (ID), ascertaining the full extent of its use within the ID population is fraught with problems. The studies are more likely to include people with ID who access or are in receipt of services, either in hospitals or within the community. A 1988 review of 35 such surveys in the former setting (mainly from the USA), concluded that typically 30–35 per cent received psychotropic medications on a regular basis (1). A census in England in 2013 found that over two-thirds of those in hospital care had been given an antipsychotic during the week leading up to census day (2). Amongst those compulsorily detained in hospital under the English Mental Health Act, 86 per cent of patients were prescribed at least one antipsychotic to be given on a regular basis with 18 per cent being prescribed more than one. When 'as required' medication was included, 57 per cent were prescribed more than one psychotropic with 40 per cent prescribed five or more (3). A study from Israel of approximately 10,000 people living in residential care centres during the period 1998–2008 showed a steady increase in the number of residents receiving psychotropics (45%-54%) and the number of doses of 'as required' psychotropics administered each year rising from 1,500-6,300 (4). Regarding surveys of those living in community care, it has been reported that those living in residential facilities are more likely to be prescribed psychotropics than those in family settings (5,6).

With the move to close institutions, the expectation was that the need for psychotropics would be reduced. However, studies suggest that the rate of prescribing has remained similar over time and for those living in residential facilities to increase. In addition to the increased use of psychotropics has been the increase of multiple psychotropic prescribing (called polypharmacy by some authors) (7–11).

Access to large prescription databases of General Practitioners (GPs) in England has enabled clearer understanding of the prescribing for larger populations who live in the community. Public Health England published in 2015 the results from a GP database study covering approximately 7.8 per cent of the entire English population of people with an ID and reported that 41.3 per cent of adults and 14.7 per cent of children and young people were receiving a psychotropic. If those receiving antiepileptics were excluded (because of epilepsy as a confounder), the figures were 29.5 per cent of adults and 6.8 per cent of children and young people. Antipsychotics were prescribed for 17.0 per cent of adults and 2.4 per cent of children and young adults, medications used in mania and hypomania for 7.1 per cent and 0.3 per cent respectively, antidepressants for 16.9 per cent and 1.2 per cent, anxiolytics for 4.2 per cent and 0.6 per cent, hypnotics for 2.7 per cent and 4.1 per cent. For most groups of psychotropics, exposure rates rose through adult life. The rate of prescribing antipsychotics in people aged 65 and over was 3.3 times the rate in those aged 18 to 24 (12). A similar study of 571 general practices contributing data to The Health Improvement Network clinical database included 33,016 adults (58% male) with ID who contributed 211,793 person years' data. Of these 49 per cent (16,242) had a record of prescription of psychotropic medication. The rate of new antipsychotic prescribing was significantly higher in people with challenging behaviour, autism, and dementia and in those of older age (13).

Why is psychotropic medication prescribed?

In general, people with an ID may be prescribed psychotropic drugs including antipsychotics in three sets of circumstances: either because they have a psychiatric diagnosis, because they have behaviour that challenges or both (18, 72, 73, 74).

A significant proportion of people with ID display behaviours that challenge. Challenging behaviour is defined as behaviour of an intensity, frequency, or duration that threatens the physical safety of the person or others, or restricts access to community facilities (75). It is a socially constructed, descriptive concept that has no diagnostic significance and makes no inferences about the aetiology of the

[†] It is with great regret that we report the death of Sabyasachi Bhaumik during the production of this textbook.

behaviour. Its definition is broad enough to cover acts of aggression towards people, aggression to property, self-neglect, self-harm, and the risk of exploitation and it therefore appears that almost anyone who has a mental health problem that reaches the threshold to need attention from primary or secondary care services would have some form of behaviour that challenges as a presenting feature (72, 73). The reverse may not be true, that is, everyone with challenging behaviour may not necessarily have a mental health problem (76).

People with ID develop mental health problems at rates similar to or higher than the general population, but it may not be recognized due to communication deficits, atypical presentations, diagnostic overshadowing, or difficulties in accessing services (72–79). Thus in clinical practice, a psychiatric diagnosis may be recorded only when the main syndromes are present (e.g. schizophrenia or bipolar disorder), while the narrative account of mental health problems (e.g. transient psychotic symptoms and affective lability in someone with milder ID and a personality disorder) is left out (72). This may contribute to under-recording of psychiatric diagnoses or indeed unnecessary prescriptions or inadequate monitoring (72).

In England, a national programme to stop over-medication of people with a learning disability (STOMP-LD) has been developed (80). While no reasonable person can be in favour of over-medication, the imperative should be to rationalize clinical practice by carefully balancing the need to stop unnecessary treatment with the possibility of exposing patients to the risk of under-treatment for legitimate indications (72–74).

Evidence from studies of the prescribing of psychotropic medication for people with ID

Evidence to support or refute the use of psychotropic medications in ID come from a limited number of studies. The huge variety of presentations within the overall category of ID and the range of behaviours studied makes it difficult to generalize from this limited number of studies. This section focuses primarily on antipsychotics which have been the most widely prescribed and most widely studied. In addition to prospective studies there are a number of studies of the withdrawal of antipsychotics.

Antipsychotics

Antipsychotics have been widely prescribed for this group since the introduction of chlorpromazine in the 1950s. Anecdotal evidence would suggest that for much of the first 40 years the antipsychotic Thioridazine was very widely prescribed and studied. Whether the profile of Thioridazine was of particular benefit in ID compared to the other available antipsychotics remains unclear. It had a lower incidence of extrapyramidal side effects than other older antipsychotics but a similar rate of the development of the irreversible long term effect of tardive dyskinesia. Concerns about these and other side effects led to the view that people with ID were more sensitive to such side effects and at greater risk (14). However, studies comparing people with ID on antipsychotics with those not failed to demonstrate higher rates of such side effects.

In the late 1990s Thioridazine was withdrawn from the market due to concerns about QTc prolongation and risk of death from Torsades de Pointes. The older antipsychotics were over a period of time mostly replaced by a new family of antipsychotics called 'atypicals', so named because of their lack of extrapyramidal side effects and reduced risk of tardive dyskinesia. The leading antipsychotic used in ID became risperidone, followed by other newer antipsychotics such as olanzapine, quetiapine and aripirazole. These newer antipsychotics however have presented with a different set of side effects and there are concerns associated with weight gain, diabetes, and metabolic syndrome following long-term use. Again, the view is held that people with ID are at greater risk of such metabolic side effects, but studies have failed to demonstrate this (15).

Antipsychotics for mental illnesses

Antipsychotics are used for a wide range of conditions including schizophrenia and bipolar mania. A Cochrane review in 2004 found no randomized controlled trial evidence to guide the use of antipsychotics for people with both ID and schizophrenia (16) although there were a number of case series such as that of clozapine that demonstrates improvement (17).

More recent guidelines have emphasized clearly however, the need to actively treat any co-existing mental illness including schizophrenia using the same treatment modalities applied to people without an ID (72, 73, 74). However, before starting medication, one has to take account of potential medication interactions, the impact of medication on other health conditions, that of other health conditions on the medication, and when necessary consult with specialists (for example, neurologists providing epilepsy care when prescribing antipsychotic medication that may lower the seizure threshold), to minimize possible interactions. There is also a need to assess the risk of non-adherence to the medication regimen or any necessary monitoring tests (for example, blood tests), establish a review schedule to reduce polypharmacy, provide support to improve adherence, assess whether support from community and ID nurses is needed for physical investigations (such as blood tests) and agree monitoring responsibilities, including who will carry out blood tests and other investigations (72, 73, 74).

Antipsychotics for behaviours that challenge

The nuanced relationship between challenging behaviour as a clinical presentation and the possibility of underlying mental health pathology has already been discussed. Although the use of antipsychotics in the management of behaviours that challenge (without an identified mental illness) remains highly controversial, it still provides a considerable evidence base. Table 19.1 provides an overview of those RCT studies of antipsychotics in children and adolescents considered by NICE (18) to have sufficient data suitable for inclusion to meet their eligibility criteria for a meta-analysis.

From the analysis of the studies above, it was concluded that there was low quality evidence that risperidone was more effective than placebo in reducing the severity of targeted behaviour that challenges, more effective at improving adaptive social functioning, but increasing the risk of having elevated prolactin levels, greater weight, increased levels of sedation, and somnolence. Likewise, there was very low quality evidence that suggested that Aripiprazole was more effective in reducing the severity of targeted behaviour that challenges, more effective in increasing quality of life, but associated with greater levels of weight gain and increased risk of sedation. From other studies of antipsychotics in children and adolescents there was very low evidence to suggest that aripiprazole was less effective than risperidone in reducing the severity of targeted

Table 19.1 An overview of those RCT studies of antipsychotic in children and adolescents considered by NICE to have sufficient data suitable for inclusion to meet their eligibility criteria for a meta-analysis

Authors	Antipsychotic(s)	Population studied	Key outcome	Adverse events associated with antipsychotic
Aman et al. (2002) (20)	Risperidone vs placebo	6-week double blind parallel-group study of 118 children (aged 5–12 years). Mild to moderate ID	Risperidone group showed significantly greater improvement of conduct from week 1	Headache and somnolence. Mean weight increases of 2.2 kg
Kent et al. (2013) (21)	Low dose risperidone (0.125mg per day) Vs high dose (1.75mg per day) vs placebo	6-week, double-blind, placebo-controlled, fixed-dose, multicentre study 96 children with autism, 77% below age 12	Only high dose risperidone showed significant improvements.	Somnolence, sedation and increased appetite occurred more frequently in high dose groups
RUPP (2002) (22)	Risperidone vs placebo.	8-week study, 101 children with autism, mean age, 8.8 years, dose range, 0.5 to 3.5 mg per day	Risperidone group 56.9% reduction in the irritability score, of aberrant behaviour checklist (ABC) vs 14.1% in placebo group	Increased appetite, fatigue, drowsiness, dizziness, and drooling
Shea et al. (2004) (23)	Risperidone vs placebo	8-week, randomized, double-blind, placebo-controlled trial, solution (0.01–0.06 mg/kg/day). 79 children, mild to moderate ID aged 5 to 12 years	Risperidone group (mean dosage: 0.04 mg/kg/day; 1.17 mg/day) greater mean decrease on the irritability subscale of the ABC	Significantly greater increases in weight (2.7 vs 1.0 kg), pulse rate, and systolic blood pressure
Snyder et al. (2002) (24)	Risperidone vs placebo	6-week, double-blind, placebo-controlled trial. 110 children with mild to moderate ID (aged 5–12 years) doses 0.02 to 0.06.mg/kg per day	47.3% reduction vs placebo-treated on Conduct problem subscale of NCBRF. Between-group differences seen as early as week 1	Somnolence, headache, Appetite increase, and dyspepsia
Marcus et al. (2009) (25)	Aripiprazole vs placebo	8-week double-blind, randomized, placebo-controlled, parallel-group study. 218 children and adolescents (aged 6–17 years) autistic disorder, and with problem behaviours randomized to aripiprazole (5, 10, or 15 mg/day) or placebo	All aripiprazole doses significantly greater improvement than placebo in mean ABC Irritability subscale scores	Sedation. 1kg weight gain with all doses. Two serious adverse events: presyncope and aggression
Owen et al. (2009) (26)	Aripiprazole vs placebo	8-week, double-blind, randomized, placebo-controlled, parallel-group study (aged 6–17 years with autistic disorder). 98 children or adolescents flexibly dosed aripiprazole (target dosage: 5, 10, or 15 mg/day) or placebo	Aripiprazole significant improvement in ABC irritability subscale. Significantly greater global improvements (CGI-I) score from week 1 through week 8	Extrapyramidal symptom-related 14.9% vs 8.0%. Mean weight gain was 2.0 kg vs 0.8kg at week 8
Ghanizadeh et al. (2014) (27)	Aripiprazole or risperidone	59 children and adolescents with autism spectrum disorders were randomized to receive either for 2 months. Aripiprazole mean dose 5.5 mg/day. Risperidone 1.12 mg/day	Aripiprazole as well as risperidone lowered ABC scores during 2 months	The safety and efficacy were comparable
Longer term and withdrawal RCTs in children and adolescents				
Authors	**Antipsychotic(s)**	**Population studied**	**Outcome**	**Antipsychotic Adverse events**
RUPP (2005) (28)	Two-part study of Risperidone	Ages 5 to 17 with autism who showed positive response in earlier 8-week trial. Part 1 (63 children) 4-month open-label treatment. Part II (32 patients) an 8-week randomized, double-blind, placebo-substitution of risperidone withdrawal	Part I Mean Risperidone dose 1.96 mg/day and remained stable over 16 weeks of open treatment. Part II. Relapse rates 62.5% for gradual placebo substitution and 12.5% for continued risperidone	The subjects gained an average of 5.1 kg
Finding et al. (2014) (29)	Two part study of Aripiprazole	Phase 1, single-blind aripiprazole flexibly dosed (2–15 mg/d) for 13--26 weeks. Phase 2. 16 week 85 patients with a stable response randomized to continue aripiprazole or switch to placebo	Time to relapse not statistically significant (relapse rates at week 16 were 35% for aripiprazole and 52% for placebo)	Phase 1 weight increase somnolence vomiting; Phase 2 upper respiratory tract infection constipation movement disorder

behaviour that challenges, olanzapine was more effective than haloperidol in reducing the severity of behaviour that challenges, but increased drowsiness and weight gain to a greater extent. It was also found that participants who initially responded to treatment with risperidone or aripiprazole and were subsequently withdrawn from this intervention were at an increased risk of demonstrating the targeted behaviour that challenges when compared with participants who continued treatment.

Table 19.2 provides an overview of those RCT studies of antipsychotics in adults considered by NICE to have sufficient data suitable for inclusion to meet their eligibility criteria for a meta-analysis (18).

From the analysis of these studies, it was concluded that there was low-quality inconclusive evidence of the effectiveness of risperidone, olanzapine, or haloperidol when compared with placebo, in reducing the severity of targeted behaviour that challenges, or the quality

Table 19.2 An overview of those RCT studies of antipsychotics in adults considered by NICE to have sufficient data suitable for inclusion to meet their eligibility criteria for a meta-analysis

Authors	Antipsychotic(s)	Population studied	Outcome
Gagiano et al (2005) (30)	Risperidone vs placebo	77 adults with disruptive behaviour randomized to risperidone (n = 39) 1 to 4 mg or placebo (n = 38) 4-week double-blind treatment. After 4-week period, open-label treatment with risperidone for 48 weeks, mean dose 1.8 mg/day	Risperidone significantly greater improvement on the ABC than placebo Further significant decrease of ABC over 48-week, open-label follow-up period
Amore et al. (2011) (31)	Risperidone vs olanzapine following first generation antipsychotic (FGA)	62 adults, 2-arm, parallel group balanced randomization pragmatic trial of olanzapine and risperidone. Blind assessment of outcome at 4, 8, 12, 16, 20 and 24 weeks after a switch (cross-tapering) from a 24-week treatment with (FGA)	Risperidone and olanzapine were more effective than FGAs in reducing aggressive behaviour
Tyrer et al. (2008) (32)	Risperidone vs olanzapine vs placebo	86 non-psychotic patients with ID and aggressive challenging behaviour randomly assigned to haloperidol, risperidone, or placebo	Aggression decreased substantially with all three treatments by 4 weeks
Haessler et al. (2007) (33)	Zuclopenthixol vs placebo	49 adults, with mild to moderate ID randomized, double-blind placebo-controlled withdrawal study. Open treatment with zuclopenthixol 2–20mg for 6 weeks. Responders group (n=39) randomized to continue or discontinue for up to 12 weeks.	The proportion of participants rated as responders, was statistically significantly larger in the zuclopenthixol group (37%, n=7) than in the placebo group (5%, n=1)
Izmeth et al. (1988) (34)	Zuclopenthixol decanoate injection vs placebo	116 adults with ID with behavioural disorders double-blind zuclopenthixol decanoate injection (mean dosage 123 mg/week) and placebo. 4-week open phase followed by a 12-week double-blind phase. Approximately half of the patients were changed to placebo	14 in placebo group withdrawn because of increased frequency and severity of behavioural disorders compared to 4 in the zuclopenthixol decanoate group
Singh & Owino (1992) (35)	Zuclopenthixol tablets	52 patients with behavioural disorders. Double blind placebo. 6-week open phase followed by randomization to 12-week period of active drug vs placebo	Significant changes in favour of zuclopenthixol.

of life. They also concluded that there was very low evidence to suggest withdrawal of zuclopenthixol was less effective than continuation of zuclopenthixol, in reducing the severity of behaviour that challenges. The NICE guidelines have exacting standards in terms of assessing efficacy and to place these findings in perspective, it is worth noting that the efficacy of psychological interventions did not fare much better either.

In addition to evidence from RCTs of individual medications, Heyvaert et al. aggregated the results from several single case or small number studies in a meta-analysis and concluded that there was no overall positive effect of pharmacological interventions (19).

Antipsychotic withdrawal

A number of studies focusing on the withdrawal of antipsychotics in people with an ID have been reported. The three main problems reported have been worsening of the behaviour, emergence or worsening of dyskinesias, and autonomic instability. Branford reported an open study of a review of 198 people who live in Leicestershire and the factors associated with successful or unsuccessful withdrawal (36, 37). Another study randomly allocated 36 people to undergo four, monthly 25 per cent drug reduction stages. There were no planned drug changes for a control group (n = 20). Twelve participants (33%) completed full withdrawal and a further seven (19%) achieved and maintained at least a 50 per cent reduction. Antipsychotic reduction was associated with increased dyskinesia and higher activity engagement but not increased maladaptive behaviour (38). A 2014 Dutch study investigated the effects of controlled discontinuation of antipsychotics prescribed for behaviour that challenge. Of 98 participants, 43 achieved complete discontinuation; at follow-up seven had resumed use of antipsychotics. There were no significant differences in improvement of behavioural ratings between the two discontinuation schedules. Higher baseline problem behaviour rating predicted higher odds of incomplete discontinuation (39).

Antipsychotics for specific behaviours that challenge

The term behaviours that challenge incorporates a wide variety of problem behaviours. Rather than focus on general overall behaviours some studies have focused on specific behaviours such as aggression, self-injurious behavior, or stereotypical repetitive behaviours. According to Cooper, the most common forms of behaviours that challenge reported are aggression (7%), destructive behaviour (4%–5%), and self-injury (4%) (40)

Aggressive behaviours: Roy et al. in 2013 published a comprehensive review of all psychotropic trials that focus on aggressive behaviours (41). Specifically excluding children and autism, the conclusion was that although risperidone and lithium were the most widely studied and provided the most supportive evidence of effectiveness for aggressive behaviours the multitude of different rating scales made it difficult to make comparisons.

Self-injurious behaviours (SIB): Many guidelines suggest antipsychotics for first line treatment of SIB, however the evidence to support their use is weak. A Cochrane review failed to find any studies of antipsychotics that met their criteria for inclusion in a meta-analysis (42). Some studies of risperidone suggest that there is value for repetitive and stereotypical SIB. One retrospective review of antipsychotics suggested efficacy for aggressive behaviours but not SIB (43).

Antidepressants

Early studies of prescribing for people with ID often failed to include antidepressants because of minimal use. Those that did report indicated a prevalence of between 1–5 per cent (1). A Leicester UK study in 1994 found 6 per cent prevalence for those in hospital care and 3 per cent for those in the community (5). However the introduction of selective serotonin reuptake inhibitors (SSRIs) led to greater use and evidence to show their efficacy in a wide range of anxiety-related disorders such as general anxiety disorder (GAD), panic disorder, post-traumatic stress disorder (PTST), obsessive compulsive disorder (OCD), and social phobia (44). In addition a number of small trials within ID have suggested their value in the control of behaviours that challenge and various behaviours associated with autism (45). Recent surveys have indicated that the prescribing of antidepressants is widespread in the ID population. The 2015 GP based study showed that not only were antidepressants widely prescribed (17% of ID population receiving) but that they were commonly prescribed in combination with other psychotropics (12). The study by Sheehan et al. put antidepressants as the second most widely newly prescribed for people with ID after anxiolytics (13). This increased use of antidepressants is not without risks. Many antidepressants have a small to moderate risk of worsening seizures, hypomania, and other behaviours that challenge and there may be problems with withdrawal of the medications (46).

Antidepressants for mental illnesses

While there are no systematic controlled trials of the treatment of depression in people with an intellectual disability, there are a number of case series and case reports that suggest that the treatment of depression in ID should be similar to that advocated by the NICE guidelines (CG90) for depression (47). This ties in with the advice for other mental illnesses in this population (73).

Antidepressants for behaviours that challenge

Aggressive behaviours: In the 2013 review of medications to manage aggressive behaviours Roy (41) provided an oversight of open, prospective, and retrospective trials of a number of SSRI antidepressants. Many studies did not specifically differentiate between global measures of behaviour (including SIB and aggression) and specific behaviours. For example, the longest study was a retrospective review of 38 people with a six-year exposure to a number of different SSRIs or clomipramine. Eighteen showed a 25 per cent reduction and six a 50 per cent reduction of global behaviour ratings (48). Conversely, a Leicestershire UK study of fluoxetine and paroxetine showed no overall improvement in aggressive behaviour with 25 per cent worse with treatment (49).

Self-injurious behaviour (SIB): A Cochrane review in 2013 included five studies including one small negative study (42). Of the included studies, only the effectiveness and safety of clomipramine for SIB was a prospective, randomized, double-blind, placebo-controlled trial and had a cross-over design. The age of included participants ranged from 21 to 39 years and 38 per cent were females. All participants were diagnosed with a severe to profound ID (50). Both Cochrane and NICE considered that there was weak evidence that clomipramine was more effective than placebo for those demonstrating SIB.

Autism: NICE in its guidance advised not to use antidepressants for the routine management of core symptoms of autism in adults. In addition, it provided no advice about the use of antidepressants for challenging behaviours associated with autism (51).

Mood stabilizers (medication used for the management and prophylaxis of mania and hypomania)

Medications for the management and prophylaxis of mania and hypomania include lithium, some antiepileptics, and a number of the newer antipsychotics. The study of GP practices undertaken by Public Health England gave a prevalence of 7.1 per cent of adults with ID receiving medications for mania and hypomania (12), that by Sheehan et al. gave a prevalence of new prescribing of mood stabilizers as similar to that of antipsychotics (13). Studies of the prevalence of prescribing of antimanics are confounded by the use of antiepileptics for epilepsy and of antipsychotics for behaviour that challenge. Also with polypharmacy of psychotropics becoming a common finding of surveys it is often difficult to know whether the antipsychotics and antiepileptics are prescribed solely as mood stabilizers.

Mood stabilizers for mental illnesses

There are no specific placebo-controlled trials of mood stabilizers for the treatment and prophylaxis of mania and hypomania in ID. As previously mentioned, any co-existing mania or hypomania in people with an intellectual disability should be treated similarly as in those without an ID, abeit with the safeguards mentioned under the section on antipsychotics (73).

Mood stabilizers for behaviours that challenge

Lithium is the mood stabilizer with the most studies, the primary endpoint usually focusing on aggressive behaviours. Two older studies; an RCT and another involving lithium as an add-on to antipsychotics showed only moderate effect (52.53) Three more recent case series extending over periods of 2–10 years showed overall reductions in aggressive behaviours. However, the longer of the studies was confused by the additional prescribing of antipsychotics. Lithium has fallen out of favour as a long-term treatment for mood disorders or aggression due to concerns about kidney damage, the requirement for regular lithium blood concentration testing and other side effects. Other medications studied as mood stabilizers are carbamazepine, valproate and topiramate. An RCT of carbamazepine focused mostly on hyperactivity and those thought to respond the best were people with associated mood disturbances (54). An open label study of valproate added to antipsychotic treatment showed mixed results with a third showing no benefits (55). A longer open label retrospective study claimed benefits in 71 per cent of the population studied. A five-year retrospective study of topiramate focused on a wide range of aggressive and other problem behaviours and estimated improvements in 78 per cent (56).

Anxiolytics (Benzodiazepines)

Benzodiazepines are not recommended for long-term use for the treatment of anxiety (44). However they are the medications of choice for the short-term management of violent and aggressive behaviours (46). Most early studies of the prevalence of prescribing of psychotropics in ID indicated very low use of benzodiazepines (usually less than 5%). However more recent studies have raised concerns about both the long-term prescribing of regular and 'as required' benzodiazepines. Although the Public Health England study showed only 4 per cent regular use, the GP-based study of Sheehan et al. found anxiolytics/hypnotics to be the highest rate of new prescribing of the groups of psychotropics (12, 13). The study by the Care Quality Commission found a benzodiazepine anxiolytic either regular or 'as required' was requested in over 80 per cent of cases (3).

Hypnotics

Sleep disturbance is common in ID and a wide variety of sedatives have been used from time to time to provide short-term relief. These include low dose antipsychotics such as chlorpromazine, antihistamines such as promethazine and antidepressants such as trazodone. The lack of any particular studies in ID suggest that their use should be similar to that of the non-ID population. Sleep hygiene and associated behavioural programmes are the methods of choice with only occasional use of hypnotics if needed for short periods of time (44).

In recent years melatonin has been advocated particularly for children with autism. There have been four small RCTs of melatonin in ID, one with adults, a second with children suffering Angelman syndrome, a third with children with autism and the largest with children classified as having neurodevelopmental disorder (57-60). NICE classified the evidence supporting melatonin prescribing as very low for the following: some evidence that melatonin increases total sleep time when compared to placebo, no evidence that Melatonin reduces the numbers of wakes or duration of wakes, no evidence of improved day time behavior, and no evidence for improvement in carer quality of life (18).

Stimulants

Hyperactivity is common in people with ID and there has been much debate whether this presentation of hyperactivity and impulsivity is diagnostic of attention deficit hyperactivity disorder (ADHD) and whether the recommendations of the NICE guideline CG72 apply (61). Prior to the study by Simonoff et al. there were only a small number of case reports and retrospective studies (62). They undertook a RCT of optimal dose methylphenidate in 122 medication-free children and adolescents with hyperkinetic disorder and ID aged 7–15. They found methylphenidate was superior to placebo using the parent and teacher Conner's ADHD index. IQ and autistic symptoms did not affect treatment efficacy. Methylphenidate was associated with sleep difficulty, loss of appetite and weight loss, but there were no significant differences in pulse or blood pressure.

Cognitive enhancers for dementia in ID

Early cognitive decline is associated with Down syndrome and in addition it is thought that people with ID have a greater likelihood of suffering dementia that those without. A Cochrane study concluded that due to the low quality of the body of evidence, it was difficult to draw conclusions about the effectiveness of any pharmacological intervention for cognitive decline in people with Down syndrome (63). They examined nine studies of five medications that are, or have been used to prevent cognitive decline. All the studies compared the medicine being tested with a placebo. Generally, those who received the cognitive enhancer did no better than those who received the placebo in any of the areas assessed. The areas assessed included general functioning (including memory and thinking, speech, mood, and behaviour); cognitive functioning (including memory, following what's going on around you); adaptive behaviours (being able to do day-to-day tasks); or behaviour problems (such as being irritable or aggressive).

Prescribing practice and guidance for clinicians

Concerns about the overuse of psychotropics, particularly antipsychotics have been a common theme for much of the last 60 years since the introduction of chlorpromazine. Many guidelines have provided advice on best prescribing practice. In 1995 a guideline for the use of psychotropic medication which proposed 10 dos and 4 don'ts was developed in the USA following an international consensus conference on psychopharmacology (64). In 2000 the *American Journal on Mental Retardation* published an expert consensus guideline for the treatment of psychiatric and behavioural problems in ID (65). In 2006, Deb et al. developed a quick reference guide 'Using medication to manage behaviour problems among adults with learning disabilities' (66) and subsequently followed it up in 2009 with the collaboration: 'International guide to prescribing psychotropic medication for the management of problem behaviours in adults with intellectual disabilities'(67). The guidelines on pharmacological treatment in people with personality disorders and ID (82) emphasized that the focus must be on identifying and actively treating comorbid mental illnesses. If clinically indicated, short-term treatment to target four predominant symptom clusters—behaviour dyscontrol, affective dysregulation, anxiety symptoms, and psychotic symptoms was suggested, albeit subject to strict monitoring standards. These are dealt with in greater detail in Chapter 14 of this book. In spite of these guidelines, there is ongoing concern about potential over-medication, partly spurred by scandals of poor care and abuse (68-71).

The standards suggested by the Royal College of Psychiatrists in 2016 (72) for prescribing psychotropic medication to people with ID draws on the most up-to-date evidence base offered by NICE guidelines (51, 73) and is a useful basis for good clinical practice. Its key points are summarized below:

1. All patients for whom prescribing is considered should have a full diagnostic evaluation that covers: the degree of intellectual disability, the cause of intellectual disability (including syndromes, behavioural phenotypes, etc.), other developmental disorders (including autism spectrum disorders, hyperkinetic disorder, etc.), any mental illnesses, personality disorders, disorders related to substance misuse or dependence, physical disorders (including any of the causes of the intellectual disability), psychosocial stressors (longstanding issues as well as recent environmental changes), and types of behaviours that challenge.
2. In this diagnostic formulation, behaviour that challenges is not treated as a diagnosis, but as a presenting symptom that is placed in the context of a range of bio psychosocial factors.
3. Prescribers should accurately record all relevant diagnoses and, equally importantly, the narrative that underpin them.
4. If the diagnosis is such that there are no mental disorders and the behaviour that challenges is the result of psychosocial factors, there might be no role for prescribing other than in the very short term to alleviate a serious risk to the safety of the patient or others while other, non-pharmacological programmes are implemented to manage the behaviour.

5. On the other hand, if an independent mental illness or disorder is diagnosed, treatment should follow established guidelines for that condition.
6. Because presentations are rarely straightforward in clinical practice, there is often a combination of several symptoms and this might not clearly meet the criteria for the categorical diagnoses of a mental illness. In those cases, there should be clear identification of the affective, psychotic, and behavioural symptoms or clusters of symptoms that are the target of treatment with medication. If the identified target symptoms are not improving satisfactorily within three months, then that drug should be tapered or stopped and other options considered.
7. Clinicians should be aware that although off-label prescribing is not inappropriate, unlawful, or unethical in itself, it can be if not done properly. When prescribing off-label, they should follow guidelines that are published by regulatory bodies such as the General Medical Council and ensure that their practice would be considered to be of an adequate standard by their peers.
8. Medications are effective at the same doses as for those without an intellectual disability and there is no clear evidence that they have more side effects. However, side effects and potential drug interactions should be monitored carefully, particularly in those with more severe degrees of ID.
9. The prescribing clinician should explain the proposed treatment to patients, their families and carers, as appropriate. This may involve providing information in an easy-to-read format, making reasonable adjustments and involving independent advocates.
10. There should be a record of the patient's consent and capacity, any best-interests decisions, timeframes for reviews and the tapering off or stopping of drugs that are ineffective.
11. The medication reviews should cover not just clinical examination, but also laboratory tests as indicated.
12. The tapering off or stopping of drugs that are ineffective will be aided by a careful recording of progress (or otherwise) with medication using standardized outcome measures that can be quickly and easily rated (e.g. clinical global impression scale) (81).

This approach sets out four over-arching prescribing standards and offers a self-assessment framework for clinicians to audit their practice, in partnership with people with ID, their families, and carers (see Table 19.3).

Case study 1

- Fred's clinical diagnosis is one of Mild Learning Disability (ICD-10 Code F70.1), a Rapid Cycling Bipolar Affective Disorder (ICD10 Code F31.6), Emotionally Unstable and Dissocial Personality Disorders (ICD-10 Codes F60.3 and 60.2). He also has a 47XYY karyotype (F98.5).
- At present, Fred is on two mood stabilizers (valproate 1200mg/day and lamotrigine 150mg/day), one antipsychotic (haloperidol 20mg/day) and one anti-muscarinic (procyclidine 10mg/day). On a PRN basis, he takes up to 4mg of lorazepam for severe anxiety/agitation and up to 10mg of procyclidine for EPS.
- The environmental, psychological, and possible physical causes of aggression are addressed in Fred's Behaviour Support Plans. His aggressive outbursts are often related to the rapid cycling mood disorder—particularly the depressive/irritable spells that last a few days at a time, as well as the impulsivity and affective instability associated with his personality disorders. These are the targets of pharmacological treatment.
- On this medication regime, his arousal and manic symptoms are under control and the affective instability though present is under a better degree of control. Although the two mood stabilizers can be considered polypharmacy, this combination has been most effective in controlling his rapid cycling mood disorder.
- All drugs are within the BNF maximum limits.
- Fred does not report any major side effects other than occasional tiredness, particularly when he has the PRN lorazepam. He also has features of mild EPS and dyskinetic movements.
- A CGI rating was completed and shows that he is maintaining his improvement (global improvement score 1, efficacy index 02).
- Fred has a general understanding of the effects and side effects of the drugs and the rationale for their use. He can retain that information and use it to reach a decision to accept the drugs. I consider him to continue to have the capacity to consent to the drugs. His consent form was last completed on 01/01/2019. Fred knows he is treated as a consenting patient and that he is free to change his mind. He feels better on this regime and is happy to continue on it. He has been given easy-read information leaflets about the drugs and is quite able to ask questions.
- His drug regime is frequently explained to his nearest relative—his father (Mr Jones), who regularly attends his Care Programme Approach (CPA) meetings along with his care coordinator and social worker.

Case study 2

- Rosie is a 25-year-old woman with mild learning disability (ICD-10 code F70.1). Known to mental health services from the age of 13, with a range of 'challenging behaviours' and a very difficult family background of abuse and neglect, she has had a number of diagnoses mentioned in the past—some with ICD 10 codes and some without. This has included autistic tendencies, mixed disorder of conduct and emotions, depressive episodes, anxiety disorder unspecified, alcohol and substance abuse, personality difficulties, and psychosis.
- After a detailed diagnostic clarification, her current diagnosis is one of a mild learning disability (ICD-10 Code F70.1) and an emotionally unstable personality disorder (ICD-10 Code F60.3). At present, there is no evidence of any mental illness, although it is possible she might have had at least two depressive episodes lasting about 2–3 months in the past. When 'stressed' due to her complicated family situation, Rosie goes through spells that last 1–2 weeks when she will complain of 'hearing voices' telling her to harm herself, abuse alcohol and she will repeatedly threaten to jump off high buildings. The evaluation suggests that she does not have a chronic psychotic illness, but that these brief psychotic episodes are happening within the context of an emotionally unstable

Table 19.3 Self-assessment framework

Standards	Key lines of enquiry	Audit standard rating
1. The indication(s) and rationale for prescribing the psychotropic drug should be clearly stated, including whether the prescribing is off-label, polypharmacy or high dose	a) Is the prescribing part of a wider multidisciplinary care plan? b) Is there documentation of the indication for prescribing? (This can include the diagnoses as well as the narrative account of the target symptoms.) c) If the prescription is only for behaviour that challenges, are the NICE guidelines being followed? (Psychological interventions have not produced a change within an agreed time period or treatment of co-existing mental and physical conditions have not led to a reduction or risk to the person or others is very severe and drugs are offered only with psychological or other interventions.) d) Is there off-label prescribing? If so, is the rationale explained? e) Is there polypharmacy? If so, is the rationale explained? f) Is there prescribing over British National Formulary maximum limits (or equivalent)? If so, is the rationale explained?	
2. Consent-to-treatment procedures (or best interests decision-making processes) should be followed and documented	a) Is there evidence of a capacity assessment? b) If the patient is deemed to lack capacity, is the best interests' process followed? c) Is there evidence that the patient's views about the drug treatment are being recorded? d) Is there evidence that the carers' or family members' views about the drug treatment are being recorded? e) If patient is compulsorily detained (e.g. under the Mental Health Act 1983 in England and Wales), are the legal requirements around consent to treatment satisfied?	
3. There should be regular monitoring of treatment response and side-effects (preferably every 3 months or less, at a minimum every 6 months)	a) Is there documentation about progress on the target symptoms for treatment? b) Is there evidence of objective evaluation of treatment response (e.g. use of standardized instruments like the CGI or equivalent)? c) Is there evidence of objective evaluation of side-effects (e.g. use of standardized instruments)?	
4. Review and evaluation of the need for continuation or discontinuation of the psychotropic drug should be undertaken on a regular basis (preferably every 3 months or less, at a minimum every 6 months) or whenever there is a request from patients, carers or other professionals	a) Is there evidence of objective evaluation of treatment response (e.g. use of standardized instruments)? b) Is there evidence of objective evaluation of side-effects (e.g. use of standardized instruments)? c) Is there evidence of regular review of the need for continuation or discontinuation of the drug? (This includes discussion of risks and benefits with the patient and/or carer.)	

personality. She responds quickly to antipsychotic medication when this happens.

- The environmental, psychological, and possible physical causes of her behavioural problems are addressed in Rosie's behaviour support plans. She has been offered therapy and support from the community intellectual disability team's psychology and outreach services.
- In spite of this, there are several episodes when Rosie acts out with aggression towards her carers in the supported living environment and makes serious attempts to self-harm, putting her and others at risk.
- My impression is that Rosie's predominant mood state even when she is not having major depressive disorder is one of dysphoria with her having little interest or motivation in becoming engaged in various activities. This low mood was associated with mood swings and impulsive behaviours, particularly when stressed.
- Because of the persisting dysphoric symptoms and mood instability, she was started on paroxetine 20mg/day and there was improvement on these target symptoms. At present, Rosie is on one antidepressant (paroxetine 20mg/day). On a PRN basis, she is on one anxiolytic (up to 2mg/day of lorazepam for severe anxiety/agitation. She has used this three times in the past month).
- Rosie does not report any major side effects other than occasional tiredness, particularly when she has the PRN lorazepam.
- Rosie has a general understanding of the effects and side effects of the drugs and the rationale for their use. She can retain that information and use it to reach a decision to accept the drugs. I consider her to have the capacity to consent to the drugs. However, the prescription of the antidepressant is off-label and I have discussed this with the team, Rosie, her support staff in the community, and her independent advocate. The family is not involved in her care because of past issues. Rosie knows she is treated as a consenting patient and that she is free to change her mind. She feels better on this regime and is happy to continue on it. She has been given easy-read information leaflets about the medication and is quite able to ask questions. The last review was on 01/01/2019.
- A CGI rating has been completed and shows that she is maintaining her improvement for about 12 months now. (She had a global improvement score of two and efficacy index of 06.)

- She does continue to have 'crises', but those involved in supporting her in the community feel that these have become less in intensity and frequency than before.

(Adapted from Royal College of Psychiatrists: Faculty of Psychiatry of Intellectual Disability report (2016) Psychotropic Drug Prescribing for People with Intellectual Disabilities, mental health problems and/or behaviours that challenge: practice guidelines)

MULTIPLE CHOICE QUESTIONS

Questions

Please select the single most appropriate answer.

1. Which of the following is true?

A. There is no clear evidence that people with an intellectual disability have more antipsychotic side effects than the general population.
B. Psychosis is more infrequent in people with an ID than the general population.
C. Antipsychotic medication is contra-indicated in the treatment of schizoaffective disorders in people with an ID.
D. Clozapine is contra-indicated in people with an ID.
E. Blood tests for clozapine have to be done more frequently in people with an ID.

2. All of the following are true except:

A. Antipsychotic prescribing for behaviour that challenges (without a mental illness) is mostly off-label
B. Off-label prescribing is considered unlawful.
C. A number of randomized controlled trials have shown that antipsychotics may be effective in children with intellectual disability and behaviour that challenges.
D. Antidepressants and mood stabilizers are widely prescribed for managing behaviour that challenges.
E. Long term prescription of antipsychotic medication can have undesirable side effects.

3. Antipsychotics may be prescribed short term for challenging behaviour in adults with a learning disability if:

A. psychological interventions have not produced a change within an agreed time period
B. treatment of co-existing mental and physical conditions have not led to a reduction
C. risk to the person or others is very severe
C. It is part of a treatment package that includes psychological measures
E. All of the above

4. Studies focusing on the withdrawal of antipsychotics in people with an ID have reported all of the following complications except:

A. Worsening of the behavior
B. Emergence of dyskinesias
C. Worsening of dyskinesias
D. Emergence of diabetes
E. Autonomic instability

5. Regarding the monitoring of antipsychotic prescribing in people with ID, all of the following are true except:

A. Record the indication and target symptoms that are being treated
B. Review the need to continue medication at least every 24 months
C. Use standardized instruments like the CGI to record progress
D. Use standardized instruments to record side effects
E. Discuss risks and benefits with patient and the family, as appropriate

Answers

1. A. The prevalence of psychosis in people with ID is higher than that in the general population. Its treatment follows the same principles. While it is prudent to 'start low and go slow' with antipsychotic medication regimes, particularly in those with severe degrees of learning disability, there is no clear evidence to show that people with ID have more side effects than the general population.
2. B. Antipsychotics are used 'off label' in the treatment of challenging behavior in children and adults with an ID. While off label prescribing is not unlawful, prescribers should follow guidelines that are published by regulatory bodies like the General Medical Council and ensure that their practice would be considered to be of an adequate standard by their peers.
3. E. In the absence of co-existing psychosis, good practice would be to prescribe antipsychotics for challenging behaviour in a time-bound manner as part of a treatment package that includes psychological measures. Consent to treatment procedures should be followed and wherever appropriate, adequate discussion with the patient and family should occur.
4. D. Worsening of behaviour, emergence or worsening of dyskinesias and autonomic instability have been reported during antipsychotic withdrawal. Diabetes and metabolic syndrome are complications associated with treatment with atypical antipsychotics.
5. B. Good practice standards include recording the indications and target symptoms, following the appropriate consent to treatment procedures, using standardized instruments to monitor response and side effects. The need to continue medication should ideally be reviewed between three to six months. A minimum yearly review has also been proposed.

REFERENCES

1. Aman M, Singh N. Patterns of drug use, methodological consideration, measurement techniques, and future trends. In Psychopharmacology of Developmental Disabilities (eds M Aman and N Singh) 1988, pp 1–29 Springer Verlag, Berlin.
2. Health and Social Care Information Centre Learning Disabilities Census Report—Further analysis England, 30 September 2013. Published 29 April 2014.
3. Care Quality Commission Learning Disability: Survey of Detained Patients' Medications. 2016 CQC.

4. Sinai A, Tenenbaum A, Aspler S, Lotan M, Morad M, Merrick J. Challenging Behavior and Related Factors in People with Intellectual Disability Living in Residential Care Centers in Israel Front Public Health. 2013;1:13.
5. Branford D. A study of prescribing for people with learning disabilities living in the community and in National Health Service care. *Journal of Intellectual Disability Research*. 1994;38:577–586
6. Branford, D. A follow-up study of prescribing for people with learning disabilities previously in National Health Service care in Leicestershire, England. *Journal of Intellectual Disability Research*. 1997;41(4):339–345.
7. Spreat S, Conroy J, Fullerton A. Statewide longitudinal survey of psychotropic medication use for persons with mental retardation: 1994 to 2000. *American Journal on Mental Retardation*. 2004;109(4):322–331.
8. McGillivray J, McCabe, M. Emerging trends in the use of drugs to manage the challenging behaviour of people with intellectual disability. *Journal of Applied Research in Intellectual Disabilities*, 2006;19(2):163–172.
9. Hobden KL, Samuel PS, LeRoy BW, Lindsay D. An empirical examination of the prevalence and predictors of polypharmacy in individuals with dual diagnoses. *International Journal of Disability Communication and Rehabilitation*. 2013;12:1.
10. Etherington J, Sheppard, LC, Ballinger BR, Fenton, GW. Psychotropic drugs in a hospital for intellectual disability: The story of 18 years. *Mental Handicap Research*. 1995;8(3):184–193.
11. Lott IT, McGregor M, Engelman L, Touchette P, Tournay A, Sandman C, et al. Longitudinal prescribing patterns for psychoactive medications in community-based individuals with developmental disabilities: Utilization of pharmacy records. *Journal of Intellectual Disability Research*. 2004;48(6):563–571.
12. Public Health England Prescribing of Psychotropic Drugs to People with Learning Disabilities and or Autism by General Practitioners in England. 2015 PHE.
13. Sheehan R, Hassiotis A, Walters K, Osborn D, Strydom A, Horsfall L. Mental illness, challenging behaviour and psychotropic drug prescribing in people with intellectual disability: UK population based cohort study. *BMJ*. 2015;351: 4326.
14. Kane JM, Smith JM. Tardive dyskinesia: Prevalence and risk factors 1959–1979. *Archives of General Psychiatry*. 1982;Apr;39(4):473–481.
15. Frighi E, Stephenson MT, Morovat A, et al. Safety of antipsychotics in people with intellectual disability. *British Journal of Psychiatry*. 2011;199: 289–295.
16. Brylewski J, Duggan L. Antipsychotic medication for challenging behaviour in people with learning disability. *Cochrane Database of Systematic Reviews*. 2004;3: CD000377.
17. Thalayasingam S, Alexander RT, Singh I. The use of clozapine in adults with intellectual disability. *J Intellect Disabil Res*. 2004;Sep;48 (Pt 6):572–579.
18. NICE. Challenging Behaviour and Learning Disabilities: Prevention and Interventions for People with Learning Disabilities whose Behaviour Challenges (NG11). NICE 2015.
19. Heyvaert M, Maes B, Onghena PA. Meta-analysis of intervention effects on challenging behaviour among persons with intellectual disabilities. *Journal of Intellectual Disability Research*. 2010;54 part 7, pp. 634–649.
20. Aman MG, De Smedt G, Derivan A, Lyons B, Findling RL, Hagerman R, et al. Double-blind, placebo-controlled study of risperidone for the treatment of disruptive behaviors in children with subaverage intelligence. *American Journal of Psychiatry*. 2002;159:1337–1346.
21. Kent JM, Kushner S, Ning X, Karcher K, Ness S, Aman M, et al. Risperidone dosing in children and adolescents with autistic disorder: A double-blind, placebo-controlled study. *Journal of Autism and Developmental Disorders*. 2013;43:1773–1783.
22. Research Units on Pediatric Psychopharmacology (RUPP) Autism Network. Risperidone in children with autism and serious behavioral problems. *The New England Journal of Medicine*. 2002;347:314–321.
23. Shea S, Turgay A, Carroll A, Schulz M, Orlik H, Smith I, et al. Risperidone in the treatment of disruptive behavioral symptoms in children with autistic and other pervasive developmental disorders. *Pediatrics*. 2004;114:634–641.
24. Snyder R, Turgay A, Aman M, Binder C, Fisman S, Carroll A. Effects of risperidone on conduct and disruptive behavior disorders in children with subaverage IQs. *Journal of the American Academy of Child and Adolescent Psychiatry*. 2002;41: 1026–1036.
25. Marcus RN, Owen R, Kamen L, Manos G, McQuade RD, Carson WH, et al. A placebo controlled, fixed-dose study of aripiprazole in children and adolescents with irritability associated with autistic disorder. *Journal of the American Academy of Child and Adolescent Psychiatry*. 2009;48:1110–1119.
26. Owen R, Sikich L, Marcus RN, Corey-Lisle P, Manos G, McQuade RD, et al. Aripiprazole in the treatment of irritability in children and adolescents with autistic disorder. *Pediatrics*. 2009;124:1533–1540.
27. Ghanizadeh A, Sahraeizadeh A, Berk M. A head-to-head comparison of aripiprazole and risperidone for safety and treating autistic disorders, a randomized double blind clinical trial. *Child Psychiatry and Human Development*. 2014;45:185–192.
28. Research Units on Pediatric Psychopharmacology (RUPP) Autism Network. Risperidone treatment of autistic disorder: longer-term benefits and blinded discontinuation after 6 months. *American Journal of Psychiatry*. 2005;162:1361–1369.
29. Findling RL, Mankoski R, Timko K, Lears K, McCartney T, McQuade RD, et al. A randomized controlled trial investigating the safety and efficacy of aripiprazole in the long-term maintenance treatment of pediatric patients with irritability associated with autistic disorder. *Journal of Clinical Psychiatry*. 2014;75:22–30.
30. Gagiano C, Read S, Thorpe L, Eerdekens M, Van Hove I. Short- and long-term efficacy and safety of risperidone in adults with disruptive behavior disorders. *Psychopharmacology*. 2005;179:629–636.
31. Amore M, Bertelli M, Villani D, Tamborini S, Rossi M. Olanzapine vs. risperidone in treating aggressive behaviours in adults with intellectual disability: A single blind study. *Journal of Intellectual Disability Research*. 2011;55:210–218.
32. Tyrer P, Oliver-Africano PC, Ahmed Z, Bouras N, Cooray S, Deb S, et al. Risperidone, haloperidol, and placebo in the treatment of aggressive challenging behaviour in patients with intellectual disability: A randomised controlled trial. *Lancet*. 2008;371: 57–63.
33. Haessler F, Glaser T, Beneke M, Pap AF, Bodenschatz R, Reis O. Zuclopenthixol in adults with intellectual disabilities and aggressive behaviours: Discontinuation study. *British Journal of Psychiatry*. 2007;190:447–448.
34. Izmeth MG, Khan SY, Kumarajeewa DI, Shivanathan S, Veall RM, Wiley YV. Zuclopenthixol decanoate in the management

of behavioural disorders in mentally handicapped patients. *Pharmatherapeutica*. 1988;5:217–227.

35. Singh I, Owino WJE. A double-blind comparison of zuclopenithixol tablets with placebo in the treatment of mentally handicapped in-patients with associated behavioural disorders. *Journal of Intellectual Disability Research*. 1992;36:541–549.
36. Branford D. A review of antipsychotic drugs prescribed for people with learning disabilities who live in Leicestershire. *Journal of Intellectual Disability Research*. 1996;40(4):358–368.
37. Branford, D. Factors associated with the successful or unsuccessful withdrawal of antipsychotic drug therapy prescribed for people with learning disabilities. *Journal of Intellectual Disability Research*. 1996;40:322–329.
38. Ahmed Z, Fraser W, Kerr MP, et al. Reducing antipsychotic medication in people with a learning disability. *British Journal of Psychiatry*. 2000;176:42–46.
39. de Kuijper GI, Evenhuis H, Minderaa RB, Hoekstra PJ. Effects of controlled discontinuation of long-term used antipsychotics for behavioural symptoms in individuals with intellectual disability. *Intellect Disabil Res*. 2014 Jan;58(1):71–83.
40. Cooper SA, Smiley E, Jackson A, Finlayson J, Allan L, Mantry D, Morrison J. Adults with intellectual disabilities: Prevalence, incidence and remission of aggressive behaviour and related factors. *J Intellect Disabil Res*. 2009;53(3):217–232.
41. Roy D, Hoffman P, Dudas M, Mendelowitz A. Pharmacologic management of aggression in adults with intellectual disability. *Journal of Intellectual Disability. Diagnosis and Treatment*. 2013;1:28–43.
42. Rana F, Gormez A, Varghese S. Pharmacological interventions for self-injurious behaviour in adults with intellectual disabilities. Cochrane Database of Systematic Reviews. 2013;
43. Ruedrich SL, Swales TP, Rossvanes C, Diana L, Arkadiev V, Lim K. Atypical antipsychotic medication improves aggression, but not self-injurious behaviour, in adults with intellectual disabilities. *J Intellect Disabil Res*. 2008; 52(Pt 2):132–140.
44. British National Formulary (BNF) Section 4.3 Antidepressants Latest Edition British Medical Association, Royal Pharmaceutical Society.
45. Bhaumik S, Branford D, Barrett M, Gangadharan SK. (2015) Frith Guidelines for Prescribing in Intellectual Disability. Wiley.
46. NICE guideline (CG90) Depression in adults: Recognition and management. 2016; NICE.
47. Taylor D, Paton C, Kapur S. The Maudsley Prescribing Guidlines in Psychiatry 12th edition. 2015: Wiley.
48. Janowsky DS, Shetty M, Barnhill J, Elamir B, Davis JM. Serotonergic antidepressant effects on aggressive, selfinjurious and destructive/disruptive behaviours in intellectually disabled adults: A retrospective, open-label, naturalistic trial. *Int J Neuropsychopharmacol*. 2005; 8(1):3748.
49. Branford D, Bhaumik S. Selective serotonin re-uptake inhibitors for the treatment of perseverative and maladaptive behaviours of people with intellectual disability. *J Intellect Disabil Res*. 1998;42(4):301–306.
50. Lewis MH, Bodfish JW. Clomipramine treatment for self-injurious behavior of individuals with mental retardation: A double-blind comparison with placebo. *Am J Mental Retardation*. 1996;100(6):654–655.
51. NICE guidelines (CG142) Autism spectrum disorder in adults: Diagnosis and management. 2012: NICE.
52. Craft M, Ismail IA, Krishnamurti D, et al. Lithium in the treatment of aggression in mentally handicapped patients: A double-blind trial. *Br J Psych*. 1987;150:685–689.
53. Tyrer SP, Walsh A, Edwards DE, Herney TP, Stephens DA. Factors associated with a good response to lithium in aggressive mentally handicapped subjects. *Progr Neuro-Psychopharmacol Biol Psych*. 1984;8(4-6):751–755.
54. Reid AH, Naylor GJ, Kay DS. A double-blind, placebo controlled, crossover trial of carbamazepine in overactive severely mentally handicapped patients. *Psychol Med*. 1981;11:109–113.
55. Ruedrich S, Swales TP, Fossaceca C, Toliver J, Rutkowski A. Effect of divalproex sodium on aggression and self-injurious behaviour in adults with intellectual disability: A retrospective review. *J Intellect Disabil Res*. 1999;43:105–111.
56. Janowsky DS, Kraus JE, Barnhill J, Elamir B, Davis JM. Effects of topiramate on aggressive, self-injurious, and disruptive/destructive behaviors in the intellectually disabled: An open-label retrospective study. *J Clin Psychopharmacol*. 2003;23(5):500–504.
57. Braam W, Didden R, Smits M, Curfs L. Melatonin treatment in individuals with intellectual disability and chronic insomnia: A randomized placebo-controlled study. *Journal of Intellectual Disability Research*. 2008a;52:256–264.
58. Braam W, Didden R, Smits MG, Curfs LM. Melatonin for chronic insomnia in angelman syndrome: A randomized placebo-controlled trial. *Journal of Child Neurology*. 2008;23:649–654.
59. Cortesi F, Giannotti F, Sebastiani T, Panunzi S, Valente D. Controlled-release melatonin, singly and combined with cognitive behavioural therapy, for persistent insomnia in children with autism spectrum disorders: A randomized placebo-controlled trial. *Journal of Sleep Research*. 2012;21:700–709.
60. Gringras P, Gamble C, Jones AP et al. Melatonin for sleep problems in children with neurodevelopmental disorders: Randomised double masked placebo controlled trial. *BMJ*. 2012; 45 e6664.
61. NICE guidelines (CG72) Attention deficit hyperactivity disorder: Diagnosis and management. 2016: NICE.
62. Simonoff E, Taylor E, Baird G, et al. Randomized controlled double-blind trial of optimal dose methylphenidate in children and adolescents with severe attention deficit hyperactivity disorder and intellectual disability. *J Child Psychol Psychiatry*. 2013 May;54(5):527–535.
63. Livingstone N, Hanratty J, McShane R, Macdonald G (2015) Medications for cognitive decline in people with Down syndrome http://www.cochrane.org/CD011546/BEHAV_medications-cognitive-decline-people-down-syndrome.
64. Kalachnik JE, Leventhal BL, James DH, et al Guidelines for the use of psychotropic medication. In: Reiss S, Aman MG, eds. *Psychotropic Medication and Developmental Disabilities: the international consensus handbook*. Ohio State University, Nisonger Centre, Columbus: 1998: 45–72.
65. Rush AJ, Frances A. Treatment of psychiatric and behavioural problems in mental retardation—expert consensus guideline series. *Am J Ment Retardation*. 2000;105(3):159–227.
66. Deb S, Clarke D, Unwin G. Using medication to manage behaviour problems among adults with learning disabilities. 2006. University of Birmingham. Available online at: www. LD-Medication.bham.ac.uk.
67. Deb S, Kwork H, Bertelli M, et al. International guide to prescribing psychotropic medication for the management of problem behaviours in adults with intellectual disabilities. *World Psychiatry*, 2009;8:181–186.
68. Department of Health. Transforming care: A national response to Winterbourne View Hospital—*Department of Health Review: Final Report* (PDF 302kb). Published online 10 December, 2012.

69. NHS Improving Quality. Winterbourne Medicines Programme: Improving the Use of Medicines in People with Learning Disabilities. 2015. *NHSIQ*.
70. NHS England Stopping Over-Medication of People with a Learning Disability (STOMPLD) 2016 https://www.england.nhs.uk/wp-content/uploads/2016/06/stopping-over-medication.pdf.
71. NHS England Stopping Over-Medication of People with a Learning Disability (STOMPLD) Pledge. https://www.england.nhs.uk/2016/06/over-medication-pledge/.
72. Royal College of Psychiatrists: Faculty of Psychiatry of Intellectual Disability report. Psychotropic Drug Prescribing for People with Intellectual Disabilities, mental health problems and/or behaviours that challenge: Practice guidelines. 2016. FR/ID/09. http://www.rcpsych.ac.uk/pdf/FR_ID_09_for_website.pdf.
73. NICE guidelines (NG54) Mental Health problems in people with learning disabilities: Prevention, assessment and management. 2016. NICE.
74. Alexander RT, Shankar R, Cooper SA, et al. Challenges and pitfalls of antipsychotic prescribing in peole with learning disability. *British Journal of General practice*, 2017;67(661):372–373.
75. Bowring DL, Totsika V, Hastings RP, Toogood S, Griffith GM. Challenging behaviours in adults with an intellectual disability: A total population study and exploration of risk indices. Br J Clin Psychol. 2016.
76. Buckles J, Luckasson R, Keefe E. A systematic review of the prevalence of psychiatric disorders in adults with intellectual disability, 2003–2010. *J Ment Health Res Intellect Disabil.* 2013;6(3):181–207.
77. Cooper SA, Smiley E, Morrison J, Williamson A, Allan L. Mental ill-health in adults with intellectual disabilities: Prevalence and associated factors. *Br J Psychiatry*. 2007 Jan;190:27–35.
78. Emerson E, Hatton C. The mental health of children and adolescents with learning disabilities in Britain. *Adv Ment Health Intellect Disabil.* 2007;1(**3**):62–63.
79. Sheehan R, Hassiotis A, Walters K, Osborn D, Strydom A, Horsfall L. Mental illness, challenging behaviour, and psychotropic drug prescribing in people with intellectual disability: UK population based cohort study. *BMJ*. 2015 Sep 1;351: h4326.
80. NHS England. Urgent action pledged on over-medication of people with learning disabilities. Leeds: NHS England, 2015. https://www.england.nhs.uk/2015/07/urgent-pledge/ (accessed 15 Jan 2017).
81. Guy W (ed). Clinical Global Impression (CGI). In *ECDEU Assessment Manual for Psychopharmacology*. US Department of Health, Education, and References 22 Welfare, 1976 (http://www.psywellness.com.sg/docs/CGI.pdf).
82. Alexander R, Bhaumik S. Psychotropic medication in the treatment of personality disorders in Intellectual Disability. In Bhaumik S, Branford D, Barrett M. (Eds). *The Frith Prescribing Guidelines for Adults with Learning Disability*, 3rd Edition, 2016.

Box 20.1 Common comorbidities in people with ID related to physical health

- Poor nutritional well-being: Underweight or overweight
- Gastro-oesophageal reflux
- Constipation
- Osteoporosis
- Visual and hearing impairment
- Musculoskeletal impairment

presentation as a sign of distress related to a physical illness particularly in those with limited communication (7). Epilepsy is a common condition in people with ID, with prevalence as high as 26 per cent as well as difficulty in seizure control and associated higher rates of behavioural and psychological problems (8). Additionally, using psychotropic medication to manage neuromotor dysfunction may worsen seizures and conversely anti-seizure medication may worsen behaviour.

As a psychiatrist you may be required to undertake assessment of a patient with whom you are not familiar. This may occur out of normal office hours such as the evening or a weekend when you have limited access to records and limited access to accurate information from regular care givers. With people with mild ID you may gain some history from the individuals themselves but for people with more profound cognitive impairment you will have to rely on written information in care plans and clinical notes and those given to you by third parties such as paid care providers.

People with ID are especially prone to developing physical illness but because of communication difficulties, behavioural manifestations may be the presenting feature (see Figure 20.1). Additionally, clinicians may delay investigation or fail to appreciate symptoms by associating them with the ID, which can result in diagnostic overshadowing (9).

Identifying common sources of pain (such as ear infections, headaches, reflux oesophagitis, urinary tract infection, and constipation) may be especially difficult. This can be challenging and there may be pressure and expectations from carers to prescribe medication to possibly sedate the person with ID and or arrange an emergency alternative placement. It remains important at this time to perform a thorough mental health and physical examination as well as assessing mental capacity before making a significant intervention that could potentially worsen the situation.

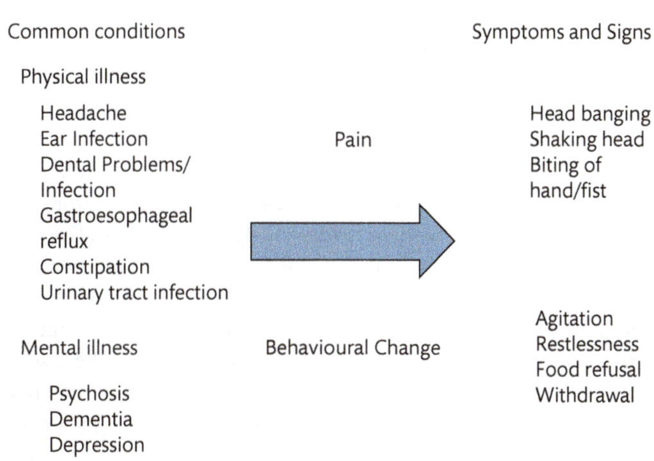

Figure 20.1 Symptoms and signs related to common conditions in ID

It is now recognized that the identification of mental health and physical problems in people with ID may be difficult due to diagnostic overshadowing, with attribution of either the physical or mental health problem to the ID, and 'normalizing' it can lead to unmet health needs. Physical health conditions may mimic, accompany, or be caused by mental health problems in people with ID. The diagnosis of a non-organic diagnosis can only be made after an appropriate physical examination and investigations. There are many positive aspects to doing a physical examination and confidence in performing them requires practice.

Clinical tips

Take a thorough history and particularly try to establish the concerns of the person with ID and their carers. If the person who is most concerned is not in attendance, consider either phoning them directly or writing to them. Use any useful information such as summary sheets from their GP with their significant past medical history and current medication. Ask to see their latest care plan and any health action plans as well as any weight charts. Before you start a physical examination, attempt to find out how the person with ID is likely to respond to touch. You will need to establish if the person with ID has capacity to consent to an examination. Find a chaperone that is trusted and well known to the person with ID. Set up the room for success by using a quiet room the person with ID is comfortable with, such as their own bedroom. Ensure there is good lighting and the room is adequately heated, especially as the person may need to remove their clothing at least partially. After washing your hands and introducing yourself, explain what you are going to do and demonstrate either on yourself or the chaperone before you proceed. The physical examination starts from the moment you first see the person as you observe their general appearance, dress, gait, repetitive movements, mobility, and how they interact with others and themselves. Continue to observe and think throughout the examination, try to examine in a respectful manner and avoid causing pain. It is always good practice when concerned about a person with an ID to try and talk to them on their own to see if there are stresses or concerns they do not want to discuss in front of carers.

In 2016 the report 'Improving the physical health of adults with severe mental illness: essential actions' was published by the Academy of Medical Royal Colleges and the Royal Colleges of General Practitioners, Nursing, Pathologists, Psychiatrists, Physicians, the Royal Pharmaceutical Society, and Public Health England (10). Among the recommendations included a requirement for mental healthcare providers to ensure National Early Warning Score (NEWS) that basic medical equipment is provided. They also recommended the use of the NEWS system in mental healthcare settings by staff trained in its use to enable the early recognition of acute illness and appropriate action to be taken in a timely way. In assessing acute illness, the NEWS (see Box 20.2), is based on a simple scoring system in which a score is allocated to physiological measurements already undertaken when patients present to, or are being monitored in hospital. In order to complete these you will need a thermometer, watch or mobile phone with second timer, sphygmomanometer, and pulse oximeter.

20

Physical Health in People with Intellectual Disabilities

Umesh Chauhan, Ken Courtenay, and Matthew Hoghton

'There has been an acceptance in society, and even in the medical profession, that people with mental health problems and intellectual disability will live shorter lives and will suffer because of unmet health needs. In the vast majority of cases, there is no good reason for this. But the voice of these vulnerable groups often goes unheard, and the status quo remains unchallenged.'

Professor the Baroness Sheila Hollins.

Reproduced with permission from the British Medical Association

Introduction

People with intellectual disabilities have a shorter life expectancy and an increased mortality rate across all ages compared to the general population. The main contributors to the health inequalities experienced by people with intellectual disabilities include:

1. Social determinants such as poverty and unemployment;
2. Health problems related to intellectual disabilities (such as congenital abnormalities related to people with moderate to profound intellectual disabilities);
3. Limited communication and health literacy skills, which may reduce their capacity to understand and convey health needs effectively to others;
4. Personal health risks related to diet and sedentary lifestyle; and
5. Organizational barriers to accessing mainstream health care (1)

People with ID continue to experience poor healthcare and social care with life expectancy at birth nearly 20 years lower than the general population (2). Potentially avoidable causes of death in people with ID include epilepsy (3.9 per cent of deaths), aspiration pneumonitis (3.6 per cent) and colorectal cancer (2.4 per cent). Analysis showed that a higher proportion of deaths from causes amenable to good medical care but a lower proportion from preventable causes compared with people without ID (2). The recent confidential inquiry into the deaths of people with a learning disability (CIPOLD), which reviewed the deaths of 247 people with ID, showed that they continue to die at a younger age from avoidable causes (3).

People with intellectual disabilities also experience higher levels of long-term conditions than the general population at a younger age. The burden of multi-morbidity is higher due to higher rates of some physical and mental health conditions and is common in all age groups in adults with ID. The pattern of disease also differs from the general population, for example, obesity affecting up to 38 per cent of people with ID compared to 25 per cent of the general population (4) (see Box 20.1).

Additionally, the prevalence of multi-morbidity does not follow the typical gradient as seen in the general population across areas of increasing neighbourhood deprivation, importantly highlighting that services are equally needed in all areas. Cooper et al. reviewed primary health-care data on 1,424,378 adults (18 years or over) registered with 314 representative Scottish practices, which included 8,014 adults with ID (5). The ID group was significantly more likely to have more health conditions, with the biggest difference found for epilepsy, constipation, and visual impairment. Hearing loss, eczema, dyspepsia, thyroid disorders, and Parkinson's disease or Parkinsonism were all more than twice as likely to be prevalent in those with ID compared to controls. Lower relative prevalence for the adults with ID was found for cardiovascular-related conditions (coronary heart disease, peripheral vascular disease, hypertension, atrial fibrillation, any cancer over the last five years, and chronic obstructive pulmonary disease (COPD)). Comorbidity increased with age but is highly prevalent at all ages, being similar at age 20–25 in those with ID to 50–54-year-olds in the general population. Similarly, in older groups of people with ID, patterns of comorbidities do not follow those seen in the general population with again relatively low levels of cardiovascular disease and higher levels of neurological conditions (6).

Symptoms and signs related to brain dysfunction can be categorized into the following: 1) cognitive dysfunction, 2) neuromotor dysfunction, 3) impulsive behaviours and 4) seizures. Cognitive dysfunction is loss of intellectual functions such as thinking, remembering, and reasoning of sufficient severity to interfere with daily functioning. Neuromotor dysfunction, particularly extrapyramidal signs and symptoms (EPSS), plays an important role in the assessment and treatment of people in the early stages of psychotic disorders such as schizophrenia and the effect of psychotropic drugs. Impulsive behaviours such as physical violence, property destruction, trichotillomania and self-injurious behaviour can be common

Box 20.2 Six simple physiological parameters form the basis of the scoring system

1. Respiratory rate
2. Oxygen saturation
3. Systolic blood pressure
4. Pulse rate
5. Level of consciousness or new confusion
6. Temperature

Reproduced from: Royal College of Physicians. National Early Warning Score (NEWS) 2: Standardizing the assessment of acute-illness severity in the NHS. Updated report of a working party. London: RCP, 2017.

After trying to establish these vital signs aim to conduct a systematic head to toe system assessment (see Box 20.3).

Assessing pain requires particular attention, as this can be difficult to ascertain and may be managed. The 'Non-Communicating Adults Pain Checklist', is an 18-item behavioral scale, which can be used to assess pain levels in adults with ID (12). The model reflects two categories of pain responses: a basic response consisting of physiological measures and body reaction and an advanced response consisting of vocal and emotional reactions and facial and protective expressions and may be a reasonable tool to assess pain.

There are certain conditions, which are more likely to occur and require proactive and regular structured assessment. For example, gastrointestinal disorders such as reflux and constipation commonly present with change in behaviour that may remain unrecognized as an underlying cause or poorly managed leading to further complications. Bowel function can be affected by underlying conditions such as Down syndrome, metabolic disorder such as hypothyroidism, but can also be a complication of medications (anticonvulsants, antipsychotics, benzodiazepines, and tricyclic antidepressants) that can reduce intestinal motility (Table 20.1).

A structured approach to reviewing a person's health requires a systematic assessment that takes into account underlying risk factors, complications of therapy, and the need for a coordinated approach across health and care settings. For example, people with ID have significant oral health problems from an early age which requires intervention at an individual/carer level through education and therapy; review of medications (for example, anticonvulsants such as phenytoin which cause gingival overgrowth and enlargement); access to regular dental assessment as well as treatment by a hygienist and appropriate surgical interventions. Targeted investigations when the clinical findings on examination cannot be explained should include the following (Box 20.4):

Box 20.3 Components of a systematic physical examination

- Body Mass Index based on up to date height and weight
- Auditory and visual assessment
- Oral health
- Dermatological assessment
- Neurological assessment
- Cardiorespiratory assessment
- Abdominal examination including genitourinary
- Musculoskeletal including postural assessment

Table 20.1 Symptoms, signs, and complications related to common causes of constipation in ID

Common Causes	Symptoms, Signs and Complications
Medications	Food refusal
Anticonvulsant	Agitation/aggression
Benzodiazepine	Bloated/tender abdomen
Antipsychotic	Irregular/infrequent bowel habit
Calcium and iron supplement	Vomiting
Antacid	Haemorrhoids
Lifestyle risk factors	Rectal bleeding
Reduced fluid/fibre intake	Obstruction
Sedentary lifestyle	
Restricted mobility	
Neuromuscular Disorders	
Spina bifida	
Megacolon	
Endocrine disorders	
Hypothyroidism	

Health promotion

Annual health checks for adults with intellectual disabilities have been shown to be effective in identifying new health needs (13), providing an opportunity to review concurrent comorbidities (e.g. epilepsy and diabetes), and to offer health promotion with information (e.g. access to dietary and smoking cessation services) as well as access to national screening programmes. In the UK, this has been an enhanced service with additional payment to GP practices to undertake but a multidisciplinary team approach involving the wider primary and community health care providers is needed to undertake health checks successfully.

Medication: The impact of medication on physical health

Drug therapy is useful in managing mental disorders, however the adverse effects of medication can have direct impacts on a person with ID and affect their physical health and their Quality of Life (QoL). Prescribing clinicians may not consider the impact of drug therapy on the person's QoL whilst seeking to treat the symptoms

Box 20.4 Targeted investigations

Blood investigations
- Full blood count and C reactive protein
- Electrolytes
- Liver function
- Random glucose and glycosylated HbA1c
- Thyroid function test
- Drug levels

Mid-stream urine sample analysis

Chest x-ray

of mental illness. As the number of psychotropic medications that a person uses increases they negatively affect the person's QoL especially where two or more drugs are prescribed (14). The impact on the person's QoL, as measured using the Intellectual Disability Quality of Life-16 Scale (IDQoL-16), does not appear to affect the care plan since the physicians do not alter the drug regimen (14).

Psychotropic medication affects physical health through metabolic and motor side effects associated with them. The metabolic side effects include weight gain, hormonal changes, abnormal blood lipid and blood sugar levels, and high blood pressure, while motor effects manifest as movement disorders. Generally, first generation antipsychotics (FGA) exert motor and hormonal effects while second generation antipsychotics (SGA) predominantly exhibit metabolic effects but not exclusively so. People with ID are especially sensitive to the adverse effects of all medication types and not just to psychotropic medication.

Motor side effects of antipsychotic medication

The motor effects are referred to as extrapyramidal side effects (EPSE) that cause dystonic reactions affecting large and small muscles of the eyes, neck, trunk, and limbs to which people with ID are especially vulnerable. Tardive dyskinesia (TD) is a known effect of FGA that results often from prolonged use of antipsychotic medication (15). The risk factors for developing TD include cognitive impairment, age, more severe ID, and chronic use of medication (16). Clinicians need to be aware that the risks are higher in people with ID and be informed about the signs of TD and how to treat it. Using SGA drugs may reduce the risk of motor side effects but not necessarily eliminate them. TD has been reported in a person with ID using aripiprazole where the mechanism of action is partial antagonism of dopamine and serotonin receptors (17). Risperidone is known to cause urinary incontinence with greater risk in people with autism and ID that can be eliminated by reducing the dose or withdrawing the drug (18). In clinical care the DISCUS (Dyskinesia Identification System: Condensed User Scale) is a useful rating scale to assess for the presence of motor side effects and TD that are found more significantly in people with ID using psychotropic medication compared with those not using medication (19).

Neuroleptic malignant syndrome

A serious and potentially life-threatening effect of psychotropic medication is Neuroleptic Malignant Syndrome (NMS) (20). ID is a recognized risk factor in developing NMS and is more likely to occur where polypharmacy, using five or more drugs, is practised (21). Clinicians working with people with ID need to be aware of and alert to the signs of NMS that include: raised temperature, fluctuating level of consciousness, aggression, variable blood pressure and heart rate, increased muscle rigidity, along with raised creatine kinase (CK) enzyme levels. The clinical signs could be attributed to other disorders, for example, delirium, infection, and heart failure, or to 'challenging behaviour' by staff not familiar with the signs of NMS. Accurate and timely diagnosis of NMS is vital to ensure appropriate treatment in hospital is instigated to reduce the high risk of death. NMS is associated with FGA but there is a growing evidence of NMS following treatment with second-generation antipsychotics such as quetiapine (22, 23).

Metabolic effects of antipsychotic medication

People with ID are more prone to being overweight and obese compared to the general population especially where the person has a mental disorder (24). There are a variety of reasons for this that includes sedentary lifestyles with few opportunities to exercise, high calorific–low nutrition diets, and using weight-inducing medication. Weight gain can be a manifestation of metabolic syndrome that increases the risk of developing diabetes mellitus, cardiovascular disease, and cancers. It is notable however; that people with severe ID are more likely to be underweight and attention should be paid to their weight status (25).

The metabolic effects of second-generation antipsychotic medication especially risperidone, include weight gain, increased cardiovascular disease risk factors, and osteoporosis related to raised prolactin levels due to dopamine D2 receptor blockade. Elevated prolactin levels over long periods of time affect sexual function manifesting as gynaecomastia or galactorrhea in men and women and amenorrhoea in women. In addition, the potential development of prolactinoma, and insulin resistance predispose people to bone fracture especially in a population that is already vulnerable to bone injury (26).

Efforts to discontinue or reduce antipsychotic medication can lead to beneficial gains in reducing weight and blood pressure (15). In practice, simple measures such as measuring weight and blood pressure and monitoring for side effects in line with practice guidance are feasible (27). Sharing written information presented in easy-read format can help people with ID and their carers to understand the importance of managing weight and its benefits and lead to reductions in body mass index (28).

Assessing for adverse effects of antipsychotic medication

For people with ID, using psychotropic medication can have potentially serious and disabling physical effects that could impair a person's level of functioning and their ability to engage in community activities. For this reason, assessment for the presence of adverse effects is good practice. Clinicians and support staff can use objective rating scales to assess for the presence of motor or metabolic side effects. The GASS (Glasgow Antipsychotic Side Effect Scale) (29) is useful in assessing for metabolic effects while the MEDS (Matson Evaluation of Drug Side effects) and DISCUS are useful for motor effects (30, 31). Incorporating assessment for side effects into clinical practice should help the detection of potentially disabling motor side effects of medication.

Physical environment and ID

Physical exercise is important in maintaining physical health in people with ID but they may not always have the opportunity to avail themselves of exercise activities. People in hospital in-patient services are at risk of developing metabolic syndrome because of the confined environment and legislative restriction on a person's liberty as part of the care plan in managing mental disorder that can limit exercise opportunities. In addition, the sedative effects of medication lead to weight gain and the possibility of poor motivation among staff to help people to exercise (32). It is essential therefore, that support staff are aware of the importance of physical exercise to a person's well-being and its beneficial effects on mental health and thus promote opportunities to exercise during in-patient admissions.

Physical activity can be incorporated into care plans that could make a difference to the person's lifestyle by using the admission as an opportunity for health promotion by introducing new activities and habits to the person. As with all of us, physical activity should be regular, fun, and socially inclusive, often working better if music is incorporated. A full review of a person's physical health while in an in-patient service is good practice to identify physical morbidity and provide an opportunity to treat physical health disorders such as long-term conditions.

Bone health in people with ID is poor especially as they age (33) and they are prone to fractures because of immobility, fewer opportunities to exercise, and low vitamin D levels (34). Prescribers may not be aware of the risk factors for osteoporosis in people with ID (35, 36) but should be informed about the impact of medication and anti-epileptic drugs (AED) in particular on bone health. In-patient admissions are likely to compound the deficiency if the person has limited access to sunlight.

People with autism are prone to sensory sensitivity affecting all the senses because of difficulties in processing sensory information (37). An environment that has hard surfaces predisposing to loud noises, or the presence of others making noise and visually uncomfortable surroundings can all directly affect a person with autism, leading to adverse changes in their behaviour. For these reasons, clinicians should be aware of the potential impact that physical environments can have on the behavioural presentation of a person with autism.

Behavioural phenotypes and physical health

Behavioural phenotypes are descriptions of behaviour associated with specific genotypes 'a characteristic pattern of social, linguistic, cognitive and motor observations consistently associated with a biological or genetic disorder' (38). They are more common among people with ID and include Prader-Willi syndrome, Down syndrome, and Williams syndrome. Behavioural phenotypes can have a constellation of multi-system physical disorders associated with them. For this reason, it is important for the clinician to consult current knowledge and evidence on physical disorders in people with behavioural phenotypes (39). In Prader-Willi syndrome obesity is directly related to the genetic microdeletion and in Smith-Magenis syndrome the pain threshold is higher posing risks to their safety. People with Down syndrome are liable to gain weight and have musculoskeletal difficulties. People with behavioural phenotypes have a greater prevalence of mental disorders and therefore likely to require drug therapy to manage the disorder potentially could affect their physical health. For the clinician, it is important to be aware of the physical characteristics of behavioural phenotypes and the impact that treatment plans could have on the person's physical health whether it is the use of drug therapy or opportunities to exercise.

Prescribing practice in ID

The prevalence of psychotropic use is high in people with ID and often without clear indications for their use where medication is prescribed 'off-licence' to manage behaviour (40, 41). Using antipsychotic medication in people with ID to manage behaviour or mental disorders is a contentious issue as evidenced by the STOMP campaign in England to reduce the prevalence of antipsychotic prescribing among people with ID (42). People with ID may require complex drug regimens to manage physical health problems along with behavioural or mental disorders and as they age, multi-morbidity is more common among older people with ID (43). Therefore people with ID are more exposed to potential side effects because of complex drug regimens. The efficacy of anti-epileptic drugs (AED) can be adversely affected by other medications interacting directly or interfering with their metabolism by the body. Prescribing errors are a risk to people with ID especially among older people using many drugs and those who are more physically and intellectually able (44). To manage drug regimens, it is advisable to use what is necessary and to review regularly the regimens to reduce the risk of adverse effects from combinations of medication (45).

A useful approach to prescribing to people with ID is to 'start low and go slow' (46). Practical guidance is available to support prescribing practice and to gain the person's consent to treatment where possible (47). Where a person does not have mental capacity to consent to treatment, prescribers should adhere to legislation or good practice guidance in effect in their jurisdiction (Box 20.5).

Liaison nursing in intellectual disability services

The role of the liaison nurse in ID Services in the UK is important where they serve as a conduit between healthcare staff in hospital settings and specialist ID services enhancing access to healthcare for people with ID. Such practitioners make a distinct contribution in raising awareness of and educating non-specialist clinicians on the health needs of people with ID that help to reduce the health inequalities that confront people with ID. Liaison nurses have been identified as key enablers in implementing strategies and policies on

Box 20.5 Good practice tips

- Assess for physical disorders
- Consider alternatives to drug therapy
- Assess potential impact of adverse effects before prescribing
- 'Start low and go slow'
- Monitor for adverse effects
- Monitor weight, BP, HR, waist circumference
- Liaise with primary care clinicians

the care of people with ID among staff in general hospitals (48). The liaison nurse in ID is a valuable resource when working with people with ID in health care settings that is appreciated by staff in hospital services (49).

Summary

People with ID have a significantly higher risk of acute and long-term physical and mental health problems that may present in complex ways including behaviours that challenge which makes it difficult for carers and clinicians to recognize. Early recognition and treatment requires a structured approach such as regular health checks, good communication and clinical skills to provide individual and systematic approach to gathering as much history and examination information before investigating and considering treatment options. Internationally, primary care remains the main point of access health care with variable provision to specialist care (50). Thus, consideration should be given to making reasonable adjustments to improve access to mainstream health care for people with intellectual disability. If the treatment is not working it remains vital to re-evaluate quickly and ask others for help in a timely manner in order to ensure distress is alleviated and the illness does not deteriorate. Carers do not usually delay seeking help for people with ID they are concerned about, but health care professionals will often delay investigating until the situation is life threatening (3). If a person with ID presents back to their GP or clinician in primary care after an initial treatment appears not to be working it is important to refer quickly to secondary care for a more detailed assessment. Practices such as 'three strikes and you are in' may lead to considerable delays in diagnosis and worsening of the person's condition. Polypharmacy and use of antipsychotics potentially contribute further to the illness burden of people with ID with FGA causing extrapyramidal side effects and newer antipsychotics increasing the risks of metabolic and cardiac side effects. Regular medication review by their GP and practice pharmacist is needed at least annually and preferably six monthly with reconciliation of medication after hospital discharge to ensure medication adjustments are safely continued in primary care. Including a clear reason for the mediation in the prescription instructions (e.g. two tablets at night for constipation) reduces the risks of medication errors.

Finally, we must all play our part in breaking down the barriers across primary and secondary health care as well as social services. Poor communication, lack of mutual respect, and professional differences between multiple agencies can lead to poor access to health care. Only then will we challenge the status quo that Baroness Hollins has highlighted and ensure both horizontal and vertical access in our health and social care systems and meet some of the unmet needs of this vulnerable group.

Case study 1

Katie is a 56-year-old woman with mild ID living in the community, where she receives 24-hour support. She has diagnoses of bipolar affective disorder with associated challenging behaviours, and memory difficulties.

Her physical health difficulties include type 2 diabetes mellitus, a diencephalic tumour, and mobility difficulties due to bunion formation. The brain tumour was an incidental finding and is kept under review. She is post-menopausal.

Drug therapy includes quetiapine for its antipsychotic properties, and lithium carbonate as a mood stabilizer. She also uses metformin and gliclazide to manage her diabetes.

Her weight is 96kg with an associated body mass index (BMI) of 38.

Clinical issues

- The impact of psychotropic medication on her physical health and quality of life
- The side effects of psychotropic medication
- The use of medication to manage physical health problems
- The psychiatric effects of a brain mass
- Monitoring of physical and mental health

Management

Drug rationalization and optimization was undertaken because of the apparent impact of quetiapine and lithium carbonate on her metabolism and weight. A fine tremor affecting her upper limbs was also evident. The fine tremor could be secondary to the use of lithium carbonate or represent a sign of changes in the brain tumour.

Quetiapine was substituted with aripiprazole, leading to a reduction in weight to 72kg with improved glycaemic control and withdrawal of hypoglycaemic medication.

Lithium carbonate was replaced with semisodium valproate with a reduction in signs of fine tremor. Semisodium valproate led to hypernatraemia that was replaced with lamotrigine for its mood stabilizing properties.

Her mobility improved with the loss of weight. Review by a podiatrist has been essential as part of monitoring Katie's hallux valgus deformity.

Thyroid levels were checked because of the thyroid effects of lithium carbonate, and were within the normal range.

The risk of memory problems and dementia are increased because of both Katie's diabetes and the presence of her brain tumour.

Regular health checks by the primary care physician and review by the psychiatrist are essential in supporting her to manage her long-term conditions.

Case study 2

Gina is a 23-year-old female with severe ID and limited verbal communication, who is cared for by her family. She was first seen by her GP on a home visit, with a two-day history of reduced mobility and apparent right knee discomfort on movement, and was struggling to walk to the bathroom. None of her family carers reported any obvious witnessed fall or injury. On examination she was walking with a slight outwardly rotation to the right side, with full range of movement of her right knee, but appeared to have some distress on movement of the joint.

Her GP referred her for an x-ray of the knee, which showed no evidence of injury. The problem persisted and her mobility reduced further, with associated pain and distress. The GP referred her to hospital services for further investigations which took a significant time to arrange (over a week). Eventually, due to escalation in concerns from the family as Gina became unable to weight bear, the GP arranged admission to the hospital's orthopaedic assessment unit.

After over two weeks in hospital she had multiple blood tests and a further x-ray revealed fracture in the distal head of her right femur. There was evidence on the x-ray of a bone cyst that was preventing the fracture from healing and a full leg cast applied to maintain the leg while the cyst was being investigated. A referral was made to a tertiary centre for an opinion on treatment.

On return from assessment in tertiary centre, Gina was transferred to her local hospital for preparation for discharge.

Clinical issues

- Communication with patient with limited verbal and non-verbal skills
- Assessment of pain and physical examination
- Coordinating health and social care in a community setting

Management

On discharge the family found they were struggling to cope with Gina's physical care. They had attempted to contact social services, as the family carers were unable to provide care due to lack of information from discharge.

The family were struggling to mobilize Gina from her bed to her wheelchair, as well as to the toilet and the sofa, as she was non-weight bearing and had a full cast on her right leg.

After discharge from hospital the Integrated Community Therapy Team visited with the following recommendations:

- Community occupational therapists (OT) assessed for outside ramps
- Leg extender fitting to her wheel chair
- Banana board provided for use from bed to wheelchair
- Social assessment for increase in care package to help with washing and personal care in bed until suitable mechanisms for moving and handing are in place.
- Therapists to assess transfers, particularly if some heights are feasible (wheelchair to sofa for example).
- OT to assess bathing options
- OT to assess feasibility of specialist seating
- Independent social care provider to support Gina and her family to commence supporting with personal care
- Community Learning Disability team for ongoing support and care coordination
- GP to review analgesic control on a regular basis using Disability Distress Assessment Tool (DISDAT)

MULTIPLE CHOICE QUESTIONS

Questions

Please select the single most appropriate answer.

1. Common causes of constipation in adults with intellectual disability include:

A. Hypercalcaemia
B. Hyperthyroidism
C. Magnesium hydroxide
D. Dhenytoin
E. All of the above

2. Tardive dyskinesia

A. Increased risk with age
B. Is less likely with SGA (second generation antipsychotics) than FGA (first generation antipsychotics).
C. Pyridoxine may be beneficial in reducing severity of symptoms
D. Quetiapine and clozapine can be used following appearance of TD
E. All of the above

3. Which of the following are metabolic side effects of SGAs?

A. Menorrhagia
B. Galactorrhoea
C. Osteoporosis
D. Insulin resistance
E. Xanthomas

4. Behaviour associated with behavioural phenotypes include:

A. Prader-Willi syndrome and obesity
B. Smith-Magenis syndrome and higher pain threshold
C. Down syndrome and musculoskeletal disorders
D. Williams syndrome and difficulty in concentration
E. Lesch-Nyhan syndrome and self-injurious behaviour
F. All of the above

5. Cardiovascular disease is NOT a common complication in the following conditions:

A. Down syndrome
B. Fragile-X syndrome
C. Turner syndrome
D. Prader-Willi syndrome
E. Williams syndrome

Answers

1. A. B and C more like to cause diarrhoea and not a common side effect with D.
2. E.
3. A. More likely to cause amenorrhea.
4. F.
5. D. Cardiovascular disease in Prader-Willi syndrome tends to be secondary to obesity.

REFERENCES

1. Emerson E, Baines S, Allerton L, Welch V. *Health inequalities and people with learning disabilities in the UK.* 2011. IHAIIDD Observatory, Public Health England, London.
2. Glover G, Williams R, Heslop P, Oyinlola J, Grey J. Mortality in people with intellectual disabilities in England. *Journal of Intellectual Disability Research.* 2016. doi: 10.1111/jir.12314.
3. Heslop P, Blair PS, Fleming P, Hoghton M, Marriott A, Russ L. The confidential inquiry into premature deaths of people with intellectual disabilities in the UK: A population-based study. *Lancet.* 2013; (published online Dec 11.)http://dx.doi.org/10.1016/S0140-6736(13)62026-7.
4. Public Health England. *Joint Health and Social Care Self-Assessment Framework* 2014. www.improvinghealthandlives.org.uk/publications/1246/Joint_Learning_Disabilities_Health_and_Social_Care_Self-Assessment_Framework_2014 (accessed 1/11/2016).
5. Cooper S-A, McLean G, Guthrie B. et al. Multiple physical and mental health comorbidity in adults with intellectual disabilities: Population-based cross-sectional analysis. BMC Fam Pract. 2015;16:110.
6. McCarron M, Swinburne J, Burke E, McGlinchey E, Carroll R, McCallion P. Patterns of multimorbidity in an older population of persons with an intellectual disability: Results from the intellectual disability supplement to the Irish longitudinal study on aging (IDS-TILDA). *Res Development Disabilit.* 2013;34:521–7. doi: 10.1016/j.ridd.2012.07.029.
7. Collacott, RA, Cooper SA Branford D McGrother C. Epidemiology of self injurious behaviour in adults with learning disabilities. *British Journal of learning Disabilities.* 1998;173;428–432.
8. McGrother CM, Bhaumik S, Thorp CF, Hauck A, Branford D, Watson JM. Epilepsy in adults with intellectual disabilities: Prevalence, associations and service implications. *Seizure,* Volume 15, Issue 6, September 2006, pages 376–386, ISSN 1059-1311, http://dx.doi.org/10.1016/j.seizure.2006.04.002.
9. Mason J and Scior K. 'Diagnostic Overshadowing' amongst clinicians working with people with intellectual disabilities in the UK. *Journal of Applied Research in Intellectual Disabilities.* 2004;17:85–90. doi: 10.1111/j.1360-2322.2004.00184.x.
10. Working Group for Improving the Physical Health of People with SMI Improving the physical health of adults with severe mental illness: essential actions (OP100). Royal College of Psychiatrists, 2016. http://www.rcpsych.ac.uk/files/pdfversion/OP100.pdf
11. Royal College of Physicians. National Early Warning Score (2012). (NEWS)https://www.rcplondon.ac.uk/projects/outputs/national-early-warning-score-news.
12. Meir L, Strand LI and Alice K. A model for pain behavior in individuals with intellectual and developmental disabilities. *Res Dev Disabil.* 2012;33:1984–1989.
13. Buszewicz M, Welch C, Horsfall L, Nazareth I, Osborn D, Hassioti A, Strydom A. Assessment of an incentivised scheme to provide annual health checks in primary care for adults with intellectual disability: Alongitudinal cohort study. *The Lancet Psychiatry.* 2014;1(7):522–530
14. Scheifes A, Walraven S, Stolker JJ, Nijman HL, Egberts TC, Heerdink ER. Adverse events and the relation with quality of life in adults with intellectual disability and challenging behaviour using psychotropic drugs. *Research in Developmental Disabilities.* 2016;49:13–21.
15. de Kuijper G, Mulder H, Evenhuis H, Visser F, Hoekstra PJ. Effects of controlled discontinuation of long-term used antipsychotics on weight and metabolic parameters in individuals with intellectual disability. *Journal of Clinical Psychopharmacology.* 2013; 33(4):520–524.
16. Matson JL, Fodstad JC, Neal D, Dempsey T, Rivet TT. Risk factors for tardive dyskinesia in adults with intellectual disability, comorbid psychopathology, and long-term psychotropic use. *Research in Disabilities.* 2010 Feb 28;31(1):108–116.
17. Lim HK, Pae CU, Lee C, Lee CU. Tardive dystonic symptoms associated with aripiprazole treatment. *Progress in Neuro-Psychopharmacology and Biological Psychiatry.* 2008; 32(2):589–590.
18. Kumazaki H, Watanabe K, Imasaka Y, Iwata K, Tomoda A, Mimura M. Risperidone-associated urinary incontinence in patients with autistic disorder with mental retardation. *Journal of Clinical Psychopharmacology.* 2014; 34(5):624–626.
19. Matson JL, Mayville EA, Bielecki J, Smalls Y, Eckholdt CS. Tardive dyskinesia associated with metoclopramide in persons with developmental disabilities. *Research in Developmental Disabilities.* 2002; 23(3):224–233.
20. American Psychiatric Association. Diagnostic and statistical manual of mental disorders (DSM-5®). *American Psychiatric Pub.* 2013.
21. Shalev A, Hermesh H, Munitz H. Mortality from neuroleptic malignant syndrome. *Journal of Clinical Psychiatry.* 1989.
22. Dan A, Bharadwaj R, Grover S. Neuroleptic malignant syndrome with use of quetiapine in mental retardation. *Psychiatry and Clinical Neurosciences.* 2009; 63(2):255–256.
23. Gortney JS, Fagan A, Kissack JC. Neuroleptic malignant syndrome secondary to quetiapine. *Annals of Pharmacotherapy.* 2009;43(4):785–791.
24. Gazizova D, Puri BK, Singh I, Dhaliwal R. The overweight: Obesity and plasma lipids in adults with intellectual disability and mental illness. *Journal of Intellectual Disability Research.* 2012; 56(9):895–901.
25. Moran R, Drane W, McDermott S, Dasari S, Scurry JB, Platt T. Obesity among people with and without mental retardation across adulthood. *Obesity Research.* 2005;13(2):342–349.
26. Hellings JA, Zarcone JR, Valdovinos MG, Reese RM, Gaughan E, Schroeder SR. Risperidone-induced prolactin elevation in a prospective study of children, adolescents, and adults with mental retardation and pervasive developmental disorders. *Journal of Child and Adoloscent Psychopharmacology.* 2005;15(6):885–892.
27. Teeluckdharry S, Sharma S, O'Rourke E, Tharian P, Gondalekar A, Nainar F, Roy M. Monitoring metabolic side effects of atypical antipsychotics in people with an intellectual disability. *Journal of Intellectual Disabilities.* 2013;17 (3):223–235.
28. Mann J, Zhou H, McDermott S, Poston MB. Healthy behavior change of adults with mental retardation: Attendance in a health promotion program. *American Journal on Mental Retardation.* 2006;111(1):62–73.
29. Waddell L, Taylor M. A new self-rating scale for detecting atypical or second-generation antipsychotic side effects. *Journal of Psychopharmacology.* 2008 1;22(3):238–243.
30. Matson JL, Mayville EA, Bielecki J, Barnes WH, Bamburg JW, Baglio CS. Reliability of the Matson Evaluation of Drug Side Effects scale (MEDS). *Research in Developmental Disabilities.* 1998;19:501–506.
31. Kalachnik J. E, Sprague R L. The Dyskinesia Identification System Condensed User Scale (DISCUS): Reliability, validity, and a total cut-off for mentally ill and mentally retarded populations. *Journal of Clinical Psychology.* 1993;49:177–189.

32. Room B, Timmermans O, Roodbol P. The prevalence and risk factors of the metabolic syndrome in inpatients with intellectual disability. *Journal of Intellectual Disability Research*. 2016; 60(6):594–605.
33. Bastiaanse LP, Mergler S, Evenhuis HM, Echteld MA. Bone quality in older adults with intellectual disabilities. *Research in Disabilities*. 2014; 35(9):1927–1933.
34. Frighi V, Morovat A, Stephenson MT, White SJ, Hammond CV, Goodwin GM. Vitamin D deficiency in patients with intellectual disabilities: Prevalence, risk factors and management strategies. *The British Journal of Psychiatry*. 2014; 205(6):458–464.
35. Burke EA, McCallion P, Carroll R, Walsh JB, McCarron M. An exploration of the bone health of older adults with an intellectual disability in Ireland. *Journal of Intellectual Disability Research*. 2016. doi: 10.1111/jir.12273.
36. Srikanth R, Cassidy G, Joiner C, Teeluckdharry S. Osteoporosis in people with intellectual disabilities: A review and a brief study of risk factors for osteoporosis in a community sample of people with intellectual disabilities. *Journal of Intellectual Disability Research*. 2011;55(1):53–62.
37. Baranek GT, David FJ, Poe MD, Stone WL, Watson LR. Sensory Experiences Questionnaire: Discriminating sensory features in young children with autism, developmental delays, and typical development. *Journal of Child Psychology and Psychiatry*. 2006;47(6):591–601.
38. O'Brien G. Behavioural phenotypes: causes and clinical implications. *Advances in Psychiatric Treatment*. 2006; 12 (5):338–348.
39. Society for the Study of Behavioural Phenotypes http://www.ssbp.org.uk/.
40. Sheehan R, Hassiotis A, Walters K, Osborn D, Strydom A, Horsfall L. Mental illness, challenging behaviour, and psychotropic drug prescribing in people with intellectual disability: UK population based cohort study. *BMJ*. 2015;351:h4326.
41. De Kuijper G, Hoekstra P, Visser F, Scholte FA, Penning C, Evenhuis H. Use of antipsychotic drugs in individuals with intellectual disability (ID) in the Netherlands: Prevalence and reasons for prescription. *Journal of Intellectual Disability Research*. 2010;54(7):659–667.
42. NHS England (2016). Stopping Overmedication in People with Learning Disability (STOMP LD) https://www.england.nhs.uk/2016/06/over-medication-pledge/.
43. Hermans H, Evenhuis HM. Multimorbidity in older adults with intellectual disabilities. *Research in Developmental Disabilities*. 2014;35(4):776–783.
44. Zaal RJ, van der Kaaij AD, Evenhuis HM, van den Bemt PM. Prescription errors in older individuals with an intellectual disability: Prevalence and risk factors in the healthy ageing and Intellectual disability study. *Research in Developmental Disabilities*. 2013;34 (5):1656–1662.
45. Mahan S, Holloway J, Bamburg JW, Hess JA, Fodstad JC, Matson JL. An examination of psychotropic medication side effects: Does taking a greater number of psychotropic medications from different classes affect presentation of side effects in adults with ID? *Research in Developmental Disabilities*. 2010;31(6):1561–1569.
46. Häßler F, Reis O. Pharmacotherapy of disruptive behavior in mentally retarded subjects: A review of the current literature. *Dev Disabil Res Rev*. 2010;16:265–272.
47. Trollor JN, Salomon C, Franklin C. Prescribing psychotropic drugs to adults with an intellectual disability. *Australian Prescriber*. 2016;39(4):126.
48. Tuffrey-Wijne I, Giatras N, Goulding L, Abraham E, Fenwick L Edwards C, Hollins S. Identifying the factors affecting the implementation of strategies to promote a safer environment for patients with learning disabilities in NHS hospitals: A mixed-methods study. *Southampton (UK): NIHR Journals Library*. 2013 (Health Services and Delivery Research, No. 1.13.) Available from: https://www.ncbi.nlm.nih.gov/books/NBK259489/ doi:10.3310/hsdr01130.
49. Brown M, MacArthur J, McKechanie A, Mack S, Hayes M, Fletcher J. Learning disability liaison nursing services in south-east Scotland: A mixed-methods impact and outcome study. *Journal of Intellectual Disability Research*. 2012; 56(12):1161–1174.
50. Bhaumik S, Kiani, R, Michael DM, et al. World Psychiatric Association (WPA) report on mental health issues in people with intellectual disability. *International Journal of Culture and Mental Health*. 2016;9:4:417–444, doi: 10.1080/17542863.2016.1228687.

21

Neurodevelopmental Disorders and Schizophrenia: Recent Developments

Kimberley Kendall, Jeremy Hall, and Sir Michael Owen

Introduction

This chapter focuses on the occurrence of schizophrenia, other psychotic disorders, psychotic symptoms in intellectual disability (ID), and autism spectrum disorder (ASD). We pay particular attention to recent developments in this area including the evidence for co-morbidity, and for shared genetic and environmental risk factors. We suggest that these findings are consistent with a recently proposed model that conceptualizes these disorders as being on a spectrum of neurodevelopmental impairment.

Evidence for increased risk of psychotic disorders in intellectual disability

Both schizophrenia and other psychotic disorders occur at increased rates in ID compared to the general population (1, 2). The degree of comorbidity varies depending on several factors including the type of psychotic disorder being considered, the inclusion of current clinical state (in remission, in episode) and the diagnostic criteria used. A longitudinal study of individuals with ID reported the point prevalence of psychosis, including schizoaffective disorder and in remission schizophrenia, to be 2.6–4.4 per cent. When the disorders examined were restricted to schizophrenia alone, regardless of current clinical state, this rate decreased to 2.4–3.4 per cent (the ranges correspond to the different diagnostic criteria used). The standardized incidence ratio for first episode psychosis, when compared with the general population, was 10.0 (1). A larger study, in which rates of comorbidity were estimated by linking population-based registers, reported a higher rate of schizophrenia diagnosis in ID (4.5–5.2%) (2). Schizophrenia and related psychotic disorders have also been reported to occur in ASD at higher rates (7.8%) than in controls (3) and up to half of cases of childhood onset schizophrenia occur in the context of pervasive developmental disorder (4). Overall, these recent studies add to a substantial body of older evidence for increased rates of schizophrenia and psychosis in ID and ASD (5–7).

Overlap of the symptoms of intellectual disability and schizophrenia

The psychopathology of schizophrenia in ID resembles that observed in schizophrenia in the general population (8)—symptoms may be classified into positive, negative, and cognitive. However, the observed frequency of symptoms in each domain may differ between schizophrenia with and without ID (9). There is conflicting evidence from studies comparing the rates of positive symptoms in these two groups with some reporting higher positive symptom ratings in individuals with ID (10, 11) and others failing to find such an association (9). Negative symptoms have been reported to occur at increased rates in schizophrenia-spectrum psychoses when ID is present (7, 10).

Eliciting positive and negative symptoms in individuals with ID can be challenging. The positive symptoms of schizophrenia are mostly based on language (12) and can therefore be difficult to elicit in individuals with poor verbal skills. Symptoms in these individuals may manifest atypically including being expressed as 'challenging behaviour', and psychosis has been reported to be one of the two psychiatric disorders with which this behaviour is most commonly associated (13). Negative symptoms can be difficult to disentangle from depressive symptoms, which are common in ID and which are also associated with 'challenging behaviour' (10, 14).

There is evidence for qualitative similarities between the cognitive phenotypes of schizophrenia and ID. In the early 1900s, Emil Kraepelin recognized that cognitive impairment was present in a substantial proportion of individuals with schizophrenia ('propfschizophrenie'). Cognitive impairment is now considered to be a core feature of the schizophrenia syndrome, and individuals with schizophrenia as a group have been reported to have mean IQ scores approximately 0.5 standard deviations below that of healthy comparison subjects (15). By definition, individuals with ID have cognitive impairment—an IQ of less than 70 is required for the diagnosis according to the International Classification of Diseases (ICD-10) (16). In both ID and schizophrenia, cognitive deficits are reported to occur across multiple domains although the extent of these deficits is generally less severe in the latter. In schizophrenia, specific cognitive domains tend to be affected more than others and a similar pattern has been observed in ASD. Deficits in attention and/or vigilance, processing speed, and executive function have been reported in both schizophrenia and ASD with studies of social cognition reporting deficits in facial recognition, emotion processing, and theory of mind performance (17–19).

The co-occurrence of schizophrenia and cognitive impairment raises questions about the relationship between the aetiologies of the two phenotypes. Does cognitive impairment mediate the risk for psychosis or do cognitive impairment and psychosis simply index the same risk factors without any mediating relationship? This question has been considered in detail elsewhere (20) and the genetic and other evidence suggests that, by and large, cognitive impairment does not mediate the risk of psychotic disorders. Rather it seems likely that both cognitive impairment and psychosis are part of the range of outcomes that can follow from disturbed brain development.

Neurological dysfunction

Neurodevelopmental disorders all feature increased rates of clinical signs suggestive of a degree of underlying neurological dysfunction. Individuals with schizophrenia, ID, and other neurodevelopmental disorders have increased rates of soft neurological signs—subtle sensory and motor impairments not localized to a particular brain region (7, 21–25). In the same vein, these disorders are also associated with increased rates of epilepsy, although the extent of this increase varies considerably between disorders (26–29). Twenty-two per cent of individuals with ASD and 26 per cent with ID are reported to have epilepsy and higher rates are observed with increasing severity of ID, whereas individuals with schizophrenia have an approximately six-fold increased risk of epilepsy compared to controls (27, 30, 31). Interestingly, individuals with epilepsy experience increased rates of schizophrenia-like psychotic symptoms and these are not always related to seizure activity (26).

Overlaps in clinical features, changes in dominant symptoms according to developmental stage, difficulties eliciting psychopathology and the hierarchical nature of diagnostic classification likely result in an underestimation of the rates of comorbidity between psychotic disorders and ID in everyday practice. Overlapping phenotypes may reflect similar underlying neurological dysfunction resulting, at least in part, from shared aetiological factors.

Neuroimaging

Neuroimaging studies have revealed overlaps between the structural and white matter abnormalities observed in schizophrenia and those observed in idiopathic ID. A study comparing structural MRI scans of individuals with ID, individuals with schizophrenia and individuals with both disorders reported that those with both disorders had brains that resembled individuals with schizophrenia rather than those with ID (32). Specific structural abnormalities reported in schizophrenia include enlargement of the lateral ventricles, agenesis of the corpus callosum, and decreases in volume in one or more parts of the temporal lobe (33, 34). Studies using diffusion tensor imaging (DTI) (which is used to examine white matter tract structure) have reported alterations in diffusion in the frontal, temporal, and parietal lobes in antipsychotic naïve patients with schizophrenia (35, 36). In individuals with chronic schizophrenia, decreased diffusion has been reported in the prefrontal region and temporal lobe along with abnormalities in the tracts connecting these regions (37), findings in keeping with the dysconnectivity hypothesis of schizophrenia.

Due to the heterogeneous nature of ID, it is not possible to list neuroimaging findings applicable to all of the disorders. We will consider the 22q11.2 deletion syndrome as an example of an ID syndrome that is associated with particularly high rates of schizophrenia (see below), the neuroimaging findings of which overlap with those reported in schizophrenia. Structural neuroimaging studies of 22q11.2 deletion syndrome have reported high rates of agenesis of the corpus callosum and other midline defects (38). Greater reductions in white matter compared to grey matter have been reported in association with this copy number variant (CNV) (38). However, in individuals with the 22q11.2 deletion and schizophrenia, the opposite is true (39), in keeping with similar studies of individuals with schizophrenia alone. DTI studies of this syndrome have reported results consistent with white matter microstructure abnormalities in the anterior limb of the internal capsule, fornix, and uncinate fasciculus (40).

Neuroimaging studies in ASD have frequently produced inconsistent results, which often depend on the age of the subjects examined. Reductions have been reported in the volume of the cerebellum and corpus callosum (41) with the latter suggested as representing decreased connectivity between the cerebral hemispheres. Abnormalities have been reported to affect white and grey matter and DTI has suggested decreased organization of tracts in the white matter of many different brain regions (42).

The overlapping neuroimaging findings described are consistent with the possibility of shared pathogenic mechanisms, particularly those impacting on the development of midline structures and connectivity within the brain.

Shared genetic risk

It has been evident for many years that genetic factors play an important role in the aetiology of ID (see Chapters 2 and 3) and also in schizophrenia and other neurodevelopmental disorders (McGuffin, Owen, and Gottesman, 2002). More recently, with the advent of data from genomics and large-scale population-based family studies, it has become apparent that these conditions share genetic risk to a degree that was initially surprising (Owen, 2014; Owen, Sawa, and Mortensen, 2016; O'Donovan and Owen, 2016). For example, family studies have shown that the children of mothers with schizophrenia, bipolar disorder and unipolar major depression are at significantly increased risk of ID reflecting genetic as well as environmental risk factors (43). Relatives of individuals with schizophrenia are at an increased risk of having ID and ADHD (44-46), and the parents of individuals with ASD or ID are at an increased risk of developing schizophrenia (46, 47). Data from genomic studies of these disorders also lend weight to the argument that these are not as aetiologically distinct as was previously assumed—here we will consider evidence for genetic overlap by focusing first on rare genetic variation, and then on common genetic variation.

Rare variation

Rare variation contributing to the risk of neurodevelopmental disorders may be broken down into copy number variants (CNVs), single nucleotide variants (SNVs) and other small variants such as indels (small insertions/deletions). CNVs are the deletion or duplication of at least 1,000 base pairs that result in altered dosage of the affected sequence. The first CNV to be associated with an increased risk of schizophrenia was the 22q11.2 deletion, a deletion on the long arm of chromosome 22 which occurs in one in ~4,000 live births (48). This CNV causes DiGeorge syndrome, also known as velocardiofacial syndrome (VCFS), which is characterized by ID, cardiac anomalies, and immune dysfunction. Approximately 30 per cent of individuals with the disorder develop schizophrenia (49). Since the original discovery of an association between the 22q11.2 deletion and schizophrenia, a further 11 CNV loci have been robustly associated with an increased risk of the disorder (50, 51) (Figure 21.1). All 12 of these loci have also been associated with an increased risk of other neurodevelopmental disorders including ID, ASD, and congenital malformations (50, 52). There are many other CNVs associated with ID syndromes, which have not yet been associated with schizophrenia. It is possible that, once large enough sample sizes are studied, more of these will be identified as also conferring risk to schizophrenia (50, 52).

The schizophrenia CNVs identified so far have variable penetrance—not everyone with these CNVs will go on to develop schizophrenia. In fact, a study of neurodevelopmental CNV penetrance found that each carried a higher risk of ID, ASD or congenital malformations than the risk of schizophrenia (52) (Figure 21.1). It is unclear exactly why two individuals with the same CNVs develop phenotypically different neurodevelopmental disorders. However, there is emerging evidence that an individual's burden of common risk alleles for schizophrenia is one important factor (53). Other possible explanations include the presence of rare modifier alleles, environmental, or stochastic factors.

SNVs are rare mutations at single DNA bases that occur within individuals. Increased rates of loss-of-function (LOF) mutations (those that effectively result in a null allele) have been reported in ID,

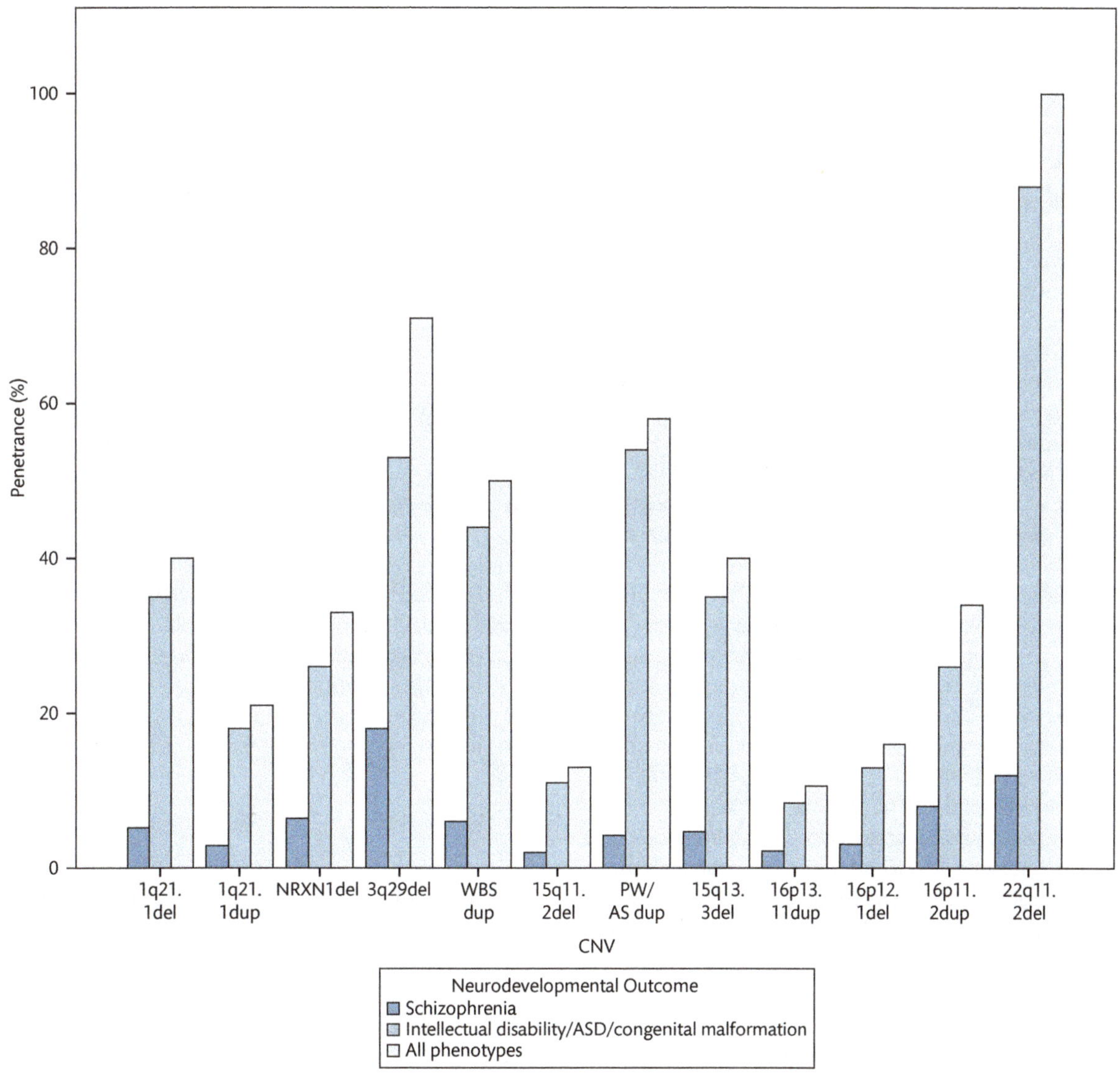

Figure 21.1 Penetrance of schizophrenia-associated CNVs for schizophrenia and intellectual disability (ID)/autism spectrum disorder (ASD)/ congenital malformations (CM).

Source data from: *Biological Psychiatry*, 75, Kirov G, Rees E, Walters JT et al, The penetrance of copy number variations for schizophrenia and developmental delay, pp. 378–385, 2014.

with damaging *de novo* mutations explaining 13–35 per cent cases of severe ID (54, 55), and have also been reported in ASD (56–59). Individuals with schizophrenia, especially those with cognitive impairment, also have an increased rate of LOF mutations, though this enrichment is not as great as that seen in ID or ASD (60). There is also an overlap in the genes affected by rare mutations in schizophrenia, ID, and ASD with genes encoding synaptic proteins particularly implicated (60). Additionally, the genes hit by *de novo* mutations and the mutation sites themselves show the highest degree of evolutionary conservation (a proxy measure of functional importance) in ID, then ASD, with mutations in schizophrenia least conserved (60). In 2016, a large sequencing study implicated rare LOF mutations in the *SETD1A* gene in schizophrenia. *SETD1A* (SET domain containing 1A) produces a protein, which is a component of a histone methyltransferase complex, a structure that catalyses the methylation of lysine residues in histone H3. LOF variants in this gene appear to play not only a role in schizophrenia but also in ID—seven of the 10 individuals with schizophrenia who carried *SETD1A* LOF variants also had learning disability and four carriers were found in a sample of children with severe neurodevelopmental disorders. These variants were rare, occurring in only two individuals out of ~45,000 people without psychiatric disorders, necessitating a large sample to detect the association (61).

Common variation

The common genetic variation contributing to an increased risk of schizophrenia consists of multiple alleles of small effect that work cumulatively to increase risk. The main method by which common variation is currently examined is genome-wide association studies (GWAS)—the genotyping of millions of DNA variants throughout the genome for association with a disorder. The largest GWAS of schizophrenia to date detected 108 independent loci associated with risk of the disorder at genome-wide levels of significance ($p < 5 \times 10^{-8}$). The study reported significant overlaps between these loci and those containing nonsynonymous variants in ID and ASD (62, 63). The heterogeneous nature of disorders that fall into the category of ID means that it would be difficult to carry out a GWAS on ID as one group. However, GWA studies have been carried out to examine intelligence. A large meta-analysis of intelligence GWAS confirmed that intelligence is heritable and that this heritability is, as expected, highly polygenic. Three loci were reported to be associated with intelligence at genome-wide levels of significance and genes at these loci had previously been associated with neuropsychiatric phenotypes (64). Only a small number of specific loci have been reported as significantly associated with the risk of ASD in GWAS (65–68), possibly due to the relatively small sample sizes studies in ASD compared to schizophrenia. However, similarly to schizophrenia, studies of the genetic architecture of ASD suggest that common genetic variation plays a sizeable role in the risk of the disorder (69). Further, the genetic correlation (based on SNPs) between ASD and schizophrenia is substantial (70), suggesting an overlap in the common variation increasing risk of the disorders.

Studies of polygenic risk have begun to illuminate the relationship between the aetiologies of schizophrenia and ID. Polygenic risk scoring (PRS) is a method used to compile disorder-specific risk profiles by adding up an individual's risk alleles weighted according to their effect sizes. PRS studies have identified an overlap between the genetics of schizophrenia and cognition. Schizophrenia PRS have been reported to be associated with lower cognitive function in the general population, and conversely PRS for cognitive function are associated with increased risk of schizophrenia (71–73). Moreover there appears to be a bi-directional relationship between schizophrenia and performance IQ but not verbal IQ and other cognitive measures that map onto the MATRICS test battery (74). In contrast, ASD PRS have been reported to be positively correlated with general cognitive ability but no relationship has been reported with ADHD PRS (75). Studies using similar approaches to PRS have reported high genetic correlations between ASD and schizophrenia (70, 76) and a study of childhood onset schizophrenia reported an association with higher polygenic risk scores for both schizophrenia and autism (77).

Biological pathways implicated by genetics

Having identified genetic risk factors associated with a disorder one can ask whether the genes implicated encode biologically-related sets of proteins (sometimes known as 'pathways'). This can point to specific areas of biology potentially implicated in the pathogenesis of the disorder. Analyses of schizophrenia-associated CNV loci have found an enrichment of genes involved in the post-synaptic density. Genes encoding the NMDA (N-methyl-D-aspartate) receptor complex mostly explained the enrichment and this included synaptic proteins, which interact with the ARC (activity-regulated cytoskeleton associated protein) complex (78). A schizophrenia exome sequencing study reported an excess of *de novo* mutations in components of the very same proteins/protein complexes (60) and an enrichment of rare mutations in voltage-gated calcium ion channels have also been reported in the disorder (79). Several studies have also reported an excess of mutations affecting targets of the FMRP (fragile X mental retardation protein), mutations in which cause fragile X syndrome, the most common inherited cause of ID (60, 79). These findings are consistent across studies. They also converge on biological processes involved in the regulation of synaptic plasticity, the process by which synapses strengthen or weaken in response to use and disuse, a process thought to be involved in learning and memory as well as in brain development (80).

Studies of gene networks have reported substantial overlaps in those implicated in schizophrenia, ID, and ASD, including chromatin remodelling and synaptic transmission (81, 82). Similarly, studies of *de novo* mutations have reported an overlap of underlying genes underlying neurodevelopmental disorders, with the largest overlap occurring between ID and ASD (83, 84). This, however, may be due to the co-occurrence of the two phenotypes (84).

Environmental overlap

All of the neurodevelopmental disorders discussed in this chapter are multifactorial—risk of the disorder is increased by both genetic and environmental risk factors. There is an overlap in the obstetric and other perinatal risk factors for schizophrenia, ID, and ASD, a finding consistent with an early neurodevelopmental origin of pathology (43, 85). A study of the high risk children of mothers with schizophrenia, bipolar disorder, and major depression reported that these risk factors operated independently of genetic risk (43). Maternal or foetal infection with specific viruses, for example, rubella or CMV, is associated with schizophrenia and is postulated as a possible explanation for winter/early spring birth being a risk factor for the disorder. Infection with the same agents is also associated with ID and ASD (86, 87). Abnormal foetal development is associated with both disorders but this may reflect underlying genetic risk factors such as pathogenic CNVs (87). In common with other neurodevelopmental disorders, schizophrenia has been reported to occur at higher rates in males than females (88–90). There is also evidence that low IQ is a risk factor for schizophrenia and psychosis (91).

As these disorder have their onset at very different points in development (ID in early development, schizophrenia in early adulthood), the overlap in environmental risk factors that occur during childhood is less than for those that occur in the perinatal period. Cognitive impairment may be caused by any traumatic injury to the brain but evidence for an association between head injury and schizophrenia is inconsistent (87).

Overall, there is considerable evidence for an overlap in the environmental risk factors for schizophrenia, ID, and ASD further supporting a neurodevelopmental pathology underpinning these disorders.

A spectrum of neurodevelopmental impairment

It is clear from the foregoing that schizophrenia, ASD, and ID share clinical features, co-occur more than would be expected by chance, and share genetic and environmental risk factors. This raises the question of the aetiological and pathogenic relationships between these disorders and whether they are best conceptualized as distinct entities. It has been proposed that it may be better to conceive of schizophrenia and the other functional psychoses as part of the group of neurodevelopmental disorders to which ID and autism belong and that these conditions might be better conceptualized as lying on a spectrum of neurodevelopmental impairment, with the final phenotype being determined by a combination of genetic and environmental risk factors and modulated by modifying and protective factors (92, 93). In this model, the position on the spectrum is determined by the degree of neurodevelopmental disruption, with more extensive impairments associated with more severe phenotypes. What is uncertain is the nature of these modifying and protective factors and exactly how genetic, environmental, modifying, and protective factors act together to determine the final phenotype. Further establishing the nature and operation of the neurodevelopmental spectrum has great potential to direct current diagnostic classification systems towards diagnostic labels based on pathogenesis. In order to fulfil these aims, there should be a greater emphasis on longitudinal studies that include detailed phenotypic analysis and that are not limited to single diagnostic categories, but cover a range of neurodevelopmental outcomes.

Clinical implications

The recent findings reviewed above indicate that there is frequent comorbidity, both at syndromic and symptomatic (e.g. psychosis, cognitive impairment) levels between schizophrenia, ID, and ASD, which is frequently overlooked because of the use of categorical classifications and diagnostic hierarchies. This is of direct relevance to clinical practice and suggests that treatments should be targeted towards the individual symptom profile of the patient and not to the categorical diagnosis. It also supports calls for more dimensional as opposed to categorical approaches to diagnosis (93).

These findings also have implications for service provision. Currently in the UK, patients with neurodevelopmental disorders can be managed by a variety of different services. In psychiatry alone this will include general adult psychiatry, the psychiatry of ID, CAMHS, and forensic services. The close relationship between these neurodevelopmental disorders would suggest the need for closer working between these specialties so that clinical care may be optimized. In particular the chronic nature of these conditions means that patients frequently transition out of child services when discontinuities of care can occur.

Finally, genetic testing for CNVs is becoming a standard diagnostic test for ID and autism, and it is being argued that serious consideration should be given to extending this to schizophrenia (94). Moreover, many of the CNVs that confer risk in ID, developmental delay, and autism are associated with a high risk of psychosis in later life. There is evidence that genetics services are ill prepared for the impact of this on genetic counselling and many families only learn of this risk from the internet (95). It seems likely that as more findings emerge from genomics there will need to be closer working between psychiatry and medical genetics.

Key points

- There is a substantial overlap between the clinical presentations of schizophrenia, ID, and other neurodevelopmental phenotypes and these disorders often co-occur in the same individual.
- There is an overlap in the genetic risk factors that predispose to schizophrenia, ID, and other neurodevelopmental disorders suggesting that at least some of the aetiology of these disorders is shared.
- Schizophrenia, ID, and other neurodevelopmental disorders may be conceptualized as lying on a spectrum of neurodevelopmental impairment. Multiple factors likely work together to determine the final phenotypic outcome.

MULTIPLE CHOICE QUESTIONS

Questions

Please select the single most appropriate answer.

1. The rate of schizophrenia in the ID population is:

A. 10–15 per cent
B. 2.4–5.2 per cent
C. 1–2 per cent
D. 18–20 per cent
E. 40 per cent

2. The main overlap in environmental risk factors for schizophrenia and ID occurs in:

A. Adulthood
B. Childhood
C. Old age

D. The perinatal period
E. Middle age

3. The neuroimaging finding most commonly seen in the 22q11.2 deletion syndrome is:
A. Hypodense lesions
B. Midline defects
C. Space occupying lesions
D. Shrunken ventricles
E. Lateral defects

4. A CNV associated with the risk of schizophrenia and ID is:
A. 3q29 deletion
B. 3p10 duplication
C. 8p25 deletion
D. 12q12 duplication
E. 1q12 deletion

5. Children of mothers with which disorder are at an increased risk of ID?
A. Post traumatic stress disorder
B. Anorexia nervosa
C. Emotionally unstable personality disorder
D. Diabetes mellitus
E. Bipolar affective disorder

Answers

1. B. Studies of schizophrenia in ID have estimated the rate to be between 2.4 per cent and 5.2 per cent (1, 2). See Evidence for Increased Risk of Psychotic Disorders in Intellectual Disability.
2. D. Consistent with an early neurodevelopmental origin of pathology, there is an overlap in the obstetric and other perinatal risk factors for schizophrenia, ID, and ASD and these risk factors appear to operate independently of genetic risk (43, 85). See Environmental Overlap.
3. B. Structural neuroimaging studies of 22q11.2 deletion syndrome have reported high rates of agenesis of the corpus callosum and other midline defects (38). See Neuroimaging.
4. A. The 3q29 deletion is associated with risk of ID and schizophrenia (51, 52). See Shared Genetic Risk—Rare Variation.
5. E. Family studies have shown that the children of mothers with schizophrenia, bipolar disorder, and unipolar major depression are at significantly increased risk of ID reflecting genetic as well as environmental risk factors (43). See Shared Genetic Risk.

REFERENCES

1. Cooper SA, Smiley E, Morrison J, Allan L, Williamson A, Finlayson J, et al. (2007): Psychosis and adults with intellectual disabilities. Prevalence, incidence, and related factors. *Soc Psychiatry Psychiatr Epidemiol.* 42:530–536.
2. Morgan VA, Leonard H, Bourke J, Jablensky A (2008): Intellectual disability co-occurring with schizophrenia and other psychiatric illness: Population-based study. *Br J Psychiatry.* 193:364–372.
3. Stahlberg O, Soderstrom H, Rastam M, Gillberg C (2004): Bipolar disorder, schizophrenia, and other psychotic disorders in adults with childhood onset AD/HD and/or autism spectrum disorders. *J Neural Transm (Vienna).* 111:891–902.
4. Rapoport J, Chavez A, Greenstein D, Addington A, Gogtay N (2009): Autism spectrum disorders and childhood-onset schizophrenia: Clinical and biological contributions to a relation revisited. *J Am Acad Child Adolesc Psychiatry.* 48:10–18.
5. Turner TH (1989): Schizophrenia and mental handicap: An historical review, with implications for further research. *Psychol Med.* 19:301–314.
6. Petty LK, Ornitz EM, Michelman JD, Zimmerman EG (1984): Autistic children who become schizophrenic. *Arch Gen Psychiatry.* 41:129–135.
7. Doody GA, Johnstone EC, Sanderson TL, Owens DG, Muir WJ (1998): 'Pfropfschizophrenie' revisited. Schizophrenia in people with mild learning disability. *Br J Psychiatry.* 173:145–153.
8. Meadows G, Turner T, Campbell L, Lewis SW, Reveley MA, Murray RM (1991): Assessing schizophrenia in adults with mental retardation. A comparative study. *Br J Psychiatry.* 158:103–105.
9. Welch K, Lawrie S, Muir W, Johnstone E (2011): Systematic review of the clinical presentation of schizophrenia in intellectual disability. *Journal of Psychopathology and Behavioral Assessment.* 33:246–253.
10. Bouras N, Martin G, Leese M, Vanstraelen M, Holt G, Thomas C, et al. (2004): Schizophrenia-spectrum psychoses in people with and without intellectual disability. *J Intellect Disabil Res.* 48:548–555.
11. Chaplin R, Barley M, Cooper SJ, Kusel Y, McKendrick J, Stephenson D, et al. (2006): The impact of intellectual functioning on symptoms and service use in schizophrenia. *J Intellect Disabil Res.* 50:288–294.
12. King BH, DeAntonio C, McCracken JT, Forness SR, Ackerland V (1994): Psychiatric consultation in severe and profound mental retardation. *Am J Psychiatry.* 151:1802–1808.
13. Holden B, Gitlesen JP (2003): Prevalence of psychiatric symptoms in adults with mental retardation and challenging behaviour. *Res Dev Disabil.* 24:323–332.
14. Moss S, Emerson E, Kiernan C, Turner S, Hatton C, Alborz A (2000): Psychiatric symptoms in adults with learning disability and challenging behaviour. *Br J Psychiatry.* 177:452–456.
15. Woodberry KA, Giuliano AJ, Seidman LJ (2008): Premorbid IQ in schizophrenia: A meta-analytic review. *Am J Psychiatry.* 165:579–587.
16. WHO (2016): International Classification of Diseases 10th Revision.
17. Millan MJ, Agid Y, Brüne M, Bullmore ET, Carter CS, Clayton NS, et al. (2012): Cognitive dysfunction in psychiatric disorders: characteristics, causes and the quest for improved therapy. *Nat Rev Drug Discov.* 11:141–168.
18. Marwick K, Hall J (2008): Social cognition in schizophrenia: A review of face processing. *Br Med Bull.* 88:43–58.
19. Harms MB, Martin A, Wallace GL (2010): Facial emotion recognition in autism spectrum disorders: A review of behavioral and neuroimaging studies. *Neuropsychol Rev.* 20:290–322.
20. O'Donovan M, Owen M (2016): The implications of the shared genetics of psychiatric disorders. *Nature Medicine.* (In Press).
21. Neelam K, Garg D, Marshall M (2011): A systematic review and meta-analysis of neurological soft signs in relatives of people with schizophrenia. *BMC Psychiatry.* 11:139.
22. Villamonte R, Vehrs PR, Feland JB, Johnson AW, Seeley MK, Eggett D (2010): Reliability of 16 balance tests in individuals with Down syndrome. *Percept Mot Skills.* 111:530–542.

23. Tavano A, Gagliardi C, Martelli S, Borgatti R (2010): Neurological soft signs feature a double dissociation within the language system in Williams syndrome. *Neuropsychologia*. 48:3298–3304.
24. Chan RC, McAlonan GM, Yang B, Lin L, Shum D, Manschreck TC (2010): Prevalence of neurological soft signs and their neuropsychological correlates in typically developing Chinese children and Chinese children with ADHD. *Dev Neuropsychol*. 35:698–711.
25. Jeste SS (2011): The neurology of autism spectrum disorders. *Curr Opin Neurol*. 24:132–139.
26. Cascella NG, Schretlen DJ, Sawa A (2009): Schizophrenia and epilepsy: Is there a shared susceptibility? *Neurosci Res*. 63:227–235.
27. McGrother CW, Bhaumik S, Thorp CF, Hauck A, Branford D, Watson JM (2006): Epilepsy in adults with intellectual disabilities: Prevalence, associations and service implications. *Seizure*. 15:376–386.
28. Canitano R (2007): Epilepsy in autism spectrum disorders. *Eur Child Adolesc Psychiatry*. 16:61–66.
29. Davis SM, Katusic SK, Barbaresi WJ, Killian J, Weaver AL, Ottman R, et al. (2010): Epilepsy in children with attention-deficit/hyperactivity disorder. *Pediatr Neurol*. 42:325–330.
30. Chang YT, Chen PC, Tsai IJ, Sung FC, Chin ZN, Kuo HT, et al. (2011): Bidirectional relation between schizophrenia and epilepsy: A population-based retrospective cohort study. *Epilepsia*. 52:2036–2042.
31. Bolton PF, Carcani-Rathwell I, Hutton J, Goode S, Howlin P, Rutter M (2011): Epilepsy in autism: Features and correlates. *Br J Psychiatry*. 198:289–294.
32. Sanderson TL, Best JJ, Doody GA, Owens DG, Johnstone EC (1999): Neuroanatomy of comorbid schizophrenia and learning disability: A controlled study. *Lancet*. 354:1867–1871.
33. McCarley RW, Wible CG, Frumin M, Hirayasu Y, Levitt JJ, Fischer IA, et al. (1999): MRI anatomy of schizophrenia. *Biol Psychiatry*. 45:1099–1119.
34. Woodruff PW, McManus IC, David AS (1995): Meta-analysis of corpus callosum size in schizophrenia. *J Neurol Neurosurg Psychiatry*. 58:457–461.
35. Peters BD, Schmitz N, Dingemans PM, van Amelsvoort TA, Linszen DH, de Haan L, et al. (2009): Preliminary evidence for reduced frontal white matter integrity in subjects at ultra-high-risk for psychosis. *Schizophr Res*. 111:192–193.
36. Szeszko PR, Ardekani BA, Ashtari M, Kumra S, Robinson DG, Sevy S, et al. (2005): White matter abnormalities in first-episode schizophrenia or schizoaffective disorder: A diffusion tensor imaging study. *Am J Psychiatry*. 162:602–605.
37. Wheeler AL, Voineskos AN (2014): A review of structural neuroimaging in schizophrenia: from connectivity to connectomics. *Front Hum Neurosci*. 8:653.
38. van Amelsvoort T, Daly E, Robertson D, Suckling J, Ng V, Critchley H, et al. (2001): Structural brain abnormalities associated with deletion at chromosome 22q11: Quantitative neuroimaging study of adults with velo-cardio-facial syndrome. *Br J Psychiatry*. 178:412–419.
39. Chow EW, Zipursky RB, Mikulis DJ, Bassett AS (2002): Structural brain abnormalities in patients with schizophrenia and 22q11 deletion syndrome. *Biol Psychiatry*. 51:208–215.
40. Perlstein MD, Chohan MR, Coman IL, Antshel KM, Fremont WP, Gnirke MH, et al. (2014): White matter abnormalities in 22q11.2 deletion syndrome: Preliminary associations with the Nogo-66 receptor gene and symptoms of psychosis. *Schizophr Res*. 152:117–123.
41. Stanfield AC, McIntosh AM, Spencer MD, Philip R, Gaur S, Lawrie SM (2008): Towards a neuroanatomy of autism: A systematic review and meta-analysis of structural magnetic resonance imaging studies. *Eur Psychiatry*. 23:289–299.
42. Anagnostou E, Taylor MJ (2011): Review of neuroimaging in autism spectrum disorders: What have we learned and where we go from here? *Mol Autism*. 2:4.
43. Morgan VA, Croft ML, Valuri GM, Zubrick SR, Bower C, McNeil TF, et al. (2012): Intellectual disability and other neuropsychiatric outcomes in high-risk children of mothers with schizophrenia, bipolar disorder and unipolar major depression. *Br J Psychiatry*. 200:282–289.
44. Keshavan M, Montrose DM, Rajarethinam R, Diwadkar V, Prasad K, Sweeney JA (2008): Psychopathology among offspring of parents with schizophrenia: Relationship to premorbid impairments. *Schizophr Res*. 103:114–120.
45. de la Serna E, Baeza I, Toro J, Andrés S, Puig O, Sánchez-Guistau V, et al. (2010): Relationship between clinical and neuropsychological characteristics in child and adolescent first degree relatives of subjects with schizophrenia. *Schizophr Res*. 116:159–167.
46. Greenwood CM, Husted J, Bomba MD, Hodgkinson KA, Bassett AS (2004): Elevated rates of schizophrenia in a familial sample with mental illness and intellectual disability. *J Intellect Disabil Res*. 48:531–539.
47. Daniels JL, Forssen U, Hultman CM, Cnattingius S, Savitz DA, Feychting M, et al. (2008): Parental psychiatric disorders associated with autism spectrum disorders in the offspring. *Pediatrics*. 121:e1357–1362.
48. Devriendt K, Fryns JP, Mortier G, van Thienen MN, Keymolen K (1998): The annual incidence of DiGeorge/velocardiofacial syndrome. *J Med Genet*. 35:789–790.
49. Murphy KC, Jones LA, Owen MJ (1999): High rates of schizophrenia in adults with velo-cardio-facial syndrome. *Arch Gen Psychiatry*. 56:940–945.
50. Rees E, Kendall K, Pardinas A, Legge S, Pocklington A, Escott-Price A, et al. (2016): Analysis of intellectual disability copy number variants implicates novel schizophrenia risk loci. *JAMA Psychiatry*. 73(9):963–969.
51. Rees E, Walters JT, Georgieva L, Isles AR, Chambert KD, Richards AL, et al. (2014): Analysis of copy number variations at 15 schizophrenia-associated loci. *Br J Psychiatry*. 204:108–114.
52. Kirov G, Rees E, Walters JT, Escott-Price V, Georgieva L, Richards AL, et al. (2014): The penetrance of copy number variations for schizophrenia and developmental delay. *Biol Psychiatry*. 75:378–385.
53. Tansey KE, Rees E, Linden DE, Ripke S, Chambert KD, Moran JL, et al. (2016): Common alleles contribute to schizophrenia in CNV carriers. *Mol Psychiatry*. 21:1085–1089.
54. de Ligt J, Willemsen MH, van Bon BW, Kleefstra T, Yntema HG, Kroes T, et al. (2012): Diagnostic exome sequencing in persons with severe intellectual disability. *N Engl J Med*. 367:1921–1929.
55. Rauch A, Wieczorek D, Graf E, Wieland T, Endele S, Schwarzmayr T, et al. (2012): Range of genetic mutations associated with severe non-syndromic sporadic intellectual disability: An exome sequencing study. *Lancet*. 380:1674–1682.
56. Neale BM, Kou Y, Liu L, Ma'ayan A, Samocha KE, Sabo A, et al. (2012): Patterns and rates of exonic de novo mutations in autism spectrum disorders. *Nature*. 485:242–245.
57. O'Roak BJ, Vives L, Girirajan S, Karakoc E, Krumm N, Coe BP, et al. (2012): Sporadic autism exomes reveal a highly interconnected protein network of de novo mutations. *Nature*. 485:246–250.

58. Sanders SJ, Murtha MT, Gupta AR, Murdoch JD, Raubeson MJ, Willsey AJ, et al. (2012): De novo mutations revealed by whole-exome sequencing are strongly associated with autism. *Nature.* 485:237–241.
59. Iossifov I, Ronemus M, Levy D, Wang Z, Hakker I, Rosenbaum J, et al. (2012): De novo gene disruptions in children on the autistic spectrum. *Neuron.* 74:285–299.
60. Fromer M, Pocklington AJ, Kavanagh DH, Williams HJ, Dwyer S, Gormley P, et al. (2014): De novo mutations in schizophrenia implicate synaptic networks. *Nature.* 506:179–184.
61. Singh T, Kurki MI, Curtis D, Purcell SM, Crooks L, McRae J, et al. (2016): Rare loss-of-function variants in SETD1A are associated with schizophrenia and developmental disorders. *Nat Neurosci.* 19:571–577.
62. Consortium SWGotPG (2014): Biological insights from 108 schizophrenia-associated genetic loci. *Nature.* 511:421–427.
63. Sullivan PF, Daly MJ, O'Donovan M (2012): Genetic architectures of psychiatric disorders: The emerging picture and its implications. *Nat Rev Genet.* 13:537–551.
64. Davies G, Armstrong N, Bis JC, Bressler J, Chouraki V, Giddaluru S, et al. (2015): Genetic contributions to variation in general cognitive function: A meta-analysis of genome-wide association studies in the CHARGE consortium (N=53949). *Mol Psychiatry.* 20:183–192.
65. Consortium C-DGotPG (2013): Identification of risk loci with shared effects on five major psychiatric disorders: A genome-wide analysis. *Lancet.* 381:1371–1379.
66. Wang K, Zhang H, Ma D, Bucan M, Glessner JT, Abrahams BS, et al. (2009): Common genetic variants on 5p14.1 associate with autism spectrum disorders. *Nature.* 459:528–533.
67. Xia K, Guo H, Hu Z, Xun G, Zuo L, Peng Y, et al. (2014): Common genetic variants on 1p13.2 associate with risk of autism. *Mol Psychiatry.* 19:1212–1219.
68. Anney R, Klei L, Pinto D, Almeida J, Bacchelli E, Baird G, et al. (2012): Individual common variants exert weak effects on the risk for autism spectrum disorders. *Hum Mol Genet.* 21:4781–4792.
69. Gaugler T, Klei L, Sanders SJ, Bodea CA, Goldberg AP, Lee AB, et al. (2014): Most genetic risk for autism resides with common variation. *Nat Genet.* 46:881–885.
70. Anttila V, Bulik-Sullivan B, Finucane H, Bras J, Duncan L, Escott-Price V, et al. (2016): Analysis of shared heritability in common disorders of the brain. *Preprint at bioRxiv*.
71. Liebers DT, Pirooznia M, Seiffudin F, Musliner KL, Zandi PP, Goes FS (2016): Polygenic risk of schizophrenia and cognition in a population-based survey of older adults. *Schizophr Bull.* 42:984–991.
72. Lencz T, Knowles E, Davies G, Guha S, Liewald DC, Starr JM, et al. (2014): Molecular genetic evidence for overlap between general cognitive ability and risk for schizophrenia: A report from the Cognitive Genomics consortium (COGENT). *Mol Psychiatry.* 19:168–174.
73. McIntosh AM, Gow A, Luciano M, Davies G, Liewald DC, Harris SE, et al. (2013): Polygenic risk for schizophrenia is associated with cognitive change between childhood and old age. *Biol Psychiatry.* 73:938–943.
74. Hubbard L, Tansey KE, Rai D, Jones P, Ripke S, Chambert KD, et al. (2016): Evidence of common genetic overlap between schizophrenia and cognition. *Schizophr Bull.* 42:832–842.
75. Clarke TK, Lupton MK, Fernandez-Pujals AM, Starr J, Davies G, Cox S, et al. (2016): Common polygenic risk for autism spectrum disorder (ASD) is associated with cognitive ability in the general population. *Mol Psychiatry.* 21:419–425.
76. Lee SH, Ripke S, Neale BM, Faraone SV, Purcell SM, Perlis RH, et al. (2013): Genetic relationship between five psychiatric disorders estimated from genome-wide SNPs. *Nat Genet.* 45:984–994.
77. Ahn K, An SS, Shugart YY, Rapoport JL (2016): Common polygenic variation and risk for childhood-onset schizophrenia. *Mol Psychiatry.* 21:94–96.
78. Kirov G, Pocklington AJ, Holmans P, Ivanov D, Ikeda M, Ruderfer D, et al. (2012): De novo CNV analysis implicates specific abnormalities of postsynaptic signalling complexes in the pathogenesis of schizophrenia. *Mol Psychiatry.* 17:142–153.
79. Purcell SM, Moran JL, Fromer M, Ruderfer D, Solovieff N, Roussos P, et al. (2014): A polygenic burden of rare disruptive mutations in schizophrenia. *Nature.* 506:185–190.
80. Hall J, Trent S, Thomas KL, O'Donovan MC, Owen MJ (2015): Genetic risk for schizophrenia: Convergence on synaptic pathways involved in plasticity. *Biol Psychiatry.* 77:52–58.
81. Hormozdiari F, Penn O, Borenstein E, Eichler EE (2015): The discovery of integrated gene networks for autism and related disorders. *Genome Res.* 25:142–154.
82. Cristino AS, Williams SM, Hawi Z, An JY, Bellgrove MA, Schwartz CE, et al. (2014): Neurodevelopmental and neuropsychiatric disorders represent an interconnected molecular system. *Mol Psychiatry.* 19:294–301.
83. Hoischen A, Krumm N, Eichler EE (2014): Prioritization of neurodevelopmental disease genes by discovery of new mutations. *Nat Neurosci.* 17:764–772.
84. Vissers LE, Gilissen C, Veltman JA (2016): Genetic studies in intellectual disability and related disorders. *Nat Rev Genet.* 17:9–18.
85. Hultman CM, Sparén P, Cnattingius S (2002): Perinatal risk factors for infantile autism. *Epidemiology.* 13:417–423.
86. Dietert RR, Dietert JM, Dewitt JC (2011): Environmental risk factors for autism. *Emerg Health Threats J.* 4:7111.
87. Dean K, Murray RM (2005): Environmental risk factors for psychosis. *Dialogues Clin Neurosci.* 7:69–80.
88. Aleman A, Kahn RS, Selten JP (2003): Sex differences in the risk of schizophrenia: Evidence from meta-analysis. *Arch Gen Psychiatry.* 60:565–571.
89. Mandy W, Chilvers R, Chowdhury U, Salter G, Seigal A, Skuse D (2012): Sex differences in autism spectrum disorder: Evidence from a large sample of children and adolescents. *J Autism Dev Disord.* 42:1304–1313.
90. Szatmari P, Offord DR, Boyle MH (1989): Ontario Child Health Study: Prevalence of attention deficit disorder with hyperactivity. *J Child Psychol Psychiatry.* 30:219–230.
91. Reichenberg A (2005): Cognitive impairment as a risk factor for psychosis. *Dialogues Clin Neurosci.* 7:31–38.
92. Owen MJ, O'Donovan MC, Thapar A, Craddock N (2011): Neurodevelopmental hypothesis of schizophrenia. *Br J Psychiatry.* 198:173–175.
93. Owen MJ (2014): New approaches to psychiatric diagnostic classification. *Neuron.* 84:564–571.
94. Baker K, Costain G, Fung WL, Bassett AS (2014): Chromosomal microarray analysis—a routine clinical genetic test for patients with schizophrenia. *Lancet Psychiatry.* 1:329–331.
95. van den Bree MB, Miller G, Mansell E, Thapar A, Flinter F, Owen MJ (2013): The internet is parents' main source of information about psychiatric manifestations of 22q11.2 deletion syndrome (22q11.2DS). *Eur J Med Genet.* 56:439–441.

22

Epilepsy in People with Intellectual Disability

Rohit Shankar and Matthew Walker

Introduction

Epilepsy is a potentially disabling, chronic and socially isolating condition. A diagnosis of epilepsy even now still carries a stigma. The individual and their family can be affected physically, psychologically and socioeconomically. Similarly, individuals with intellectual disability (ID), in broad terms a condition which occurs during the developmental period and leads to deficits in intelligence, overall development, and adaptive functioning skills or abilities, and their families and carers, experience a range of physical, social, and mental health issues. The co-existence of epilepsy and ID in an individual thus poses unique challenges (1).

Appropriate diagnosis and management of epilepsy are essential to reduce the considerable social impact, potential stigmatization, secondary handicap and low self-esteem compounded by social exclusion experienced by people with ID.

Definitions

Seizures are transient disturbed behaviour, emotional, motor or sensory symptoms or signs with or without an alteration in consciousness due to abnormal excessive or synchronous neuronal activity (2).

Epilepsy is the propensity to have recurrent unprovoked seizures. The International League Against Epilepsy (ILAE) (2, 3) state that epilepsy is a disease of the brain defined by any of the following conditions:

1. At least two unprovoked (or reflex) seizures occurring greater than 24 hours apart
2. One unprovoked (or reflex) seizure and a probability of further seizures similar to the general recurrence risk (at least 60 per cent) after two unprovoked seizures, occurring over the next 10 years
3. Diagnosis of an epilepsy syndrome

Status Epilepticus is defined by the ILAE as a condition resulting either from the failure of the mechanisms responsible for seizure termination or from the initiation of mechanisms, which lead to abnormally, prolonged seizures (after time point t1). It is a condition which can have long-term consequences (after time point t2), including neuronal death, neuronal injury, and alteration of neuronal networks, depending on the type and duration of seizures (4). For convulsive status epilepticus, t1 is about 5 minutes and t2 is of the order of 30 minutes.

Sudden Unexpected Death in Epilepsy (SUDEP): SUDEP is the sudden and unexpected death of a person with epilepsy (PWE) when complete autopsy and toxicology does not identify a cause for death. Based on this definition, SUDEP is a diagnosis of exclusion. *Definite* SUDEP requires an autopsy to confirm no anatomical or toxicological cause. *Probable* SUDEP is applied when autopsy is not performed but the circumstances of death are otherwise very suggestive and *possible* SUDEP is when autopsy is not performed and there is a potential competing cause of death (5).

Classifications

Classification of seizures

Seizures are divided into two main types, and the temrnaology has been recently revised by the International League against Epilepsy:

1. Focal-onset Seizures—The seizures arise from brain networks that are limited to one hemisphere. These seizures are divided into focal seizures with or without loss of awareness (previously termed simple partial or complex partial seizures). They are then subdivided into those with motor (e.g. automatisms, clonic) or nonmotor onset (e.g. sensory, cognitive). Secondary generalization is now referred to as focal to bilateral tonic-clonic.
2. Generalized-onset Seizures—Seizures that rapidly engage bilateral brain networks. Consciousness is impaired from the beginning, for example, absence, myoclonic, tonic-clonic, tonic, and atonic seizures. The latter seizure types are often associated with ID.

Classification of epilepsy

Similar to the classification of seizures, the ILAE has revised the classification of the epilepsies into (3):

1. The types of seizures—focal, generalized or combined focal and generalized.
2. The specific epilepsy syndrome (e.g. West syndrome, Lennox-Gastaut syndrome, Dravet syndrome etc.)
3. The presumed seizure aetiology–
   - structural, genetic, infectious, metabolic, and/or immune or unknown

Epilepsy is often caused by the same brain damage or maldevelopment that caused the ID. It is much more common in some conditions, particularly tuberous sclerosis. In people with Down syndrome, the onset of myoclonic epilepsy may herald the onset of dementia.

Epidemiology

Epilepsy

In the adult general population, epilepsy is the second commonest serious chronic neurological disorder after stroke (1). The National Institute for Health and Care Excellence (NICE) (4) stated that an accurate estimate of incidence and prevalence was difficult because of the problem in identifying and defining people who may have epilepsy. Epilepsy has been estimated to affect around 600,000 people in the UK. In addition, there will be further individuals, estimated to be 5–30 per cent, so approximately 100,000 people, who have been diagnosed with epilepsy, but in whom the diagnosis is incorrect. The incidence of epilepsy in high-income countries is estimated to be 50 per 100,000 per year (7) and the prevalence of active epilepsy in the UK is estimated to be 5–10 cases per 1000. Two-thirds of people with epilepsy can have their seizures completely controlled with anti-epileptic drugs (AEDs). Optimal management improves health outcomes and can also help to minimize other, often detrimental, impacts on social activities, education, and employment. However, a third of people with epilepsy do not achieve complete seizure control despite trying multiple medications.

Epilepsy and intellectual disability

Both epilepsy and ID may be caused by a range of pathological processes (8, 9, 10). Among people known to ID services in the UK, the prevalence of epilepsy is 20–30 per cent and possibly higher in the residual populations of long-stay institutions (11). The prevalence of epilepsy in ID is between 22–26 per cent and increased with increasing level of ID (12, 13). The estimated prevalence for mild ID is around 10 per cent compared to 30 per cent for those with moderate, severe or profound ID (14). Two-thirds of people with ID and epilepsy are considered to show a poor response to anti-epileptic medication (13). People with ID and epilepsy have more physical impairments than those with ID but not epilepsy(12). However, whilst psychiatric or behavioural co-morbidity is common in people with ID, rates were not necessarily higher than in those with ID without epilepsy (12). It is associated with high healthcare costs and increased mortality (12). It was noted that in the UK convulsions and epilepsy were the most frequent cause of what were considered as potentially avoidable hospital admissions in people with ID, accounting for approximately 6,000 admissions a year, equivalent to 40 per cent of all emergency admissions for ACSCs in adults with ID (15). This is representative of the problem worldwide (16).

The co-existence of ID, drug refractory epilepsy, and neurological deficits are often associated with genetic/chromosomal abnormalities or with structural brain pathology (either damage or maldevelopment of the brain) (17). The known single gene mutations associated with ID and epilepsy is expanding; some of these are important for treatment strategies and so should always be considered. For example, SCN1A mutations are associated with Dravet syndrome, characterized by febrile and non-febrile seizures beginning in the first 12 months of life, episodes of status epilepticus, initial normal development, but intellectual decline in the second year of life. This syndrome can respond poorly to drugs that block sodium channels (e.g. lamotrigine, carbamazepine and phenytoin) (18). Tuberous sclerosis may respond well to vigabatrin (19). GLUT1 deficiency, which is associated with seizures in the first four months of life, dystonia (in particular exercise induced dyskinesia), and ID, may respond particularly well to a ketogenic diet (20). Supporting people with ID and epilepsy especially those with poorly controlled epilepsy requires high levels of competence and confidence in staff in community settings (21, 22).

Seizures in people with ID are commonly of multiple types and resistant to drug treatment (23, 24, 25). This is especially true in severe and profound ID. Uncontrolled epilepsy can have serious negative consequences on both quality of life and mortality (26, 27). There is very poor understanding and evidence base supporting suitable prescribing in this vulnerable population (28).

The management of epilepsy is also particularly important because of the risk of SUDEP. The incidence of sudden death appears to be 20 times higher in patients with epilepsy compared to the general population, and SUDEP is the most important directly epilepsy-related cause of death (29). People with drug resistant epilepsy are particularly at risk of SUDEP (29, 30). NICE (6) recommends that patients, carers and families need to be counselled using information tailored to the patient's relative risk of SUDEP. An evidence-based risk factor checklist to engage patients in such a person-centred discussion which includes people with ID has been developed (29). There is evidence that a bespoke service taking into account the current good practice for supporting people with ID and amalgamating it with good practice for managing epilepsy can reduce deaths in ID (31, 32). This is further highlighted by the recent ILAE special report, published in 2016 (33). It is important to mention that ID and epilepsy are also associated with various other syndromes, both epileptic (such as epileptic encephalopathies), whose discussion is beyond the scope of this chapter, and non-epileptic (Table 22.1).

Table 22.1 Common ID syndromes associated with epilepsy

ID Syndrome	Percentage of Patients Diagnosed With Epilepsy
Autism	30%
Autism with severe intellectual disability and cerebral palsy	67%
Degenerative disorders	70%
Rett syndrome	70–90%

Diagnosis

The diagnosis of epilepsy is clinical, and usually established by a specialist medical practitioner with training and expertise in epilepsy. Obtaining a good history of a patient with epilepsy and ID is very important and must cover information about when the epilepsy started and its progress over time(34). Detailed description of the seizures including duration, frequency, daytime/night time, abnormal movements, abnormalities of tone, any warning signs, events, and/or behaviours leading up to the seizure (pre-ictal), after the seizure (postictal), seizure hazards such head injuries, difficulty in breathing etc., triggers for the seizure, and any family history of neurological and psychiatric disorders is needed.

An eyewitness account of the episode is important and collateral information from family and carers is of critical importance. If appropriate, a request to have a video clip of the episode having ensured adequate security and protection is taken, not only to help the patient in the acute state but around the material collected can be a valuable asset for diagnosis. This can be obtained with patient's consent where an individual has the capacity to provide this, or through a formal best interest process using family/carers or an independent mental capacity advocate. It can be difficult to obtain sufficient information about early development in people with ID, especially in people with severe ID.

Allied professional staff in day and residential services commonly attempt to classify seizures rather than describing them. They often use the out-dated terms 'grand mal' and 'petit mal'. 'Petit mal' is technically an earlier name for 'absences' and is all too often misused to cover any seizure or event that is not a typical tonic clonic seizure. Hence it is important that a description is obtained or recorded. When possible a video of the seizure by carers should be obtained as described above.

The clinical decision or diagnosis of an epileptic seizure should be based on the combination of the description of the attack and different symptoms. Diagnosis should not be based on the presence or absence of single features. If a definite diagnosis of epilepsy is not possible or cannot be clearly established, further investigations and/or referral to a tertiary epilepsy specialist should be considered. Follow-up should always be arranged (6). The diagnosis of epilepsy can be life changing, so there is a need for optimal diagnostic accuracy.

Differential diagnosis

Not all that shakes is epilepsy (35). The distinction is usually made on history (36). The differential diagnosis can include, syncope (e.g. vasovagal, orthostatic, cardiac arrhythmia), psychogenic states (e.g. panic attacks, dissociative disorders, affect disorders, psychosis), behavioural disorders (e.g. stereotypies, head banging, head rolling, body rocking obsessions, compulsions, self-injurious behaviour, self-stimulating behaviour), vascular pathology (e.g. migraine, transient ischemic attacks, transient global amnesia), sleep disorders (e.g. enuresis, nightmares, parasomnia, narcolepsy/cataplexy), metabolic (e.g. hypoglycaemia, hypernatremia, insulinoma, hypocalcaemia), migraine, movement disorders (e.g., paroxysmal dyskinesia), and toxic states (e.g. drugs, alcohol). The most common non-epileptic seizure is syncope caused by sudden decrease in perfusion of oxygenated blood throughout the brain(37). Table 22.2 provides the salient differences between seizures and syncope. Psychogenic non-epileptic seizures are discussed later in the chapter.

Investigations

Electroencephalography (EEG) through the use of electrodes placed on the scalp records electrical changes produced by the superficial cerebral cortex. It helps in identifying the location of any epileptic focus. A normal EEG between seizures does not rule out epilepsy. Unless an actual seizure is captured on the recording, an EEG can only support a clinical diagnosis of epilepsy and should not be used in isolation. 'Epileptiform' activity on an EEG does not necessarily mean that the diagnosis is epilepsy; even 0.5 per cent of aircrew have an abnormal EEG (38) and this percentage is much higher in people with ID, psychiatric disease, and/or brain damage, especially when on anti-psychotics. Most people with ID will be able to co-operate with an EEG but would need to have it explained to them

Table 22.2 Differences between seizures and syncope

	Seizures	Vasovagal Syncope
History of seizures	Yes	No
Onset	Sudden	Sudden
Prodromal mood changes	Associated	Unusual, but presyncopal features are common including light-headedness, sweating, clamminess, nausea, and/or blurred vision
Precipitating factors	Rare. Flashing lights (rare, less than 5%)	Unpleasant physical or emotional stimuli (pain, fright etc.)
Incontinence	Associated	Unusual
Pulse rate	Often elevated but may be normal	Slow at onset, later rapid and weak
Respiratory rate	Depends on phase and type of seizure	Normal
Tone	Increased	Floppy
Tongue bitten or scarred	Associated	Unusual
Appearance	Cyanosed or normal	Pale and sweaty
Recovery phase	Post ictal	Rapid recovery on assuming the supine position

in terms they understand, and consented appropriately (including explaining the risks of seizures with activating procedures such as sleep deprivation, photic stimulation, or hyperventilation). Steps to examine mental capacity and consenting are provided in pathway 1 (see box 22.1).

Sleep deprived EEG, repeat EEG, long-term video, or ambulatory EEG increase the EEG yield. Video telemetry, which combines EEG and video recording is invaluable in determining whether an identified behaviour is epileptic or not.

Box 22.1 Pathway 1 Consenting process for investigations for an individual with ID designed using the Mental Capacity Act UK 2005

1. Presume the person to have capacity to make an informed decision.
2. If the individual has ID, be sensitive to the possibility of the person needing more support in receiving and processing the information.
3. Consider utilizing a communication specialist (speech and language therapist) and suitable communication medium, that is, visual, tablet, social story etc.
4. Ensure there are no other deficits such as hearing or visual deficits.
5. Environment needs to be stress free and the patient should be relaxed.
6. If needed arrange for a visit to the centre. People with ID and their carers appreciate having the opportunity to make a reconnaissance pre-visit to the hospital EEG and scan rooms and meet key personnel.
7. Ask for feedback on understanding of key points and feedback on visit.
8. Be flexible to provide reasonable adjustments at the centre, for example, having a double appointment space.
9. Little issues such as parking availability and an identified co-ordinator such as a liaison nurse who knows the setting being there to support the person from start to finish could be invaluable.
10. Be prepared to call off the process if the individual becomes distressed as the trauma can have long-standing influence on the person with ID and negatively affect their future access to health care.
11. If the person lacks capacity to make an informed decision on the investigations then a formal best interest meeting would need to be held.
12. The best interest meeting would need to involve all key stakeholders including family, carers, patient's GP, social worker, and other relevant people such as key workers and hospital staff who conduct the procedure. If there is no family member or friend who can represent the patient an independent mental capacity advocate needs to be sought. Care should be taken that even if the patient lacks capacity their wishes, if any, on the situation can be considered suitably.
13. The best interest meeting needs to consider how relevant and important the investigation is to the individual in the context of the patient's compliance and distress potential to it. If it is felt absolutely necessary but there is a significant likelihood of patient distress the possibility of doing the process under sedation or general anaesthetic (GA) needs exploring. The risk of the GA or sedation should be factored into the relevance of the assessment.
14. An attempt to explain the final decision to the patient needs to be made.
15. Proactive planning for the procedure such as organization of ambulances, minimizing delay, ensuring medication is given etc. must be care planned along with relevant risk assessments and contingency plans.
16. Throughout the pathway it is imperative good records be kept and information communicated clearly between all parties.

Neuroimaging of the brain routinely includes Computed Tomography (CT) Scanning and Magnetic Resonance Imaging (MRI). CT scanning is readily available and can provide information on brain symmetry and on large potentially epileptogenic lesions like infarction or tumours. It is particularly useful where there are calcified abnormalities and skull changes. However, CT is insufficiently sensitive to use as definitive imaging in most people with epilepsy. MRI has essentially replaced CT as the imaging of choice for epilepsy because of its sensitivity and specificity in identifying structural lesions that could be the origin of epileptic discharges. However, MRI is not always widely available, making CT sometimes still the appropriate initial investigation especially during emergencies. With careful preparation many people with ID can have an MRI scan, but some will need heavy sedation or a general anaesthetic and in such instances, the yield of MRI and the clinical impact have to be weighed against the risk of such a procedure. Pathway 1 (Box 22.1) highlights the processes which need to be considered in consenting people with ID.

Electrocardiogram (ECG) is an important investigation to exclude possible heart conditions that could resemble epilepsy or when an individual is reported to have experienced blackouts and falls of unknown cause.

Laboratory studies are useful in excluding metabolic or toxic causes of seizures (e.g. hypernatremia, hypoglycaemia, drugs).

Management

As antiepileptic medication is the most important and relevant method to ensure control of seizures. It is important to get the treatment right in this vulnerable group to prevent avoidable harm. There is very little evidence-based research for AED prescribing in people with ID (28).

People with epilepsy and ID should have the same access to a specialist (epilepsy) service and have a comprehensive care plan agreed (6). As already mentioned, epilepsy is not only more common in people with ID but can also be more difficult to treat, so both the regular treatment and focus on the emergency treatment of acute seizures in this group is important (39). People with ID are at higher risk of being on concomitant medications that lower the seizure threshold, increasing their risk of seizure occurrence (40).

There are multiple outcomes that might be the focus of treatment. The principle aims of management are for the patient to be seizure free and free from any adverse medication effects. However, often this cannot be fully realized, especially given the difficulties in diagnosis and higher potential of treatment resistance. In such a situation it would be good to help the patient make informed choices on what are realistic outcomes. Where the patient is lacking the mental capacity to make or participate in these choices, a best interest meeting (as per the Mental Capacity Act 2005 in the UK) with key stakeholders should be held to provide guidance and goals for seizure management, using similar principles outlined in pathway 1.

The current management can comprise of pharmacological treatment in the form of antiepileptic drugs (AED), vagus nerve stimulation (VNS), and resective surgery. The ketogenic diet has been shown in randomized controlled trials to be effective in children with refractory epilepsy, but this class of evidence is, at present, lacking in adults.

The management approach must be centred on the needs and wishes of the person with epilepsy and take into account their experiences and social context. Education about epilepsy is important for all those with epilepsy, as well as those who support them. Video, pictures and photographs can be used to support education, which should be directed towards families and care staff as well as the person with epilepsy. Language, sequencing and memory difficulties may contribute to poor adherence to a treatment regime, and thus these need to be considered actively when planning a treatment strategy.

It must be kept in mind that a 'one size fits all' approach using 'easy read' or communication via videos etc. has its limitations, and possible use of communication experts such as speech and language therapists can be useful. People with ID and epilepsy have typically experienced very little control of their own lives. Resentment over this may also lead to difficulties, especially with adherence to complex drug treatment.

It is also worth bearing in mind that 'improvement' in seizures does not always translate as an 'improvement' for the individual and their carers. There are not only individual expectations but carer expectations to contend with. A principal example is the emergence of behavioural and cognitive side effects to AED treatment. This is usually reported by family or carers. A Cochrane Review (41) found that the majority of studies in this field typically used no or nonreplicable measures of behavioural exacerbation, were uncontrolled, and were mostly retrospective in nature. A systematic review reported no difference in rates of behavioural problems between individuals with ID who have epilepsy and those who do not (12). Specifically regarding AEDs, research indicates that some AEDs may have both positive and negative behavioural side effects. Research in this area is, however, significantly limited.

When assessing for presence of a potential behavioural side effect, careful consideration needs to be given to the following questions:

1. Is it a side effect that has been described for the drug (Table 22.3)?
2. Would this side effect be expected in someone with the same nature and degree of ID? This information is limited due to lack of evidence at the present time.
3. Could it be that the improvement in seizure control has enabled the person with epilepsy to be better able to express their opinion?
4. Is this a problem that is due to the personality, cognitive deficit, and/or social skills of the individual as opposed to side effects of the medication?
5. Is this the result of drug interactions due to polypharmacy, as occurs in many people with ID? (42).
6. How accurate is the information from carers?
7. Would therapy be useful for behavioural management?

An enquiry into the family or social dynamics of the individual, the nature and type of behaviour and the involvement of behavioural, communication, and occupational therapists would be helpful in developing a coherent formulation. Attempts should be made to retain the medication if it has been efficacious, and withdrawal should only be considered if there is a clear indication of an association of the side effect to behaviour or mental state. Often reduction of dose rather than withdrawal of the medication may be sufficient to address such side effects.

Behaviour and its manifestations have a pervasive impact on people with ID and epilepsy. Both ID and epilepsy vary by nature and severity with little evidence on how they associate. Any person with an ID, epilepsy, and behavioural disorder should be provided with multidisciplinary care (33).

Table 22.3 Behavioural and mental side effects associated with AEDs

Anxiety/nervousness	Psychosis/psychotic symptoms	Aggression/hostility
Clobazam*†	(Carbamazepine)	(Carbamazepine)
Clonazepam	Clobazam*†	Clobazam*†
Eslicarbazepine acetate	Clonazepam	Clonazepam
Gabapentin	Eslicarbaepine acetate	Ethosuximide
Levetiracetam	Etho suximide	**Gabapentin**
Oxcarbazepine	Lacosamide	Lacosamide
Perampanel	Levetiracetam	**Lamotrigine**
Topiramate	Topiramate	**Levetiracetam**
Vigabatrin	Vigabatrin	**Perampanel**
Zonisamide	**Zonisamide**	**Pregabalin**
		Topiramate*
		Valproate
		Vigabatrin
		Zonisamide

*†Especially in paediatric or elderly population. Brackets indicate rare/very rare (<0.1%). Bold indicates common (≥1% to <10%). Remainder are uncommon (≥0.1% to <1%) or rates are not given (clobazam, clonazepam).

Source data from the Summary of Product Characteristics.

Electronic Medicines Compendium (eMC) https://www.medicines.org.uk/emc/ (Accessed 12/06/2018). © Datapharm.

Pharmacological treatment

AEDs are the mainstay treatment for epilepsy. Pathway 2 (Box 22.2) lists the considerations needed to prescribe to people with ID. However, the level of evidence of individual AEDs to specific groups of people with ID is limited (28). Treatment should be individualized, starting with a single AED (monotherapy) wherever possible at a low initial dose with slow titration, unless rapid control of seizures is required (6). Should this be unsuccessful, another AED (monotherapy) should be tried. This is when the primary monotherapy is unsuccessful or the patient develops adverse effects, the second AED is introduced and built up to a therapeutic or tolerable dose before the first AED is slowly withdrawn. Combination therapy should only be considered if monotherapy fails. Though some AEDs work best against particular seizure types, several AEDs may have to be tried (28, 43, 44). There is also a significant lack of evidence of the use of individual AEDs in different subsets of ID.

A popular choice are benzodiazepines (e.g. clonazepam, clobazam, clonazepam, diazepam and midazolam), which are used as both rescue medication and as an effective add-on treatment in refractory epilepsy, especially prevalent in people with an ID (28). Clobazam in particular is recognized as being especially useful as intermittent rescue treatment, given in short courses to break up clusters of seizures or to provide short-term break to help develop more robust treatment strategies. Clobazam is considered appropriate to use regularly as second line or adjunct therapy for all major seizure types, and is of particular value in refractory epilepsy (28). Tolerance is a major issue, particularly in ID populations, although it is speculated that around 30 per cent of PWE on clobazam could continue without encountering long-term tolerance (28). The potential negatives of tolerance include the distress of changing medication and the need to reduce the drug slowly. The other risk is that significant numbers of PWE and ID find themselves on various benzodiazepines to handle behaviour, mood, or anxiety. There needs to be awareness of the overall 'benzodiazepine load' by clinicians who are prescribing and monitoring clobazam for seizures.

Box 22.2 Pathway 2 Considerations to prescribing in people with ID

1. Attempt to ensure good clinical practice for investigation and diagnosis of epilepsy is implemented.
2. Each person with ID is different and it is important to gauge the level of understanding of the individual to make informed choices around benefits and risks of medication.
3. Consider providing more clinic time for appointments for people with ID.
4. Attempt to provide individuals and carers with suitable information at a level they can comprehend—easy read literature etc.
5. If the individual lacks the mental capacity to make informed choices consult with key stakeholders in the patient's best interest and provide relevant information on medication especially impact and side effects.
6. Define seizure improvement to the individual and agree on a method of monitoring and reporting.
7. Look to make medication choices based on evidence base as described in the paper, syndrome diagnosis, comorbidities, and other current medication.
8. Gain feedback appropriately including impact on mood, behavior, and social activity
9. If noted resistance to medication consider alternatives including the possibility of the movements/seizure description being due to other conditions which mimic seizure presentations such as tics, stereotypes in people with ID, and autism.
10. Arrange for structured reviews and feedback.

Benzodiazepine treatments have been criticized for potential adverse side effects, including cognitive impairment in long-term use in both general and ID populations, and as a result are favoured more for use as rescue medication (28). There are no definitive studies or guidelines to manage treatment using this group of drugs.

At present it is advised that people with an ID, especially those susceptible to balance problems, are not prescribed phenytoin. It is also not recommended for long-term use, as it can lead to marked cognitive impairment or symptoms and signs of cerebellar disease (28). Preventing phenytoin intoxication and subsequent phenytoin-induced encephalopathy remains dependent upon very careful monitoring of people and frequent monitoring of drug levels (28). This would prove difficult in people with ID given their distress potential to recurrent venepuncture and difficulties to fully comprehend the need for monitoring. The available literature highlights the complexity of using phenytoin in ID populations and the lack of systematic evaluation.

Gabapentin and lamotrigine are broadly considered safe treatment for epilepsy in people with an ID (28). Lamotrigine has been investigated in various studies in people with ID and found to be broadly of positive benefit. However, the study designs and selection of ID populations prevent robust conclusions of side effect and efficacy profiles. A single study looked at topiramate and found that it is generally well tolerated and did not have a negative impact upon behaviour. This study concluded that topiramate reduced seizure rates in patients with epilepsy and ID without compromising quality of life (28).

Sodium valproate has been widely used as a broad-spectrum treatment option anticonvulsant drug for over 40 years with a good safety profile (28). Some research has demonstrated that due to this it is recommended for use in patients with seizures which are challenging to classify and thus those with treatment-resistant epilepsy with an ID may be more responsive to valproate treatment (28). Limitations for the use of valproate in the general population are that although it is first choice it is teratogenic and often causes significant weight gain. Furthermore, in some people (in particular those with urea cycle deficits or mitochondrial disease), valproate therapy can increase plasma ammonia, sometimes leading to encephalopathy and a paradoxical worsening of seizures.

Studies of tolerability of AEDs such as ethosuximide, carbamazepine, sodium valproate, eslicarbamazepine, lacosamide, retigabine, zonisamide, levetiracetam, and perampanel in ID populations are extremely limited. To date, the tolerability and efficacy of these AEDs has not been evaluated in any suitable fashion amongst ID populations. The UK Ep-ID research Register is a National Institute of Health Research adopted project whose design is of a retrospective cohort real world study looking at outcomes of tolerability and efficacy of various AEDs in people with ID based on their nature and severity of ID (28). A recent enquiry into perampanel by the Register has highlighted that people with moderate to profound ID are less likely to drop out possibly due to their inability to report or communicate subjective side effects and higher rates of seizure improvement due to higher rates of retention and compliance (45).

A problem uncommonly encountered in ID populations is of pregnancy when on AEDs. A recent study identified 217 pregnancies to mothers with recorded ID of 245,007 births 1970–1989 in Oxford (population: 850,000). No major differences were seen in offspring of mothers with ID (28).

No studies have looked at teratogenic effects of AEDs specifically in mothers with ID and epilepsy. It would be expected that the impact of AEDs on pregnancy and their children would be no different in mothers with ID as in the general population. There could, however, be additional confounders such as genetic disorders to which the foetus might be more vulnerable. Given the significantly low numbers expected of mothers with ID on AEDs (statistically less than one/year for one million populations) there would be an expectation that such a pregnancy and post birth would be managed with highest levels of monitoring and surveillance [28].

Patients on AEDs need to be monitored for adverse effects. All AEDs by necessity cross the blood brain barrier. All therefore have the potential to produce adverse effects on alertness, cognition, and mental state. These effects may be particularly pronounced in people with ID (46).

Evidence, such as it is, indicates that lamotrigine should be considered first-line therapy for focal epilepsy and valproate should be considered first-line for generalized epilepsy (47). However, in view of its teratogenic potential, valproate should be avoided in women of child-bearing age, unless the woman is using appropriate contraception. This might be an academic issue in women in the moderate to profound ID range. However, there is now an increase in pregnancies in women with mild ID. For this population the complexity of teratogenic risk may prove beyond their comprehension (48) and these women would benefit from proactive management, including ensuring that valproate is not used.

Blood monitoring does not need to be routinely done unless clinically indicated (e.g. breakthrough seizures or unexpected occurrence of side effect) or to manage phenytoin doses; nevertheless, baseline blood levels for some drugs are helpful when people are on stable doses. AEDs should be introduced and withdrawn slowly with the aim of achieving the lowest effective dose. It is dangerous to stop AEDs suddenly, because this may precipitate status epilepticus even when the AED has not apparently been effective.

People with ID and their carers may not understand the importance of adhering to a treatment regime. A simple regime, the use of pictures, and close liaison with the pharmacist all help. The use of pictures to communicate with people with ID can help (49). Healthcare professionals have a role in educating patients, carers, and family members in understanding epilepsy, the rationale for treatment, reducing the stigma attached, and developing positive relationships (6).

If a patient is seizure free for a period of two years whilst on AED then withdrawal of AED can be considered. This should however be discussed with patient, their carers, and/or family where possible, and actions done with the best interest of the patient in mind. Withdrawal of the AED should be monitored and under the guidance of a specialist (6). Withdrawal of AEDs, even when optimally undertaken, can be associated with re-emergence of seizures. In people with ID a decision to withdraw AEDs need to be taken alongside consideration of the likelihood of the benefits the medication is offering versus the fact that people with ID can be more likely to be treatment resistant, thus possibly being at higher risk of a relapse.

Status epilepticus

Individuals with ID are more likely to develop status epilepticus (50). The mortality risk is also increased for this patient group. The treatment of status epilepticus is considered a medical emergency. Treatment should be given if the individual has a prolonged (convulsive) seizure that lasts for five minutes or more or if seizure occurs three or more times in an hour (6). Treatment options available in the community include buccal midazolam (first-line treatment) and rectal diazepam (if midazolam is not suitable). The administration of rectal diazepam in the community raises dignity issues. Other medications can be prescribed within the hospital setting. Depending on the individual's personalized care plan and their response to their rescue treatment an ambulance needs to be called if seizure carries on after the administration of treatment and/or if there are concerns about their breathing, airway, or other vital signs.

Carers and family need to be appropriately trained in the administration of these rescue medications. Standards of training however vary across the UK, with potential consequences that could be serious for the individual patient given the risk of brain damage and mortality (51). Shortly there is to be released new national guidance on training and good practice of administering midazolam as an update from the previous Joint Epilepsy Committee guidance (52). There is a development to also have a standardised e-test to ensure safe and consistent practice.

Vagus nerve stimulation (VNS)

Although AEDs remain the main treatment for intractable epilepsy, a significant proportion of people with ID will respond poorly to AEDs, with up to 40 per cent on polytherapy but poor seizure control (46, 53), which means that alternatives need to be considered. VNS is indicated for use as an adjunctive therapy in reducing the frequency of seizures in adults who are refractory to AED and are not suitable for resective surgery. There is some evidence that VNS can be effective in multiple seizure types, including drop attacks, which carry a high morbidity (54). VNS is a relatively safer surgical option for patients with ID (55). One should be mindful of short- and long-term side effects, including rare presentations such as an impact on heart conduction (56). Where there are communication and capacity issues, in-depth consenting processes need to be addressed prior to surgery.

Resective surgery

Epilepsy in people with ID can be refractory to AEDs and so can be potentially suitable for resective surgery. The main role of epilepsy surgery is to achieve seizure freedom or a significant reduction in seizure frequency, without producing adverse cognitive or psychological effects (57). ID is not a contraindication to surgery (33), and surgery can be considered even when multiple lesions are present, as in tuberous sclerosis. The risks to the patient of on-going refractory epilepsy and the impact that it could have on quality of life should be considered when contemplating the possibility of epilepsy surgery. Issues such as mental capacity and ability to make informed choices on the advantages, and disadvantages of surgery can sometimes be challenging.

Psychological impact

Cognitive activity is affected by the underlying brain pathology, by the effects of repeated interruptions in consciousness, and by AEDs. All tend to reduce cognitive function. This may lead to sedation and poor motivation, or it may be expressed as irritability, impulsiveness, and disinhibition (58).

Repeated disruption of consciousness interrupts memory and learning. This is a particular problem in 'absence' seizures, where the seizures are brief and may be unrecognized, but are often frequent, especially in children. A person with undiagnosed nonconvulsive status epilepticus may resemble someone with severe ID or autism, and can sometime explain deterioration in cognition or behaviour. An EEG is necessary for diagnosis of this under-diagnosed condition. When their epilepsy is treated, their whole demeanour may change dramatically.

Epilepsy can have a negative effect on self-esteem. It is a hidden disability, but one that can be internally stigmatizing (59).

Many AEDs, particularly but not exclusively, vigabatrin, can produce behaviour problems and even psychosis. As previously mentioned, valproate can be associated with a metabolic encephalopathy, presenting as worsening of seizures or deterioration in mental capacity.

Psychological disturbance may occur before, during, or after a seizure. People with focal seizures commonly experience a warning or aura, which may take the form of a particular emotional state or a hallucinatory experience. Some seizures, particularly focal seizures affecting the temporal or frontal lobes result in the person behaving in a bizarre and stereotyped way without full awareness, though they may exhibit apparent conscious behaviour. After a seizure many people sleep, some have headaches, and many are irritable or confused (60). Post-ictal psychosis can also rarely occur, usually after a lucid interval of hours to days, and lasts from days to weeks. This is usually associated with disordered thought, paranoia, and aggressive behaviour.

An EEG should be considered when there is any enduring change in mental capacity, state, or behaviour or unexplained deterioration to exclude non-convulsive status epilepticus.

Detailed discussion on behavioural issues, ID, and epilepsy has been presented earlier in the chapter.

Social impact

Watching a person have a convulsive seizure can be frightening. People unfamiliar with epilepsy can think the person is dying. For some relatives/carers, and some people with epilepsy, this fear persists. There are also real risks of serious injury, for example by drowning during a bath or falling downstairs or in front of traffic. Services are afraid of litigation. It is not surprising that people with epilepsy and ID are sometimes offered more protection than they need. Risk management is an important aspect of epilepsy but could come at the cost of access to community or impact on quality of life (for example stopping swimming or hydrotherapy). One needs to be mindful, especially if the concerned individual has limited ability to make informed choices, that the risk management needs to be tempered by pragmatism, and the least restrictive frameworks of care balanced against possible risk needs to be established.

People with epilepsy are usually allowed to drive if they have been free of seizures for a year as per UK law (61). However, it is important that if this is an issue the latest advice is taken from the GP and/or the DVLA. Most people with ID do not drive. However transport can still be a problem, especially if the individual is on a rescue medication protocol. Practical issues such as lack of an escort or frequent public transport can impact heavily on the individual's quality of life. Seizures further limit access to employment, leisure, and sporting activities (62). They therefore contribute to poverty and social isolation. This in turn contributes to a sense of powerlessness and low self-esteem.

In some cultures, epileptic seizures are seen as evidence of demonic possession or of infection. This can mean that people are reluctant to touch or share cutlery with anyone who has seizures. People with ID from such cultures can be highly vulnerable to prejudice and discrimination.

Rescue medication administration, such as buccal midazolam or rectal diazepam can pose particular difficulties. It is useful in the prevention of status epilepticus in vulnerable individuals and can be given by specially trained, but otherwise unqualified people. It can enable people with ID to avoid frequent in-patient admissions. However staff may be reluctant to use it. They may fear injuring the person or that there could be accusations of sexual abuse especially with rectal diazepam use.

An individually based person-centred assessment at regular intervals of the real risks of particular activities and treatments will often allow the person to lead a much fuller life. Such a plan needs to consider suitability of the residential placement and access to activities and services suitable to the individual's needs and recreation. An epilepsy care plan, centred on the person with epilepsy and involving everyone with a responsibility to care for them, is helpful. Such a plan should form part of the Health Action Plan recommended by the UK White paper, Valuing People Now (2009) (63).

Risk management

This will usually involves assessing the patient's level of risk and depends on the individual, their environment, frequency, and severity of epilepsy (64). Professionals need to be aware of the higher risk held by individuals with ID and epilepsy and that these be discussed with the individual, their families, and/or carers (6). It is also recommended that a risk assessment takes place and includes bathing and showering, preparing food, using electrical equipment, managing prolonged or serial seizures, the impact of epilepsy in social settings, SUDEP, and the suitability of independent living (6, 65, 66).

The SUDEP and seizure safety checklist is a 10 minute evidenced-based risk communication tool which is available free to download and use (29, 31, 32, 67).

Various national and international charities issue excellent leaflets on various activities and epilepsy, for example, sport, leisure, employment, and computers. The emphasis should be on having strategies in place to prevent injury from occurring if the person has a seizure, rather than restricting their activities (65, 66).

Psychogenic non-epileptic seizures (PNES)

The misdiagnosis rate of epilepsy is considered to be around 25–30 per cent. It is considered that around 90 per cent of the misdiagnosis is PNES when seizure presentation is co-related with EEGs (68). To diagnose PNES can be difficult, as it usually involves overturning an existing diagnosis. It is made more problematic as there are no diagnostic tests or cluster of symptoms that are completely reliable. It is a diagnosis of exclusion.

The patient's history may suggest the diagnosis. Certain clinical features and presenting symptoms should raise the suspicion that seizures may be psychogenic rather than epileptic (Table 22.4).

Resistance to antiepileptic drugs (AEDs) is usually the first clue, though epilepsy in people with ID can be difficult to treat. Approximately 80 per cent people with PNES have been treated with AEDs before the correct diagnosis is made. A psychogenic aetiology should be considered when AEDs have no effect on the reported frequency of seizures.

Specific psycho-social triggers such as stress, fibromyalgia, chronic pain, chronic fatigue, somatization, and environmental situations need to be considered. PNES rarely occurs in sleep and is more frequent in the presence of other people (audience). A psycho-social history with evidence of maladaptive behaviours or associated psychiatric diagnoses should raise the suspicion of PNES. A mental status exam, highlighting soft signs such as the presenting general demeanour of the person and their carers, appropriateness of the level of concerns, over dramatization, hysterical features and in particular looking to 'scapegoat' seizures as explanation for relationship dysfunction is helpful. In people with ID, especially those with mild ID, where there could be a degree of suggestibility, it is important to assess if their 'seizures' are facilitating a 'sickness role' which stands to the benefit of the individual and/or carer.

It is not uncommon for a detailed seizure history to reveal characteristics not consistent with epileptic seizures. An episode captured on EEG would provide significant insight to the diagnosis however this could be difficult to achieve, especially in people with ID. A resistance to gainfully make inroads towards validating the diagnosis such as refusing to bring a video sample or an alternative carer are also soft signs suggestive of PNES.

It is expected that the episodes would have been investigated as seizures.

The following categories are suggested for a diagnosis of PNES (69):

- Documented PNES—confirmed by clinical history plus EEG video monitoring
- Clinically established PNES—defined by clinical history, clinician witness, and EEG recording of habitual events without video
- Probable PNES—determined by clinical history, clinician witness of video or live events, and a normal EEG
- Possible PNES—relies on patient's self-report of clinical events and a normal EEG

The main obstacle to effective treatment is effective delivery of the diagnosis. Delivering the diagnosis of PNES, especially to a person who has received a diagnosis of an organic illness such as epilepsy

Table 22.4 Psychogenic non-epileptic seizures

	Seizure	Non Epileptic Attack
Precipitating cause	Rare	Common: stress and emotion
Location	Can happen in sleep and when alone	Occur in wakefulness, but can happen from sleep. Often occurs in company
Onset	Usually short	Variable
Aura	Usually stereotyped—various	Fear, panic, altered mental state, and dissociation
Duration	Few minutes	Variable
Consciousness	Complete loss in generalized tonic clonic seizures; may be incomplete in complex partial seizures	Is variable and often inconsistent with the considered seizure type
Movement	Consistent with seizure type, synchronous, small amplitude jerks	Asynchronous, opisthotonous, flailing of limbs, pelvic thrusting
Speech	Grunt at onset; word automatisms, cry	Unintelligible, semi-voluntary
Response to stimulation	None in generalized tonic-clonic; may respond in complex partial and postictal	Often reacts and this may terminate episode
Incontinence	Common	Sometimes
Injury	Tongue bite (usually side), fall, directed violence rare	Tongue biting is usually tip and rarely draws blood Carpet burns are not uncommon Directed violence not uncommon
Recovery	Dependent of seizure type—few minutes with or without confusion Possible tiredness and need to sleep	May be rapid or very prolonged. Tearfulness often occurs

Reproduced from National Guideline Centre (2012) Epilepsies: diagnosis and management, Clinical guideline 137.

could be challenging. The patient reaction could be adversarial in the form of disbelief, denial, anger, and hostility. Patients who accept their diagnosis and follow through with therapy are more likely to experience a successful outcome; therefore, patient education is crucial. It is important that the patient recognize that the diagnosis is incidental and change in symptom profile would require alternative strategies. In people with ID a communication specialist might be of benefit, to help provide the information in a manner the patient can comprehend.

Treatment of PNES varies and can include psychotherapy and use of adjunctive medications to treat coexisting anxiety or depression. Evidence exists that indicates that Cognitive Behaviour Therapy (CBT) significantly reduces psychogenic seizure frequency compared to standard medical care (70). This was further reinforced in a study that showed CBT and sertraline (an antidepressant) together provided better outcomes for seizure control than the sertraline only group (71). However a recent Cochrane review concluded that there is little reliable evidence to support the use of any treatment, including CBT, in the treatment of non-epileptic seizures (72).

The counter issue of misdiagnosis of epilepsy by not diagnosing epilepsy needs to be considered. A systematic review showed that between 32–38 per cent of people with ID were diagnosed as not having epilepsy or as having nonepileptic events (73). The main reason for misdiagnosis was the misinterpretation of behavioural, physiological, syndrome-related, medication-related, or psychological events by parents, paid carers, and health professionals. The review indicates high levels of non-epileptic events which have the potential to be misdiagnosed as epileptic events in people with and without ID. The occurrence of seizures may be both over-estimated and under-recognized. People may experience a combination of epileptic and non-epileptic events, and in some cases it may not be possible to reach a diagnosis. The knowledge of family members, support workers and a range of health staff also affects whether events are correctly diagnosed as epileptic or not. These issues are not unique to people with ID. However, the findings do suggest that people with ID are likely to face additional barriers to receiving an accurate diagnosis. The review establishes that cognitive issues, behavioural problems, communication difficulties, motor problems, and side effects of medication experienced by people with ID may be misinterpreted as epileptic events.

Seizures, intellectual disability and challenging behaviour

Epilepsy and behavioural disturbances are closely associated and have multiple possible associations. This is a complex area which has been poorly researched.

1. Seizures can cause behavioural disturbance as part of the seizure phenomenology.
2. Seizures can lead to brain damage which can result in personality change and maladaptive behaviours.
3. Seizures can co-exist with mental illness which can then have a symbiotic effect of influencing behaviour.
4. Medication especially first generation and third generation AEDs can have a negative impact on behaviour.
5. Successful treatment of seizures can still leave a damaged or under-developed personality which would lack social skills to cope and live in their environment. This can result as challenging behaviour.

It is important that any challenging behaviour assessment be person centred and include the diagnosis and impact of seizures in the formulation. It is important to separate primary associations such as direct organicity and medication impact on behaviour from secondary links where the behaviour is a function of frustration, communication, poor coping mechanisms, or habituation to get specific responses. The cause and effect needs to be understood. It is critical that the overall best interest of the individual be considered and not have a piecemeal approach of treating only the epilepsy or the behaviours separately. Management strategies should be on the lines identified in recent good practice documents(74).

Conclusion

Managing epilepsy in people with ID is not only challenging but requires a diverse skill set. Complexities encountered in the routine management of epilepsy in the general population such as compliance, alcohol, and recreational drug issues, driving concerns, and pregnancy are more limited in the ID population. However, there is higher representation of communication deficits, lack of informed decision-making, physical and mental health comorbidity, side-effect sensitivity and higher levels of total drug prescribing, which bring their own challenges. Lately there has been the development of good practice guidance reports from the Royal College of Psychiatrists UK on the delivery of epilepsy care (75) for this vulnerable population and on prescribing (74). Further, in the field of epilepsy there is a rapid growth of technology (76), understanding of influence of genetics and improved characteristics of seizures and risk (77, 78, 79). It is hoped that such documents and the attention they bring will help stimulate more research to improve understanding of this complex area as research in ID and epilepsy still remains significantly lower than other clinical areas (80).

Case study 1

Mary, a 46-year-old who has moderate ID with seizures in remission for over five years and on sodium valproate 2000mgs/day and haloperidol presented with five month history of lassitude, tiredness, falls, and minor confusion having had three episodes of respiratory infections requiring antibiotic care. There was a recurrence of seizures with the infection which was perceived by the general practitioner to be secondary to the high temperature occurring with the infection. Initially there was consideration of her going through menopause. On being reviewed, full blood count among other bloods was requested. It revealed thrombocytopenia. Sodium valproate was then gradually reduced to 1500mg/day and a re-test of full blood count in three months' time showed full recovery. Along with it her problems of tiredness, infections, seizures, and falls stopped

Case study 2

Jason is 20 and has mild ID, transient mood disorder, and Down syndrome. He was diagnosed with epilepsy and started on levetiracetam without full consideration of his psychological issues at his local hospital. The levetiracetam with each increase in dose as advised by the BNF improved his seizures but worsened his mood and behaviours. He became aggressive and violent and was commenced on risperidone by his GP which had an impact of improving his behaviours but again causing a worsening of his seizures. Eventually when referred to a specialist in ID and epilepsy, sodium valproate was commenced and titrated and on stabilization both the risperidone and levetiracetam withdrawn gradually one by one.

Case study 3

Rachel has a Rett's syndrome and severe to profound ID. She presented with brief apnoea attacks with no associated symptomology to aid diagnosis of whether these attacks were of seizure origin. She would not co-operate to have an ambulatory EEG. As there is seizure association of >90 per cent with Rett's a trail of AED was attempted. Rachel's apnoea attacks receded with each dose increase and went to complete cessation.

MULTIPLE CHOICE QUESTIONS

Questions

Please select the single most appropriate answer.

1. The prevalence of epilepsy in people with ID is approximately

A. 10 per cent
B. 20 per cent
C. 30 per cent
D. 40 per cent

2. Which of these statements about SUDEP is false?

A. SUDEP is more common in general population than people with ID
B. SUDEP is linked to having frequent generalized seizures
C. Duration of poorly treated epilepsy is associated with increased SUDEP risk
D. QTc prolongation and other cardiac irregularities are associated with higher risk of SUDEP

3. Which one of these statements on investigations is true?

A. EEGs are essential in people with ID as they can definitely confirm presence of seizures
B. It is important to investigate irrespective of the distress caused to the patient
C. A 'best interest' process to investigations is essential for an individual with ID who cannot consent and could get distressed by attempts to do so
D. It is not important to consider a head MRI in a new patient presenting with episodes suggestive of seizures

4. Which of these should be avoided in managing epilepsy in people with ID?

A. Slow titration of AED possibly at half or quarter of the suggested rates for general population
B. If reported behavioural side effects immediately stop the AED
B. While swapping ideally build up an alternate AED then withdraw the other
D. The risks of having more than two regular AEDs could significantly outweigh the benefits of their positive effects

5. Which of these combinations is considered to be a beneficial one?

A. Phenytoin—Carbamazepine
B. Carbamazepine—Lamotrigine
C. Clobazam—Zonisamide
D. Lamotrigine –Sodium valproate

Answers

1. B. Robertson et al (https://www.ncbi.nlm.nih.gov/pubmed/26076844) in their systematic review identified the pooled estimate for epilepsy in people with ID from 38 studies was 22.2 per cent (95% CI 19.6-25.1). A population-based study by McGrother et al. (https://www.ncbi.nlm.nih.gov/pubmed/16782360) highlighted prevalence of epilepsy in people with ID to be 26 per cent
2. A. In the overall epilepsy population, mortality rates are approximately 2.5-fold higher than in the general population Cockerell et al. (https://www.ncbi.nlm.nih.gov/pubmed/7934347), and Hauser et al. (https://www.ncbi.nlm.nih.gov/pubmed/7398606). A US population-based study by Ficker et al. (https://www.ncbi.nlm.nih.gov/pubmed/9818844) showed SUDEP rates in the epilepsy population exceeded the expected rate of sudden death in the general population by 24 times. Sillanpaa et al. https://www.nejm.org/doi/full/10.1056/NEJMoa0911610) in their cohort study of following 245 children with epilepsy for 40 years reported 24 per cent mortality of which 30 per cent were classified as SUDEP.
3. C. While all reasonable attempts need to be taken to encourage the individual to participate in investigations to help identify and assess for seizures consideration needs to be given to the potential for distress and the benefits one gains from an investigation by subjecting a non-capacitous individual through the process. If the person requires to be sedated for a brief EEG then the risks of the sedation, the impact of the sedation on the EEG activity, and the potential lack of any obvious seizure activity at the time of investigation and overall utility should be weighed in balance to the potential iatrogenic trauma to the individual.
4. B. Abrupt withdrawal of AED can lead to significant increased risk of SUDEP and higher recurrence rates of seizures.
5. D. There is a significant synergistic drug interaction with valproate (valproate is an enzyme inhibitor, lamotrigine clearance is reduced, and thus lamotrigine levels are higher. There is evidence to suggest valproate and lamotrigine combine positively and synergistically offering improved results in

refractory epilepsy; Brodie et al. https://www.ncbi.nlm.nih.gov/pubmed/9127723) and Pisani et al. https://www.ncbi.nlm.nih.gov/pubmed/10448829).

REFERENCES

1. Prasher VP, Kerr MP. *Epilepsy and Intellectual Disabilities.* 2008 Springer.
2. Fisher SF, Acevedo C, Arzimanoglou A et al A practical clinical definition of epilepsy. *Epilepsia.* 2014;55(4):475–482.
3. Scheffer IE, Berkovic S, Capovilla G et al. ILAE classification of the epilepsies: Position paper of the ILAE Commission for Classification and Terminology. *Epilepsia.* 2017;58(4):512–521.
4. Trinka E, Hesdorffer D, Rossetti AO et al. Definition and classification of status epilepticus—report of the task force on classification of status epilepticus. *Epilepsia.* 2015;56(10):1515–1523.
5. Nashef L, So E, Ryvlin P et al. Unifying the definitions of sudden unexpected death in epilepsy. *Epilepsia.* 2012;53(2):227–233.
6. The National Institute for Health and Care Excellence (NICE). The epilepsies: The diagnosis and management of the epilepsies in adults and children in primary and secondary care. 2012 NICE clinical guideline 137 guidance.nice.org.uk/cg137.
7. Sander JW, Shorvon SD. Epidemiology of the epilepsies. *J Neurol Neurosurg Psychiatry.* 1996;61:433–443.
8. Forsgren L, Edvinsson S-O, Blomquist HK et al. Epilepsy in a population of mentally retarded children and adults. *Epilepsy Res.* 1990;6:234–238.
9. Bowley C, Kerr M. Epilepsy and intellectual disability. *J Intellect Disabil Res.* 2000;44(5):529–543.
10. Lhatoo SD, Sander JWAS. The epidemiology of epilepsy and learning disability. *Epilepsia.* 2001;42(Suppl. 1):6–9.
11. Bell GS, Sander JW. The epidemiology of epilepsy: The size of the problem. *Seizure.* 2001;10(4):306–314.
12. Robertson J, Hatton C, Emerson E et al. Prevalence of epilepsy among people with intellectual disabilities: A systematic review. *Seizure.* 2015;29:46–62.
13. McGrother CW, Bhaumik S, Thorp CF et al. Epilepsy in adults with intellectual disabilities: Prevalence, associations and service implications. *Seizure.* 2006;15:376–386.
14. Robertson J, Baines S, Emerson E et al. Service responses to people with intellectual disabilities and epilepsy: A systematic review. *J Appl Res Intellect Disabil.* 2015 doi:10.1111/jar.12228.
15. Glover G, Evison F. Hospital admissions that should not happen. *Improving Health and Lives: Learning Disabilities Observatory*; 2013 ([Available from:https://www.improvinghealthandlives.org.uk/publications/1169]).
16. Balogh R, Brownell M, Ouellette-Kuntz H, Colantonio A. Hospitalization rates for ambulatory care sensitive conditions for persons with and without an intellectual disability: A population perspective. *Journal of Intellectual Disability Research.* 2010;54:820–832.
17. Busch RM, Najm I, Hermann B, Eng C. Genetics of cognition in epilepsy. *Epilepsy and Behavior: E&B.* 2014;0:297–306.
18. Catterall WA. Sodium Channel Mutations and Epilepsy. In: Noebels JL, Avoli M, Rogawski MA, et al., editors. *Jasper's Basic Mechanisms of the Epilepsies* [Internet]. 4th edition. Bethesda (MD): National Center for Biotechnology Information (US); 2012.
19. Curatolo P, Verdecchia M, Bombardieri R. Vigabatrin for tuberous sclerosis complex. *Brain Dev.* 2001; 23(7):649–653.
20. Klepper J, Scheffer H, Leiendecker B et al. Seizure control and acceptance of the ketogenic diet in GLUT1 deficiency syndrome: A 2- to 5-year follow-up of 15 children enrolled prospectively *Neuropediatrics.* 2005;36(5):302–308.
21. Kerr M, Linehan C, Thompson R et al. A white paper on the medical and social needs of people with epilepsy and intellectual disability: The Task force on intellectual disabilities and epilepsy of the international league against epilepsy. *Epilepsia.* 2014;55:1902–1906.
22. Thompson R, Kerr M, Glynn M et al. Caring for a family member with intellectual disability and epilepsy: Practical, social and emotional perspectives. *Seizure.* 2014;23:856–863.
23. Amiet C, Gourfinkel-An I, Bouzamondo A, Tordjman S, Baulac M, Lechat P, et al. Epilepsy in autism is associated with intellectual disability and gender: evidence from a meta-analysis. *Biological Psychiatry.* 2008;64:577–582.
24. Branford D, Bhaumik S, Duncan F. Epilepsy in adults with learning disabilities. *Seizure.* 1998;7:473–477.
25. Matthews T, Weston N, Baxter H, Felce D, Kerr M. A general practice-based prevalence study of epilepsy among adults with intellectual disabilities and of its association with psychiatric disorder, behaviour disturbance and carer stress. *Journal of Intellectual Disability Research.* 2008;52:163–173.
26. Kerr M, Bowley C. Evidence-based prescribing in adults with learning disability and epilepsy. *Epilepsia.* 2001;42(Suppl. 1):44–45.
27. Kerr M, Bowley C. Multidisciplinary and multiagency contributions to care for those with learning disability who have epilepsy. *Epilepsia.* 2001; 42(Suppl. 1):55–56.
28. Doran Z, Shankar R, Keezer MR, et al. Managing anti-epileptic drug treatment in adult patients with intellectual disability: A serious conundrum. *Eur J Neurol.* 2016;23:1152–1157.
29. Shankar R, Cox D, Jalihal V et al. Sudden unexpected death in epilepsy (SUDEP): Development of a safety checklist. *Seizure.* 2013;22:812–817.
30. Hesdorffer DC, Tomson T, Benn E et al. Commission on Epidemiology. Subcommission on mortality combined analysis of risk factors for SUDEP. *Epilepsia.* 2011;52(6):1150–1159.
31. Shankar R, Jalihal V, Walker M et al. A community study in Cornwall UK of sudden unexpected death in epilepsy (SUDEP) in a 9-year population sample. *Seizure.* 2014;23(5):382–385.
32. Shankar R, Walker M, McLean B et al. A step to modify and prevent SUDEP. The validity of risk factors in the SUDEP and Seizure Safety Checklist: A case control study. *Journal of Neurology* DOI 10.1007/s00415-016-8203-3.
33. Kerr M, Linehan C, Brandt, C et al. Behavioral disorder in people with an intellectual disability and epilepsy: A report of the Intellectual Disability Task Force of the Neuropsychiatric Commission of ILAE. *Epilepsia Open.* 2016. doi:10.1002/epi4.12018.
34. Bowley C, Kerr M. Epilepsy and intellectual disability. *J Intellect Disabil Res.* 2000;44(Pt 5):529–543.
35. Rothner AD. 'Not everything that shakes is epilepsy'. The differential diagnosis of paroxysmal nonepileptiform disorders. *Cleveland Clinic Journal of Medicine.* 1989;56 Suppl Pt 2:S206–S213.
36. Hopkins A, Shorvon S, Cascino G. *Epilepsy.* 2 ed. 1995 London: Chapman & Hall.
37. Crompton D, Berkovic S. The borderland of epilepsy: Clinical and molecular features of phenomena that mimic epileptic seizures *The Lancet Neurology.* 2009;Volume 8, Issue 4, 370–381.

38. Gregory RP, Oates T, Merry RTG. EEG epileptiform abnormalities in candidates for aircrew training. *Electroenceph Clin Neurophysiol.* 1993;86:75–77.
39. Pellock JM, Morton LD. Treatment of epilepsy in the multiply handicapped. *Ment Retard Dev DR.* 2000;6: 309–323.
40. http://www.rcpsych.ac.uk/pdf/FR_ID_09_for_website.pdf (accessed 22/10/2016).
41. Beavis J, Kerr M, Marson AG. Pharmacological interventions for epilepsy in people with intellectual disabilities. *Cochrane Database Syst Rev.* 2007;(3):CD005399.
42. Camfield PR, Bahi-Buisson N, Trinka E. Transition issues for children with diffuse cortical malformations, multifocal postnatal lesions (infectious and traumatic), and Lennox-Gastaut and similar syndromes. *Epilepsia.* 2014;55:24–28.
43. Feely M. Drug treatment of epilepsy. *BMJ.* 1999;318 (9 January):106–109.
44. Livanainen M, Alvarez N. Drug treatment of epilepsy in people with intellectual disability. *JIDR.* 1998;42 Suppl 1:iv.
45. Shankar R, et al. Presented at ECE 2016, Prague, Czech Republic, September 11–15.
46. Espie CA, Gillies JB, Montgomery J M. Antiepileptic polypharmacy, psychosocial behaviour and locus of control orientation among mentally handicapped adults living in the community. *J Ment Defic Res.*1990;34:351–360.
47. Marson, A et al. The SANAD study of effectiveness of valproate, lamotrigine, or topiramate for generalised and unclassifiable epilepsy: An unblinded randomised controlled trial. *The Lancet*, Volume 369, Issue 9566, 1016–1026.
48. Porter E et al., Developing the pregnancy support pack for people who have a learning disability *British Journal of Learning Disabilities.* 2012;40: 310–317.
49. Hollins, S. *Books Beyond Words: Telling the Whole Story in Pictures.* 2003. Available: http://www.intellectualdisability.info/how-to../books-beyond-words-telling-the-whole-story-in-pictures. Last accessed 22/10/2016.
50. Pellock JM, Morton LD. reatment of epilepsy in the multiply handicapped. Ment Retard Dev D R 6. 2000:309–323.
51. Rohit Shankar Testing Competency in Delivering Epilepsy Protocol Medication. Advances in clinical neuroscience and rehabilitation: ACNR 06/2014; 14(2):31.
52. Joint Epilepsy Committee. *Buccal Midazolam Guidelines.* 2014. Available: http://www.jointepilepsycouncil.org.uk/resources/buccal_midazolam.html. Last accessed 22/10/2016.
53. Singh BK, Towle P O. Antiepileptic drug status in adult outpatients with mental retardation. *Am J Ment Retard.* 1993;98: 41–46.
54. Zamponi et al. *Seizure* 2011;20(6):468–474.
55. Prasher VP. Furlong E, Weerasena L. Vagus Nerve Stimulation Therapy: An Intellectual Disabilities Perspective. In: Prasher VP Kerr MP. *Epilepsy and Intellectual Disabilities.* 2008. London: Springer. Pp. 109–128.
56. Shankar R, Olotu V, Cole N, Sullivan H, Jory C. Case report: Vagal nerve stimulation and late onset asystole. *Seizure.* 2008;22 (4):312–314.
57. Nicolson, A. Resective Surgery for Patients with Epilepsy and Intellectual Disabilities. In: Prasher V Kerr, M. *Epilepsy and Intellectual Disabilities.* 2008. London: Springer. Pp. 129–151.
58. Espie CA, Pashley AS, Bonham KG, Sourindhrin I, O'Donovan M. The mentally handicapped person with epilepsy: A comparative study investigating psychosocial functioning. *Journal of Mental Deficiency Research* 1989;33:123–135.
59. Scambler G. Stigma and disease: changing paradigms. *Lancet.* 1998;352(9133):1054–1055.
60. Fenwick P. (1995). Psychiatric Disorder and Epilepsy. In: Hopkins A, Shorvon SD, Cascino G, editors. *Epilepsy.* London: Chapman Hall, pp. 453–502.
61. Shorvon SD. Epilepsy and driving. *BMJ.* 1995;310:885–886.
62. Scambler G, Hopkins A. Generating a model of epileptic stigma: The role of qualitative analysis. *Soc Sci Med.* 1990;30(11):1187–1194.
63. Department of Health. Valuing People Now: A new three year strategy for people with learning disabilities. *Department of Health*, London, 2009.
64. International Association of the Scientific Study of Intellectual Disabilities (IASSID). Clinical guidelines for the management of epilepsy in adults with an intellectual disability. *Seizure* 2001;10:401–409.
65. Forjuoh SN, Guyer B. Injury prevention in people with disabilities. *BMJ.* 2001;322:940–941.
66. Besag F. Lesson of the week: Tonic seizures are a particular risk factor for drowning in people with epilepsy. *BMJ.* 2001;322:975–976.
67. https://sudep.org/checklist accessed 22/10/2016.
68. Benbadis SR. Errors in EEGs and the misdiagnosis of epilepsy: Importance, causes, consequences, and proposed remedies. *Epilepsy Behav.* 2007;11(3):257–262.
69. LaFrance WC Jr, Baker GA, Duncan R, Goldstein LH, Reuber M. Minimum requirements for the diagnosis of psychogenic nonepileptic seizures: A staged approach.A report from the International League Against Epilepsy; Nonepileptic Seizures Task Force. *Epilepsia.* 2013;54(11):2005–2018.
70. Goldstein LH, Chalder T, Chigwedere C, Khondoker MR, Moriarty J, Toone BK et al. Cognitive-behavioral therapy for psychogenic nonepileptic seizures: A pilot RCT. *Neurology.* 2010;74(24):1986–1994.
71. LaFrance WC Jr, Baird GL, Barry JJ, Blum AS, Frank Webb A, Keitner GI et al. Multicenter pilot treatment trial for psychogenic nonepileptic seizures: A randomized clinical trial. *JAMA Psychiatry.* 2014;71(9):997–1005.
72. Martlew J, Pulman J, Marson AG. Psychological and behavioural treatments for adults with non-epileptic attack disorder. *Cochrane Database of Systematic Reviews.* 2014, Issue 2. Art. No.: CD006370. DOI: 10.1002/14651858.CD006370.pub2.
73. Chapman Melanie et al. The misdiagnosis of epilepsy in people with intellectual disabilities: A systematic review. *Seizure* 20 2011:101–106.
74. Prescribing Antiepileptic Drugs for people with epilepsy and Intellectual Disability. Royal College of Psychiatrists College Report 206. 10/2017.
75. Management of Epilepsy in people with Intellectual Disability. Royal College of Psychiatrists College Report 203. 05/2017.
76. Mclean B, Shankar R Hanna J et al. SUDEP—Measures to reduce risk Pract Neurol. 2017;17:13–20
77. Watkins L, Shankar R, Sander JW. Identifying and mitigating. Sudden Unexpected Death in Epilepsy (SUDEP) risk factors. 2018. Expert Rev Neurotherapeutics. DOI: 10.1080/14737175.2018.1439738.
78. Watkins L Shankar R. Reducing the risk of Sudden Unexpected Death in Epilepsy. *Curr Treat Options Neurol.* 2018;20: 40. https://doi.org/10.1007/s11940-018-0527-0.
79. Young C, Shankar R, Henley W, et al. SUDEP and seizure safety communication: Assessing if people hear and act. *Epilepsy Behav.* 2018. https://doi.org/10.1016/j.yebeh.2018.06.040.
80. Shankar R, Rowe C, Van Hoorn A et al. Under representation of people with epilepsy and ID in research. *PLOS One.* June 21, 2018. 10.1371/journal.pone.0198261.

23 Behavioural Phenotypes

Anthony Holland

Introduction

This chapter has three main aims. The first is to examine how the concept of the behavioural phenotype has developed over time, giving examples of where genetically-determined neurodevelopmental syndromes have been found to be associated with particular developmental trajectories and specific comorbid risks for challenging behaviour or mental ill-health. The second is to move from descriptive studies that have characterized such relationships to considering examples of potential neural and other mechanisms that might explain the observed genotype/phenotype associations. The third is to consider the implications for intervention and how an understanding of neural mechanisms might lead to novel syndrome-specific treatments.

To achieve these aims key terms are defined and principles set out that underpin the concept of behavioural phenotypes, and the potential for incorporating these understandings into clinical practice are considered. As is discussed, the term 'behavioural phenotype' is used to refer to specific and obvious 'behaviours' (e.g. self-injury, aggression, repetitive, and ritualistic etc.). However, the use of this term has expanded over time and there is inevitably a blurring of boundaries between different phenomena. Some of these are obvious behaviours; others may be the manifestation of a cluster of signs and symptoms that meet the diagnostic criteria for a specific mental disorder; and yet other observations are better described as abnormal mental or emotional states, or refer to specific patterns of cognitive, linguistic, social, or functional abilities. Furthermore, there is an inevitable overlapping of the physical and the psychological. An examination of this concept of behavioural phenotypes crosses many disciplines, not least developmental biology, developmental and clinical psychology, various disciplines in clinical medicine, and molecular biology. For a more complete understanding of how behavioural phenotypes arise it would be necessary to set it within the context of the complex field of child development, and particularly the theories of brain development and associated cognitive, language, motor, social, and emotional development. This is beyond my own expertise and outside the scope of this chapter. However, the Cambridge Encyclopedia of Child Development (1) provides detailed overviews of the relevant topics from many different perspectives.

The chapter is primarily aimed at trainees, clinicians, and clinical researchers and, for this reason, is about those aspects of the behavioural phenotypes that impinge negatively on a person's health, well-being, and quality of life. This is not in any way to deny the very positive characteristics that may also be part of the phenotype of children and adults with the neurodevelopmental syndrome. It is, however, these former aspects that bring individuals to the attention of clinical services and for which help is requested. Furthermore, whilst research into behavioural phenotypes focuses on groups of individuals defined by their genotype, in clinical practice it is the individual who is the focus of attention. The skills required of the clinician is to integrate what is known about the individual and his or her circumstances in order to arrive at an understanding of the problem that led to the referral. Where it is appropriate, this should include considering the relevance or not of the cause of his/her intellectual disability (ID).

Not every possible neurodevelopmental syndrome associated with an ID and related behavioural phenotypes is listed. Most, if not all, neurodevelopmental syndromes will have a particular physical phenotype and may well also have a cognitive and behavioural phenotype characteristic of the syndrome. Where examples are given, the main focus will be when the nature and extent of the relationship between the syndrome and its behavioural phenotype has clinical utility. In such circumstances clinicians and social care providers will benefit from knowing when such relationships exist, particularly when there are implications for intervention, prognosis, and treatment. The nature and extent of the clinical utility in any given syndrome may be fluid in nature, changing with future medical advances. Many reputable syndrome-specific websites and published papers on given syndromes now provide such information.

Background

Children and adults defined as having an ID on the basis of their developmental delay and intellectual and functional impairments are, as a group, very heterogeneous, varying in the nature and extent of their intellectual and cognitive impairments and functional disabilities, and over time, in their developmental trajectories and risk for physical and sensory comorbidities. Population-based studies have also identified high prevalence rates of comorbid mental ill-health, autism spectrum disorder, and of what is now most commonly referred to as 'challenging behaviour' (2, 3). The major impact of such behaviours and/or of comorbid autism spectrum disorders on the wellbeing and quality of life of those affected, and that of their families, together with the transactional nature of the relationship between family stress and the challenging behaviour, has highlighted the need for effective and informed interventions directed both towards the individual and his/her family or the support network (4–6).

A major focus of clinical research has been on better understanding the developmental, biological, psychological, and environmental factors that might predispose to, precipitate, or maintain particular behaviours, such as self-injury and aggression. In this context, the use of the term 'challenging behaviour' is not strictly a diagnosis, rather it is descriptive, and by itself implies no understanding as to the aetiology of the behaviour. When such behaviour is present, what is required is an understanding of that behaviour as it affects an individual, set out in a formulation and in the context of an appropriate research-informed theoretical context. Within the field of ID, three broad and overlapping conceptual models have informed our understanding of challenging behaviour, and these continue to guide clinical practice. These are: a) applied behavioural analysis (ABA) based on learning theory; b) the impact of the development of comorbid mental and physical illness on mental functioning and behaviour; and c) the recognition that some behaviours may be characteristic of a particular stage of development and their persistence is a direct manifestation of delayed or atypical development. As set out below, in the last of these it may now be argued that the concept of syndrome specific risks for particular behaviours and/or mental-ill health should be included.

Ideas based on the first of these models, learning theory, have dominated thinking in this field, and since the early work of Iwata and colleagues, there have been many studies that have demonstrated how the occurrence of particular adaptive or maladaptive behaviours can be shaped by past and present circumstances, and, for example, how aggression or self-injurious behaviours may be reinforced by particular contingencies and may be under the influence of internal or external setting conditions (7). Given this understanding of how behaviours are shaped and learned, positive behavioural support has been seen as key to the provision of good services. However, what has also become increasingly apparent is that there may be very specific profiles of risk that are dependent on the particular, usually genetic, cause of a person's ID. Where a specific profile of adaptive and maladaptive behaviours are consistently present in children and/or adults with a particular cause for their ID, this relationship cannot be explained fully by learning theory and must be considered to relate more directly to the biological cause of that person's ID.

Although the relationship between a particular genotype and physical characteristics has long been recognized, the link between genotype and an aspect of the phenotype that is 'a behaviour', came to prominence with the observations of Lesch and Nyhan in 1964 (8). They described a group of males with a clear developmental syndrome specifically associated with a characteristic and severe pattern of early onset self-injurious behaviour. In an address to the American Pediatric Association in 1971 Nyhan used the phrase 'a behavioural phenotype in organic genetic disease' to describe this phenomena and stated that self-injurious behaviour was a key part of the phenotype of those males who were born with what became known as Lesch-Nyhan syndrome (9). This concept of behavioural phenotypes within a specific syndrome focused on the relationship between a particular cluster of adaptive and maladaptive behaviours (phenotype) in a syndrome, the cause of which was, in this case, mutations in a particular gene (genotype) coding for hypoxanthine phosphoribosyltransferase (HPRT1). It is the disruption of this particular pathway that results, directly or indirectly, in the manifestation of the characteristic clinical features of the syndrome, which include various movement disorders, a particular form of self-injurious behaviour in which self-restraint is a feature, and high levels of uric acid in the blood. Nyhan argued that this behaviour of self-injury was 'self-programmed'. These observations in this group of children were important because, by ultimately understanding causal pathways, it held out the possibility that novel syndrome-specific treatments could be developed. Furthermore, this new perspective could still allow for the fact that maladaptive behaviours, such as severe self-injury, can be shaped by events and circumstances, but such observations as those of Nyhan clearly indicated that there also has to be a syndrome-specific explanation as to why certain behaviours are so common in people with ID due to particular causes and not others, even though levels of intellectual and functional impairments and disabilities may be similar.

Flint (10) referred to observations of such links between genetically determined neurodevelopmental disorders and behavioural phenotypes as providing 'a window on the biology of behaviour', potentially leading to insights into those problems as they occurred in the typically developing population. However, initially, this concept of a genotype/phenotype relationship as applied to behaviour, was not readily taken up by those working in the ID field. One can speculate that this was at least partially because of skepticism of what could be seen as an over-reductionist approach to understanding behaviour, something that would normally be considered complex and multifaceted in its aetiology. This neglect may also have been due to echoes of the Eugenics movement. At the time, when these observations were first being made, there was also the danger that something seen as being genetically determined would be considered to be irremediable. O'Brien (11) argued that attitudes began to change in the 1990s as observations were increasingly made and syndrome support groups were similarly describing relationships between a specific syndrome and a particular behaviour. Furthermore, these various concerns can now be effectively countered. There are strong international human rights conventions and, in many countries, national anti-discrimination laws that protect against any re-emergence of a eugenic approach. Also, with advances in both genetics and the neurosciences, there is a new emphasis on, and potential for new therapies for disorders of genetic origin and a nihilistic approach to symptoms of genetic origin is no longer warranted. There are examples of how increasing knowledge of syndromes is leading to potential novel treatments. Two examples of syndrome-specific pharmacological approaches include using mTor inhibitors designed to reduce the tubers in tuberous sclerosis (12) and the use of mGluR5 antagonist to reduce symptoms associate with fragile-X syndrome (13). Although such trials have highlighted serious challenges they are illustrative of this new thinking and approach. In addition, as is discussed later, understanding of the mechanisms that underpin specific behavioural phenotypes may lead to more nuanced psychological interventions or to completely novel treatments.

Defining a behavioural phenotype

One of the challenges in this field has been, and remains, agreeing a definition of a behavioural phenotype that is not so broad so as to have little utility, but is wide enough that it captures meaningful relationships where they exist, and which, in turn, have clinical and scientific relevance. The term 'phenotype' generally has been taken to refer to the total observable physical characteristics of an organism given the environment in which the organism is living. The phenotype is a manifestation of an interaction between genetics (genotype) and, to a varying extent, environmental influences. Examples of obvious physical phenotypes manifest in individuals include skin, hair, and eye colour and also those characteristics that may also be under significant environmental influence, such as weight. The term phenotype is also used to refer to markers that are not immediately visible, such as biochemical indices. As is discussed later, when it comes to underlying markers of behavioural traits, the term 'endophenotype' has been suggested. In the case of people born with a specific syndrome, the phenotype of that syndrome will be those characteristics found in excess in people with that syndrome. Some characteristics may be required for the syndrome to be confirmed; others may be considered as supportive diagnostic criteria. The term 'phenotype' therefore refers to certain characteristics of an individual and also to the characteristics that define a group of people, for example, according to gender, race, or people with a specific neurodevelopmental syndrome.

The concept of a 'behavioural phenotype', as applied to people with specific neurodevelopmental syndromes, has been widened beyond the original description of Nyhan or that given by Harris in 1987 (14) (see Box 23.1). First, Flint and Yule (15) in their definition acknowledged that environmental causes of significant disability, such as maternal alcohol abuse leading to foetal alcohol syndrome, could also be associated with a particular behavioural phenotype. Subsequent studies have suggested a deficit in complex cognitive processing (16). Secondly, the term 'behavioural phenotype' has been expanded to also include a specific developmental course, cognitive profile, and/or social and functional abilities. Some examples of neurodevelopmental syndromes and their behavioural phenotypes are given in Table 23.1. Importantly, as is illustrated in the definition by Dykens (17), when it comes to a specific behaviour, that characteristic of the phenotype may not be inevitable, but rather there may be an increased probability of occurrence in people with that particular syndrome in the context of specific environmental conditions.

Determining whether a particular characteristic should be thought of as a behavioural phenotype may not easy. By definition neurodevelopmental syndromes represent a class of disorders in which there are abnormalities of brain development and in the functioning of underlying neural networks. Impairments in intellectual functioning, in skills development and in various cognitive abilities such as memory, executive functioning, and attention will be common. In this context, challenging behaviours may arise as a consequence of general abnormalities of brain function, such as impairments in emotional regulation, or disturbances in executive abilities to regulate behaviour. In addition, the frequency and severity of such behaviours, may also have been shaped by environmental circumstances and subsequent observations may indicate that they have a functional significance, such as being demand-avoidant or attention-maintained. Thus, determining whether or not people with a particular syndrome should be described as having a 'behavioural phenotype' will depend upon whether or not the associated pattern of behaviours or mental ill-health and its prevalence is the same or different when compared to other groups with similar levels of impairments and disabilities. For example, in people with Down syndrome it is generally agreed that congenital heart disease is common, although not universal and it is accepted as part of the physical phenotype. Similarly, the high risk of developing dementia due to Alzheimer's disease is clearly specific to individuals with Down syndrome; other people with intellectual disabilities may of course develop dementia but it is much less likely at the relatively young age it is observed to occur in people with Down syndrome. When it is a particular behaviour, such as aggression or self-injurious behaviour, or the presence of an autism spectrum disorder, the population to be compared against will be influenced by the level of intellectual disability, and this needs to be controlled for when determining whether these behaviours truly occur with an increased prevalence. Furthermore, self-injurious behaviour is more common in people with autistic spectrum disorders and, for this reason, where high rates of such behaviour occurs, this may be best understood as a secondary consequence of the autistic spectrum disorder, rather than necessarily a direct consequence of having the syndrome (18).

In clinical practice it is a detailed and often multi-disciplinary assessment of the individual informed by these research observations, not just an understanding of the syndrome, which informs intervention.

Box 23.1 Definitions of 'behavioural phenotypes'

- Behavioural phenotypes are stereotypic patterns of behaviour that are reliably identified in groups of individuals with known neurodevelopmental disorders and which are not learnt (14).
- Behavioural phenotypes are a characteristic pattern of motor, cognitive, linguistic, and social abnormalities that is consistently associated with a biological disorder (15).
- A behavioural phenotype is a heightened probability that people with a given syndrome will exhibit certain behavioural sequelae relative to those without the syndrome (17).

Endophenotypes

The widening of the definition of the term behavioural phenotype has included incorporating particular characteristics that are not immediately apparent when observing someone or are not obvious from their history, but instead have to be measured. Although the term 'phenotype' can be used to encompass this wider concept, when it comes to behaviour or mental health the term 'endophenotype' has come to be used to refer to these measurable characteristics that are linked to a particular phenotypic trait, and which are usually under some degree of genetic control. They have been conceptualized as 'an internal phenotype that lie on the pathway between genes and

Table 23.1 A summary of key, potentially clinically significant, features of specific neurodevelopmental syndromes. A more extensive description is given in Udwin and Kuczynski (19)

Syndrome/birth incidence	Genotype	Behavioural phenotype
Angelman syndrome population prevalence 1:40,000 to 1:10,000	Deletion or mutation UBE3A 15q.11-13, chromosome 15 paternal disomy	Significant developmental delay and ID. Happy and excitable disposition, paroxysmal giggling and laughing, hand flapping, inattention and hyperactivity, some aggressive behaviours reported.
Cornelia de Lange syndrome 1:50,000 to l:15,000	Genetically heterogeneous	Significant phenotypic heterogeneity, gastro-oesophageal reflux, mild self-injury, risk of significant physical abnormalities.
Down syndrome birth incidence 1:700–1000	Trisomy 21, rare translocation and mosaic DS	Early decelerating developmental trajectory. Behavioural, memory and functional decline in mid-life and increased age-related risk of dementia (Alzheimer's disease).
Fragile-X syndrome birth incidence 1: 3,600	Increased number of CCG repeats (usually 50–200) in the FMR-1 gene on the long arm X chromosome. Males most severely affected.	Profile of autistic-like behaviours, particularly social avoidance (poor eye gaze) and repetitive behaviours. Oversensitivity to stimuli and shyness and social anxiety described.
Lesch Nyhan syndrome birth incidence 1:380,000 (X-linked affecting males only)	Mutation HPRT gene Xq26-Xq27.2	Early development of hypertonia and spasticity, involuntary movements, characteristic bouts of severe self-injurious behaviour with attempts at self-restraint, verbal and physical aggression.
Prader-Willi syndrome birth incidence 1:24,000	Paternal 15q11-13 deletion, maternal 15 UPD, IC defect	Hyperphagia, temper outburst, repetitive and ritualistic behaviours, mood disorder, psychotic illness primarily in mUPD.
Rett syndrome birth incidence 1:12,000 females	MeCP2 gene Xq28	Early regression, epilepsy, stereotypic hand movements, inappropriate laughing and screaming, self-injurious behaviour in response to change/noise.
Smith-Magenis syndrome 1:25,000	17p11.2 deletion	Hyperactive, impulsiveness, self-injurious behaviour and aggression and destructive behaviours, severe sleep disturbance.
Tuberous sclerosis complex birth incidence 1:6,000	Genetic mutations in one of two genes at the following loci TSC1 9q34, TSC2 16p13.3	Varied cognitive abilities, autism spectrum disorder, severe epilepsy, potential for changing brain and other organ systems pathology leading to deteriorating abilities and physical health.
Velocardiofacial syndrome populations prevalence 1:200 to 1:7000	22q11.2 deletion	ADHD, psychosis and affective disorders. Increasing risk of neuropsychiatric disorder with age.
Williams syndrome population prevalence 1:7,500 to 1:10,000	7q11.23 deletion	Relatively good verbal skills, excessive sociability, difficult maintaining social relationships, anxiety and specific fears, hyperacusis.

disease' (20) and may be neurophysiological, biochemical, endocrinological, neuroanatomical, cognitive, or neuropsychological. Walters and Owen (21), in an editorial, review the criteria for psychiatric endophenotypes. When applying these to neurodevelopmental syndromes, for a particular measured characteristic to be classed as an endophenotype, it should be consistently associated with that syndrome and specifically with the presence of the behavioural phenotype in question.

The importance of the concept of endophenotypes is twofold. First, their identification can provide insights into the mechanism underpinning the behavioural phenotype in question. Secondly, they may themselves be a useful proxy marker for determining the efficacy of any given intervention. Particularly in neurodevelopmental syndromes, they may also be useful in determining whether a mental state, such as anxiety, in one syndrome has the same underlying mechanism as that of an apparently similar phenotype in another. In those with neurodevelopmental syndromes, differences in interrelationships of phenotype, endophenotype, and genotype are likely to be increasingly important clinically as endophenotype-informed treatments are developed. For the above reasons it is more appropriate to talk about 'behavioural endophenotypes and phenotypes in organic genetic disease'. Considering the definitions given earlier, the criteria that have to be met to define a behavioural phenotype and endophenotype are summarised in Box 23.2.

The concept of behavioural phenotypes therefore has become more layered, moving beyond descriptions of behaviour. First, there are observable manifestations including: the presence of a particular behaviour, for example, characteristic hand movements in children with Rett syndrome, self-injurious behaviour in people with Lesch Nyhan and other syndromes, easily provoked bouts of laughter in children with Angelman syndrome, aggression in children with Smith Magenis syndrome, gaze avoidance in people with fragile-X syndrome, and hyperphagia in people with Prader-Willi syndrome, or it may include an unusual style of communication as in people with William's or fragile-X syndromes. Secondly, in some cases the 'behaviours' so observed will be part of a wider group of signs and symptoms that indicate the presence of a specific developmental or comorbid diagnostic entity, such as an autistic spectrum disorder; the manifestations of an anxiety disorder in various forms, as in people with Williams syndrome (22); a particular mental illness, as in one genetic type of Prader-Willi Syndrome (23) or in adults with velo-cardio-facial syndrome (24); or dementia as in people with Down syndrome (25). These are all phenomena that are detectable through history-taking and observation. The

Box 23.2 Criteria to be met to determine the validity of a claim for a behavioural phenotype or endophenotype associated with a specific neurodevelopmental syndrome

a The manifestation of a particular behaviour, or combinations of behaviours, or of comorbid mental illness occurring during the lifespan of individuals associated with a recognized syndrome, usually of known aetiology.
b Through clinical, psychological and/or biological investigations the identification of markers (endophenotypes) consistently associated with a particular syndrome and its behavioural phenotype, including unique patterns of cognitive, language, and/or social functioning, and/or biological markers, and measures of cerebral functioning using technologies such as neuroimaging.
c 'a' and 'b' occur consistently in excess in children and/or adults with that syndrome compared to others with neurodevelopmental syndromes.
d 'a' and 'b' are broadly consistent in their characteristics in those with the same syndrome, such as the age of onset and course of the observed behavioural phenotype over the lifespan, and, for example, any specific cognitive and/or linguistic profiles or identified biological markers
e 'a' and b' cannot be accounted for by other variables that independently would increase the risk of their occurrence, for example, the level of functioning and its impact on behaviour, or the presence of an autism spectrum disorder.
f Even if not immediately apparent or proven, the existence of hypothesized mechanism open to testing, which may account for the observed relationship and which are consistent with genetic, neuroscience, and/or psychological theories.

next layer down comprises the endophenotypes. These might include those characteristics identified through the use of specific psychological or language assessments, such as the recognition, for example, of an unusual language and cognitive profile, and abnormalities of attention and of theory of mind as observed in children with fragile-X syndrome (26, 27); or neuroimaging findings such as impaired satiety and abnormal neural response to food intake in people with Prader-Willi syndrome (28); neural abnormalities in people with tuberous sclerosis (29); or physical abnormalities outside of the central nervous system associated with the behaviour in question such as gastro-oesophageal reflux in people with Cornelia de Lange syndrome (30). With advances in different forms of neuroimaging and other investigations these endophenotypic markers will increasingly be identified at the structural and functional levels. The complex challenge is to then identify and map such markers against the background of development and to move from an understanding of underlying brain mechanisms to treatment developments.

Mechanisms linking genotypes to behavioural phenotypes

In the majority of neurodevelopmental syndromes it is the atypical expression of a specific gene or genes or the production of an aberrant gene product that ultimately results in a delayed and/or atypical pattern of development, atypical neural functioning, and in some syndromes in the emergence of the behavioural phenotype characteristic of that syndrome. The loss of one copy (allele) of a particular gene, the phenotypic effect of which may be dose sensitive, may have a particular deleterious effect in the development and functional organization of the brain (31). In the case of syndromes, such as Down syndrome, or where there are chromosomal interstitial duplications (copy number variants) it may be the excess of any given gene product that directly or indirectly gives rise to the resultant phenotype, either directly or through its effects on other genes. For those syndromes where the genetics are known, variation at the level of the syndrome genotype is frequently found to be present. For example, this may include different mutations and/or copy number variants associated with specific syndromes (32); more than one genetic loci for a similar syndrome as in the case with tuberous sclerosis complex with loci at 9q34 and 16p13.3 (33), in Prader-Willi syndrome with the 15q11-13 deletion of paternal origin and the maternal chromosome 15 uniparental disomy, and also in Angelman syndrome with mutations in the UBE3A gene or the presence of a deletion of maternal origin or uniparental paternal disomy of chromosome 15. In each of these examples individuals will share the core features of that particular syndrome but there may be important differences, depending on the exact genotype. In addition, as is the case with all of us, background genetics and the past and present environment may influence the way such behaviours may present, and when, during the life-course.

With the sequencing of the human genome many common and rare copy number variations are being identified and the genetics of identifiable syndromes are increasingly well characterized. However, it is in the area of epigenetics that advances are being made in terms of understanding the link between genotype and phenotype. Epigenetics is the term given to the regulation of gene expression in the absence of changes in the DNA, and is concerned with, for example, differences in gene expression at the level of different organ systems, how gene expression is modified during the course of development, and how 'imprinting' (switching off) of particular genes contributes to neurodevelopmental disorders such as Prader-Willi and Angelman syndromes and also in disease states (34). The challenge for behavioural phenotype research is, that to advance our understanding of mechanisms that link genotype to behavioural phenotype, it is an understanding of gene expression in the brain that is likely to be required. This is clearly problematic during life. The development of stem-cell technologies and the ability to convert pluripotential stem cells to neurons (35), together with the investigation of genetically altered mouse and other animal models of syndromes (see Moy and Nadier (36) for review of mouse models of autism and of neurodevelopmental syndromes associated with autism) are now providing the tools to address such issues. Many of the well-known neurodevelopmental syndromes, such as fragile-X, Williams, and Prader-Willi syndromes, have genetic mouse models, which have enabled detailed neurobiological investigation. For example, in Williams syndrome, earlier clinical descriptions of the behavioural phenotype has led to mechanistic studies and to more informed treatment recommendations (37). Neuroimaging is also an increasingly important tool for investigating brain mechanisms. Lesch-Nyhan syndrome was one of the early examples of using ligand-based PET neuroimaging to identify, in this case, significant reductions in dopamine transporter density in the putamen and caudate nuclei in the brain (38). Other examples are given later in the chapter. These are exciting times, as clinical, neuroscientific, and laboratory-based technologies are allowing questions to be addressed that previously could not have been. This is explored further using the following four examples.

Williams syndrome: an example of a complex endophenotype and phenotype

In considering the potential reasons why a particular behaviour or mental state may have a high prevalence in those with a specific neurodevelopmental syndrome, it is necessary to characterize the nature of the behavioural phenotype. As mentioned earlier in the chapter, not all apparently similar behaviours or mental states are the same. The physical characteristics of Williams syndrome include hypercalcaemia, supravalvular aortic stenosis, and a characteristic craniofacial dysmorphology, together with developmental delay and connective tissue abnormalities (39). One significant outward manifestation of the behavioural phenotype is severe anxiety, which may occur as part of a more general impairment in mood regulation (22). Anxiety has been reported in over 60 per cent of people with the syndrome, and the anxiety observed is not a generalized anxiety disorder, but closer to a phobia, with fears, for example, of thunderstorms. Anticipatory anxieties also occur and, although social anxiety disorders are rare in people with Williams syndrome, they may have anxieties of a more social kind, for example, if people like them or not. The criteria of markedly increased prevalence of anxiety compared to general population rates and to other groups with neurodevelopmental syndromes, together with the presence of a characteristic 'anxiety phenotype' in people with Williams syndrome, supports the case for anxiety, along with other features, such as a characteristic cognitive profile and pattern of language development, being called a behavioural phenotype and endophenotype. Leyfer et al (40) have argued that the Williams syndrome chromosome deletion at 7q11-13 could be a locus for a gene in which the deletion of one allele predisposes to this type of anxiety. In contrast, in fragile-X syndrome anxiety takes a very different form and is closer to a genuine social anxiety. The specificity of a phenotype (in this case anxiety) is quite striking. It is reasonable, therefore, to assume that there will be different psychological mechanisms and neural pathways that underpin the anxiety disorders of these two syndromes. By extension, it is also likely that approaches to treatment may differ.

Jarvinen-Pasley et al (41) have extensively reviewed the literature on Williams syndrome. They explore the relationships between the genetics of Williams syndrome and cognitive, language, and social functioning across ages. They demonstrate how the links between genes and behaviour, and particularly social functioning can be studied and how differences in social networks in the brain have been reported, including the observation of a large amygdala and augmented volume and grey matter densities in other parts of this network. Their paper seeks to take us from the characteristic 1.5 to 1.8 megabase chromosomal deletion at 7q11-23 of usually 25 genes, to considering the consequential atypical developmental trajectory, and the cognitive profiles and functional manifestations of this atypical development. Relevant to development in general and to neurodevelopmental syndromes in particular, they argue that early brain development shows considerable plasticity, and it is in this context that unique patterns of development occur and that the cognitive strengths that are an outcome of development in Williams syndrome are best considered as due to altered neuro-computational constraints. They argue that relatively genetically homogenous syndromes, such as Williams syndrome, provide 'an experiment of nature', which allows the neural pathways and psychological processes that underpin typical and atypical development to be explored. What is also striking about people with Williams syndrome is the unusual social behaviour described as indiscriminate friendliness, enhanced emotional empathy, and loquaciousness (see 42 and 43 for reviews). From the perspective of the cognitive (endo)phenotype, it is the profile of the cognitive function with lower performance than verbal scores on IQ that is striking. Older children are observed to be proficient in language and facial processing, but major deficits are observed in aspects of general intellectual functioning, such as in planning and problem solving. Observational studies have shown how children with Williams syndrome, even with such cognitive deficits, engage in social contact and show more frequent approaches to strangers compared with other atypically developing children. Paradoxically, children with Williams syndrome, although showing increased sociability, have substantial difficulties with social adjustment and sustaining relationships with peers.

Velo-Cardio-Facial Syndrome: insights into the aetiology of a psychotic illness

In terms of mechanistic studies Velo-Cardio-Facial syndrome illustrates the challenges of linking genotype to phenotype (see 24 for review). The chromosomal deletion on chromosome 22 (this syndrome is also known as 22q deletion syndrome) may vary from 1.5 to 3 megabases. It is estimated that the common larger deletion is the locus for at least 40 genes, all of which will be hemizygous given that one allele is deleted. From a phenotypic perspectives, 180 characteristics of the syndrome have been described, involving all organ systems. The neuropsychiatric phenotype has received considerable attention with rates of serious mental illness (schizophrenia and bipolar disorder) increased 25 times compared to the general population. Murphy et al (44) reported that 42 per cent of a cohort of 50 adults with VCFS had a major psychotic illness. Thus, this syndrome has been seen as a model for studying psychotic illness with attention focused, from a genetic perspective, on the catechol-O-methyltransferase (COMT) gene, which is situated at the 22q locus. There have also been studies investigating structural brain abnormalities, given the mid-line deficits observed in those with the syndrome. Abnormalities of the corpus callosum, the amygdala, the caudate nucleus, and temporo-parietal regions have all been described. In their review Murphy and Owen (45) consider if the risk for psychotic illness is best conceptualized as neurodevelopmental or neurochemical. They suggest that findings from different studies have found facial and brain abnormalities and in people with schizophrenia and those in VCFS that are similar. They therefore propose that it is the impact of the deletion on neural development, rather than the impact of the deletion of an allele of the COMT gene affecting the catecholamine pathway that is likely to be the most significant aetiological factor. At present therefore these observations have not resulted in significant treatment developments, but they have highlighted the need to be aware of the risk to those with the syndrome and to diagnose and treat any comorbidity as it arises. As is described below Prader-Willi syndrome also offers the potential for insights into the aetiology of psychotic illnesses.

Prader-Willi syndrome (PWS): an example of a complex behavioural endophenotype and phenotype

Many studies of children and adults with Prader-Willi syndrome have identified a physical and behavioural phenotype that changes and develops during childhood and across the lifespan. The most striking feature is the development of hyperphagia in childhood following a period of hypophagia and failure to thrive after birth and in infancy (46). These polar extremes of eating with reversal after infancy, are universally present. Other studies have found that particular behaviours (e.g. temper outbursts, skin picking) are not universal but occur with increased frequency (47), and yet further studies have found high rates of psychotic illness within one genetic type of PWS (those with a maternal uniparental disomy of chromosome 15 as opposed to those with 15q11-13 deletions of paternal origin (23, 48, 49). In addition, although varying in intensity, hyperphagia (and the associated risk of obesity), and the other behaviours when they occur are similar in their characteristics across all people with PWS. Temper outbursts may be triggered by change and usually have a characteristic course and pattern of resolution. The approach in the case of PWS has been to focus on the mechanisms that underpin specific aspects of the behavioural phenotype and to seek to develop individual treatments, for example, for the hyperphagia, temper outbursts, and comorbid mental health problems. Neuroimaging studies have focused on better understanding the hyperphagia and, together with observational studies, have shown impairment in the satiety cascade and the brain's response to food intake (28, 50). Similarly, studies using functional MRI have shown that different areas of the brain are recruited when undertaking attention-switching tasks. Tunnicliffe et al. (51) proposed that temper outbursts in PWS may be triggered by the cognitive demands of attention-switching when change occurs. Self-injurious behaviour in PWS is very characteristic and takes the form of skin-picking, which may result in serious complications and may extend to anal poking. Interestingly, Hall et al. (52) has shown that there is a significant environmental influence on the likelihood of such behaviour, the behaviour being more marked when the patient is without social contact. Using fMRI Klabunde et al. (53) compared people with PWS who did or did not skin-pick finding that there was increased activation of those areas of the brain most associated with interoceptive, motor, attention, and somatosensory processing in those who skin-picked. Improvements with the administration of N-acetylcysteine, whose action is on the glutaminergic pathways in the brain (54), provides some evidence that such behaviour also has a biological basis.

A further striking finding in PWS has been the observation of high rates of affective psychotic illness (60%) that preferentially affect those with PWS due to the uniparental disomy. From a mechanistic perspective, this observation suggests that the two genetic forms of PWS (15q11-13 deletion and chromosome 15 maternal uniparental disomy), although sharing the features of PWS, must differ in their subsequent neural development in a manner that results in this propensity to psychotic illness. Aman et al. (55) have proposed a model linking genetics to brain and cognitive function, arguing that a combination of affective instability, common to both genetic types of PWS and impairments in sensory processing, which are most marked in those with the disomy, might account for this high risk for psychosis.

Down syndrome and dementia: a behavioural phenotype of later life

The focus on behavioural phenotypes has tended to be on children or young adults. However, observations first made in the early twentieth century reported that people with Down syndrome inevitably developed the neuropathology characteristic of Alzheimer's disease (25). Many studies since have reported that age-specific rates of clinically diagnosed dementia in people with Down Syndrome increase from 1 or 2 per cent in their 30s to 50 per cent or more in their 50s (56). A recent follow-up study of a cohort of people with DS has suggested that almost all people with Down syndrome develop the clinical features of dementia if they survive into, what for them, given the reduced life-expectancy, is later life (57). With the gene coding for the Amyloid Precursor Protein being located on chromosome 21 (58) and, given other observations on the role of amyloid in the aetiology of Alzheimer's disease in the general population, the amyloid cascade hypothesis has been seen as the most likely explanation of this relationship between a neurodevelopmental syndrome apparent at birth (Down syndrome) and a disorder of later life (Alzheimer's disease). The onset of dementia may be atypical, with evidence of behavioural and personality changes prior to functional memory impairments, however, the subsequent course of dementia is characteristic with a profound loss of functional abilities (59). Significant advances are being made in our understanding of Alzheimer's disease in people with Down syndrome with the use of both PET and MRI neuroimaging. Such studies are now able to map the relationship between clinical change, amyloid binding in the brain, and structural brain changes (60–62). The earlier clinical studies very importantly raised the profile of this relationship between the two disorders and the onset of dementia is now more readily recognized, and appropriate assessments used to ensure an accurate diagnosis and the implementation of support strategies to help maintain dignity and wellbeing. As discussed later in the chapter the long-term aim is the development of effective preventative treatments.

The treatment implications of the identification of behavioural phenotypes

How might the recognition that a particular neurodevelopmental syndrome has a behavioural phenotype help? First, knowledge about such relationships may in itself be crucial and lead to early informed interventions. A very obvious example is in Prader-Willi syndrome. Early diagnosis, combined with an understanding of the development of hyperphagia, has meant that parents can limit access to food and prevent severe obesity. Secondly, as the psychological and neural bases that underpin such relationships are elucidated, these, in turn, will result in more nuanced assessments and interventions of the individual. Examples include more detailed assessments of executive functioning or of language of individuals with fragile-X or Williams syndrome where social impairments and language abnormalities are known to be characteristic of those with the syndrome. The findings from such assessments may then directly inform how support is provided and specifically the communication environment where the person lives. Thirdly, with an increasing recognition of the clinical relevance of this behavioural phenotype perspective, in the context of the wider theoretical framework of our understanding of challenging behaviour, this has perhaps led to a greater acceptance of the value of this approach alongside others. For example, an understanding of the behavioural phenotype may result in a better understanding of how behaviours may be triggered and shaped in those with a particular syndrome. Similarly a knowledge of the behavioural phenotype of a given syndrome may make families and others providing support aware of the risks of specific psychiatric comorbidity and thereby ensuring the treatment of such illnesses as and when they arise. Finally, this perspective has highlighted the complexity of this population and the importance of bio-psych-social and developmental perspectives. The challenge of research is to move from observation to understanding causality, and then to developing and implementing specific interventions. The prevention and treatment of the outward manifestations of what has become known as the 'behavioural phenotype of organic genetic disease' is increasingly a realistic possibility.

When a child or adult with an ID is referred because of concerns about their behaviour, the aim of any assessment is to identify the reasons for such behaviour, usually within the framework of one or more of the theoretical models described at the beginning of the chapter. The subsequent formulation should include a statement about whether the cause of the person's ID is known and if it is, whether or not the clinical picture might be wholly or partially explained by the known phenotype of the syndrome in question. If that is the case, this knowledge should inform subsequent assessments and guide intervention. Knowing the association of a specific syndrome to the frequent presence of, for example, an autistic spectrum disorder, can lead to the necessary assessments to determine whether this is the case or if it is, autism informed educational and support strategies may then be helpful.

The broader concept of behavioural phenotypes provides a useful research perspective when seeking to understand the relationship between genetic abnormalities and development. However, from a clinical perspective some associations may not be of clinical value at this point in time. For example, since Langdon Down first described Down syndrome, there has been an assumption that this group of people have a particularly happy demeanor. Such an observation may have little clinical utility in contrast to observations of the risk of dementia, or, for example, high anxiety, in people with Williams or fragile-X syndrome, or hyperphagia in people with Prader-Willi syndrome. It is the outward manifestation of those aspects of a behavioural phenotype that impacts on health, well-being, and/or quality of life that is the clinical problem to be addressed. However, from a treatment perspective, the endophenotype may provide the clues that both guide research into mechanisms and may also guide interventions. For example, the behavioural phenotype of self-injurious behaviour is characteristic of several different neurodevelopmental syndromes (63, 64) (e.g. Lesch Nyhan, fragile-X, Prader-Willi, Smith Magenis, Cornelia de Lange syndromes). In each syndrome there are considerable differences in the nature of the self-injurious behaviour, including its topography, the presence or absence of self-restraint, the age of onset, etc. In such cases the psychological and neurobiological underpinnings (endophenotypes) of the behaviour are likely to be very different, and there will be no single 'treatment' for self-injurious behaviour. Rather, further research will be needed and clinical skills required, to identify the causative mechanisms before interventions are developed and applied. Studies are seeking to establish the nature of these relationships and the underlying mechanisms and the implications for treatment (65). A striking example of causative mechanisms outside of the brain is oesophageal reflux in people with Cornelia de Lange syndrome. Someone with this syndrome may not be able to articulate his/her experience of pain and the onset of, or deterioration in, a specific pattern of self-injurious behaviour may be an indication of pain from reflux. In this case the treatment for self-injurious behaviour is treatment for the reflux (66).

Prader-Willi syndrome particularly illustrates the importance of behavioural phenotypes. First, the recognition that the hyperphagia has its basis in impairments in the neural circuits that underpin satiety has emphasized the importance of food security to prevent life-threatening obesity. Although there are no specific treatments for hyperphagia, treatment trials of agents acting on feeding pathways are underway (67). Secondly, studies in PWS have shown how investigations of cognitive abilities can inform intervention and how serendipitous observations can advance knowledge. Temper outbursts are common among children and adults with this syndrome. It has been argued that the characteristics of these outbursts are not dissimilar to those observed as part of typical development in early childhood (47). Woodcock et al (68) found that people with PWS have particular difficulties in switching attention to recruiting different areas of the brain than aged-matched typically developing people when asked to do such a task. They have argued that the cognitive demands required to switch attention causes anticipatory anxiety which, in turn, leads to repetitive questioning and ultimately to an outburst. Whilst the normal recommendations have been to try and support people with PWS in a predictable environment, Bull et al. (69) have proposed a different view as that approach may make things worse, that is, the use of strategies, such as a prompt card, to help those with PWS to better manage change (70). From a very different perspective, in a proof of concept trial using vagus nerve stimulation from an implanted device to try and improve the hyperphagia, it was found that, although eating behaviour did not change, unexpectedly temper tantrums were observed to be markedly reduced in number and severity (71). This would suggest that there may be an impairment of autonomic regulation and emotional control. Through the initial recognition of the association between this syndrome and temper outbursts, an understanding of the reasons are emerging and, as a result, psychological and other treatment approaches are being established. Thirdly, given that affective psychotic illness has been found to be common by early adult life, predominately in those with the rarer disomy (UPD) form of the syndrome, this alerts those providing support and clinicians as to this possibility. One small follow-up study has reported positive outcomes for the treatment of the psychotic illness (72).

Down syndrome and the high risk for dementia due to Alzheimer's disease is another example where this association is leading not only to better recognition of the problem but also to the possibility of preventative treatments (73). As described earlier, the use of neuroimaging and other techniques is giving rise to a better understanding of the role of amyloid deposition in the brain. At present knowledge of the particular risk for Alzheimer's disease in people with Down syndrome has led some services to advocate cognitive screening in nearly adult life to provide a baseline to enable the detection of later deterioration in cognitive and functional abilities and diagnostic instruments and guidance are available to support the making of an accurate diagnosis and informed support (74).

Conclusion

As research in this field has accumulated, some general clinical principles have become apparent, which guide thinking. First, a developmental perspective is essential, as particular behaviours in any given syndrome may develop at specific ages or developmental stages in the context of an already atypical pattern of development. For example, self-injurious behaviour in people with Lesch-Nyhan syndrome develops in very early childhood, as does the hyperphagia in people with PWS. However, in contrast, it is not until age 50 and over that the specific risk of dementia due to Alzheimer's disease first becomes apparent in people with Down syndrome. Secondly, from a research perspective, phenotypic and endophenotypic analysis needs to be fine grained. Terms such as aggression, self-injury, anxiety, obesity, etc. are insufficient. Self-injury, for example, may take many forms and may or may not be associated with self-restraint; anxiety may be generalized or specific. In each case the mechanisms underpinning the phenotype are likely to be different. Thirdly, having characterized the behavioural phenotype, it is an understanding of the cognitive and other characteristics of the endophenotype that will inform our understanding of causation and ultimately treatment. Fourthly, the concept of a behavioural phenotype in organic genetic disease is one perspective in helping to identify the reasons for challenging behaviour. Integration with other conceptual frameworks is essential, that is what is required from skilled clinicians. Finally, whilst research may identify key pathways to the behaviour associated with a particular neurodevelopmental syndrome, in any given individual with that syndrome there will be other inherent and acquired influences that affect how that behaviour presents and when. Knowing about a behavioural phenotype is no substitute for individual assessment and knowing the individual.

MULTIPLE CHOICE QUESTIONS

Questions

Please select the single most appropriate answer.

1. Lesch Nyhan syndrome is associated with all of the following except:

A. Hypotonia
B. Spasticity
C. Involuntary movements
D. Self-injurious behaviour
E. Aggression

2. Autistic spectrum traits are associated with:

A. Down syndrome
B. Fragile X syndrome
C. Cornelia de Lange syndrome
D. All of the above
E. None of the above

3. All of the following are endophenotypic markers except:

A. Abnormalities of attention and of theory of mind on psychometric testing in children with fragile-X syndrome
B. Neuroimaging finding of impaired satiety in people with Prader-Willi syndrome
C. Observed hyperphagia and self-injurious behaviour in people with Prader-Willi syndrome
D. Imaging findings of neural abnormalities in people with tuberous sclerosis
E. Abnormal neural response to food intake in people with Prader-Willi syndrome

4. Behavioural phenotype for Prader Will syndrome includes all of the following except:

A. Hyperphagia
B. Psychosis
C. Paroxysmal laughter
D. Mood disorders
E. Ritualistic behaviour

5. Velo-Cardio-Facial syndrome is associated with all of the following except:

A. ADHD
B. Psychosis
C. Affective disorders
D. A decreasing risk of neuropsychiatric disorder with age
E. A deletion on Chromosome 22

Answers

1. A. Hypertonia is observed in people with Lesch Nyhan Syndrome.
2. D. All the above syndrome, to varying degrees, have been reported to have increased rates of autistic spectrum disorder.
3. C. The features described in people with PWS are all apparent from observation or from the history whereas the others will only be fully apparent on formal assessment.
4. C. Paroxysmal laughter is associated with Angelman's syndrome not PWS. These two disorders are both associated with abnormalities on chromosome 15. The very different phenotypes are a consequence of different gender of origin imprinting of specific genes.
5. D. The risk of psychiatric disorder increases, not decreases, with age.

REFERENCES

1. Hopkins B, Geangu E, and Linkenauger S (Editors). *Cambridge Encyclopedia of Child Development*. Cambridge University Press. 2017.
2. Cooper SA, Smiley E, Morrison J, Williamson A, Allan L. Mental ill-health in adults with intellectual disabilities: prevalence and associated factors. *The British Journal of Psychiatry*. 2007;190(1):27–35.
3. Matson JL, Shoemaker M. Intellectual disability and its relationship to autism spectrum disorders. *Research in developmental disabilities*. 2009;30(6):1107–1114.
4. Baker BL, Blacher J, Crnic KA, Edelbrock C. Behavior problems and parenting stress in families of three-year-old children with and without developmental delays. *American Journal on Mental Retardation*. 2002;107(6):433–444.
5. Totsika V, Hastings RP, Emerson E, Lancaster GA, Berridge DM. A population-based investigation of behavioural and emotional

problems and maternal mental health: Associations with autism spectrum disorder and intellectual disability. *Journal of Child Psychology and Psychiatry*. 2011 1;52(1):91–99.
6. Woodman AC, Mawdsley HP, Hauser-Cram P. Parenting stress and child behavior problems within families of children with developmental disabilities: Transactional relations across 15 years. *Research in developmental disabilities*. 2015;36:264–276.
7. Iwata BA, Dorsey MF, Slifer KJ, Bauman KE, Richman GS. Toward a functional analysis of self-injury. *Journal of Applied Behavior Analysis*. 1994;27(2):197–209.
8. Lesch M, Nyhan WL. A familial disorder of uric acid metabolism and central nervous system function. *The American Journal of Medicine*. 1964;36(4):561–570.
9. Nyhan WL. Behavioral Phenotypes in organic genetic disease: Presidential Address to the Society for Pediatric Research, *Pediatric Research*. 1972;6:1–9.
10. Flint J. Annotation—behaviour phenotypes: A window on to the biology of behavior. *Journal of Child Psychology and Psychiatry*. 1996;37(4):355–367.
11. O'Brien G, editor. Behavioural phenotypes in clinical practice. *Cambridge University Press*. 2002.
12. Sahin M. Targeted treatment trials for tuberous sclerosis and autism: No longer a dream. *Current Opinion in Neurobiology*. 2012;22(5):895–901.
13. Jacquemont S, Berry-Kravis E, Hagerman R, Von Raison F, Gasparini F, Apostol G, Ufer M, Des Portes V, Gomez-Mancilla B. The challenges of clinical trials in fragile X syndrome. *Psychopharmacology*. 2014;231(6):1237–1250.
14. Harris JC. Behavioral phenotypes of neurodevelopmental disorders: Portals into the developing brain. Chapter in *Neuropsyhopharmacology: The fifth generation of progress*. Lippincott, Williams & Wilkins, Philadelphia. 1987.
15. Flint J and Yule W. Behavioural phenotypes. In: Rutter M, Taylor E, Hersov L. Editors. *Child and Adolescent Psychiatry: Modern Approaches*. 3rd edition. London: *Blackwell Scientific*. 1994, 666–687.
16. Kodituwakku PW. Defining the behavioral phenotype in children with fetal alcohol spectrum disorders: A review. *Neuroscience and Biobehavioral Reviews*. 2007;31(2):192–201.
17. Dykens EM. Measuring behavioral phenotypes: Provocations from the 'new genetics'. *American Journal on Mental Retardation*. 1995.
18. Minshawi NF, Hurwitz S, Fodstad JC, Biebl S, Morriss DH, McDougle CJ. The association between self-injurious behaviors and autism spectrum disorders. *Psychology Research and Behavior Management*. 2014;7:125.
19. Udwin O, Kuczynski A. Behavioural phenotypes in genetic syndromes associated with intellectual disability. *The Handbook of Intellectual Disability and Clinical Psychology Practice*. 2007:447–487.
20. Gottesman II, Gould TD. The endophenotype concept in psychiatry: Etymology and strategic intentions. *American Journal of Psychiatry*. 2003;160(4):636–645.
21. Walters JT, Owen MJ. Endophenotypes in psychiatric genetics. *Molecular psychiatry*. 2007;12(10):886.
22. Dykens EM. Anxiety, fears, and phobias in persons with Williams syndrome. *Developmental Neuropsychology*. 2003;23(12):291–316.
23. Boer H, Holland A, Whittington J, Butler J, Webb T, Clarke D. Psychotic illness in people with Prader Willi syndrome due to chromosome 15 maternal uniparental disomy. *The Lancet*. 2002;359(9301):135–136.
24. Shprintzen RJ. Velo-cardio-facial syndrome: 30 years of study. *Developmental Disabilities Research Reviews*. 2008;14(1):3–10.
25. Oliver C, Holland AJ. Down's syndrome and Alzheimer's disease: A review. *Psychological Medicine*. 1986;16(2):307–322.
26. Cornish K, Sudhalter V, Turk J. Attention and language in fragile X. *Developmental Disabilities Research Reviews*. 2004;10(1):11–16.
27. Cornish K, Burack JA, Rahman A, Munir F, Russo N, Grant C. Theory of mind deficits in children with fragile X syndrome. *Journal of Intellectual Disability Research*. 2005;49(5):372–378.
28. Hinton EC, Holland AJ, Gellatly MS, Soni S, Patterson M, Ghatei MA, Owen AM. Neural representations of hunger and satiety in Prader-Willi syndrome. *International Journal of Obesity*. 2006;30(2):313.
29. Grajkowska W, Kotulska K, Jurkiewicz E, Matyja E. Brain lesions in tuberous sclerosis complex. Review. *Folia neuropathologica*. 2010;48(3).
30. Luzzani S, Macchini F, Valade A, Milani D, Selicorni A. Gastroesophageal reflux and Cornelia de Lange syndrome: Typical and atypical symptoms. *American Journal of Medical Genetics* Part A. 2003119(3):283–287.
31. Fisher E, Scambler P. Human haploinsufficiency—one for sorrow, two for joy. *Nature Genetics*. 1994 May;7(1):5.
32. Grayton HM, Fernandes C, Rujescu D, Collier DA. Copy number variations in neurodevelopmental disorders. *Progress in Neurobiology*. 2012 ;99(1):81–91.
33. Leung AK, Robson WL. Tuberous sclerosis complex: A review. *Journal of Pediatric Health Care*. 2007;21(2):108–114.
34. Nature Insight: *Epigenetics*. 2007;447 (7143):396–440.
35. Telias M, Ben-Yosef D. Modeling neurodevelopmental disorders using human pluripotent stem cells. *Stem Cell Reviews and Reports*. 2014;10(4):494–511.
36. Moy SS, Nadler JJ. Advances in behavioral genetics: Mouse models of autism. *Molecular Psychiatry*. 2008;13(1):4.
37. Morris CA, Mervis CB. Williams syndrome and related disorders. *Annual Review of Genomics and Human Genetics*. 2000;1(1):461–484.
38. Wong DF, Harris JC, Naidu S, Yokoi F, Marenco S, Dannals RF, Ravert HT, Yaster M, Evans A, Rousset O, Bryan RN. Dopamine transporters are markedly reduced in Lesch-Nyhan disease in vivo. *Proceedings of the National Academy of Sciences*. 1996;93(11):5539–5543.
39. Morris CA, Mervis CB. Williams syndrome and related disorders. *Annual Review of Genomics and Human Genetics*. 2000;1(1):461–484.
40. Leyfer O, Woodruff-Borden J, Mervis CB. Anxiety disorders in children with Williams syndrome, their mothers, and their siblings: Implications for the etiology of anxiety disorders. *Journal of Neurodevelopmental Disorders*. 2009;1(1):4.
41. Järvinen-Pasley A, Bellugi U, Reilly J, Debra L, Galaburda A, Reiss AL, Korenberg JR. Defining the social phenotype in Williams syndrome: A model for linking gene, the brain, and behavior. *Development and Psychopathology*. 2008;20(1):1–35.
42. Jones W, Bellugi U, Lai Z, Chiles M, Reilly J, Lincoln A, Adolphs R. II. Hypersociability in Williams syndrome. *Journal of Cognitive Neuroscience*. 2000;12(Supplement 1):30–46.
43. Mervis CB, Klein-Tasman BP. Williams syndrome: Cognition, personality, and adaptive behavior. *Developmental Disabilities Research Reviews*. 2000;6(2):148–158.
44. Murphy KC, Jones LA, Owen MJ. High rates of schizophrenia in adults with velo-cardio-facial syndrome. *Archives of General Psychiatry*. 1999;56(10):940–945.

45. Murphy KC, Owen MJ. Velo-cardio-facial syndrome: A model for understanding the genetics and pathogenesis of schizophrenia. *The British Journal of Psychiatry*. 2001;179(5):397–402.
46. Butler JV, Whittington JE, Holland AJ, McAllister CJ, Goldstone AP. The transition between the phenotypes of Prader-Willi syndrome during infancy and early childhood. *Developmental Medicine and Child Neurology*. 2010 ;52(6).
47. Holland AJ, Whittington JE, Butler J, Webb T, Boer H, Clarke D. Behavioural phenotypes associated with specific genetic disorders: Evidence from a population-based study of people with Prader-Willi syndrome. *Psychological Medicine*. 2003;33(1):141–153.
48. Soni S, Whittington J, Holland AJ, Webb T, Maina E, Boer H, Clarke D. The course and outcome of psychiatric illness in people with Prader-Willi syndrome: implications for management and treatment. *Journal of Intellectual Disability Research*. 2007;51(1):32–42.
49. Soni S, Whittington J, Holland AJ, Webb T, Maina EN, Boer H, Clarke D. The phenomenology and diagnosis of psychiatric illness in people with Prader-Willi syndrome. *Psychological Medicine*. 2008;38(10):1505–1514.
50. Holsen LM, Zarcone JR, Chambers R, Butler MG, Bittel DC, Brooks WM, Thompson TI, Savage CR. Genetic subtype differences in neural circuitry of food motivation in Prader-Willi syndrome. *International Journal of Obesity*. 2009;33(2):273.
51. Tunnicliffe P, Woodcock K, Bull L, Oliver C, Penhallow J. Temper outbursts in Prader-Willi syndrome: Causes, behavioural and emotional sequence and responses by carers. *Journal of Intellectual Disability Research*. 2014 ;58(2):134–150.
52. Hall SS, Hustyi KM, Chui C, Hammond JL. Experimental functional analysis of severe skin-picking behavior in Prader-Willi syndrome. *Research in Developmental Disabilities*. 2014;35(10):2284–2292.
53. Klabunde M, Saggar M, Hustyi KM, Hammond JL, Reiss AL, Hall SS. Neural correlates of self-injurious behavior in Prader-Willi syndrome. *Human Brain Mapping*. 2015;36(10):4135–4143.
54. Miller JL, Angulo M. An open-label pilot study of N-acetylcysteine for skin-picking in Prader-Willi syndrome. *American Journal of Medical Genetics Part A*. 2014;164(2):421–424.
55. Aman L, Manning K, Whittington J, Holland A, (in press). A major genetic cause for affective psychotic illness: Mechanistic insights from Prader-Willi Syndrome. *Lancet Psychiatry*.
56. Holland AJ, Hon J, Huppert FA, Stevens F, Watson P. Population-based study of the prevalence and presentation of dementia in adults with Down's syndrome. *The British Journal of Psychiatry*. 1998;172(6):493–498.
57. McCarron M, McCallion P, Reilly E, Dunne P, Carroll R, Mulryan N. A prospective 20-year longitudinal follow-up of dementia in persons with Down syndrome. *Journal of Intellectual Disability Research*. 2017;61(9):843–852.
58. Goldgaber D, Lerman MI, McBride OW, Saffiotti U, Gajdusek DC. Characterization and chromosomal localization of a cDNA encoding brain amyloid of Alzheimer's disease. *Science*. 1987;235(4791):877–880.
59. Ball SL, Holland AJ, Treppner P, Watson PC, Huppert FA. Executive dysfunction and its association with personality and behaviour changes in the development of Alzheimer's disease in adults with Down syndrome and mild to moderate learning disabilities. *British Journal of Clinical Psychology*. 2008;47(1):1–29.
60. Handen BL, Cohen AD, Channamalappa U, Bulova P, Cannon SA, Cohen WI, Mathis CA, Price JC, Klunk WE. Imaging brain amyloid in nondemented young adults with Down syndrome using Pittsburgh compound B. *Alzheimer's and Dementia: The Journal of the Alzheimer's Association*. 2012;8(6):496–501.
61. Annus T, Wilson LR, Hong YT, Acosta-Cabronero J, Fryer TD, Cardenas-Blanco A, Smith R, Boros I, Coles JP, Aigbirhio FI, Menon DK. The pattern of amyloid accumulation in the brains of adults with Down syndrome. *Alzheimer's and Dementia: The Journal of the Alzheimer's Association*. 2016;12(5):538–545.
62. Annus T, Wilson LR, Acosta-Cabronero J, Cardenas-Blanco A, Hong YT, Fryer TD, Coles JP, Menon DK, Zaman SH, Holland AJ, Nestor PJ. The Down syndrome brain in the presence and absence of fibrillar β-amyloidosis. *Neurobiology of Aging*. 2017;53:11–19.
63. Arron K, Oliver C, Moss J, Berg K, Burbidge C. The prevalence and phenomenology of self-injurious and aggressive behaviour in genetic syndromes. *Journal of Intellectual Disability Research*. 2011;55(2):109–120.
64. Huisman S, Mulder P, Kuijk J, Kerstholt M, van Eeghen A, Leenders A, van Balkom I, Oliver C, Piening S, Hennekam R. Self-injurious behavior. *Neuroscience and Biobehavioral Reviews*. 2017.
65. Waite J, Heald M, Wilde L, Woodcock K, Welham A, Adams D, Oliver C. The importance of understanding the behavioural phenotypes of genetic syndromes associated with intellectual disability. *Paediatrics and Child Health*. 2014;24(10):468–472.
66. Oliver C, Arron K, Hall S, Sloneem J. The behavioural phenotype of Cornelia de Lange syndrome. *The British Journal of Psychiatry*. 2008;193:466–470.
67. Miller JL, Strong TV, Heinemann J. Medication trials for hyperphagia and food-related behaviors in Prader-Willi syndrome. *Diseases*. 2015-;3(2):78–85.
68. Woodcock KA, Oliver C, Humphreys GW. Task-switching deficits and repetitive behaviour in genetic neurodevelopmental disorders: Data from children with Prader-Willi syndrome chromosome 15 q11-q13 deletion and boys with Fragile X syndrome. *Cognitive Neuropsychology*. 2009;26(2):172–194.
69. Bull LE, Oliver C, Callaghan E, Woodcock KA. Increased exposure to rigid routines can lead to increased challenging behavior following changes to those routines. *Journal of Autism and Developmental Disorders*. 2015;45(6):1569–1578.
70. Bull LE, Oliver C, Woodcock KA. Signalling changes to individuals who show resistance to change can reduce challenging behaviour. *Journal of Behavior Therapy and Experimental Psychiatry*. 2017;54:58–70.
71. Manning KE, McAllister CJ, Ring HA, Finer N, Kelly CL, Sylvester KP, Fletcher PC, Morrell NW, Garnett MR, Manford MR, Holland AJ. Novel insights into maladaptive behaviours in Prader-Willi syndrome: Serendipitous findings from an open trial of vagus nerve stimulation. *Journal of Intellectual Disability Research*. 2016;60(2):149–155.
72. Larson FV, Whittington J, Webb T, Holland AJ. A longitudinal follow-up study of people with Prader-Willi syndrome with psychosis and those at increased risk of developing psychosis due to genetic subtype. *Psychological Medicine*. 2014;44(11):2431–2435.
73. Castro P, Zaman S, Holland A. Alzheimer's disease in people with Down's syndrome: The prospects for and the challenges of developing preventative treatments. *Journal of Neurology*. 2017;264(4):804–813.
74. Royal College of Psychiatrists and British Psychological Society. Guidance on the assessment, diagnosis, treatment and support of people with learning disabilities who develop dementia. CR196, Co-published by *The British Psychological Society and the Royal College of Psychiatrists*. 2015.

24

Visual and Hearing Impairments and their Impact on the Mental Health of Adults with Intellectual Disability

Reza Kiani and Sugato Bhaumik

Introduction

Intellectual Disability (ID) is a lifelong condition with the onset in the developmental age consisting of global impairment of intellectual, adaptive and social functioning. Although there is variation in reporting, a meta-analysis of 52 studies (1), reported an overall ID prevalence of 10.37/1000, with the highest rates seen in low- and middle-income countries, children, and in those studies that used psychological assessments for case identification.

The Government's 2001 White Paper '*Valuing People*', specifically for people with ID, initiated a commitment to inclusion and enabled people with ID to 'make use of mainstream services' (2). Since then, a number of policy initiatives have focused on the need to improve access to generic services for people with ID, so that they remain independent and integrated in their communities without suffering from social isolation.

The provision of high-quality healthcare for people with ID is a national priority, as highlighted by '*Valuing People Now*' (3). The follow-up report to '*Death by Indifference*', '*Six Lives: The Provision of Public Services to People with Learning Disabilities*' (4), raised serious questions and concerns about how well-equipped the NHS and local authorities were to plan for and provide services tailored to the needs of people with ID.

The Department of Health (5) has made it explicit that all healthcare providers should make reasonable adjustments to service delivery to meet the complex needs of vulnerable groups of service users in accordance with the Equality Act. Following one of the recommendations of the '*Healthcare for All*' (5), the Learning Disabilities Observatory was established to provide better and more accessible information on the health of people with ID. The observatory aims to help hospitals and other providers to better understand the complex needs of people with ID and their carers which, in turn, should improve outcomes for this vulnerable client group (6).

A better understanding of the challenges and barriers (Box 24.1) (7) to the delivery of better healthcare to people with ID will, therefore, enable clinicians to assess and treat various health difficulties in people with ID more effectively.

Visual and hearing impairments are more commonly seen in those with ID than the general population, and therefore reasonable adjustments for these groups of individuals are important to consider. Professional teams, at best, have few professionals with very basic awareness and knowledge of communicating with individuals with ID who have accompanying visual and hearing impairment. Furthermore, teams usually do not include professionals with sensory impairment, or those who have a working knowledge of blindness and/or deafness and know how to facilitate access to appropriate services (8).

People with ID and sensory impairments have complex needs, which can be missed in clinical practice owing to diagnostic overshadowing and lack of awareness and training on the part of the healthcare professionals (Box 24.1).

This chapter will describe the prevalence and clinical presentations of visual and hearing impairments in people with ID and their impact on psychosocial development and mental health. It will also provide information on the management strategies and the necessary reasonable adjustments appropriate for these individuals that will be needed for improved service delivery.

Epidemiology of sensory impairment in people with ID

Hearing impairment

Hearing impairment is the most common sensory disorder in humans, with approximately 1–2 per 1000 children born deaf or developing deafness during early childhood (9, 10, 11, 12, 13).

In the UK, 1 in 7–8 people (over 10 million) have a hearing loss, and there are around 45,000 children who are deaf. Effective communication in the healthcare setting is, therefore, a priority for people with hearing impairment (14, 15). Degree of hearing impairment

Box 24.1 Barrier to accessing services by people with Intellectual Disability (ID)

Barriers related to service users

- Comorbid physical disability, physical and mental ill health, and autism.
- Severity of ID and communication difficulties.
- Atypical presentation of physical ailments through changes in behaviour.
- Fear of hospital and investigation.
- Some people with ID might not understand the importance of their symptoms or hide them from healthcare professionals for a variety of reasons.

Barriers related to service provision

- Lack of accessible/pictorial information.
- Underfunding/lack of resources.
- Poor access to the clinics and general hospitals.
- Environmental barriers (e.g. lack of user friendly sign postings).
- Disconnection between teams (social and health services).
- Not taking into consideration needs of individuals with special needs for appointments (e.g. no flexible appointments, no waiting time for someone with autism, not offering a quiet waiting area etc.).

Barriers related to healthcare professionals and carers

- Attitudes and assumptions.
- Individuals with disability considered as low priority.
- Lack of awareness and training.
- Institutional discrimination.
- Marginalized status of sensory work.

can be classified by audiometry (Table 24.1), which measures the intensity of a sound (decibel; dB) required for someone to hear at a particular frequency (Hertz; Hz). A person with normal hearing ability can hear sounds as low as 0–20 dB (a whisper is about 10–20 dB) (16, 17, 18, 19).

Prevalence of hearing impairment is considerably higher in individuals with ID compared with the general population. One study found a prevalence of 3.4 per cent for severe to profound deafness in 18,657 people with ID in England and Wales (Kropka, 1984) (20). Another study at the *German Special Olympics Summer Games 2006* showed a high proportion of undetected hearing impairment, even among those with a mild or moderate ID who were otherwise physically fit (21).

Visual impairment

According to the World Health Organization (WHO), a visual acuity of less than 0.3 (a normal visual acuity is 1.0) or a visual field of below 30 degrees (a normal visual field is 180 degrees) is an indicator of visual impairment (22). Blindness is an inability to see with a visual acuity of less than 3/60 and a visual field of fewer than 10 degrees (23).

While the prevalence of visual impairment has been reported to be 0.5–2.0 per cent in the general population (22), a number of studies have shown that this is several times higher in people with ID (24, 25).

Evenhuis (26, 27) reported that the prevalence of visual impairment was at least 10 times higher in people with ID compared with the general population. Similarly, van Splunder (28) and van Splunder et al. (29, 30) found that 5 per cent of people with ID in Holland were blind and 14 per cent were partially sighted.

The estimated prevalence of blindness and partial sightedness in the adult ID population has been reported to be 9.3 per cent (31).

Table 24.1 Degree of hearing impairment based on audiogram

Degree of hearing impairment	Hearing loss in decibel (dB)
Mild	20–39
Moderate	40–69
Severe	70–94 (difficulty even with a hearing aid)
Profound	>95 (no perception)

Conjoined visual and hearing impairments

It is estimated that there are about 365,000 people with some level of combined hearing and sight loss in the UK (31). The prevalence of deaf-blindness is about 1 in 10,000 in school-age children in the UK (32). The aetiologies of deaf-blindness are usually extreme prematurity, congenital rubella syndrome, meningo-encephalitis, Usher and other rare genetic syndromes, for example, CHARGE syndrome. Approximately 40–50 per cent of congenitally blind children have additional disability, including hearing impairment and ID (33). One visual screening programme of deaf students found that almost half (48 per cent) also had significant eye problems (34). A study in the USA reported that 27 per cent of their deaf and hard-of-hearing students (6–19 years old) had additional disabilities, for example, ID 9 per cent and visual impairment 4 per cent (35).

Most cases of deaf-blindness in people with severe to profound ID could easily go undetected if no objective assessment tools were used (36). Fellinger et al. (36) reported a rise in the prevalence of deaf-blindness from 3.6 per cent to 21.4 per cent in their study population of adults with ID (n = 224) following completion of objective assessments for both hearing and visual impairment.

Deaf-blindness has a huge impact on cognitive, psychosocial, and language development to the extent that the behavioural and social manifestations can be very similar to ASD (37). Deaf-blind people are highly reliant on carers to actively participate in activities; therefore, interventions to engage this group of service users in social interaction and to promote their independence are extremely important to avoid isolation and social exclusion (38).

For more information on this subject readers are advised to look at a literature review by the National Deaf Children's Society published in 2012 (www.ndcs.org.uk/professional_support/news/healthy_minds.html).

Factors that influence the prevalence of sensory impairment

Age

Using data from a New York register of 45,000 adults (aged 35 years and older) with ID, Janicki and Dalton (39) found that prevalence of hearing impairment increased significantly with age. Thus, studies on older sample populations yield higher prevalence estimates of

Table 24.2 Examples of genetic syndromes associated with sensory impairment

Genetic syndrome	Examples of signs and symptoms
Alport	Kidney abnormalities, deafness, ocular abnormalities
CHARGE	Coloboma, heart defects, atresia choanae, retardation of growth, ear anomalies, deaf-blindness
Coffin Lowry	Hypotonia and short stature, hearing impairment
Jervell and Lange-Nielson	Fainting and long QT interval in ECG, deafness
Klippel Feil	Short webbed neck, visual and hearing impairment
MELAS	Myopathy, encephalitis, lactic acidosis, and stroke, associated with hearing impairment
Neurofibromatosis	Café au lait spots, visual and hearing impairment
Pendred	Hypothyroidism, deafness
Stickler	Joint hyperflexibility, cataract, glaucoma and retinal detachment, visual and hearing impairment
Treacher Collins	Facial dysmorphology and coloboma, visual and hearing impairment
Usher	Retinitis pigmentosa, deaf-blindness
Waardenburg	Blue iris and white forelock, deafness
Down	Heart and digestive system defects, visual and hearing impairment

sensory impairment (40, 26, 27); for example, studies in Holland reported a prevalence of 16.7 per cent for blindness and 67 per cent for partial visual impairment in adults with Down syndrome who were aged 50 years or over (28, 29, 30).

Degree of ID

The more severe the degree of ID, the higher would be the prevalence of sensory impairment (16, 22).

Study population

Studies using ID case registers, inpatient units or on those in receipt of specialist social and healthcare services are unable to accurately measure the prevalence of mild ID in the general population. However, such studies tend to comprise a representative sample of people with moderate to profound ID because they have additional support and healthcare needs (41). Therefore, studies in this population tend to render relatively high prevalence rates of sensory impairment.

Methods of case ascertainment

Warburg (24) found that the concordance rate in diagnosing visual impairment between carers' report (questionnaire) and objective clinical assessment was less than one-third (32 per cent). Similarly, it has been reported that the prevalence of hearing impairment is lower if cases are identified by subjective reports from carers (9.4 per cent), as opposed to objective clinical assessments (38.9 per cent) (42).

Ethnicity

Deafness and blindness may be more prevalent among the immigrant population. This can be a consequence of marriage within close family networks, greater chance of poverty and inadequate access to healthcare and immunization in this population (43, 14, 44).

Aetiology of sensory impairment

In addition to usual causes of visual impairment (e.g. cataract, glaucoma, diabetic retinopathy, etc.) and hearing impairment (e.g. related to noise exposure, ageing, and chronic infection, etc.), there are other specific conditions that cause both ID and sensory impairment (Table 24.2) such as Waardenburg syndrome, Usher syndrome, Down syndrome, and congenital rubella syndrome (45, 46, 47, 48). The aetiology of hearing impairment, based on whether it is congenital or acquired, ranges from genetic conditions to infectious causes (43). Approximately half of cases of congenital deafness are due to genetic causes, mainly recessive genes (e.g. gene GJB2 for Connexin 26 protein) (49, 50), mitochondrial syndromes (e.g. MELAS syndrome, MERRF syndrome and Kearns-Sayre syndrome), and other genetic syndromes (51, 52, 53).

Cerebral palsy (CP) is another cause of sensory impairment and ID. CP occurs in approximately two per 1,000 live births in developed countries, and is an umbrella term used for a group of conditions that cause movement problems, ID, epilepsy, and sensory impairment (54).

Structural anomalies of sensory organs, such as narrowed ear canals and Keratoconus, are common in people with Down syndrome. As a result, age-related hearing loss (presbycusis) occurs several decades earlier in people with Down syndrome compared with the general population (55, 56, 57). Adults with Down syndrome have anomalies of the ear, with a predisposition to infection, which needs aggressive treatment to avoid irreversible hearing loss (58). Hearing impairment due to impacted earwax is relatively common. A study on people with Down syndrome also found that 57 per cent of those aged 35–62 had a bilateral loss greater than 40dB and only 25 per cent had been diagnosed before the study (16).

Usher syndrome is one of the most common causes of deaf-blindness in adults, causing 5–10 per cent of cases of deafness, 18 per cent of cases of retinitis pigmentosa and visual impairment, and over 50 per cent of cases of deaf-blindness. The prevalence in the general population is 3–5 per 100,000 (59). Usher syndrome causes gradual loss of vision due to progressive retinitis pigmentosa. Retinitis pigmentosa, which is essential for diagnosis, can be confirmed by electro-retinography. The visual impairment usually starts with night blindness during adolescence and progresses to tunnel vision and blindness. Rubella in pregnancy can cause sensorineural deafness, central auditory imperceptions, visual impairment, and developmental delay, all of which may be under-diagnosed in people with ID. Chess (45, 60) and Chess et al. (61) studied 243 preschool children with congenital rubella syndrome and found that 37 per cent had ID, 15 per cent had reactive behaviour disorder, and 7 per cent had autism. When followed up at the age of 8–9 years, the prevalence of ID had decreased; however, challenging behaviours (i.e. behavioural problems) had increased owing to neurological damage. The authors also reported new cases of autism spectrum disorder (ASD) and few remissions at follow up and hypothesized that the course of ASD was that of a chronic infection, with remission and delayed emergence of symptoms. In an update of the literature on congenital rubella, Berger and colleagues (62) concluded that the measles, mumps, and rubella (MMR) vaccine had, between 2001 and 2010, prevented several thousand cases of ASD, ID, and sensory impairment in the USA. In addition to the above, it is recognized in the literature that other adverse events during pregnancy can also cause sensory impairment and ASD including infection with cytomegalovirus (63).

Clinical assessment of sensory impairment

An undiagnosed sensory impairment in people with ID may impair their ability to carry out activities of daily living (64). One study showed that 39 per cent of people with ID received less eye care than those in the general population (65). Another study reported that 30 per cent of people with ID and hearing impairment had never had their hearing tested (66). Deficits in communication in people with ID pose a significant challenge to the assessment of sensory impairment. In practice, diagnostic overshadowing may occur, whereby changes in behaviour and loss of skill may be attributed to ID, dementia, or a mental illness rather than to a sensory impairment. In such cases, the underlying health needs of an individual may not be addressed and treated appropriately and accurately (67). Carers may perceive a person to be non-cooperative when, in reality, they cannot hear or see properly; alternatively, some people will try to cover up their sensory loss which can be misinterpreted by carers, leading to statements such as 'he can hear/see when he wants to' (68). Therefore, when there is a clinical suspicion of a visual or hearing impairment, it is extremely important that a referral is made to the speech and language therapist colleagues for an initial assessment of communication skills and development of an individualized communication passport.

McGlade et al. (69) reported that for a quarter of their cases with ID, they needed three or more sessions to complete their optician assessment, reflecting the complexity of the client group. Over 50 per cent of their study population needed glasses for refractive error. It is therefore imperative that adults with ID have access to specialist sensory assessment in order to help with the identification of sensory impairment, which may go unrecognized by carers. Furthermore, it is vitally important to ensure that carers have training in blind and deaf awareness and are able to access appropriate aids (hearing aids or eye glasses) and environmental adaptations if needed. Training carers and staff can help them to identify sensory impairment, which can then be followed up by specialist assessment. Specialist assessment can provide service users and carers with information on what a service user can and cannot see or hear; it also ensures that they have access to appropriate aids and services (70, 71).

Yeates (72, 73, 74) found that, given access to specialist audiology services, 56 per cent of adults with ID were able to complete a pure tone audiometery. She concluded that people with a deficit or lack of linguistic abilities should not be considered as unable to benefit from diagnosis of their hearing loss. She also emphasized that it would be ideal for adults with ID to have access to specialist audiology services, as generic audiology services are too busy to meet these service users' needs. Meuwese-Jongejeugd and colleagues (56, 75) set up a prospective study of a new audiological rehabilitation programme designed to meet the needs of people with ID with a recently diagnosed hearing loss. They implemented a detailed, well-thought and thorough multidisciplinary protocol for audiological rehabilitation in ID and audiological services. Even with all this in place, they were able to rehabilitate successfully only three of 31 adults with ID, because they found that screening adults with ID revealed a huge amount of unmet needs for which services were not ready, and that rehabilitation required coordinated work between different agencies and professionals. They concluded that, for successful rehabilitation, there should be changes in both.

If it is decided that an individual needs to undergo specialist assessment, the process of desensitization and preparation should be started as soon as possible. By law, hospitals are required to make reasonable adjustments for people with ID to access health services. This includes access to hearing and visual services. More information on this topic is provided on the Public Health England website (6). Boxes 24.2, 24.3 and 24.4 provide further details on assessing individuals with sensory impairment. The following provision of information is extremely helpful if used well in advance to prepare service users for their appointment:

- Use of illustrated information leaflets, audio materials or information in Braille and other alternative communication strategies to take into account sensory impairment, before attending audiology or ophthalmology clinic.
- Use of text and audio messages.
- Information in DVD or CD format.
- Role play

Box 24.2 Points to consider when taking a service user's history to assess visual and hearing impairment*

- Family history of sensory deficits and genetic disorders.
- History of kernicterus, peri-natal asphyxia, and in utero exposure to TORCHES (Toxoplasmosis, Other infections, Rubella, CMV, Herpes Simplex, and Syphilis).
- Childhood history of meningo-encephalitis.
- Developmental milestones.
- Any recent change in behaviour.
- Previous injury to ears/eyes.
- Discharge, itchiness and pain in sensory organs.
- Problems with earwax.
- Dizziness, vertigo, loss of balance, and tinnitus.
- Double vision or blurred vision.
- Previous assessments and provision of hearing aids or eyeglasses.
- Past operations on sensory organs.
- Past or current use of medication affecting sensory organs (e.g. aminoglycosides).
- Motor abnormalities.

Adapted from *Oxford Desk Reference: Clinical Genetics*, Firth H, Hurst J, Hall, J (eds), 2005.

Box 24.3 Assessment of visual impairment

Examples of functional assessment

- External appearance of the eyes (coloboma, squint).
- Abnormal eye movements.
- Watching from angle of eyes.
- Head tilting.
- Finger flicking in front of the eyes.
- Eye poking.
- Bringing objects very close to eyes.
- Not recognizing familiar faces.
- Groping to find things.
- Preference for bright objects.
- Bumping into things.
- Difficulty using steps.
- Not looking confident when walking.

Examples of specialist assessment

- Visual acuity tests*.
- Visual field tests.
- Ophthalmoscopy.
- Contrast sensitivity tests.
- Binocular vision tests.

*During examination of visual acuity, Kay pictures (http://www.kaypictures.co.uk/) and the Cardiff Acuity Test (preferential looking pictures) can be used instead of the Snellen chart: http://www.cardiff.ac.uk/optom/eyeclinic/downssyndromegroup/thecardiffacuitytest.html.

History taking in acquired hearing loss, or when a hearing impairment deteriorates, includes determining: (i) whether the hearing loss is unilateral or bilateral, sudden onset or gradual, fluctuating or progressive; (ii) whether it is associated with symptoms such as vertigo, tinnitus etc. and (iii) its effect on quality of life, communication/work, and family life (76).

Clinical examination should include examining external ears, wax impaction, tympanic membrane, head and neck, and then cranial nerve examination. The whispered voice test is a very simple screening test and can be used at arm's length behind the service user, occluding the contra-lateral ear. Tuning fork (512 Hz) test can also be used (Rinne and Weber tests) to distinguish between conductive hearing loss (CHL) and sensorineural hearing loss (SNHL) (76).

The same principles could be adopted when assessing a visual impairment (Box 24.3). The invisible nature of some of these problems often complicates investigation in people with ID. For example, in this population there is also a high prevalence of central (cortical) auditory processing disorders, which are difficult to diagnose in a person with an otherwise normal ear anatomy and structure (77). People with central auditory processing problems may not be recognized as having hearing difficulties because they do not have trouble detecting sound or recognizing speech in ideal listening situations. Since they appear to 'hear normally', the difficulties these individuals experience are often assumed to be the result of an attention deficit, a behaviour problem, lack of motivation, or depression. For more information on this subject please refer to a review article by Hitoglou et al. (78).

Health guidelines, published by the International Association for the Scientific Study of ID (IASSID) (79) recommend that specialist screening for age-related visual and hearing loss in people with ID, especially in those with Down syndrome, should be started at an earlier age and on a regular basis thereafter. For more details on the assessment of sensory impairment in people with ID, refer to (80) and the Health Guidelines published by the IASSID (79).

People with ID are able to express their wishes and ideas regarding hearing aids, provided that they are given sufficient information tailored to their cognitive abilities. Several elements (e.g. cosmetics, sound quality, and comfort/ease of use) may play a role in satisfaction with hearing aids (82, 56, 75), but research shows that while 70 per cent of the service users had been seen by audiology services at some time in their life, only 24 per cent had ongoing assessments and hearing-aid maintenance (66). The latter study also showed that only 20 per cent of them wore their hearing aids regularly and that only 2 per cent of care home staff had received training on maintaining hearing aids despite the positive effect of hearing aids on communication and behavior. Boxes 24.5 and 24.6 show the reasons for and ways to improve non-compliance with wearing hearing aids and glasses (81, 82).

Box 24.4 Assessment of hearing impairment*

Examples of functional assessment

- Size and shape of the ears (absent or very small ears).
- Talking unusually loudly or in a whisper.
- Not taking notice of prolonged or loud noises such as fire alarms.
- Startled by people approaching who are not in sight.
- Liking TV/radio on louder than normal.
- Responding only to certain voices (inconsistent in response).
- Misunderstanding instructions.
- Covering, poking, slapping ears.
- Experimenting with noises.
- Getting close to sounds.

Examples of specialist assessment

- Otoscopy.
- Pure tone audiometry.
- Warble tone audiometer.
- McCormick Toy Discrimination Test.
- South London Object Test.
- Tympanometry.
- Otoacoustic emission.
- Brainstem evoked response.

Adapted from: Hindley P and Kitson N, *Mental health and deafness*,2000; Austen S and Crocker S (eds), *Deafness in mind: working psychologically with deaf people across the life span*, 2004.

Box 24.5 Reasons* for non-compliance with hearing aids or eyeglasses

- Badly fitting or painful device.
- Broken or lost device.
- Poorly maintained device.
- Ineffectual device owing to wrong assessment/diagnosis.
- Feeling stigmatized.
- Teasing by others.

Adapted from: Austen S, Crocker S (eds), *Deafness in mind: working psychologically with deaf people across the life span*, 2004.

Box 24.6 Ways* to improve compliance with hearing aids and eyeglasses

- Allow clients to choose their preferred model and colour.
- Gradually extend usage from one setting to another.
- Give the client the responsibility for using and cleaning them.
- Positive reinforcement and lots of praise.
- Integrate devices into everyday life.
- Establish a routine around them.
- Practice role-play and modelling.

Adapted from: Austen S, Crocker S (eds), *Deafness in mind: working psychologically with deaf people across the life span*, 2004.

Impact of sensory impairments on psychosocial development and mental health

People with sensory impairment do suffer from a whole range of mental health problems commonly seen in the general population; however, they are more vulnerable to develop certain categories of mental health disorders.

Association with neurodevelopmental disorders

ASD is highly prevalent in individuals with ID compared with the general population (83). Prevalence rates vary between 8 per cent and 27 per cent (84, 85, 86, 87, 88), depending on diagnostic criteria used and ID severity in the sample population. ASD is more prevalent as the severity of ID increases (85, 89, 90) and in men, although the sex differences do not appear to be as pronounced as in the general population (89, 90). Pre-lingual and profound sensory deficits are reported to adversely affect acquisition of theory of mind and abstract thinking, either independently or through accompanying brain damage, which might result in ASD/autistic-like symptoms (71, 37).

Hearing impairment and ASD

Delayed access to sign language in deaf children has negative impacts on language development and this, along with loss of access to incidental learning, are known to affect cognitive abilities, development of theory of mind and social problem solving adversely (91, 92, 93, 94, 95, 96). Children with an existing ID are at a higher risk of such developmental delays (97, 98).

This might explain why ASD has been reported higher in congenitally deaf children (99, 100). In contrast, in deaf children who are born in deaf families where the parents are signing, or in those who are born to hearing families where parents have learned to sign, theory of mind develops normally (101, 102, 103, 95, 96).

A number of studies describing the relationship between ASD and deafness have reported different results. For example, in 1999, Rosenhall et al. (104) reported on the presence of hearing impairment in those with a diagnosis of ASD and found that 9.5 per cent (19 out of 199 autistic children) had a hearing impairment. In 1991, Jure (99) and colleagues reported a 4 per cent prevalence of ASD (n = 46) in a sample of 1,150 children with hearing impairment, with a male to female ratio of 2:1. They reported that this comorbidity had led to a delay of approximately several years in diagnosis of either condition. Jure and colleagues (99) showed that one-third of their sample (35%) had accompanying visual impairment. The authors also found a relationship between the degree of ID (not degree of deafness) and prevalence of ASD, therefore it was argued that the high prevalence of ASD reported was mediated through accompanying brain damage (a literature review on the following website provides more information on this topic: http://www.aucd.org/).

The 2009–10 Annual Survey of Deaf and Hard of Hearing Children and Youth in the US reported a comorbidity of ASD with hearing impairment at an approximate rate of 1.9 per cent (105). Kancherla et al. (106) using data from the population-based Metropolitan Atlanta Developmental Disabilities Surveillance Program, reported a co-existing diagnosis of ASD in approximately 6–7 per cent of 8-years-old children with hearing and visual impairment.

In 2004, Kielinen et al. (107) carried out a population-based survey among 152,732 Finnish children and adolescents aged less than 16 years and found that 187 of them fulfilled DSM-IV criteria for a diagnosis of ASD. They reported that 8.6 per cent of their autistic sample had a hearing impairment and 3.7 per cent of children with ASD had severe accompanying visual impairment.

In brief, children with congenital deafness may present with symptoms very similar to ASD (93, 94, 95, 108) but in congenital deafness, the main psychopathology is insufficient access to language exposure, while in ASD the main psychopathology seems to be genetically/neurologically determined (96, 103, 109). It is therefore paramount for those who embark on assessing ASD in congenitally deaf people to have a specialist knowledge of the normal development, communication skills, sign language, and behavioural characteristics of this population, so that in clinical practice misdiagnosis and inappropriate management strategies are avoided (93, 94, 95, 96, 110, 111, 112).

Visual impairment and ASD

Congenitally blind children also miss out on incidental learning. Blind children have basic difficulties in knowing about the existence, nature, and permanence of objects and their relationships (113). They cannot see others, therefore they face a challenge to internalize what is happening around them and to understand the actions of others and their roles (71, 113, 114, 115, 116, 117, 118, 119).

Blind children are usually delayed in perceiving the holistic picture of the environment around them, as they are limited to their other senses to experience things from a close distance, whereas sighted children experience these things quickly from a distance without any need to learn. Blind children, therefore, need to learn sequentially, slowly and step-by-step (113, 120, 121).

Congenitally blind children could therefore present with symptoms similar to ASD (71, 117, 118, 122, 123, 124). Although common in congenitally blind children, these symptoms do not amount to a formal ASD diagnosis and were known in the literature as 'blindism' (125, 126). Warren (127) described blindism as a result of somatosensory deprivation and social isolation in congenitally blind children.

Studies of speech development in blind children and autistic sighted children have shown that both groups use highly imitative, repetitive, and stereotypical (modelled) speech, known as echolalia (117, 118, 123, 128, 129, 130, 131). However, in blind children without accompanying disabilities, this modelled speech seems to be more meaningful and positively related to language development in serving a communication purpose (118, 132).

In the majority of cases, however, blind children overcome these difficulties over time, albeit with delay, by compensating blindness with other senses (118). However, in some children with blindness there is a significant degree of qualitative impairments in social and language skills that might qualify for a diagnosis of ASD (133, 124, 71).

Although some researchers argue that a congenital lack of visual experience early on in life causes an autistic-like presentation that is qualitatively different from the neurologically determined ASD (or Kanner's autism), it is quite challenging to ascertain with certainty whether these features in blind children are due to classical autism or are directly as a result of a pre-lingual visuo-social deprivation. One of the main reasons behind this controversy is the fact that any research on development of theory of mind or ASD in congenitally blind children is extremely difficult to carry out (134, 135).

There is also presence of an accompanying brain damage in congenital blindness that makes studying its association with ASD development a challenge. For example, in 2014, Begeer et al. (136) showed that performances of children with congenital blindness who had accompanying damage to their central nervous system (n = 22), were delayed compared with children with congenital blindness without an accompanying neurological deficit (n = 9) and sighted children (n = 103) on theory of mind tasks.

The association of congenital blindness and ASD/autistic-like features has also been noted in congenital blindness due to various neurological conditions, for example, congenital rubella syndrome (45, 60, 61).

Cass et al. (137) studied 102 infants with congenital blindness and found that 11 per cent showed set-back in their development. Nearly one-third (31%) of those with profound visual impairment (10 out of 32) developed a developmental set-back at 15–27 months, compared with 1 in 72 of children with severe visual impairment (those who had form vision) who developed the developmental set-back. The set-back phenomenon occurred regardless of the aetiology of congenital blindness but was related to its severity (138). The authors concluded that even slight form vision, particularly where present from the first few months of life, seemed to be a protective factor for developmental set-back. Other risk factors reported for this developmental set-back were the number of lesions in the brain magnetic resonance imaging (MRI), failure in or lack of the brain myelination process (139) degree of abnormal connectivity (140), ID, deprivation of visual input negatively affecting the functional systems of the brain (138), and qualitative factors within the family environment (138, 141). Given the latter risk factor, it has been suggested that early intervention starting within the first two years of life might be beneficial to improve development (137, 138, 140, 142). However, it has been argued that this reversibility cannot take place with a neurodevelopmental condition such as ASD, as symptoms by definition have a life-long course (117, 118). Perez-Pereira and Conti-Ramsden (118) argued that the majority of blind children studied by Cass et al. (137) were not autistic and those who had ASD had additional disabilities such as brain damage and ID. They concluded therefore that visual impairment per se did not cause the autistic symptoms.

On the other hand, some researchers argued that a pure blindness (i.e. without accompanying brain damage) could be an independent risk factor for ASD. For example, in 1977, Fraiberg (125) suggested that some of the autistic symptoms seen in congenitally blind service users were as a result of gross impoverishment in the development of sensorimotor skills.

In 1997, Brown and colleagues (143) carried out a study at several special schools for blind children and found out that the majority had autistic-like features. The authors subsequently compared nine of these children with nine sighted autistic children who had been matched on age and IQ (all had IQ<70) and determined that blind children had autistic-like symptoms that were qualitatively different in comparison to the sighted autistic children. They reported that blindness had added to the ASD symptomatology. According to Hobson and Bishop (144) and Hobson (145, 146) there are several explanations as why this might be the case: one of the reasons is an inability to see the physical characteristics of the items or people. Blind children also struggle to have mutual conversations because of their inability to see and read non-verbal cues. They are unaware of events, items, and other peoples' attitudes towards each other and themselves and how things are being experienced by others because it is impossible for them to see other people. This makes it very challenging for them during their development to learn how to relate to others and understand how other people's point of view could be different from their own. These all can result in deficits in social and communication skills which are similar to that seen in sighted autistic children (144, 145, 146).

For more detailed information on the association of ASD and visual impairment, readers are advised to look at the following websites:

http://ianpbell.com/visual-impairment-autism/.

http://www.ssc.education.ed.ac.uk/resources/vi&multi/boyce.html

http://icevi.org/publications/ICEVI-WC2002/papers/03 topic/03brandsborg.htm

http://www.focusfamilies.org/focus/docs/blindnessandautism.pdf

http://icevi.org/publications/ICEVI-WC2002/papers/07-topic/07-ingsholt2.htm

http://www.tsbvi.edu/autism-in-the-visually-impaired-child

Deaf-blindness, mental illness, and ASD

In one study, five deaf-blind service users with a clinical consensus diagnosis of ASD were compared with five service users without a clinical consensus diagnosis of ASD (37). Even with the additional measures, diagnosis of ASD in deaf-blind people with ID was found to be a challenge, primarily because their communication skills were impaired as a result of their dual sensory loss. The situation was worse for those who had an additionally significant ID. However, despite a large overlap in symptom presentation of those who were deaf-blind with those who were both deaf-blind and autistic, it was possible to diagnose ASD by thorough consensus assessment.

In children with deaf-blindness, development of language first and then other skills such as cognitive ability, socio-emotional development and motor development are affected most (147, 148). People with deaf-blindness with or without ASD can present with stereotyped behaviours as a compensation for social and sensory deprivation. However, over time and as children with deaf-blindness grow older, these behaviours tend to reduce in frequency and intensity if children are offered more opportunities to communicate with others and explore the environment around them (147, 149, 150, 151). Many symptoms in deaf-blind children such as lack of initiation and social withdrawal are secondary to their dual sensory loss and their dependence on carers (152). These symptoms do not differentiate between autistic and non-autistic deaf-blind children. Although communication and social interaction are impaired in all people with deaf-blindness, these impairments are more prominent and have a greater adverse effect on the quality of life of people when there is a comorbid ASD (37).

Those with CHARGE syndrome, one of the most common causes of deaf-blindness, have been reported to have more delayed language development and autistic symptoms when compared with those who have other developmental conditions, such as Down syndrome and Williams Syndrome (153, 154).

In 2002, Carvill and Mraston reported (155) a high rate of ASD (n = 15; 83%) in their sample of 18 adults with sensory impairment referred to their service for self-injurious or aggressive behaviours. Of these, 11 had deaf-blindness, four were blind (but not deaf) and three were deaf (but not blind). The aetiology of sensory impairment was congenital rubella syndrome in 12 of their sample (67%). Those remaining had Joubert syndrome (n = 1), infection during infancy (n = 1), Leber's congenital amaurosis (n = 2), self-injury (causing blindness; n = 1), and rhesus haemolytic disease (n = 1). The majority were males, with an average age of 31-years-old. The authors reported that it was challenging to reach a final psychiatric diagnosis owing to their subjects' unusual presentations, with only seven cases being diagnosed with postulated depression and four with a definite diagnosis of depression. Service users responded to a variety of treatment strategies including medication, staffing support, and environmental adaptation. The authors (155) reported that the majority of individuals (n = 15; of which 10 were deaf-blind, three were blind, and two deaf) had atypical ASD or autistic-like features based on ICD-10 criteria (156); they concluded that this high rate was less of a clinical concern and more of academic interest, since the management of all these presentations were the same in clinical practice. Psychotic symptoms have also been reported in the context of deaf-blindness in people with Usher syndrome (157).

Relationship between sensory impairment and mental ill-health

Being deaf in a hearing world can results in discrimination; people who are deaf are less likely to have appropriate jobs and more likely to have restricted access to education and social and health services. Deaf people tend to use more body contact and appear to be more direct and abrupt with their comments, mainly trying to gain the attention of others. Miscommunication is therefore very common between deaf people and hearing people. Sign language is not commonly used among services such as education and health and social services. Therefore, deaf people experience more barriers in accessing services, which can be extremely frustrating for them. In addition, deaf children commonly experience marginalization, scapegoating, physical, emotional, and sexual abuse which are all risk factors for mental illness. Deaf people's language, whether in sign, speech, or writing, may be limited and their written English can be poorly presented in British Sign Language (BSL) word order, which gives the appearance of formal thought disorders. For professionals who are not 'deaf aware', features of deaf culture and sign language might be therefore misinterpreted as challenging behaviour or mental illness, though under diagnosis of mental illness is also common and various personality traits such as immaturity, egocentricity, lack of empathy, lability, and explosive personalities have all been unfairly attributed to deaf people (surdophrenia) (8, 14, 20, 81, 82, 95, 96, 110, 158, 159, 160).

Being born in a hearing family, which is the case for 90–95 per cent of congenitally deaf children, appears to be a risk factor for the development of mental illness and emotional problems, because hearing parents with deaf children are usually communicating through speech which adversely affect language development in children with deafness (101, 161, 162, 163). It has been found that delayed language development (either speech or sign language) increases the likelihood of mental illness. In contrast, deaf children, born to deaf families or to hearing families with signing parents, develop language (sign language) in time, and research shows that in contrast to those deaf children with delayed language development, these children have a similar risk of developing mental illness as their hearing counterparts (164, 165, 166, 167). Using sign language early on in the family environment helps to facilitate development of speech as well as psychosocial and emotional development in deaf children; these are all protective factors against mental health problems (82, 95, 96, 160,168, 169, 170).

If no remedial measures are taken early in life, congenital deafness can adversely affect language, identity, and psychosocial/cognitive development (171, 172). Research shows that between 40–50 per cent of deaf children suffer from mental illness and emotional or behavioural problems, in comparison to 25 per cent of their hearing peers (173). The prevalence of attention deficit hyperactivity disorder (ADHD) in children who are deaf from non-inherited causes is reported to be higher than that of hearing children (174, 175). A study on deaf adolescents and young children has shown an excess of behavioural and emotional problems (176) mediated through difficulties in communication and experience of stigma and oppression in a predominantly hearing world. Some of the causes of challenging behaviour and mental illness in deaf children, however, might be due to associated ID, co-existing physical health problems, including the genetic syndrome causing the deafness, and environmental issues in relation to communication breakdown (32, 82, 95, 96, 160, 170,176).

Studies of the effects of deafness on mental health in adult populations have rendered different outcomes (81). Earlier studies reported lower rates of depression and anxiety in the deaf population; however, later studies argued that an absence of appropriate service provision for this population may have caused this reduction. The rate of schizophrenia in the deaf population is similar to that of hearing people and it is believed that schizophrenia in this population is less responsive to antipsychotic medication and may require higher dosages and augmentation with a mood stabilizer (9, 81, 82, 159, 175).

Previous reports also suggest an association between acquired deafness with psychotic illness (late paraphrenia) (177) and acquired blindness with visual hallucinations (Charles Bonnet syndrome) (178) in elderly people.

A population-based study in Scotland (179) however found no independent association between mental illness and sensory impairment in people with ID. Challenging behaviours may also be common in deaf adults with ID. A community-based study found that 62 per cent of deaf adults with ID living in the community displayed challenging behaviours (66). One population study of people with ID (both deaf and hearing) found that people who displayed challenging behaviours tended to have more restricted expressive and receptive communication (180). In 1959, Hallgren (181) reported an association between deaf-blindness in Usher syndrome and psychosis in up to 23 per cent of people. In this study, most of the individuals with psychosis had ID. A follow-up study of young adults in a birth cohort who experienced in utero exposure to rubella in the 1964 rubella epidemic, found a five-fold increase in non-affective psychosis (182).

Management strategies for people with ID and sensory impairment

It has been argued that better management of service users with multi-morbidities requires putting greater emphasis on: (i) clinical judgement when assessing service users and their carers' needs and (ii) coordination of care that can promote good therapeutic relationship. In this model, it is important that a generalist's skills are used by the specialist team for the better management of problems in the community (183). Effective management in people with ID is challenging as medical treatments form only one component of the management strategy (Table 24.3) (68).

Early identification of sensory impairment and ASD and early intervention is the key to success. These are crucial in reducing a feeling of isolation and will eventually result in better communication and development of social skills. For those who are deaf, this can be achieved through access to schools and colleges that allow them to mix with a more able group of deaf students who can sign fluently (95, 96, 184). For blind children, non-visual communications could be promoted to compensate for blindness and help them to develop joint attention and shared interest (184, 185, 186, 187, 188).

Experts in the field of visual impairment advise mothers to use other senses and activities such as touch, feel, smell, swinging, and tickling to make up for the lack of eye contact between themselves and their children so that babies could be engaged in joint attention. It is also important that the blind person's learning partner takes on a greater role in ensuring that tactile information is mediated to meet the person's needs though exploratory strategies (189). The learning partner has the responsibility of employing a range of prompts to facilitate engagement and participation of the person in structured activities (189).

Most people with ID who are deaf use a very simple version of sign language. Some might know Makaton or Signalong, which have basic sign language vocabulary and structure. The Picture Exchange Communication System (PECS) can also be used to facilitate service users' autonomy by showing pictures of the items they need. For people who are blind, communication can be via Braille, Moon, objects of reference, or audio materials. For those who are deaf-blind, it is essential to communicate through the deaf-blind manual, hands-on signing, visual frame signing, or block alphabet. A person with dual sensory loss experiences a greater degree of impairment than the sum of the visual impairment and hearing impairment alone. Dual sensory loss is a major risk factor for falls and injuries; therefore, the environment should be adapted in a way that those with a dual sensory loss can orientate themselves through touch and smell (190).

Some of the autistic-like features in the context of a congenital blindness could improve over time as blind children grow older, provided that they can be offered more exposure and further enjoyable sensory and motor activities. It is reported that with staff input, further exposure to various opportunities and appropriate sensory activities, autistic-like symptoms could be reduced through therapeutic relationship (118, 124, 191, 192).

Both service users with deafness and blindness with similarities and differences in their communication and language development regardless of whether they have ASD or not, also benefit from similar autism-friendly environment and approaches (e.g. the need for predictable routines and structured activities) (193). This will help them to gather the environmental information, step by step and sequentially, and convert them into a holistic manner and offer them an opportunity to learn from experiences (194, 195, 196). Use of remaining eyesight should be encouraged by reducing the glare and providing appropriate lighting and contrasting colours (190). An occupational therapist or charity organization (Box 24.7) could be consulted for the environmental adaptation of a day centre or the home.

Table 24.3 Management strategies for people with sensory impairment and ID

Medical	Environmental	Psychosocial	Communication	Other
Medication	Appropriate lighting and contrast colouring	Social skill training (e.g. social stories)	PECS†	TEACCH†
Eye glasses	Consistency of rooms	Psycho-education	Braille and Moon	Sensory integration
Hearing aids	Uncluttered rooms Railing for stair or driveways (outside the house) Adapted bathroom	One-to-one support from a support worker conversant in sensory impairment	Sign language and Makaton	Irlen tinted Glasses (for SS*)
Surgery	Light or vibrating alarms and clocks Pagers for doorbells and calendar boxes Use of special carpet and audio, touch and smell orientation Good signage, big calendar and clock and use of magnifying lenses, loop system	Commissioning structured day time and leisure activities Access to sensory room	Deaf-blind manual and block alphabet Objects of reference	ABA Intensive interaction

ABA: Applied Behavioural Analysis (200); PECS: Picture Exchange Communication System; SS: Scotopic Sensitivity or Irlen syndrome; TEACCH: Treatment and Education of Autistic and related Communication handicapped Children.

*An article by Williams (201) questioned the validity of Irlen syndrome and prescription of filtered lenses.

†PECS and TEACCH can be adapted for people with visual impairment by replacing pictures with tactile symbols and objects of reference (202) (203).

Box 24.7 Charity organizations for people with sensory impairment

Look Up	www.lookupinfo.org
SeeAbility*	www.seeability.org.uk
Deafblind UK	www.deafblind.org.uk
VISTA	www.vistablind.org.uk
Sense	www.sense.org.uk
Royal National Institute of Blind People†	www.rnib.org.uk
Royal National Institute for Deaf People‡	www.rnid.org.uk

*Seeability is a web-based charity organization providing training and consultancy services for people with ID and visual impairment. It provides accessible information for patients and those who are involved with their care (www.seabaility.org).

†RNIB Technology support squad can help clients to regain their independence through provision of support and use of new technology (www.rnib.org.uk/techsupport). Action for blind people (part of the RNIB group) (www.actionforblindpeople.org.uk) provides advice and support in dealing with employment issues, financial entitlement, social activities, events, and sport opportunities. There is also an Eye Clinic Liaison Officer (ECLO) service, which help people access their appointments in hospitals.

‡RNID has now changed to Action on Hearing Loss.

Table 24.4 'Dos' and 'Do nots' when communicating with people with sensory impairment

Do:	Do not:
Always tell them where you are, and where you are going to go.	Assume the person is totally blind and deaf. They may have some residual visual or hearing ability.
Consider supplementing verbal communication with simultaneous signs and symbols.	Shout or speak very loudly unless you are asked to do so.
Facilitate lip reading by allowing them to see your mouth clearly.	Misinterpret head tilt for extra-pyramidal symptoms; they may be using their better ear to listen to you!
Encourage those with macular degeneration to look at objects through the angle of their eyes and teach them to use magnifying lenses.	Assume the service user lacks eye contact (e.g. as in autism and fragile X syndrome); they may be looking slightly off-axis due to loss of central vision.
Respect confidentiality by not talking too loudly.	Mumble or exaggerate your lip movements.

Management requires an approach that is not simply multi-modal and multi-disciplinary, but also multi-agency and trans-disciplinary (197), combining education, social services, and other agencies such as charity organizations to ensure a holistic response to service users' difficulties. Input from the speech and language therapy colleagues is paramount as part of a multidisciplinary approach in managing sensory impairment. Psychological approaches (e.g. psycho-education), tailored to the individual service user's level of language and cognitive ability, are important to help clients make sense of the social world around them. These can be complemented with social skills training (e.g. social stories) to improve the service user's understanding of other people's emotions and minds as well as their own. Occupational therapists commonly use sensory integration approach, which helps individuals to integrate their senses so that the individual can use more than one sense at a time. For some people with severe ASD and ID, intensive interaction has also been helpful in establishing attention and emotional engagement (198). Educational approaches like Treatment and Education of Autistic and related Communication Handicapped Children (TEACCH) can reduce anxiety by providing a structured and predictable daily timetable for different activities (199). Objects of reference are taught by pairing an event with an object to facilitate the learning process, for example handing a cup to a deaf-blind service user when it is time for a drink.

More information on education of sensory impaired children and young people can be found on the website of the Scottish Sensory Centre: http://www.ssc.education.ed.ac.uk/library/publications/retrospective.pdf

and the Texas school for the blind and visually impaired: http://www.tsbvi.edu/.

The National Autistic Society's recommendations for teaching children with ASD uses five principles: structured, positive, empathic, low arousal, and links (acronym of SPELL). This can be adjusted for children with sensory impairment (195).

Communication with people with ID who have sensory impairment is challenging and complex. Staff working in such settings must receive regular training and be given the opportunity to practice, in order to be able to communicate effectively with service users (Table 24.4).

To provide additional guidance for professionals, the RNIB developed the Visual Impairment and Autism Project's resource pack in 2011 which consisted of a CD-ROM and booklet. The material is now freely available at the RNIB website: www.rnib.org.uk/autism. Bell (204) provides more information about this project and also on communication issues in people with ASD and visual impairment at: http://ianpbell.com/communication-in-vi-children/.

The Royal College of Ophthalmologists has also created a Best Practice Guide for GPs on visual impairment in people with ID, which was launched in June 2012, highlighting key areas to ensure this group of service users has access to appropriate eye health care. VISION 2020 UK also facilitates collaboration and cooperation between organizations that focus on visual impairment (205). Kendall et al. (206) and Pilling et al. (207) have summarized the NICE and SCIE guidance on management of ASD in children and young adults. These also apply to those who have additional disabilities such as sensory impairment or ID, albeit with some modifications.

The National Autistic Society also provides information on the association of hearing and visual impairment with ASD:

http://www.autism.org.uk/about-autism/related-conditions/visual-impairment-and-autism-spectrum-disorders.aspx

http://www.autism.org.uk/about-autism/related-conditions/asds-and-hearing-impairments.aspx

Conclusion

Research into sensory impairments and ASD has the potential to improve service provision for people with ID. There are, however, potential challenges and barriers to the design of research investigating presence of sensory impairment and ASD in this population. These include the heterogeneity of people with ID, sensory impairment, and ASD, difficulties in finding a relatively large sample size and appropriate control group and presence of additional comorbidities (e.g. epilepsy) (71, 208, 209). The research methodology should be therefore appropriate when assessing the ID service users with sensory impairment, that is, they need to be given adequate time, experience, and opportunity (118) so that they can show their abilities and that reliable conclusions can be drawn from the results: as Lewis and Collins (210) put it, the research methods should be fit for purpose.

Observations from follow-up work by Hobson and Lee (211) and Jure et al. (212) suggest that symptoms of ASD may improve in blind children. It is therefore important to carry out follow-up studies on congenitally blind children with ASD to find out more about any differences in presentation over time during their adulthood.

Another interesting research project on the same topic has been the recent development of a new assessment tool (Observation of Autism in People with Sensory and Intellectual Disability; OASID) for diagnosing ASD in people with ID and accompanying sensory impairment (213, 214) as, in spite of its high prevalence, ASD is often overlooked in this population in clinical practice. Improving diagnosis facilitates early access to services which has been advocated by the National Institute for Health and Care Excellence (NICE) (215).

In addition, the paucity of evidence in determining association between mental illness in people with ID and sensory impairment warrants further well-designed research in both children and adults. The finding from these studies will determine the model of care and service provision for these marginalized groups of individuals and improve the quality of care they receive.

MULTIPLE CHOICE QUESTIONS

Questions

Please select the single most appropriate answer.

1. Barriers to accessing services in people with ID are related to:

A. Service users and their carers
B. Health care services
C. Health care professionals
D. All the above
E. Only options B and C

2. Prevalence of visual or hearing impairment in people with ID is:

A. Lower than the general population
B. Higher than the general population
C. The same as in the general population
D. Higher in males
E. Higher in females

3. Prevalence of visual and hearing impairment is influenced by:

A. Age
B. Severity of ID
C. Aetiology of ID
D. Ethnicity
E. All the above

4. A visual or hearing impairment can present with:

A. Challenging behaviours
B. Loss of skills
C. Symptoms similar to dementia
D. Symptoms similar to mental illness, for example, depression, anxiety
E. All the above

5. Assessment and management of visual and hearing impairment should be:

A. Medically oriented
B. Led by the occupational therapist
C. Multidisciplinary
D. Led by the speech and language therapist
E. None of the above

Answers

1. D. Barriers to accessing services can be generally grouped into three categories in relation to (1) services (e.g. no access to loop system for those who are using hearing aids), (2) professionals (e.g. prejudice) and (3) patients themselves (e.g. being unable to express their discomfort due to communication difficulties).
2. B. Prevalence of sensory impairment is higher in those with intellectual disability than the general population because of the higher rate of accompanying brain damage in the former. There is no association between these and gender.
3. E. Research shows that sensory impairment is much more common in older people and if they have a more severe form of intellectual disability or an underlying condition as a cause of their intellectual disability (e.g. Down syndrome). These have also been reported more common in those from the ethnic minority background.
4. E. This can happen due to people with intellectual disability having communication difficulties and being unable to complain of their visual and hearing impairment; therefore manifestation of these could be similar to mental health problems or dementia.
5. C. Assessment and management of sensory impairment in people with intellectual disability should involve members of the multidisciplinary/multi-agency team (e.g. hearing services, optician, speech and language therapist, occupational therapist etc.) to successfully address these issues in clinical practice.

REFERENCES

1. Maulik PK, Mascarenhas MN, Mathers CD et al. (2011). Prevalence of intellectual disability: A meta-analysis of population-based studies, *Research in Developmental Disabilities*, 32 (2), pp. 419–436.
2. Department of Health (2001). *Valuing People. A new strategy for Learning Disability for the 21st century.* White Paper, London: HMSO. (www.archive.official-documents.co.uk/document/cm50/5086/5086.pdf). [Accessed June 2013].

3. Department of Health (2009). *Valuing people now: A new three-year strategy for people with learning disabilities.* London: HMSO.
4. Local Government Ombudsman and Health Service Ombudsman (2009). *Six Lives: The Provision of Public Services to People with Learning Disabilities.* London: The Stationery Office.
5. Michael J (2008). *Healthcare for all: Report of the independent inquiry into access to healthcare for people with learning disabilities*, London: Department of Health.
6. Public Health England (2015). Reasonable adjustments. Available at: (http://www.improvinghealthandlives.org.uk/projects/reasonableadjustments). [Accessed on: 1 Oct 2009].
7. Marston G and Perry D (2013). Intellectual disabilities. In Cormac I, Gray D (eds.). *Essentials of physical health in psychiatry.* Glasgow: Bell & Bain Ltd, *The Royal College of Psychiatrists Publication*, pp. 372–382.
8. Miller H. and Courtenay, K (2006). *Towards equity and access? Newsletter of the Faculty of Learning Disability: Psychiatry.*
9. Kitson N and Fry R (1990). Pre-lingual deafness and psychiatry, *British Journal of Hospital Medicine*, 44 (5), pp. 353–356.
10. Morton NE (1991). Genetic epidemiology of hearing impairment, *Annals of the New York Academy of Sciences*, 630 (1), pp.16–31.
11. Fortnum H and Davis A (1997). Epidemiology of permanent childhood hearing impairment in Trent Region, 1985–1993. *British Journal of Audiology*, 31 (6), pp. 409–446.
12. Fortnum HM, Summerfield AQ, Marshall DH et al. (2001). Prevalence of permanent childhood hearing impairment in the United Kingdom and implications for universal neonatal hearing screening: Questionnaire based ascertainment study, *British Medical Journal*, 323 (7312), pp. 536–540.
13. Agrawal Y, Platz E, Niparko JK (2008). Prevalence of hearing loss and differences by demographic characteristics among US adults, *Archive of Internal Medicine*,168 (14), pp.1522–1530.
14. Royal National Institute for Deaf People. (2003) Available at: (http://www.actiononhearingloss.org.uk/your-hearing/about-deafness-and hearing-loss/statistics.aspx). [Accessed on: 1 Oct 2009].
15. Middleton A, Niruban A, Girling G et al. (2010). Communicating in a healthcare setting with people who have hearing loss, *British Medical Journal*, 341, c4672.
16. Evenhuis HM, Theunissen M, Denkers I et al. (2001). Prevalence of visual and hearing impairment in a Dutch institutionalised population with learning disability, *Journal of Learning Disability Research*, 45 (5), pp. 457–464.
17. Acker T and Crocker S (2004). Tip-toeing through technology. In Austen S Crocker S. (eds.). *Deafness in mind: Working psychologically with deaf people across the lifespan.* London: John Wiley & Sons, pp. 53–72.
18. Graham J (2004). Medical and psychological aspects of deafness, in: Austen S. Crocker S (eds.). *Deafness in mind: Working psychologically with deaf people across the life span.* London and Philadelphia: *Whurr Publishers*, pp.37–52.
19. Baines D (2007). Unravelling the anomaly of deafness. In Austen S, Jeffery D. (eds.). *Deafness and challenging behaviour: The 360° perspective.* London: John Wiley & Sons, pp. 17–32.
20. Carvill S (2001). Sensory impairment, learning disability and psychiatry, *Journal of Intellectual Disability Research*, 45 (6), pp. 467–483.
21. Hild U, Hey C, Baumann U et al. (2008). High prevalence of hearing disorders at the special Olympics indicate need to screen persons with intellectual disability, *Journal of Intellectual Disability Research*, 52 (6), pp. 520–528.
22. van den Broek EGC, Janssen, CGC, van Ramshorst T et al. (2006). Visual impairment in people with severe and profound multiple disability: An inventory of visual functioning, *Journal of Learning Disability and Research*, 50 (6), pp. 470–475.
23. World Health Organisation (2007). Vision 2020, *The Right to Sight, Global initiative for the elimination of avoidable blindness. Action plan 2006–2011.* Available at: (https://www.who.int/blindness/Vision2020_report.pdf) [Accessed on 20 Jan 2019].
24. Warburg M (1994). Visual impairment among people with developmental delay, *Journal of Learning Disability Research*, 38 (4), pp. 423–432.
25. Warburg M (2001). Visual impairment in adult people with intellectual disability: Literature review, *Journal of Intellectual Disability Research*, 45 (5), pp. 424–438.
26. Evenhuis HM (1995). Medical aspect of ageing in a population with intellectual disability: I. Visual impairment, *Journal of Intellectual Disability Research*, 39 (1), pp.19–25.
27. Evenhuis H, Henderson CM, Beange H et al. (2000). *Healthy Ageing. Adults with Intellectual Disabilities: Physical Health Issues.* Geneva: WHO.
28. van Splunder J (2003). *Visual Impairment, Prevalence and Causes of Visual Impairment in Adult with Intellectual Disability.* Utrecht: Universiteit Utrecht.
29. van Splunder J, Stilma JS, Bernsen RMD et al. (2004). Prevalence of ocular diagnoses found on screening 1539 adults with intellectual disabilities, *Ophthalmology*, 111 (8), pp. 1457–1463.
30. van Splunder J, Stilma JS, Bernsen RMD et al. (2006). Prevalence of visual impairments in adults with intellectual disabilities in the Netherlands: Cross-sectional study, *Eye*, 20 (9), pp. 1004–1010.
31. Robertson J and Emerson E (2010). *Estimating the Number of People with Co-occurring Vision and Hearing Impairments in the UK.* Lancaster, Centre for Disability Research: Lancaster University.
32. Bond DE (2000). Mental health in children who are deaf and have multiple disabilities. In Hindley P, Kitson N (eds.). *Mental health and deafness.* London and Philadelphia: *Whurr*, pp. 127–148.
33. Hirst C, Poole JJ, Snelling G S (1993). Liverpool visual assessment team 1985–1989: 5 years on, *Child: Care, Health and Development*, 19 (3), pp. 185–195.
34. Brinks MV, Murphey WH, Cardwell W et al. (2001). Ophthalmologic screening of deaf students in Oregon, *Journal of Paediatric Ophthalmology and Strabismus*, 38 (1), pp. 11–15.
35. Gallaudet Research Institute (2008). *Regional and National Summary of Report Data from the 2006–2007 Annual Survey of Deaf and Hard of Hearing Children and Youth.* Gallaudet University.
36. Fellinger J, Holzinger D, Dirmhirn A et al. (2009). Failure to detect deaf-blindness in a population of people with intellectual disability, *Journal of Intellectual Disability Research*, 53 (10), pp. 874–881.
37. Hoevenaars-van den Boom MA, Antonissen AC, Knoors H, Vervloed MP (2009). Differentiating characteristics of deaf-blindness and autism in people with congenital deaf-blindness and profound intellectual disability, *Journal of Intellectual Disability Research*, 53 (6), pp. 548–558.
38. Prain M, McVilly K., Ramcharan P. et al. (2010). Observing the behaviour and interactions of adults with congenital deaf-blindness living in community residences, *Journal of Intellectual and Developmental Disability*, 35 (2), pp. 82–91.
39. Janicki MP, Dalton AM (1998). Sensory impairments among older adults with learning disability, *Journal of Intellectual and Developmental Disability*, 23 (1), pp. 3–11.

40. Cooke L (1989). Hearing loss in the mentally handicapped. A study of its prevalence and association with ageing. *The British Journal of Mental Sub-normality*, 34, pp. 112–116.
41. Smiley E (2005) Epidemiology of mental health problems in adults with learning disability: An update, *Advances in Psychiatric Treatment*, 11 (3), pp. 214–222.
42. Lavis D, Cullen P, Roy A (1997). Identification of hearing impairment in people with a learning disability: From questioning to testing, *British Journal of Learning Disability*, 25, 100–105.
43. Admiraal RJC, Huygen PLM (2000). Changes in the aetiology of hearing impairment in deaf-blind pupils and deaf infant pupils at an institute for the deaf, *International Journal of Pediatric Otorhinolaryngology*, 55 (2), pp.133–142.
44. Gilbert CE, Shah SP, Jadoon MZ et al. (2008). Poverty and blindness in Pakistan: Results from the Pakistan national blindness and visual impairment survey, *British Medical Journal*, 336 (7634), pp. 29–32.
45. Chess S (1971). Autism in children with congenital rubella, *Journal of Autism and Childhood Schizophrenia*, 1 (1), pp. 33–47.
46. Jones KL (1997). *Waardenburg syndrome. Smith's recognizable pattern of human malformation*. 5th Edition. Philadelphia, PA: WB Saunders Company, pp. 248–249.
47. Toriello HV, Reardon W, Gorlin RJ (eds.) (2004). Hereditary hearing loss and its syndromes. Oxford: Oxford University Press.
48. Firth H, Hurst J, Hall J (eds.) (2005). *Severe deafness in early childhood. Oxford desk reference Clinical Genetics*. Oxford University Press, pp. 91–92.
49. Marazita ML, Ploughman LM, Rawling, B et al. (1993). Genetic epidemiological studies of early-onset deafness in the U.S. school-age population, *American Journal of Medical Genetics*, 46 (5), pp. 486–491.
50. Steel KP, Bussoli TJ (1999). Deafness genes: Expressions of surprise, *Trends in Genetics*, 15 (6), pp. 207–211.
51. Hutchin TP, Thompson KR, Parker M et al (2001). Prevalence of mitochondrial mutations in childhood/congenital onset non-syndromal sensorineural hearing impairment, *Journal of Medical Genetics*, 38 (4), pp. 229–231.
52. Cryns K, Van Camp G (2004). Deafness genes and their diagnostic applications. *Audiolgy Neurootolarngology*, 9, pp. 2–22.
53. Hsu CH, Kwon H, Perng CL et al. (2005). Hearing loss in mitochondrial disorders, *Annals of New York Academy of Sciences*, 1042, pp. 36–47.
54. Rosenbaum P (2014). What causes cerebral palsy? A genetic or familial component now looks likely, *British Medical Journal*, 349, g4514.
55. Prasher V, Janicki M (eds.) (2002). *Physical Health of Adults with Intellectual Disabilities*, Oxford: Wiley-Blackwell.
56. Meuwese-Jongejeugd A, Harteloh P, Verschuure H et al. (2005). Audiological rehabilitation in adults with intellectual disability: Why does it fail? *Journal of Policy and Practice in Intellectual Disabilities*, 2 (1), pp. 66–67.
57. Meuwese-Jongejeugd A, Vink M, van Zanten B et al. (2006). Prevalence of hearing loss in 1598 adults with an intellectual disability: Cross-sectional population-based study, *International Journal of Audiology*, 45 (11), pp. 660–669.
58. Shott SR, Joseph A, Heithaus D (2001). Hearing loss in children with Down syndrome, *International Journal of Paediatric Otorhinolaryngology*, 61 (3), pp. 199–205.
59. Rosenburg T, Haim M, Hauch AM et al. (1997). The prevalence of Usher syndrome and other retinal dystrophy hearing impairment associations, *Clinical Genetics*, 51 (5), pp. 314–321.
60. Chess S (1977). Follow up report on autism in congenital rubella, *Journal of Autism and Childhood Schizophrenia*, 7 (1), pp. 69–81.
61. Chess S, Fernandez P, Korn S (1978). Behavioural consequences of congenital rubella, *Journal of Paediatrics*, 93, pp. 699–703.
62. Berger BE, Navar-Boggan AM, Omer SB (2011). Congenital rubella syndrome and autism spectrum disorder prevented by rubella vaccination—United States, 2001–2010, *BMC Public Health*, 11, p. 340.
63. Sweeten TL, Posey D.J, McDougle CJ (2004). Autistic disorder in three children with cytomegalovirus infection, *Journal of Autism and Developmental Disorders*, 34 (5), pp. 583–586.
64. Evenhuis HM, Sjoukes L, Koot HM et al. (2009). Does visual impairment lead to additional disability in adults with intellectual disabilities? *Journal of Intellectual Disability Research*, 53 (I), pp. 19–28.
65. Starling S, Willis A, Dracup M et al. (2006). Right to sight, *Journal of Intellectual Disabilities*, 10 (4), pp. 337–355.
66. Timehin C, Timehin E (2004). Prevalence of hearing impairment in a community population of adults with Learning Disability: Access to audiology and impact on behaviour, *British Journal of Learning Disabilities*, 32 (3), pp. 128–132.
67. Lindsey M (2002). Comprehensive health care services for people with learning disabilities, *Advances in Psychiatric Treatment*, 8 (2), pp. 138–147.
68. Kiani R and Miller H (2010). Sensory impairment and intellectual disability. *Advances in Psychiatric Treatment*,16 (3), pp. 228–235.
69. McGlade A, Bickerstaff D, Lindsay J et al. (2010). Making a difference. Visual health needs of people with a learning disability, *British Journal of Learning Disabilities*, 38 (3), pp. 187–193.
70. Domokos, A. (2000) *An evaluative study of a specialist training course as a means of changing and improving staff practice in the care of people with profound and multiple disabilities*. B Phil dissertation, University of Birmingham.
71. Pring L (ed.) (2005). *Autism and Blindness, Research and Reflections*, London and Philadelphia: *Whurr*.
72. Yeates S (1991). Hearing loss in adults with learning disability, *British Medical Journal*, 303 (6800), pp. 427–428.
73. Yeates S (1995). The incidence and importance of hearing loss in people with severe learning disability: The evolution of a service, *British Journal of Learning Disabilities*, 23 (2), 79–84.
74. Yeates S (2000). Audiological assessment of people with special difficulties. In Hindley P, Kitson N (eds.). *Mental Health and Deafness*, London and Philadelphia: *Whurr*, pp. 25–41.
75. Meuwese-Jongejeugd A, Verschuure H, Evenhuis HM (2007). Hearing aids: Expectations and satisfaction of people with an intellectual disability, a descriptive pilot study, *Journal of Intellectual Disability Research*, 51 (11), pp. 913–922.
76. Edmiston R, Mitchell C (2013). Hearing loss in adults, *British Medical Journal*, 346, f2496.
77. Neumann K, Hey C, Ludwig A et al. (2007). *High prevalence of hearing disorders indicate need to screen persons with intellectual disability*. Available on line at: (www.egms.de/en/meetings/dgpp2007/07dgpp70.shtml). [Accessed on: Oct 2013].
78. Hitoglou M, Ververi A, Antoniadis A et al. (2010). Childhood autism and auditory system abnormalities, *Pediatric Neurology*, 42 (5), pp. 309–314.
79. International Association for the Scientific Study of Intellectual Disabilities (2002). Health Guidelines for Adults with an Intellectual Disability. IASSID, Available at: (http://www.iassid.org/pdf/healthguidelines-2002.pdf). [Accessed on: 1 Oct 2008].

80. Northfield J (2008). *Visual impairment and people with learning disabilities*, NLH Learning disabilities Specialist Library.
81. Hindley P, Kitson N (2000). *Mental health and deafness*, London and Philadelphia: *Whurr*.
82. Austen S, Crocker S (eds.) (2004). *Deafness in mind: Working psychologically with deaf people across the life span*. London: John Wiley & Sons.
83. Bhaumik S, Branford D, McGrother C et al. (1997). Autistic traits in adults with learning disabilities, *British Journal of Psychiatry*, 170 (6), pp. 502–506.
84. Wing L, Gould J (1979). Severe impairments of social interaction and associated abnormalities in children: Epidemiology and classification, *Journal of Autism and Childhood Schizophrenia*, 9 (1), pp. 11–29.
85. Deb S, Prasad KB (1994). The prevalence of autistic disorder among children with a learning disability, *British Journal of Psychiatry*, 165 (3), pp. 395–399.
86. Beadle-Brown J, Murphy, GH, Wing L et al. (2002). Changes in social impairment for people with intellectual disabilities: A follow-up of the Camberwell Cohort, *Journal of Autism and Developmental Disorders*, 32 (3), pp. 195–206.
87. de Bildt A, Systema S, Kraijer D et al. (2005). Prevalence of pervasive developmental disorders in children and adolescents with mental retardation, *Journal of Child Psychology and Psychiatry*, 46 (3), pp. 275–286.
88. Bhaumik S, Tyrer, F, McGrother C et al. (2008). Psychiatric service use and psychiatric disorders in adults with intellectual disability, *Journal of Intellectual Disability Research*, 52 (11), pp. 986–995.
89. Brugha ST, McManus S, Bankart J et al. (2011). Epidemiology of autism spectrum disorders in adults in the community in England, *Arch Gen Psychiatry*, 68 (5), pp. 459–465.
90. Brugha T, Cooper SA, McManus S et al. (2012). *Estimating the Prevalence of Autism Spectrum Conditions in Adults: Extending the 2007 Adult Psychiatric Morbidity Survey*. Leeds: The Health and Social Care Information Centre.
91. Lundy JEB (2002). *Age and Language Skills of Deaf Children in Relation to Theory of Mind Development*, Oxford University Press.
92. Mayberry RI, Lock, E (2003). Age constraints on first versus second language acquisition: Evidence for linguistic plasticity and epigenesist, *Brain and Language*, 87 (3), pp. 369–384.
93. Edwards L (2004). Neuropsychological development of hearing impaired children, in: Austen S Crocker S (eds.). *Deafness in mind, working psychologically with deaf people across the life span*, London and Philadelphia: *Whurr*, pp. 127–143.
94. Edwards L, Crocker S (eds.) (2008). *Psychological processes in deaf children with complex needs: An evidence-based practical guide*. London and Philadelphia: *Jessica Kingsley Publishers*.
95. Gentili N, Holwell A (2011). Mental health in children with severe hearing impairment, *Advances in Psychiatric Treatment*, 17 (1), pp. 54–62.
96. Sessa B, Sutherland H (2013). Addressing mental health needs of deaf children and their families: The National Deaf Child and Adolescent Mental Health Service, *The Psychiatrist*, 37 (5), pp. 175–178.
97. Peterson CC, Siegal M (1995). Deafness, conversation and theory of mind, *Journal of Child Psychology and Psychiatry*, 36 (3), pp. 459–474.
98. Peterson CC, Siegal M (2000). Insights into theory of mind from deafness and autism, *Mind and Language*, 15 (1), pp.123–145.
99. Jure R, Rapin I, Tuchman RF (1991). Hearing-impaired autistic children, *Developmental Medicine and Child Neurology*, 33 (12), pp. 1062–1072.
100. Newschaffer CJ, Croen LA, Daniels J et al. (2007). The epidemiology of autism spectrum disorders, *Annual Reviews Public Health*, 28, pp. 235–258.
101. Lederberg AR, Everhart VS (1998). Communication between deaf children and their hearing mothers: The role of language, gesture and vocalization, *Journal of Speech, Language and Hearing Research*, 41, pp. 887–899.
102. Spencer PE (2000). Looking without listening: Is audition a prerequisite for normal development of visual attention during infancy? *Journal of Deaf Studies and Deaf Education*, 5 (4), pp. 291–302.
103. Schick B, de Villiers P, de Villiers J et al. (2007). Language and theory of mind: A study of deaf children, *Child Development*, 78 (2), pp. 376–396.
104. Rosenhall U, Nordin V, Sandstrom M et al. (1999). Autism and hearing loss, *Journal of Autism and Developmental Disorders*, 29 (5), pp. 349–357.
105. Szymanski CA, Brice PJ, Lam KH et al. (2012). Deaf children with autism spectrum disorders, *Journal of Autism and Developmental Disorder*, 42(10), pp. 2027–2037.
106. Kancherla V, Van Naarden Braun K, Yeargin-Allsopp M (2013). Childhood vision impairment, hearing loss and co-occurring autism spectrum disorder, *Disability Health Journal*, 6 (4), pp. 333–342.
107. Kielinen M, Rantala H, Timonen E et al. (2004). Associated medical disorders and disabilities in children with autistic disorder: A population-based study, *Autism* 8 (1), pp. 49–60.
108. Roper L, Arnold P, Monteiro B (2003). Co-occurrence of autism and deafness: Diagnostic considerations, *Autism*, 7 (3), pp. 245–253.
109. Baron-Cohen S, Tager-Flusberg H and Cohen DJ (eds.) (1993). *Understanding other minds: Perspectives from autism*. Oxford: Oxford University Press.
110. Austen S, Jeffery D (eds.) (2007). *Deafness and challenging behaviour: The 360° perspective*. Chichester: John Wiley & Sons.
111. Collins PCarney S (2007). Autistic spectrum disorder, deafness and challenging behaviour. In Austen S Jeffery D (eds.). *Deafness and challenging behaviour, the 360° perspective*. London: Wiley Publishers, pp. 125–143.
112. Szymanski CA Brice PJ (2008). *When autism and deafness coexist in deaf children. Odyssey: New Directions in Deaf Education* 9 (1), pp. 10–15.
113. Boyce F, Hammond, F (1996). Autism and visual impairment—Making sense, Scottish Sensory Centre: Autism and Visual Impairment Conference, Edinburgh, 27 March. Available at: (www.ssc.education.ed.ac.uk/resources/vi&multi/boyce.html). [Accessed on: 2 February 2011].
114. Millar S (1983). Language and active touch: Some aspects of reading and writing by blind children. In Mills A. (ed.). *Language acquisition in the blind child: Normal and deficient*. San Diego: *College-Hill Press*.
115. Kekelis L, Sacks S (1992). The effects of visual impairment on social interactions in regular education programmes. In Sacks S, Kekelis L, Gaylord-Ross R (eds.). *The development of social skills by blind and visually impaired students: Exploring studies and strategies*. New York: *AFB Press*.
116. Warren D (1994). *Blindness and children: An individual differences approach*. Cambridge: Cambridge University Press.
117. Perez-Pereira M, Castro J (1992). Pragmatic functions of blind and sighted children's language: A twin case study. *First Language*, 12 (34), pp. 17–37.

118. Perez-Pereira M, Conti-Ramsden G (2005). Do blind children show autistic features? In Pring L (ed.). *Autism and Blindness, Research and Reflections*. London and Philadelphia: *Whurr*, pp. 99–127.
119. Lechelt EC, Hall DL. (n.d.). *The Impact of vision loss on the development of children from birth to 12 Years: A Literature review*. Ottawa: The Canadian National Institute for the Blind. Available at: (http://martintolley.com/DevChild/documents/Blindness%20and%20Development.pdf). [Accessed on: 1 Oct 2014].
120. Bishop V (1991). Preschool children with visual impairments. *Texas School for the Blind and Visually Impaired*. Available at: (http://www.tsbvi.edu/curriculum-a-publications/3/1069-preschool-children-with-visual-impairments-by-virginia-bishop). [Accessed on: 1 Oct 2015].
121. Sugden J, Duthie A, Lee M et al. (2012). Early years visual impairment education: A retrospective, The Scottish Sensory Centre (SSC) 21st Anniversary. Available at: (http://www.ssc.education.ed.ac.uk/library/publications/retrospective.pdf). [Accessed on: 1 Oct 2014].
122. Preisler G (1991). Early patterns of interaction between blind infants and their sighted mothers, *Child: Care, Health and Development*, 17 (2), pp. 65–90.
123. Mills A (1993). Visual Handicap. In Bishop D, Mogford K (eds.). *Language development in exceptional circumstances*. Hove: Laurence Erlbaum Associates.
124. Gense M, Gense D (2002). *Autism spectrum disorder in learners with blindness/vision impairments: Comparison of Characteristics*.US: Focus Families. Available online at: (http://www.focusfamilies.org/focus/docs/blindnessandautism.pdf). [Accessed on: Oct 2011].
125. Fraiberg S (1977). *Insights from the Blind: Comparative Study of the Blind with Sighted Children*. New York: *Basic Books, Souvenir Press*.
126. Hobson RP, Lee A, Brown R. (1999). Autism and congenital blindness, *Journal of Autism and Developmental Disorders*, 29 (1), pp. 45–56.
127. Warren DH (1986). *Blindness and early childhood development*. University of California at Riverside, Riverside, CA: American Foundation for the Blind.
128. Frith U (1989). A new look at language and communication in autism, *British Journal of Disorders of Communication*, 24 (2), pp. 123–150.
129. Webster A, Roe J (1998). *Children with visual impairments: Social interaction, language and learning*. London: Routledge.
130. Tager-Flusberg H.(1999). Language development in atypical children. In Barrett M (ed.). *The development of language*. Hove: *Psychology Press*, pp. 311–348.
131. Ingsholt A (2002). Blindness, mental retardation and—or autism. *New Visions: Moving Toward an Inclusive Community*. Proceedings, 11th ICEVI World Conference: Leeuwenhorst Congress Centre, Netherlands, 27 July—2 August. Available at: (www.icevi.org/publications/ICEVIWC2002/papers/07-topic/07-ingsholt2.htm). [Accessed on: 1 Oct 2011].
132. Kehoe, T. (2012) The role of repetitive questioning in a pupil with visual impairment and autism. Available at: (http://ianpbell.wordpress.com/visual-impairment-autism/). [Accessed on: 1 Oct 2013].
133. Loftin, M. (1999) Pervasive developmental disorders in children with visual impairments. *See/Hear*; 4 (2), pp. 22–4. Available at: (www.tsbvi.edu/Outreach/seehear/spring99/devdisorders.htm). [Accessed on: 1 Oct 2011].
134. Hobson R P, Brown, R, Minter, ME et al. (1997). Autism revisited: The case of congenital blindness. In Lewis V, Collis MG (eds.). *Blindness and psychological development in young children*, Leicester, UK: *British Psychology Society Books*, pp. 99–115.
135. Minter M., Hobson RP, Bishop M (1998). Congenital visual impairment and theory of mind, *British Journal of Developmental Psychology*, 16 (2), pp. 183–196.
136. Begeer S, Dik, M., Marieke J et al. (2014). A new look at theory of mind in children with ocular and ocular-plus congenital blindness, *Journal of Visual Impairment and Blindness*, 108 (1), pp. 17–27.
137. Cass H, Sonksen P.M, McConachie HR (1994). Developmental set back in severe visual impairment, *Archives of Disease in Childhood*, 70 (3), pp. 192–196.
138. Dale N (2005). Early signs of developmental setback and autism in blind infants. In Pring L (ed.). *Autism and Blindness, Research and Reflections*. London and Philadelphia: *Whurr*, pp. 74–98.
139. Waugh MC, Chong WK, Sonksen PM (1998). Neuroimaging in children with congenital disorders of the peripheral visual system, *Developmental Medicine and Child Neurology*, 40 (12), pp. 812–819.
140. Sonksen PM, Dale N (2002). Visual impairment in infancy: Impact on neurodevelopmental and neurobiological processes, *Developmental Medicine and Child Neurology*, 44 (1), pp. 782–791.
141. Dale N, Salt A (2008). Social identity, autism and visual impairment (VI) in the early years, *British Journal of Visual Impairment*, 26 (2), pp. 135–146.
142. Dale N, Sonksen P (2002). Developmental outcome, including setback, in young children with severe visual impairment. *Developmental Medicine and Child Neurology*, 44 (9), pp. 613–622.
143. Brown R, Hobson P, Lee A et al. (1997). Are there 'autistic-like' features in congenitally blind children?, *Child Psychology and Psychiatry*, 38 (6), pp. 693–703.
144. Hobson RP, Bishop M (2003). The pathogenesis of autism: Insights from congenital blindness, *Philosophical Transactions of the Royal Society of London: Series B: Biological Sciences*, 358 (1430), pp. 335–344.
145. Hobson RP (2002). *The cradle of thought*. Basingstoke, UK: Macmillan.
146. Hobson RP (2005). Why connect? On the relationship between autism and blindness. In Pring L (ed.). *Autism and Blindness, Research and Reflections*. London and Philadelphia: *Whurr*, pp. 10–25.
147. van Dijk J, Janssen M (1993). Doofblinde kinderen [Deafblind children], in: Nakken H (ed.). *Meervoudig gehandicapten:een zorg apart* [Multiply Handicapped: an Unusual Care], Rotterdam: Lemniscaat, pp. 34–73.
148. Gense MH, GenseDJ (2005). *Autism spectrum disorders and visual impairment: Meeting students' learning needs*, New York: *American Foundation for the Blind Press*.
149. Murdoch H (2000). Repetitive behaviours in children with sensory impairment and multiple disabilities, *DBI Review*, 26, pp. 7–111.
150. Frith Uta (2003). *Autism: Explaining the enigma*. Cambridge, MA: *Blackwell Pub*.
151. Hartshorne TM, Grialou TL, Parker KR (2005). Autistic-like behaviour in CHARGE syndrome, *American Journal of Medical Genetics*, 133A (3), pp. 257–261.
152. Knoors H, Vervloed MPJ (2003). Educational programming for deaf children with multiple disabilities. In: Marschark M,

Spencer PE (eds.). *Oxford Handbook of Deaf Studies, Language and Education*. New York: Oxford University Press, pp. 82–94.

153. Graham JMJ, Rosner B, Dykens E et al. (2005). Behavioral features of CHARGE syndrome (Hall-Hittner syndrome) comparison with Down syndrome, Prader-Willi syndrome, and Williams syndrome. *American Journal of Medical Genetics*, 133A (3), pp. 240–247.
154. Peltokorpi S Huttunen K (2008). Communication in the early stage of language development in children with CHARGE syndrome, *British Journal of Visual Impairment*, 26 (1), pp. 24–49.
155. Carvill S, Marston G (2002). People with learning disability, sensory impairments and behavioural disorder: A case series, *Journal of Intellectual Disability Research*, 46 (3), pp. 264–272.
156. World Health Organisation (1992). *The ICD-10 International statistical classification of diseases and related health problems. Classification of mental and behavioural disorders: Clinical descriptions and diagnostic guidelines. Tenth revision (ICD-10)*, Geneva: WHO.
157. Hess-Rover J, Crichton J, Byrne K, et al. (1999). Case report: Diagnosis and treatment of a severe psychotic illness in a man with dual severe sensory impairments caused by the presence of Usher syndrome, *Journal of Intellectual Disability Research*, 43 (5), pp. 428–434.
158. Basilier T (1964). Surdophrenia. The psychic consequences of congenital or early acquired deafness. Some theoretical and clinical considerations, *Acta Psychiatrica Scandinavica*, 39 (S180), pp. 363–372.
159. du Feu M, Fergusson K (2003). Sensory impairment and mental health. *Advances in Psychiatric Treatment*, 9 (2), pp. 95–103.
160. Fellinger J, Holzinger D, Pollard R (2012). Mental health of deaf people, *Lancet* 17; 379 (9820), pp. 1037–1044.
161. Moores DF (1987). *Educating the Deaf: Psychology, Principles and Practices (3rd edition)*. Houghton Mifflin.
162. Lederberg AR, Everhart VS (2000). Conversations between deaf children and their hearing mothers: Pragmatic and dialogic characteristics, *Journal of Deaf Studies and Deaf Education*, 5 (4), pp. 303–345.
163. Meadow-Orlans K, Erting C (2000). Deaf people in society. In Hindley P, Kitson N (eds.). *Mental Health and Deafness*. London and Philadelphia: *Whurr*, pp. 3–24.
164. Bishop DVM (1983). Comprehension of English syntax by profoundly deaf children. *Journal of Child and Psychological Psychiatry*, 24 (3), pp. 415–434.
165. Sinkkonen J (1994). Hearing impairment, communication and personality development, PhD thesis, Department of Child Psychiatry, University of Helsinki (cited in Hindley PA (1997). Psychiatric aspects of hearing impairment, *Journal of Child Psychology and Psychiatry*, 38 (1), pp. 101–117.
166. Sutton-Spence R, Woll B (1998). *The Linguistics of British Sign Language: An Introduction*. Cambridge: Cambridge University Press.
167. Strong M (2007). *Language Learning and Deafness*. Cambridge: Cambridge University Press.
168. Mahshie S (1995). *Educating Deaf Children Bilingually*, Laurent Clerc National Deaf Education Center.
169. Pickersgill M, Gregory S (1998). *Sign Bilingualism—A Model, Laser Publications*.
170. Wright B (2011). The cognitive and behavioral complications of deafness, in: Nass., R, Frank Y (eds.). *The Cognitive and Behavioral Abnormalities of Pediatric Diseases*. Oxford: Oxford University Press, pp. 544–562.
171. Hauser PC, Wills KE, Isquith PK (2006). Hard-of-hearing, deafness and being deaf. In Farmer JE, Donders J, Warschausky S (eds). *Treating neurodevelopmental disabilities: Clinical research and practice*. Guilford Press, pp. 119–131.
172. Woll B (2008). Mental capital and wellbeing: Making the most of ourselves in the 21st century. *State-of-Science Review: SR-D5 Deafness and Hearing Impairment*. Foresight, UK Government Office for Science.
173. Vostanis P, Hayes M, Du Feu M et al (1997). Detection of behavioural and emotional problems in deaf children and adolescents: Comparison of two rating scales. *Child: Care, Health and Development*, 23 (3), pp. 233–246.
174. Hindley PA, Kroll L (1998). Theoretical and epidemiological aspects of attention deficit and over-activity in deaf children, *Journal of Deaf Studies and Deaf Education*, 3 (1), pp. 64–72.
175. Hindley PA (2005). Mental health problems in deaf children, *Current Paediatrics*, 15 (2), pp. 114–119.
176. van Gent T, Goedhart AW, Hindley PA et al. (2007). Prevalence and correlates of psychopathology in a sample of deaf adolescents, *Journal of Child Psychology and Psychiatry*, 48 (9), pp. 950–958.
177. Eastwood MR, Corbin SL, Reed M et al. (1985). Acquired hearing loss and psychiatric illness: An estimate of prevalence and co-morbidity in a geriatric setting, *British Journal of Psychiatry*, 147, pp. 552–556.
178. Jacob A, Prasad S, Boggild M et al. (2004). Charles Bonnet syndrome—elderly people and visual hallucinations, *British Medical Journal*, 328 (7455), pp. 1552–1554.
179. Cooper SA, Smiley E, Morrison J et al. (2007). Mental ill-health in adults with intellectual disabilities: Prevalence and associated factors, *British Journal of Psychiatry*, 190 (1), pp. 27–35.
180. Emerson E, Kiernan C, Alborz A et al. (2001). The prevalence of challenging behaviours: A total population study, *Research in Developmental Disabilities*, 22 (1), pp. 77–93.
181. Hallgren B (1959). Retinitis pigmentosa combined with congenital deafness; with vestibulecerebellar ataxia and mental abnormality in a proportion of cases: A clinical and geneticostatistical study, *Acta Psychiatrica Scandinavica*, 34 (Suppl 138), pp. 1–101.
182. Brown AS, Cohen P, Greenwald S et al. (2000). Non-affective psychosis after prenatal exposure to rubella, *American Journal of Psychiatry*, 157 (3), pp. 438–443.
183. Rolan M, Paddison C (2013). Better management of patients with multimorbidity, *British Medical Journal*, 346, f2510.
184. Akers A (2011). *Augmenting the awareness of social communication in a congenitally blind child: A case study*. BSc dissertation in Human Communication (Speech and Language Therapy), De Montfort University.
185. Moore V, McConachie H (1994). Communication between blind and severely visually impaired children and their parents, *British Journal of Developmental Psychology*, 12 (4), pp. 491–502.
186. Edlund M, Tobiason Jackson G, Lönngren G (2002). Using sound to understand the environment and to be able to handle the surroundings for a person with severe visual impairment and autism. *New Visions: Moving Toward an Inclusive Community*. Proceedings, 11th ICEVI World Conference: Leeuwenhorst Congress Centre, Netherlands, 27 July—2 August. Available at: (www.icevi.org/publications/ICEVIWC2002/papers/02-topic/02-edlund.htm). [Accessed on: Oct 2011].
187. Loots G, Devise I, Sermijn J (2003). The interaction between mothers and their visually impaired infants: An intersubjective

developmental perspective, *Journal of Visual Impairment and Blindness*, 97 (7), pp. 403–417.

188. Clarke A (2010). Visual impairment and autistic spectrum condition: Learning braille, *Insight*, 30, pp. 17–18.
189. McLinden M (2012). Mediating haptic exploratory strategies in children who have visual impairment and intellectual disabilities, *Journal of Intellectual Disability Research*, 56 (2), pp. 129–139.
190. Butler S (2004). *Hearing and Sight Loss: A Handbook for Professional Carers.* London: Age Concern.
191. Adelson E, Fraiberg S (1976). Sensory deficit and motor development in infants blind from birth. In Jasterzembska ZS (ed.). *The Effects of Blindness and Other Impairment on Early Development.* New York: *American Foundation for the Blind*, pp. 75–111.
192. Barrett M (2014). *Changes of autistic traits in adults with learning disability over time,* MSc project: University of Birmingham.
193. Preisler GM (1995). The development of communication in blind and deaf infants—similarities and differences, *Child: Care, Health and Development*, 21 (2), pp. 79–110.
194. Howley M, Preece D (2003). Structured teaching for individuals with visual impairments, *British Journal of Visual Impairment*, 21 (2), pp. 78–83.
195. Gibbons R (2005). Guidelines for teaching students with visual impairment and autistic spectrum disorders. In Pring L (ed.). *Autism and Blindness, Research and Reflections*, London and Philadelphia: *Whurr Publishers*, pp. 158–180.
196. Stevens T (2010). Gentle teaching: A positive approach to visual impairment children with autism and their staff, *Insight*, 30, pp. 15–16.
197. Jordan R (2005). Educational implications of autism and visual impairment. In Pring L (ed.). *Autism and Blindness, Research and Reflections,* London and Philadelphia: *Whurr*. pp. 142–157.
198. Caldwell P, Horwood J. (2008). *Using intensive interaction and sensory integration, a handbook for those who support people with severe autistic spectrum disorder.* London: *Jessica Kingsley Publishers.*
199. Schopler E, Mesibov GB (1995). *Structured teaching in the TEACCH system. Learning and cognition in autism.* New York: *Plenum Press.*
200. Lovaas OI (1987). Behavioural treatment and normal educational and intellectual functioning in young autistic children, *Journal of Consulting and Clinical Psychology*, 55 (1), pp. 3–9.
201. Williams GS (2014). Irlen syndrome: Expensive lenses for this ill-defined syndrome exploit patients, *British Medical Journal*, 349, g4872.
202. Lund SK, Troha JM (2008). Teaching young people who are blind and have autism to make requests using a variation on the picture exchange communication system with tactile symbols: A preliminary investigation, *Journal of Autism and Developmental Disorders*, 38 (4), pp. 719–730.
203. Taylor K, Preece D (2010). Using aspects of the TEACCH structured teaching approach with students with multiple disabilities and visual impairment Reflections on practice, *British Journal of Visual Impairment*, 28 (3), pp. 244–259.
204. Bell I (2013). The Visual Impairment and Autism Project. Available at: (http://ianpbell.com/visual-impairment-autism/). [Accessed on: 1 Oct 2014].
205. VISION 2020 UK (2012). Available at: (www.vision2020uk.org.uk). [Accessed on: 1 September 2012].
206. KendallT, Megnin-Viggarsm O, Gould N et al. (2013). Management of autism in children and young people: Summary of NICE and SCIE guidance, *British Medical Journal*, 347, f4865.
207. Pilling S, Baron-Cohen S, Megnin-Viggars O et al. (2012). Recognition, referral, diagnosis, and management of adults with autism: Summary of NICE guidance, *British Medical Journal*, 344, e4082.
208. Tager-Flusberg H (2005). Reflection on the connections between autism and blindness. In Pring L (ed.). *Autism and Blindness, Research and Reflections,* London and Philadelphia: *Whurr*, pp. 181–188.
209. Salt A (2010). Visual impairment and autism: Diagnostic approaches. In *Children who have visual impairment and autism* conference. London, Thursday 18 and Friday 19 November 2010. Available at: (http://www.autism.org.uk/about-autism/related-conditions/visual-impairment-and-autism-spectrum-disorders.aspx). [Accessed on: 1 Oct 2013].
210. Lewis V, Collins G (2005). Research methods fit for purpose. In Pring L (ed.). *Autism and Blindness, Research and Reflections,* London and Philadelphia: *Whurr*, pp.128–141.
211. Hobson RP, Lee A (2010). Reversible autism among congenitally blind children? A controlled follow-up study, *Journal of Child Psychology and Psychiatry*, 51 (11), pp. 1235–1241.
212. Jure R, Pogonza R, Rapin I (2016). Autism Spectrum Disorders (ASD) in blind children: Very high prevalence, potentially better outlook, *Journal of Autism and Developmental Disorder*, 46 (3), 749–759.
213. de Vaan G, Vervloed M, Peters-Scheffer NC, van Gent T., Knoors H, Verhoeven L (2016). Behavioural assessment of autism spectrum disorders in people with multiple disabilities. *Journal of Intellectual Disability Research*, 60 (2), 101–112.
214. de Vaan G, Vervloed M, Peters-Scheffer NC, van Gent T, Knoors H, Verhoeven L (2018). Assessing autism spectrum disorder in people with sensory impairments combined with intellectual disabilities. *Journal of Developmental and Physical Disabilities*, 30 (4), 471–487.
215. National Institute of Clinical Excellence (2012). Autism: Recognition, referral, diagnosis and management of adults on the autism spectrum, *NICE Clinical Guideline*, CG142.

25

Family Experiences of Psychiatric Services for their Relative with Intellectual and Developmental Disabilities

Verity Chester, Neil James, Ian Rogers, Jackie Grace, and Regi Alexander

Introduction

When a relative develops a mental or behavioural issue that requires the support of services, it can be highly distressing for their families and carers. If that relative also suffers from an intellectual or developmental disability (DID), this can be even more difficult, due to problems accessing services adapted to their loved one's needs. There is strong recognition of the important role that families can play in patients' recovery. Many people with intellectual disability have small social networks (1) and therefore their family members are intensely important to them. Contact with and support from families is often a key factor in sustaining a patient's motivation and sense of self-worth. Recent National Institute for Clinical Excellence (2015) guidelines (2) recommend that services and professionals work in partnership with family carers, and UK policies advocate the need to consult with carers when planning and delivering services. In a King's Fund report, Foot et al. (3) noted that involving families and carers is an essential part of good patient care, acknowledging the diverse number of roles, including:

- providing emotional, social, and financial support
- domestic assistance
- monitoring health and wellbeing
- providing basic health and personal care
- helping to provide professionals with information about the individual
- advocating for individuals
- proactively seeking out care and treatment options.

Meaningfully involving families is associated with positive outcomes for patients, carers, and service quality (3). Patient outcomes include increased knowledge, confidence, and understanding of their health problems, reduced rates of relapse and admissions to hospital. Involvement can enhance self-confidence, and provide carers with the opportunity to learn new skills, which supports their caring role. Organizational benefits include improved staff confidence and teamwork, and reduced numbers of complaints. The authors discuss the 'triangle of care' concept, a holistic approach that brings together carers, patients, and health professionals, and which aims to promote safety and recovery for people with mental health issues by including and supporting carers. Foot et al. (3) outline that the involvement of families and carers should be considered at all stages of care-planning, decision-making, and delivery, with the same thought and attention as for the patient.

Unfortunately, families often report that their experiences do not reflect this guidance, that they have had to 'fight' to access services, and once they have accessed care, their liaison with professionals and services has been challenging (4), an experience that is very often described in other healthcare settings too. This chapter will review the literature on the experiences of carers preceding and during psychiatric care for their relative with DID, including a case study written by a father with direct experience of seeking support for his daughter with Down Syndrome who developed mental health issues. Barriers to family involvement will be discussed, in addition to the developments of some good practice standards, in order for clinicians and services to begin establishing and nurturing positive relationships with patients' families.

Family experiences of a relative with DID and mental health/behavioural issues

Research has typically framed the experiences of families with a relative with DID negatively, in terms of stress and burden (5). Indeed, some families report lower levels of psychological wellbeing (6, 7), self-esteem (8), and chronic levels of stress (9). Family carers report experiencing a lack of acceptance, negative attitudes, feeling blamed for their relatives behaviour, and being stared at in public, therefore restricting their activities; and thus loneliness, isolation, stigma, and reduced quality of life (10–15). Emotional issues such as grief, loss, causation, guilt, and worry about who will look after their relative when they pass away (16, 17) are common.

However, overemphasizing stress and burden creates an overly negative perception of having a relative with DID. Further research has attempted to redress this balance, and provide a more balanced perspective, highlighting that many families talk about their child with DID in exactly the same terms as their children without DID, as a source of joy and happiness (5). Families have reported expanded personal and social networks and community involvement, an increased sense of purpose, personal growth and strength, strengthening of family unity and closeness, increased tolerance and understanding (5). Therefore it is important to recognize that all families are different. Children and adults with DID have highly heterogenous levels of disability and associated needs and behaviours. Accordingly, their relatives have varying degrees of coping skills, and levels of personal support. Furthermore, caring evolves through several transition periods of stability and change—starting and leaving school, adolescence and leaving home, with differing degrees of challenges and predictability.

People with DID are equally, or more likely, than the general population to experience mental health problems (20). Lives can alter immeasurably when a close relative develops mental health difficulties (16). The illness can mean the person experiences personality changes, becomes unpredictable, and in a minority of cases, violent (19). Families can suffer financially, due to being unable to work due to their caring commitments (19). However, people with DID often face additional difficulties in obtaining mental health treatment. These difficulties include problems establishing a reliable psychiatric diagnosis, due to receptive and expressive language deficits that limit the ability of an individual to articulate their internal experience and emotions (20). Some people with DID actively attempt to hide their symptoms, to appear competent (20). People with DID find it difficult to navigate through services and to negotiate the care they need (21). Mental disorders among people with a DID often present in atypical ways and coexist more frequently with autism, epilepsy, and other neurological disorders (22). Diagnostic overshadowing is another issue, where psychopathology is attributed to the DID, and the potential for comorbid mental illness overlooked, a phenomena discussed further in our case study. This is important, as diagnosis is often key to accessing services, and providing a basis for treatment (20). Therefore, family members are heavily relied upon to provide a pivotal advocacy role in alerting professionals to changes in their relatives presentation (15).

A further barrier to mental health treatment for people with DID can be ongoing disagreements about whether care is provided by generic/mainstream, or specialist services. There is wide international variation in provision, with the UK and The Netherlands having the most developed specialist services. In Scandinavia, the USA, Australia, and most of Western Europe, care is mainly provided by general psychiatric wards or services (23, 24). While this debate is beyond the scope of this chapter, it is relevant due to the impact on patients and their families. Care may suffer because of boundary disputes between specialist and general services—with possible exclusion from both (24). Indeed, families have reported difficulties accessing support, getting the GP to refer them to a specialist, and then facing long waiting lists (25). Parents have described services often as fragmented, uncompromising, hard to reach, and not in accordance with their needs (26). Carers frequently report 'fighting' to obtain services, noting that situations need to reach crisis point before help is provided (27, 28).

Research exploring the carer perspectives on their relative's admission to in-patient settings highlighted that this can be a disempowering experience, especially if unplanned, due to professionals assuming the role of experts and having control over decisions and care of their relative. Carers can become uncertain regarding the definition of their role and how they fit into the care being provided (29). Therefore, while their relative is now being cared for outside the family home, families may remain in a crisis state due to the uncertainty and continuing concern (30), particularly about their child's vulnerability and that they will not be cared for in the same way that their family would (29). A further difficulty is the 'language of mental health'. Staff are so well versed with diagnoses, processes, procedures, and acronyms used within their practice they can forget that this may not be accessible to carers. Families have described concerns around transitions, and lacking coordination of care when an individual is ready for discharge into the community from inpatient services (31, 32), with the prospect of discharge leading to increased uncertainty and anxiety about reduced levels of support for their relative (33). This is not because staff do not care, rather that they inevitably become occupied by tasks, demands, and focus on the patient.

In a systematic review investigating family involvement in the treatment of patients with psychosis, Eassom et al. (32) highlighted the systemic reasons for poor involvement of families. Staff overwhelmingly reported on the practical aspects of family work: that it requires time, resources, and funding and is difficult to integrate with other clinical casework, particularly in areas with high demands and clinical crises. Specific needs reported for family work included flexible hours and the accommodation of family requirements such as childcare facilities or home visits. These issues were compounded by reports of services and managers not making time allowances for family work, for example, not providing time in lieu for out of hours work, or obstructing time use, for example, by refusing the release of staff for training. Relatedly, all mental health services in the UK are experiencing significant financial cuts to their funding, which impacts on quality of care across all aspects of service provision, including family involvement. However, cultures in which family involvement is not promoted are not conducive to quality care. Indeed, the public inquiry into the care failings and substandard care at Mid Staffordshire NHS Foundation Trust noted that a significant factor within the events which occurred was that relatives felt excluded from effective participation in the patients' care (34).

Case study 1: A parent's perspective

My daughter Emma was born with Down syndrome. Emma developed into a contented, fun loving, young lady who enjoyed music, cinema, swimming, and family time. However as Emma entered adulthood, things began to change. She began to withdraw to her bedroom offering no contact with family or friends, became physically tired and collapsed on one occasion, and refused to engage in social activities previously enjoyed. She became very angry and sometimes physical when challenged about her behaviour, increasingly refused to communicate verbally, became increasingly anxious, and developed a hysterical fear of flying insects. Emma's GP undertook a physical examination and blood tests which revealed nothing physiologically awry and referred her to the specialist DID support service. A psychologist visited but said that 'she couldn't connect with Emma to draw any firm conclusions', taking no further action. In the meantime, our own research led us to believe that Emma may be displaying signs of a depressive mental illness. We expressed our concerns to professionals, but got the impression that they thought that Emma's condition was more related to her Down syndrome than a mental health issue.

Emma's condition then further deteriorated. She withdrew completely, and barely spoke. She lost her appetite, refused to leave her bedroom and withdrew into a fantasy world with her dolls (with whom she spoke quite loudly). We immediately contacted our community care worker, who requested an urgent appointment with a psychiatrist. We heard nothing for a few weeks; then received a call inviting Emma for an appointment that afternoon. Ignoring Emma's semi-mute state, the psychiatrist increasingly 'talked over' Emma about her condition to us. After increasing distress for Emma, we stopped the interview and asked if we could speak in private. In this discussion, the psychiatrist conceded that he had not read Emma's notes and had little background knowledge. I gave a full briefing detailing Emma's rapid decline and mental health. Following the consultation, the psychiatrist wrote a report to our GP, expressing the opinion that Emma's condition was due to the upheaval of a recent house and geographical area move, providing no diagnosis or prescription. We challenged this outcome with the GP on the grounds that it did not take into account Emma's progressive symptoms and the unsatisfactory consultation. The GP supported our view and referred Emma back to the psychiatrist.

Weeks after the psychiatric consultation, we were invited to a multidisciplinary review of Emma's condition attended by the psychiatrist, psychologist, community care worker and the life skills centre manager, who knew Emma very well. There was an agreed support process, but still no firm diagnosis or medication. Emma had settled into a 'withdrawn' lifestyle, with her only regular trip out being a weekly visit to the life skills centre. We continued to press for a firm diagnosis of her mental health condition, having taken advice from specialist charities. Finally, the psychiatrist prescribed medication to assist Emma, pending an assessment of Emma's decision-making capacity.

Matters came to a head almost six months after we first sought support. Emma began refusing to eat or drink, would not speak to anyone, and passively sat on her bed, moving only to go to the bathroom. The GP visited and examined Emma, confirming no physiological obstruction and tried to persuade her to eat and drink, to no avail. After two days, Emma conceded to take a little milk from the tip of my wife's finger, and on the third day took some milk on a dessert spoon, but nothing more. This coincided with a multidisciplinary meeting where I was able to report the current crisis in Emma's health. We were told that Emma would probably start eating soon when hunger demanded. It was agreed that medication should now be prescribed (fluoxetine) on a 'best interests' basis.

Emma continued refusing to eat, drinking minimal liquids. The GP explained that if this situation continued, Emma may have to be admitted to hospital for feeding. We became desperate for assistance, but heard nothing from the psychologist or psychiatrist despite placing a number of calls. I phoned Emma's life skills centre to send her apologies on the day she would normally attend. On the phone I broke down, explaining that we were desperate for contact from the specialist team, and practically begged the support worker to get us some help. An emergency meeting was arranged, with a liaison nurse sent to visit in the meantime, which provided moral support. We nursed Emma, spoon feeding her about 800mls of milk per day. We could see no end to the situation and feared that Emma may have to be admitted to hospital.

The cycle was thankfully broken, when staff from the life skills centre visited Emma at home to see if 'they could get through to her'. Emma knew that these care workers 'loved her to bits' and, utilizing this level of trust, they very skilfully persuaded her to start eating and drinking again that day. This proved to be the turning point. Over the following few weeks, Emma slowly began to eat and drink normally, became less anxious, and regained self-confidence. After a few months, she began to communicate, came off medication, started attending the cinema and swimming, and was living partly with us (three nights a week), and happily in a supported living house for the rest of the week. We had our daughter back!

Improving family experiences of accessing and engaging with mental health/ID services

A developing body of research has sought to understand what families expect from services caring for their relative. This literature, and Emma's case study, illustrates a number of issues which carers commonly raise as unsatisfactory in relation to their interactions with professionals and services. The case study particularly highlights that while families do want to have adequate access to services that listen to their concerns, they are also keen to have a diagnosis that explains their relative's current difficulties and informs the treatment plan that is proposed.

These issues are summarized in Table 25.1, alongside strategies which can be considered in order to improve practice. While not all of the issues are viewed as a core aspect of the psychiatrist's role, such as the provision of pleasant environmental facilities for families, they remain important for the psychiatrist to be aware of in relation to influencing the broader service quality in their respective organizations.

Foot et al. (3) set out some broad standards outlining how to achieve meaningful family involvement in health services:

- Organizations should have a carer policy that is well communicated to staff, with training programmes and specific remits for staff around involving carers.
- Health professionals need to identify carers, and then keep this information up to date in medical records.
- Involving carers requires the agreement of the individual who they are caring for.
- Subject to consent, information should be shared with the carer, including details of services, diagnosis, treatment options, and support mechanisms.
- Carers should be involved in care-planning and discharge plans from hospital, as team members.
- Carers should receive adequate support with their own needs. This can range from arranging appointments at times of the day when carers can get cover, through to providing formal periods of respite care. In the UK, the Care Act 2014 mandates that carers have the legal right to an assessment and support from their local authority.

Within these broad standards, there are some important areas to consider. For example, when identifying carers, it may be that the patient's closest familial bond is not with parents, but a grandparent,

Table 25.1 Improving family experiences of accessing and engaging with mental health/ID services

Capacity assessments and ascertaining patient's wishes regarding family involvement.	While this can be a source of contention for families, the patient's wishes regarding their family involvement must be sought and respected.	Prior to initiating contact or sharing information with an adult patient's family, a capacity assessment should be undertaken. If: a) the patient has capacity, their consent is required in order to involve their families in their care, what information they are happy to share with their relatives, and what level of contact they would like. b) the patient does not have capacity, there should be a 'best interests' decision regarding family involvement. This process can be supported by an independent advocate, who listens to and supports the person at the heart of the decision to make their opinions heard, and resolve any conflicts between stakeholders. Capacity should be reviewed regularly, according to the patient's presentation or the family situation.
Proactive and meaningful inclusion and involvement.	Carers most satisfied with the service their relative receive, report being an active participant within, and 'member of the care team'.	Consider and treat your patient's relative as a member of the team, or colleague. Recognize and respect their expertise and knowledge on their relative's history, current presentation, past and present response to treatment, and what is likely to work in regards to future plans.
Good quality, inclusive information.	In Emma's case study, her family were not provided with any information about mental health, and had to undertake their own research. This is an additional burden for carers already experiencing difficulties, will not be possible for all carers, and the quality of the information accessed could be of variable quality.	Provide carers with information on: • the signs and symptoms of mental ill health • the current and developing needs of their relative • how to manage their relative's condition • their relative's rights whilst within services • available services and financial support This should be both prior to accessing a service (e.g. with an appointment letter) and during care, and might involve signposting to evidence-based and accessible websites, or services developing their own.
Accessibility: a) **Of services.**	Carers often do not have knowledge of the services available to their relative, and rely on referrals from general practitioners.	Services should be 'joined up' and easily accessible to patients and carers. Access procedures should be reviewed from the point of view of families.
b) **Of clinicians.**	In Emma's case, it proved difficult to her family to access expert support when it was needed. Telephone calls were not returned and her parents had no emergency contact numbers to alert professionals to her symptoms worsening, and delaying her care.	When meeting and communicating with families, be friendly and approachable. Outline your contact preferences and availability, e.g. 'I always respond to emails' or 'I am usually office based on Tuesday afternoons'. Set 'out of office' messages on both email and telephone systems informing families of your return to work dates and details of cover in your absence. Consider providing a 'key worker' to each case who could be easily accessed by carers and responsible for ensuring that appropriate parties are alerted to and respond to any changes.
c) **Of procedures.**	Procedures and processes followed within services can be counterintuitive and alienating for carers. Carers often complain they are left waiting for long durations for assessment results, meeting conclusions, etc.	Explain the background to procedures and processes to help understanding, e.g. 'the CPA—Care Programme Approach Meeting—was established so that everyone involved in patient's care can regularly get together, review progress and plan for the future. They happen every six months and you will be invited by the clinical secretary once we have set the date'. Provide carers with information on what to expect following an assessment or meeting, i.e. 'you will receive a letter within five working days' or 'we will send you a copy of the assessment report within two weeks'.
d) **Of language.**	Language, e.g. complex diagnostic terms and acronyms can exclude families.	All information provided to families, whether written or verbal, should be inclusive and accessible. Remember your first week in a new job or service and the process of learning the terminology and incorporate this into your interactions with families. Provide full explanations of acronyms and complex terms, e.g., 'we think your son may be showing signs of autism spectrum disorder, or ASD. This is a condition which affects the way a person interacts socially... Here is a leaflet about the condition. Please feel free to ask any questions, either now, or once you have had chance to read up a little more'.
Diagnostic overshadowing.	Families often report that initially, all of their relatives problems were attributed to their DID, with no exploration of the possibility of a co-occuring mental illness. This limits the opportunity for early intervention, prolongs symptoms and delays care.	Do not assume any issue arising is due to the DID. The reason for seeking treatment will usually be due to a change or deterioration in presentation which has been observed by those around the patient. Undertake a full mental health assessment, seeking support from a DID specialist, if available.

Table 25.1 Continued

Develop the knowledge.	In Emma's case, information was provided about her presentation which was not reviewed prior to her consultation. This meant the consultation caused distress to Emma and her family. Understanding of both the patient and their family should be developed through the review of available information, such as referral letters, case files, and the developing working relationship.	Take the time to review any information which has been provided prior to consultations. When time is scarce in a busy clinic, patients would prefer to be kept waiting an extra five minutes while you read the referral letter or scan the case file. This can make the consultation more efficient and tailored to the patient's needs, and develop a more positive relationship. Write detailed notes about your consultations with patients in order to share your developing knowledge with the team, and review others notes and reports.
Listening	Emma's case study evidences how family members' opinions can be dismissed and not listened to.	Remember that families know their relative the best and are the most familiar with their history and behaviours over many years. As such they are often well placed to report on any changes in health or behaviour. Acknowledge and listen to families views and manage any disagreements professionally, highlighting the reasons for your opinion or decision in a transparent manner.
Welcoming environment.	Environments within services accessed by families, such as reception areas, meeting and visitors rooms can be intimidating. This can affect the experience of consultations and visits. Families are often central to recovery and if they are not comfortable in the service it can cut short or discourage visits.	Review the environment from the point of view of a family member. Do they create a good first impression? Are facilities well signposted? Is it too hot or too cold? The environment should be made welcoming and accommodating of visitors, with comfortable facilities, considering temperature, seating, and provision of refreshments.
Support for carers.	Carers receive minimal formal support from governmental agencies. This can mean they suffer from stress, which negatively affects themselves and their ability to provide good care.	Consider providing a support group/online network for carers. Signpost to relevant local/national services or groups. Be supportive and respectful and all times.
Auditing carer experience and satisfaction.	If feedback is not sought from carers on their experience and satisfaction levels, problems can get hidden and services may be operating under a false sense of competency in this area.	Family and carer experience should be measured routinely as part of the annual audit cycle, and any positive or negative comments and suggestions considered and acted upon, as necessary.

sibling, or cousin, or for those have grown up in local-authority/state care, a foster carer. Furthermore, some patients do not have a carer. Cheshire, Chester, Graham, Grace, and Alexander (36) reported that approximately 20 per cent of patients detained within in-patient specialist forensic DID services were not in contact with their families. Some patient's relatives had passed away, and others related to families being unable to cope with their relative's offence history, or being the victim of the relative's offence. Therefore, it should be recognized that families are not monolithic; each of its members have their own individual characteristics, needs, and differing levels of knowledge and involvement. This highlights the need for an individualized approach, and to develop knowledge and understanding of each individual patient's family context.

It is important to obtain consent from the patient as to whether they wish for their family to be involved in their care, and specify what this contact will look like, particularly in terms of the information patients wish to be shared with family. This is a decision which requires an assessment of the patient's capacity, a process enshrined in Mental Capacity Act (2005) legislation in England and Wales. If the patient is assessed as lacking capacity then any action taken, or any decision made on behalf of that person, must be made in their 'best interests'. This process may involve an independent mental capacity advocate (IMCA) who fulfils the role of a statutory safeguard and supports those lacking capacity to make important decisions. A further consideration at this stage is to assess whether any safeguarding issues are present. People with DID are vulnerable to abuse (37), because of dependence on other people for personal care; 'imbalances of power' between the carer and the person being cared for; communication difficulties; lack of sexual knowledge and assertiveness; and guilt and shame at being disabled (38). Research has suggested that many people with DID in in-patient services experience painful relationships with family, and histories of conflict and abuse (39). Alexander et al. (40) reported that as many as 50 per cent of patients within forensic DID settings have experienced abuse. Furthermore, this abuse may be the reason services are required, with victims of sexual abuse having higher rates of mental illness, behavioural disturbance, and post traumatic stress disorder, with the severity of the effects related to the severity of abuse (41). If abuse is uncovered, or disclosed by the patient, safeguarding processes are activated to protect against further abuse.

This process can be frustrating for family members, with the perception that confidentiality is used by professionals as a way to not share information (32). However, patients emphasize how important the opportunity to consent is to them, strongly linked to self-esteem, privacy, personal choice, independence, autonomy, general wellbeing, and empowerment (42). Therefore, the only situation in which information should not be shared with family, is if a patient with capacity, has requested it be kept private, or if the capacity assessment has deemed family contact is not in the patient's best interests. This situation is very difficult for relatives, particularly if a relative is withholding contact and information. There are a number of reasons why patients may not wish their relative(s) to be involved in their care, including privacy concerns (keeping the extent of the illness from the family), fears of placing relatives in a position of power, or of exposing their vulnerability (28). The rationale for withholding any information should therefore be explained in a transparent manner to relatives. Furthermore, it is important to outline that consent will be reviewed regularly, and so the situation may change in the future.

Once consent has been obtained and the patient's wishes ascertained, the process of information sharing and involvement can begin. A useful starting point is if the main professionals involved introduce themselves to their patient's relatives, describe their role in the team, their practice remit in relation to policy, legislation, accountability, professional codes, organizational boundaries and resource availability. There is no prescriptive guidance as to the frequency, or modes of contact, as this will depend on the individual situation of the carer and their other commitments, among other factors, and may also evolve over time. However, it is important for agreed contact times and methods to be adhered to, and to make contact at the next opportunity, if for example, something comes up which affects whether an agreed telephone call can be made. While information is provided from the care team to the carer(s), such as revisions to the working diagnosis and care plan, discussions around visits, meetings, and progress, a lesser discussed role of the family is the value of the information they provide on their relative, which is crucial to numerous aspects of assessment and treatment, such as; the 'getting to know you' process, developing a diagnosis, and to assess levels of risk. Ideally, a patient's family are contacted at an early stage of the patient's contact with services. Family members ore often pleased to supply a full account of the patient's life, which is hugely valuable, providing a full picture of their life and who they are, their behaviour across contexts, and key events and timeline. This information should be recorded carefully, taking care on clarity, chronology, names of schools, details of different placements, etc.

The National Institute for Health and Care Excellence (NICE) (2015) (2, 18) emphasize the importance of professionals, services, and family carers working in partnerships for involvement to be meaningful. Consideration needs to be given as to how families are involved, so that they do not feel sidelined, powerless or overwhelmed, but fundamental to the care process. For example, some carers have reported being invited to particular sections of meetings, and gaining the impression that decisions have been made prior to their attendance. Good communication processes, such as information sharing and joint working between professionals, agencies, and relatives are also important. This could include, regular multiagency care reviews, joint strategy meetings, and a shared list of all agencies/professionals involved with an individual and their family. Providing validation about their knowledge, positive feedback, and treating carers as members of the care team, supports the development of positive relationships (3, 43, 44). Identifying a key worker, who acts as a single point of access to a service and professionals can ensure carers are empowered and kept involved by co-ordinating meetings, assessments and contact (25). On occasions, there may be disagreements on diagnostic, management, and treatment decisions between relatives and others within the team. This may be because carers and professionals recognize and understand the needs of the individual differently based on their relationship, knowledge, and experience. Conversely, relatives can experience denial about the extent of their relative's difficulties. Carers may be concerned about the use of medication or other treatments they perceive as restrictive and potentially harmful (45). As a consequence, conflict may occur and professionals need to manage this disagreement and try to find a pragmatic resolution which benefits the patient.

A developing area of practice is in the provision and evaluation of groups for family members. Chiocchi and colleagues (46) described a carer-led programme for mental health carers co-delivered over 20 two-hour training sessions. Sessions included mental health psychoeducation, family skills, and problem-solving sessions. There was a high number of referrals to the programme, and an evaluation indicated improved well-being, reduced burden, and increased family empowerment in carers. Smallwood et al. (47) described a caregiver support service, which offered individual and group psychoeducation, practical advice, and emotional support, working alongside usual community mental health provision for people with established psychosis. The evaluation suggested improvements in wellbeing, and in caregiving experiences. Rye et al. (35) described a group for young people with a sibling having a disability, which aimed to increase understanding about disability, provide a space for peer support and skills development, for self care, and care of their siblings. These groups show promise in providing support for a diverse group of family carers. However, such interventions may not be accessible to all, and further research should explore innovative methods of providing support to family carers.

Conclusion

This chapter has considered the experiences of relatives and carers in accessing and using psychiatry or behavioural services for their loved one with DID. Families go through a lot to support their relative, forgoing their own needs, and experience significant stresses and traumatic experiences to do so. It is therefore imperative that professionals working in services do their utmost to support this group, alongside providing quality care for their relative. The literature review, and our case study, written by a father with direct experience of attempting to access the right care for his daughter highlighted a number of common themes consistently raised by the families of those with DID accessing services. While it must be acknowledged that services are generally more likely to receive criticism than praise (48), there are a number of recommendations which can be adopted by all services which can support the provision of good quality care across the lifetime of people with DID.

One relates to the prevention of development and worsening of mental health and behavioural problems in people with DID, via the provision of good quality information to those caring. This information needs to be provided sensitively, and in a timely manner, so as not to frighten families about all the potential negative outcomes facing their child, whilst giving an indicator of what signs to look for so that help can be obtained. Relatedly, the need for the right diagnosis at the right time, has implications for services. Following the aftermath of the Winterbourne View abuse scandal in the UK, some have questioned the need for specialism, and indeed psychiatry in the care of people with DID (49). While a mainstream model of care may be preferable to some, it is clear that the diagnosis of mental health problems in this population requires a degree of specialist expertise, preferably from an expert in the mental health of people with DID or alternatively from staff who have had equivalent training. It is this professional expertise that guarantees an equity of treatment outcome for a vulnerable patient group.

The recommendation of a key worker, or a named point of contact is one that many families would value. One only needs to reflect on a personal dissatisfaction with being unable to access the same GP or specialist doctor to recognize this basic need to develop a relationship with a professional with ongoing understanding and knowledge of your, or your relative's case history and current treatment. On the other hand, this should be managed in a flexible way, so that one professional does not 'own' the relationship with a particular relative, and therefore the relative receives no contact when that staff member goes on holiday or sick leave.

The need for carers to be listened to, is a recurrent theme which crops up in most family narratives. If the starting point is honest, and collaborative relationships between families and services, this should not be a problem. However as noted, staff working within services can be known to take the line 'we know best'. In some cases, the service will know best, and in others, the family will, and in the majority, the truth will lie somewhere in between. Sometimes the only way to ascertain the best diagnosis or approach is for one party to try to listen to the other's suggestion and vice versa. It is important that a respectful culture is fostered so that any disagreements can be managed positively. If these recommendations are practised, it is likely that positive relationships can be developed between services and patient's relatives and carers, improving outcomes for all parties.

Undoubtedly, there is currently a lack of social and professional support for families of relatives accessing services. While generic carer services are of some utility for practical information and support, newly developed specific services which are linked to the service their relative is receiving have been rated positively by families (16, 47). These services are in their infancy and will only succeed if substantially funded by governments.

MULTIPLE CHOICE QUESTIONS

Questions

Please select the single most appropriate answer.

1. All of the following about the triangle of care concept are true except:

A. Includes patients
B. Protects health professionals against claims
C. Supports carers
D. Promotes patient safety
E. Promotes recovery

2. Regarding requirements for meaningful involvement of families in healthcare, all of the following are true except:

A. Carers have to be identified correctly by healthcare professionals
B. Carers should be offered support for their needs
C. Relevant information should be shared with the carer
D. Getting patient consent is less important in this context
E. Healthcare organizations should have a carer policy

3. People with an intellectual or developmental disability may be more vulnerable to abuse because of:

A. Dependence on others for personal care
B. Communication difficulties
C. Lack of assertiveness
D. Lack of sexual knowledge
E. All of the above

4. Patients may not want carers or family members to be given information about their condition because of:

A. Not wanting them to know the extent of their illness
B. Fear of placing carers in a position of power
C. Exposing vulnerabilities
D. Privacy concerns
E. All of the above

5. To improve the experience of families in accessing healthcare for their relatives in mental health services, all of the following are true except:

A. Stating that appointment times are beyond clinical control
B. Providing written information before and after consultations
C. Families feeling that they are part of the care team
D. Signposting to the evidence base
E. Measuring carer experience

Answers

1. B. The triangle of care concept is a holistic approach that brings together carers, patients, and health professionals, and which aims to promote safety and recovery for people with mental health issues by including and supporting carers. The involvement of families and carers should be considered at all stages of care-planning, decision-making, and delivery.
2. D. Organizations should have a carer policy that is well communicated to staff, with training programmes and specific remits for staff around involving carers. Health professionals need to identify carers, and then keep this information up to date in medical records. Involving carers does require the agreement of the individual who they are caring for. Subject to consent, information should be shared with the carer, including details of services, diagnosis, treatment options, and support mechanisms.Where the patient lacks the capacity to consent, best interest decisions may have to be taken. Carers should receive adequate support with their own needs—ranging from arranging appointments at convenient times to providing formal periods of respite care.
3. E. People with intellectual and developmental disabilities may be vulnerable to abuse because of dependence on other people for personal care, 'imbalances of power' between the carer and the person being cared for, communication difficulties, lack of sexual knowledge, and assertiveness and guilt and shame at being disabled.
4. E. The process of needing patient consent to share information can sometimes be frustrating for family members, with the perception that confidentiality is used by professionals as a way to not share information. However, the opportunity to consent is strongly linked to self-esteem, privacy, personal choice, independence, autonomy, general wellbeing, and empowerment. If any information is not being shared, the rationale for that should be explained in a transparent manner to relatives. It should also be explained that consent will be reviewed regularly and hence this situation may change.
5. A. These factors are summarized in Table 25.1. Some of these such as appointment timings that are convenient for families and the physical environment of the consultation space may

be beyond the control of individual clinicians. However a willingness to listen carefully, be accommodating, and show flexibility wherever possible while acknowledging limitations in a transparent and sympathetic way tends to be more helpful.

REFERENCES

1. Forrester-Jones R, Carpenter J, Coolen-Schrijner P, Cambridge P, Tate A, Beecham J, et al. The social networks of people with intellectual disability living in the community 12 years after resettlement from long-stay hospitals. *J Appl Res Intellect Disabil* [Internet]. 2006 Dec [cited 2017 7 Mar];19(4):285–295. Available from: http://doi.wiley.com/10.1111/j.1468-3148.2006.00263.x.
2. The National Institute for Health and Care Excellence (NICE). Challenging behaviour and learning disabilities: Prevention and interventions for people with learning disabilities whose behaviour challenges [Internet]. 2015. Available from: https://www.nice.org.uk/guidance/ng11.
3. Foot C, Gilburt H, Dunn P, Jabbal J, Seale B, Goodrich J, et al. People in control of their own health and care: The state of involvement [Internet]. 2014. Available from: https://www.kingsfund.org.uk/sites/default/files/field/field_publication_file/people-in-control-of-their-own-health-and-care-the-state-of-involvement-november-2014.pdf.
4. James N. Supporting carers during assessment and treatment unit admissions. *Adv Ment Heal Intellect Disabil* [Internet]. 2016 Mar 7 [cited 2017 13];10(2):116–127. Available from: http://www.emeraldinsight.com/doi/10.1108/AMHID-08-2015-0039
5. Stainton T, Besser H. The positive impact of children with an intellectual disability on the family. *J Intellect Dev Disabil* [Internet]. 1998 Jan [cited 2017 23 Aug];23(1):57–70. Available from: http://informahealthcare.com/doi/abs/10.1080/13668259800033581.
6. James N. Enhancing relationships between family carers and professionals. *Learn Disabil Pract* [Internet]. 2013 Jul [cited 2017 8 Mar];16(6):34–37. Available from: http://rcnpublishing.com/doi/abs/10.7748/ldp2013.07.16.6.34.e1444.
7. Dawson F, Shanahan S, Fitzsimons E, O'Malley G, Mac Giollabhui N, Bramham J. The impact of caring for an adult with intellectual disability and psychiatric comorbidity on carer stress and psychological distress. *J Intellect Disabil Res* [Internet]. 2016 Jun [cited 2017 8 Mar];60(6):553–563. Available from: http://www.ncbi.nlm.nih.gov/pubmed/27028105.
8. Emerson E, Hatton C, Llewellyn G, Blacker J, Graham H. Socio-economic position, household composition, health status and indicators of the well-being of mothers of children with and without intellectual disabilities. *J Intellect Disabil Res* [Internet]. 2006 Dec [cited 2017 8 Mar];50(12):862–873. Available from: http://www.ncbi.nlm.nih.gov/pubmed/17100947.
9. Griffith GM, Hastings RP. 'He's hard work, but he's worth it'. The experience of caregivers of individuals with intellectual disabilities and challenging behaviour: A meta-synthesis of qualitative research [Internet]. Vol. 27, *Journal of Applied Research in Intellectual Disabilities*. 2014 [cited 2017 23 Feb]. pp. 401–419. Available from: http://www.ncbi.nlm.nih.gov/pubmed/24105755.
10. Scior K, Werner S. Changing attitudes to learning disability [Internet]. London; 2015 [cited 2017 Feb 23]. Available from: https://www.mencap.org.uk/sites/default/files/2016-08/Attitudes_Changing_Report.pdf
11. Ngo H, Shin JY, Nhan NV, Yang LH. Stigma and restriction on the social life of families of children with intellectual disabilities in Vietnam. *Singapore Med J* [Internet]. 2012 Jul [cited 2017 23 Feb];53(7):451–457. Available from: http://www.ncbi.nlm.nih.gov/pubmed/22815013.
12. Busner J, Targum SD. The clinical global impressions scale: Applying a research tool in clinical practice. *Psychiatry (Edgmont)* [Internet]. 2007 Jul [cited 2016 13 Jul];4(7):28–37. Available from: http://www.ncbi.nlm.nih.gov/pubmed/20526405.
13. Ryan S. 'Busy Behaviour' in the 'Land of the Golden M': Going out with learning disabled children in public places. *J Appl Res Intellect Disabil* [Internet]. 2005 Mar [cited 2017 23 Feb];18(1):65–74. Available from: http://doi.wiley.com/10.1111/j.1468-3148.2004.00225.x.
14. Kenny K, McGilloway S. Caring for children with learning disabilities: an exploratory study of parental strain and coping. *Br J Learn Disabil* [Internet]. 2007 Dec [cited 2017 8 Mar];35(4):221–228. Available from: http://doi.wiley.com/10.1111/j.1468-3156.2007.00445.x.
15. Mitter N, Ali A, Scior K. Stigma experienced by family members of people with intellectual and developmental disabilities: multidimensional construct. *BJPsych Open* [Internet]. 2018 Sep 15 [cited 2019 24 Mar];4(5):332–338. Available from: https://www.cambridge.org/core/product/identifier/S205647241800039X/type/journal_article.
16. Smallwood J. Who cares for the carers.pdf. *Psychologist* [Internet]. 2016 [cited 2017 22 Feb];29(9):698–699. Available from: https://thepsychologist.bps.org.uk/volume-29/september/who-cares-carers.
17. Brennan D, Murphy R, McCallion P, McCarron M. 'What's going to happen when we're gone?' Family caregiving capacity for older people with an intellectual disability in Ireland. *J Appl Res Intellect Disabil* [Internet]. 2018 Mar 1 [cited 2019 24 Mar];31(2):226–35. Available from: http://doi.wiley.com/10.1111/jar.12379.
18. The National Institute for Health and Care Excellence (NICE). Mental health problems in people with learning disabilities: prevention, assessment and management [Internet]. 2016. Available from: https://www.nice.org.uk/guidance/ng54.
19. The Princess Royal Trust for Carers. 5 Key Facts about Mental Health Carers [Internet]. 2007. Available from: https://professionals.carers.org/sites/default/files/media/5-key-facts-on-mh-carers-final-2825.pdf.
20. Fletcher RJ, Barnhill J, Cooper S-A. Diagnostic Manual—Intellectual Disability (DM-ID-2). New York: *NADD Press*; 2016.
21. Royal College of Psychiatrists. Enabling People with Mild and Mental Health Problems to Access Healthcare Services. 2012.
22. Cumella S. Mental health services for people with a learning disability. *Adv Ment Heal Learn Disabil* [Internet]. 2009 Jul 16 [cited 2017 13 Mar];3(2):8–14. Available from: http://www.emeraldinsight.com/doi/10.1108/17530180200900014.
23. Chaplin R, Flynn A. Adults with learning disability admitted to psychiatric wards. *Adv Psychiatr Treat* [Internet]. 2000 Mar 1 [cited 2017 13];6(2):128–134. Available from: http://apt.rcpsych.org/cgi/doi/10.1192/apt.6.2.128.
24. Chaplin R. General psychiatric services for adults with intellectual disability and mental illness. *J Intellect Disabil Res* [Internet]. 2004 Jan [cited 2017 13 Mar];48(1):1–10. Available from: http://doi.wiley.com/10.1111/j.1365-2788.2004.00580.x.
25. Foundation for People with Learning Disabilities. Feeling Down: Improving the mental health of people with learning disabilities. London; 2014.
26. Ingólfsdóttir JG, Egilson ST, Traustadóttir R. Family-centred services for young children with intellectual disabilities and their families: Theory, policy and practice. *J Intellect Disabil* [Internet].

2018 Dec 22 [cited 2019 24 Mar];22(4):361–77. Available from: http://journals.sagepub.com/doi/10.1177/1744629517714644.
27. McGill P, Cooper V, Honeyman G. Developing better commissioning for individuals with behaviour that challenges services—a scoping exercise. [Internet]. Canterbury/Chatham; 2010. Available from: https://www.challengingbehaviour.org.uk/learning-disability-files/Better-Commissioning-full-report.pdf
28. McKenzie K, Mayer C, Whelan KJ, McNall A, Noone S, Chaplin J. The views of carers about support for their family member with an intellectual disability: With a focus on positive behavioural approaches. *Health Soc Care Community* [Internet]. 2018 Jan 1 [cited 2019 24 Mar];26(1):e56–63. Available from: http://doi.wiley.com/10.1111/hsc.12475.
29. James N. Family carers' experience of the need for admission of their relative with an intellectual disability to an Assessment and Treatment Unit. *J Intellect Disabil* [Internet]. 2016 Mar 1 [cited 2017 8 Mar];20(1):34–54. Available from: http://jid.sagepub.com/cgi/doi/10.1177/1744629515592073.
30. Gavois H, Paulsson G, Fridlund B. Mental health professional support in families with a member suffering from severe mental illness: A grounded theory model. *Scand J Caring Sci* [Internet]. 2006 Mar [cited 2017 13 Mar];20(1):102–109. Available from: http://doi.wiley.com/10.1111/j.1471-6712.2006.00380.x.
31. Devapriam J, Gangadharan S, Pither J, Critchfield M. Delayed discharge from intellectual disability in-patient units. *Psychiatr Bull* [Internet]. 2014 Oct [cited 2017 13 Mar];38(5):211–215. Available from: http://www.ncbi.nlm.nih.gov/pubmed/25285218.
32. Eassom E, Giacco D, Dirik A, Priebe S. Implementing family involvement in the treatment of patients with psychosis: a systematic review of facilitating and hindering factors. *BMJ Open* [Internet]. 2014 Oct 3 [cited 2017 8 Mar];4(10):e006108–e006108. Available from: http://bmjopen.bmj.com/lookup/doi/10.1136/bmjopen-2014-006108.
33. Chester V, Geach N, Morrissey C. Treatment outcomes from forensic intellectual disability services: The perspectives of patients and their family/carers. *J Intellect Disabil.* 2017 5 Sep
34. Francis R. Report of the Mid Staffordshire NHS Foundation Trust Public Inquiry: Executive summary. London; 2013.
35. Rye K, Hicks S, Falconer C. Evaluating a group for young people who have a sibling with a disability. *Learn Disabil Pract* [Internet]. 2018 May 29 [cited 2019 24 Mar];21(3):17–23. Available from: https://journals.rcni.com/doi/10.7748/ldp.2018.e1901.
36. Cheshire L, Chester V, Graham A, Grace J, Alexander RT. Home visits: A reflection on family contact in a specialist forensic intellectual disability service. Jane McCarthy and Dr John Devapriam, eds. *Adv Ment Heal Intellect Disabil* [Internet]. 2015 Jul 6 [cited 2017 23 Feb];9(4):186–195. Available from: http://www.emeraldinsight.com/doi/10.1108/AMHID-02-2015-0010.
37. Brown H, Craft A. *Thinking the unthinkable: Papers on sexual abuse and people with learning difficulties.* London; 1989.
38. Cooke LB, Sinason V. Abuse of People with Learning Disabilities and Other Vulnerable Adults. *Adv Psychiatr Treat* [Internet]. 1998 Mar 1 [cited 2017 23 Feb];4(2):119–125. Available from: http://apt.rcpsych.org/cgi/doi/10.1192/apt.4.2.119.
39. Chinn D, Hall I, Ali A, Hassell H, Patkas I. Psychiatric inpatients away from home: Accounts by people with intellectual disabilities in specialist hospitals outside their home localities. *J Appl Res Intellect Disabil* [Internet]. 2011 Jan 1 [cited 2017 24 Aug];24(1):50–60. Available from: http://doi.wiley.com/10.1111/j.1468-3148.2010.00572.x.
40. Alexander R, Hiremath A, Chester V, Green F, Gunaratna I, Hoare S. Evaluation of treatment outcomes from a medium secure unit for people with intellectual disability. *Adv Ment Heal Intellect Disabil.* 2011;5(1):22–32.
41. Sequeira H, Howlin P, Hollins S. Psychological disturbance associated with sexual abuse in people with learning disabilities: Case-control study. *Br J Psychiatry* [Internet]. 2003 Nov 1 [cited 2017 13 Mar];183(5):451. Available from: http://bjp.rcpsych.org/cgi/doi/10.1192/bjp.183.5.451.
42. Slade M, Pinfold V, Rapaport J, Bellringer S, Banerjee S, Kuipers E, et al. Best practice when service users do not consent to sharing information with carers: National multimethod study. *Br J Psychiatry* [Internet]. 2007 [cited 2017 2 Aug];190(FEB.):148–155. Available from: http://bjp.rcpsych.org/content/190/2/148.
43. Hiebert-Murphy D, Trute B, Wright A. Parents' definition of effective child disability support sServices: Implications for implementing family-centered practice. *J Fam Soc Work* [Internet]. 2011 Mar [cited 2017 8 Mar];14(2):144–158. Available from: http://www.tandfonline.com/doi/abs/10.1080/10522158.2011.552404.
44. Seddon D, Robinson C, Tommis Y, Woods B, Perry J, Russell I. A study of the carers strategy (2000): Supporting carers in Wales. *Br J Soc Work* [Internet]. 2010 Jul 1 [cited 2017 13 Mar];40(5):1470–1487. Available from: https://academic.oup.com/bjsw/article-lookup/doi/10.1093/bjsw/bcp081.
45. Sheehan R, Kimona K, Giles A, Cooper V, Hassiotis A. Findings from an online survey of family carer experience of the management of challenging behaviour in people with intellectual disabilities, with a focus on the use of psychotropic medication. *Br J Learn Disabil* [Internet]. 2018 Jun 1 [cited 2019 24 Mar];46(2):82–91. Available from: http://doi.wiley.com/10.1111/bld.12216.
46. Chiocchi J, Lamph G, Slevin P, Fisher-Smith D, Sampson M. Can a carer (peer) led psychoeducation programme improve mental health carers well-being, reduce burden and enrich empowerment: A service evaluation study. *J Ment Heal Training, Educ Pract* [Internet]. 2019 Mar 11 [cited 2019 24 Mar];14(2):131–140. Available from: https://www.emeraldinsight.com/doi/10.1108/JMHTEP-10-2018-0057.
47. Smallwood J, Jolley S, Makhijani J, Grice S, O'Donoghue E, Bendon P, et al. Implementing specialist psychological support for caregivers in psychosis services: a preliminary report*. *Psychosis* [Internet]. 2016 Dec 12 [cited 2017 8 Mar];1–10. Available from: https://www.tandfonline.com/doi/full/10.1080/17522439.2016.1259647.
48. House of Commons Health Committee. Patient and public involvement in the NHS: Third Report of Session 2006–07. London: The Stationery Office Ltd; 2007.
49. Royal College of Psychiatrists' Faculty of Psychiatry of Intellectual Disability. People with learning disability and mental health, behavioural or forensic problems: The role of in-patient services. Faculty Report (FR/ID/03). 2013.

26

Current and Future Research Priorities in the Psychiatry of Intellectual Disability

Rupert Thurston, Samuel Tromans, Verity Chester, Sally-Ann Cooper, Andre Strydom, Sabyasachi Bhaumik†, and Dheeraj Rai

Introduction

This chapter will provide an overview of current areas of interest for research in the field of intellectual disability (ID) and consider future directions. The chapter is divided into the following broad headings: understanding the causes of ID, outcomes, and comorbidities of ID, pharmacological and psychological interventions, service models and health services research, and a final section on building capacity and overcoming barriers to research in ID. While it is impossible to provide an exhaustive summary within a single book chapter, focus will be directed to areas most relevant to practice of ID psychiatry. Within United Kingdom policy, distinctions are made between research, and other best practice activity, such as service evaluation and clinical audit (1). This policy defines research as 'the attempt to derive generalisable or transferable new knowledge to answer or refine relevant questions with scientifically sound methods'. Table 26.1 summarizes the differences between research, service evaluation, and audit. However, while service evaluation and audit are of value, particularly when assessing the current standards and outcomes of care, this chapter is concerned with the current state of research in regards to the field of ID. The chapter should be read in conjunction with others in the book, where important current and future challenges for research are also highlighted.

Understanding the causes of intellectual disability

Despite the many advances in medicine over the past decades, causal factors remain unidentified in a large proportion of individuals with ID. However, it is well established that ID may result from many different causes. The practical benefit of research on the aetiology of ID is sometimes questioned, and discussion of causation or prevention often raises complex ethical issues, although conflating these with eugenicist ideologies is overly simplistic (3). Here, we argue that there are many reasons why an improved understanding of aetiology has the potential to help improve clinical practice and clinical care for our patients. For example, consider the condition phenylketonuria (PKU), a rare but preventable cause of ID. In this congenital condition, a defect in the phenylalanine hydroxylase (PAH) gene on chromosome 12 leads to an error in metabolism, resulting in the accumulation of phenylalanine, leading to neurotoxicity and detrimental effects on cognitive development. In the early 1960s, a restriction of phenylalanine in the diet was found to be effective in preventing the impaired cognitive development associated with the condition (4). This led to national neonatal screening programmes for PKU across the world and a successful public health strategy through a dietary intervention. Advances in genomics and further understanding of pathways leading to development of ID may identify conditions where successful interventions could potentially be developed. We will broadly use the term 'stratified medicine' to discuss this idea below and this may be interchangeably used with other recent terms such as 'precision medicine'.

Genomic medicine and the promise of stratified approaches

The rapidly advancing field of genomics offers major opportunities for identifying currently unknown causes of ID, and will enhance understanding of targets for prevention or treatment. Among the most important recent advances has been the discovery of changes in chromosome structure, leading to alterations in sections of DNA with deletions or duplications of greater than 1,000 base pairs known as copy number variants (CNVs). Some genetic loci (such as 1q21.1, 3q29, 15q11.2, 15q13.3, 16p11.2, 16p13.1 and 22q11), have been shown to have rare but recurrent CNVs that are important risk factors for several neurodevelopmental and neuropsychiatric disorders including ID, autism, epilepsy, and schizophrenia (5, 6). Microarray-based methods to identify CNVs are now in clinical use and could facilitate earlier detection and treatment of at-risk individuals, as well as help understand comorbidity with other conditions (7).

Recent studies have highlighted the potential for identifying genetic causes of ID in individuals where this was previously unknown. A recent study using genome-wide chromosomal microarray analysis of 202 adults with idiopathic ID found an 11 per cent yield of

† It is with great regret that we report the death of Sabyasachi Bhaumik during the production of this textbook.

Table 26.1 Comparison between research, audit and service evaluation.

Research	Service Evaluation*	Audit
The attempt to derive new knowledge, including studies that aim to generate hypotheses as well as studies that aim to test them.	Designed and conducted solely to define or judge current care.	Designed and conducted to produce information to inform delivery of best care.
Quantitative research—designed to test a hypothesis. Qualitative research—identifies or explores themes following established methodology.	Designed to answer 'what standard does this service achieve?'	Designed to answer '"does this service reach a predetermined standard?'
Addresses clearly defined questions, aims and objectives.	Measures correct service without reference to a standard.	Measures against a standard.
Quantitative research—may involve evaluating or comparing interventions, particularly new ones.	Involves an intervention in use only.	The choice of treatment is that of the clinician and patient according to guidance, professional standards and/or patient preference.
Usually involves collecting data that are additional to those for routine care, but may include data collected routinely. May involve treatments, samples or investigations additional to routine care.	Usually involves analysis of existing data but may include administration of interviews or questionnaires.	Usually involves analysis of existing data but may include administration of a simple interview or questionnaire.
Quantitative research study design may involve allocating patients to intervention groups. Qualitative research uses a clearly defined sampling framework underpinned by conceptual or theoretical justifications.	No allocation to intervention: the health professional and patient have chosen intervention before service evaluation.	No allocation to intervention: the health professional and patient have chosen intervention before audit.
May involve randomization.	No randomization.	No randomization.
Normally requires Research Ethics Committee (REC) review.	Does not require REC review.	Does not require REC review.

likely pathogenic CNVs, most frequently at recurrent loci, including the 15q11-q13 and 16p11.2-p13.11 regions (8). In another study, involving using whole-genome sequencing in a well characterized cohort of 50 individuals with severe ID, pathogenic CNVs were found to account for approximately 12 per cent of cases, and whole exome sequencing identified the causal genetic mutation in a further 27 per cent of individuals (9). These studies show that a genetic aetiology may be identifiable in a significant proportion of individuals in contact with ID services, and are suggestive of microarray or sequencing methods playing an increasing role in clinical practice. Routine genetic testing in clinical populations may also offer opportunities for future research. Although providing sufficient sample sizes to obtain meaningful results may prove challenging; multi-centre-based collaboration likely represents the best approach to address this issue. Beyond gene discovery, the biological mechanisms underpinning pathways through which mutations lead to the development of ID are an area of further work and may lead to major advances in both the understanding of pathophysiological mechanisms, as well as development of novel treatment options (10).

The identification of potential brain circuitry or molecular pathways which may be targeted, and the possibility of a personalized approach in the event of biomarkers being identified continues to be a research priority (11). The initial stages of this approach have been successful in some conditions related to ID. For example, Sturge-Weber syndrome is a neurocutaneous syndrome associated with epilepsy and ID, due to a somatic mutation in the GNAQ gene. This mutation has since been associated with overactivation of specific biological pathways (the Ras-Raf-MEK-ERK and Hippo-YAP pathways); drugs which inhibit such pathways represent novel potential therapeutic targets (12). In tuberous sclerosis complex, another condition associated with ID, the identification of the mTOR signalling pathway and targeted drug therapy has been shown to be effective in treatment of associated tumours, such as subependymal giant cell astrocytomas and angiomyolipomas (13). Another avenue which appears to show promise is 'early intervention' with anti-epileptics in individuals at risk of epilepsy associated with the tuberous sclerosis complex. It has been suggested that electroencephalography (EEG) could be used to screen individuals and initiate early treatment even before developing clinical symptoms, possibly leading to improved outcomes including intellectual disability (14).

Beyond genomics, the emergence of high-throughput techniques applying other 'omics' technologies, including epigenomics, metabolomics, proteomics, and transcriptomics, will also open new frontiers for the understanding of the causes and pathways pertaining to ID.

Environmental risk factors

Apart from genetic factors, it is known that the environment may be important in the development of ID. A range of prenatal environmental risk factors have been suggested, and a recent systematic review by Huang et al. highlighted the prenatal factors that have been investigated, including advanced maternal age, low maternal education, exposure to toxins such as alcohol and smoking, and of maternal physical health conditions, including hypertension, diabetes, asthma, and epilepsy (15). The review also concluded that epidemiological studies have focused less on perinatal or neonatal factors, and that little is known about the combinations and interactions of factors that might point to mechanisms in development of ID.

Some knowledge gaps regarding environmental risk factors may be addressed by large population-based studies. For example, studies have reported that gestational age and birthweight could account for 27 per cent of intellectual disabilities (16), and that season of conception is related to intellectual disabilities (highest rates in January–March) (17), such that 15 per cent of intellectual disabilities is potentially preventable if the risk throughout the year was reduced to that in the third quarter (July–September). Biologically plausible causes for this are infections and maternal vitamin D levels, which are potentially amenable to intervention. There has been an exponential increase in register-based epidemiology of other neurodevelopmental conditions, such as autism. International consortia, most notably using data sources from Scandinavian countries and Western Australia (18), have also emerged. Epidemiological studies of autism, where it has been possible to differentiate between autism with or without ID have found stronger associations for advancing parental age (19), poor fetal growth (20), parental migration (21), vitamin D deficiency (22), and maternal hospitalization for infections during pregnancy (23), for autism with ID relative to higher functioning autism. This raises the question of whether such factors are associated with ID more generally, rather than autism specifically. Such record linkage cohorts, where it may be able to identify non-syndromic forms of ID, could significantly advance the understanding of contributory environmental factors. For example, a recent large Swedish population-based study using sibling comparisons to strengthen causal inference reported that birth at non-optimal gestation duration may be causally associated with non-syndromic intellectual disability (24).

Outcomes and comorbidities

Although understanding of aetiology is important, clinicians will often intuitively be more interested in the outcomes for people with ID, as this is often of greater focus in day-to-day clinical practice.

Physical health and mortality

The physical health of people with ID has been of long-standing concern (25). This is broadly due to people with ID having higher rates of adverse health conditions, because of health inequalities and disparities, due to people with ID receiving poorer care from health providers. A learning disabilities observatory report on health inequalities (26) highlighted that health conditions such as gastrointestinal cancer, leukaemia, respiratory disease, osteoporosis, sensory impairment, dementia, epilepsy, oral health problems, mental health problems, and challenging behaviour, occurred more often or more seriously in people with ID than the general population. Additionally, there are a number of so-called 'lifestyle' risk factors, and many with ID are at significant risk of deviating from normal weight and to lead sedentary lives (27). However, it is important to note that many of these factors may not be within the individual's control, due to dependency needs on family or paid carers. Furthermore, many of these factors are interrelating, for example, people with ID are more likely to be prescribed psychotropic medication, which can produce negative side effects such as metabolic syndrome and weight gain (27) due to the higher rates of challenging behaviour or higher rates of mental health issues (28). There is also some research that reports higher rates of hospital admissions for ambulatory care-sensitive conditions in people with intellectual disabilities, which may indicate poorer health care management (29, 30).

The UK-based Confidential Inquiry into the Premature deaths of People with Learning Disabilities (CIPOLD) reported that the median age at death for people with ID was 13 and 20 years below that of the general (non-ID) population of males and females respectively (31). Over a third of the deaths in this population were deemed avoidable, which was significantly greater than that of the general population. The confidential inquiry provided a stark reminder of the inequalities in life expectancies faced by people with ID, and has focused priority for further research in the understanding of the determinants of early mortality, as well as preventable causes and interventions to mitigate against them. It has led to further investigation of this issue, using contemporary sources of data to further assess this question (32–34). It has been suggested that 37 per cent of deaths in people with ID may be classified as 'amenable to good medical care' (34) and additionally, as the Office of National Statistics definitions of amenable deaths do not include several causes of death common in people with intellectual disabilities such as deaths from urinary tract infections and aspiration pneumonia, this figure is likely to be an underestimate.

A range of factors which would fall under this umbrella have been highlighted by previous research, which can be at both the public health, and local service/individual practitioner level. At the public health level, Burtner and colleagues (35) suggested that many people with ID are unable to access health messages about smoking because of difficulties in reading, interpreting, and understanding product labelling and health campaigns, as well as reduced capacity to understand the complications and implications of smoking. To this date, little emphasis is placed on the accessibility of health messaging for all population subgroups, and this would be an important area for future research. At the local service and individual practitioner level, it has been suggested that knowledge of people with ID, and their additional needs is poor, in part due to this group's historical segregation from society (36). Many professional groups report being ill-equipped to care for people with ID, with knowledge of how to adapt their verbal and written communication, and to understand the differential presentation of certain conditions in people with ID. For example, research has suggested that people with ID can struggle to communicate that they are in pain, and therefore may present with a deterioration in behaviour (37).

Similarly, patients can find it difficult for services to take responsibility for their care, with reports of being turned away from both 'mainstream' or 'specialist' services. Attitudes and beliefs are a key factor, with many patients reporting that practitioners erroneously attribute symptoms to the ID, rather than exploring a possible health comorbidity, known as 'diagnostic overshadowing'. It has been suggested that people with ID are not screened for common behaviours and habits associated with poorer health outcomes, such as smoking (38), alcohol, or substance misuse (39) due to prevailing beliefs that people with ID do not smoke or take drugs (40).

In response to these issues, in the UK, the Equality Act (2010) mandated that services must make 'reasonable adjustments' in order to remove the barriers faced by people with disabilities. An important research priority would therefore be to identify how people with ID could receive better quality care. In England and Wales, the development and implementation of the annual health check has been a promising advance. An evaluation of an incentivized scheme for general practitioners to provide health checks for people with ID appears to have led to greater rates of a range of investigations than non-incentivized practices (41) and an intervention based on practice nurse health checks was found to be clinically and cost effective (42). These studies suggest that such schemes may be useful in reducing health inequalities in people with ID within a primary care setting.

Mental disorders

A body of literature now exists that appears to suggest a greater burden of a range of mental disorders in people with ID relative to the general population. A landmark study by Cooper et al. found a point prevalence of 40.9 per cent for mental ill-health (based on clinical diagnosis) among a sample of 1,023 persons with ID (43). This included prevalence rates of 4.4 per cent for psychotic disorders, 6.6 per cent for affective disorders, 3.8 per cent for anxiety disorders and 7.5 per cent for autistic spectrum disorder. Additionally, burden of mental ill-health increased with increasing severity of ID. An earlier study by Deb et al. (44) found a point prevalence of 14.4 per cent for functional psychiatric illness in persons with ID according to ICD-10 criteria (95% confidence interval = 7.4–21.4%), similar to the rate of 16 per cent reported in the general population. This included rates of 4.4 per cent for schizophrenia, 2.2 per cent for depressive disorder and 2.2 per cent for anxiety disorder. A systematic review pertaining to mental disorder prevalence studies in individuals with ID reports wide-ranging prevalence estimates for presence of mental disorder (from 13.9–75.2 per cent), citing differences in sampling and diagnostic criteria across studies as contributory factors underpinning such variation (45).

It is recognized that the presentation of mental illness in people with ID may be different to the general population, with the general extent of such difference increasing with increasing severity of ID (46). Additionally, patterns of symptoms of mental disorder in persons with ID may differ from the non-ID population, as demonstrated by Bouras et al. (47), who found that patients with ID and psychotic disorders had higher levels of observable psychopathology, negative symptoms, and functional impairment relative to their non-ID counterparts.

For these reasons, specific classification systems for assessment of mental disorder in persons with ID have been developed. These include the diagnostic criteria for psychiatric disorders for use with adults with learning disabilities (DC-LD), based on the international classification of diseases (48, 49), and the diagnostic manual—intellectual disability (DM-ID currently DM-ID2), based on the diagnostic and statistical manual of mental disorders (DSM) (50).

As the classification of mental disorders evolves with new iterations of the DSM (currently DSM-5) and the international classification of diseases and related health problems (ICD-11 under development), refining the diagnostic criteria to measure mental health in people with ID, including research reliability, would help underpin robust measurement protocols in randomized controlled trials (RCTs)(51). As well as accurate measurement in relation to the identification of mental illness, including brief measures suitable for use in primary care, it is also important to design instruments which can accurately and sensitively measure change in symptoms, which could be used to measure treatment outcomes in both trials and clinical practice. Additionally, large sample sizes achieved through multi-centre collaboration and widespread consensus regarding diagnostic criteria[1] would help yield further high quality research to add to the current evidence base on the epidemiology of mental disorder among persons with ID.

1. Or at least separate prevalence measurements according to different diagnostic criteria within the same study.

Behavioural phenotypes

Apart from mental illness, a related important area for further research is to better understand key behavioural profiles associated with recognized syndromes. There already exists a significant body of work in the literature in relation to behavioural phenotypes (52). There are numerous examples of how identifying underlying syndromes and their behavioural phenotypes can positively impact care. For example, a systematic review and meta-analysis by Royston et al. found a higher prevalence of anxiety disorders in patients with Williams syndrome (53), directing a stratified approach to assessing such patients. Identifying that overeating is a feature of Prader-Willi syndrome (54) ensures that measures can be put in place to safeguard the physical health of those with the condition. Similarly, the knowledge that autistic-spectrum disorder (ASD) and an ADHD overactivity are common features of fragile X syndrome means that regimens of ADHD psychotropic medication can be considered, in addition to multimodal assessment and programmed intervention relating to the autistic features of the condition, such as speech therapy and ongoing social skills education (54). O'Brien identifies the most prominent benefits of diagnosing and labelling behavioural phenotypes, including that practitioners can draw on a long history of observations from other clinicians, and the generation of a widely corroborated framework within which clinicians can identify and manage typical medical and behavioural features (54). O'Brien notes that phenotype research has encouraged an academic interest in disability, and that anticipation of behaviours and complications increases predictive validity and facilitates early intervention and treatment (54). However, these advantages are balanced against a number of possible drawbacks, which include the possibility of stigma, that the idea of eugenics might be revisited, that phenotypes may become a self-fulfilling prophecy, or that phenotypes encourages therapeutic nihilism, or give patients and their families the idea that the course and characteristics of the syndrome are unchangeable. Behavioural phenotypes may also be interacting with mental illness in a way which modifies their clinical presentation, impacting on the clinical usefulness of traditional diagnostic criteria. Work in this area may be useful in accurately identifying underlying mental illness which may manifest as episodes of behaviour that challenge, hence reducing inappropriate and potentially harmful prescribing. The advances in genetic technologies detailed above may increase opportunity for further research in this area.

Behaviours that challenge

Behaviours that challenge are one of the most common reasons for referral to community teams working with people with ID. It is clear that such behaviours are not always attributable to mental illness, and may be caused by numerous underlying physical, psychological, and social factors. The process of systematically assessing behaviour which challenges and the identification and management of underlying causes continues to be a priority for research.

In residential or nursing care settings within the community, it may be a challenge to objectively assess and monitor behaviours consistently due to shift changes and staff turnover. Understanding the most effective measure for assessment of behaviours that challenge across different settings is therefore an important area for further work, as there is currently a lack of high quality clinical evidence pertaining to this issue (55). Additionally, reliable and valid tools for the identification and measurement of behaviours that challenge, such as the aberrant behaviour checklist (56), are likely to help in the design of large-scale pragmatic trials into appropriate intervention and management.

The National Institute for Health and Care Excellence (NICE) guidelines for behaviours that challenge in people with ID (55) recommended several areas as research priorities, including prevention of behaviours that challenge from developing in children with ID aged under five years, interventions[2] to reduce the frequency and intensity of behaviours that challenge in the community setting, comparing locally accessible care with out-of-area placements, and understanding the factors contributory to sustained, high quality residential care provision.

Neurodevelopmental comorbidities

Although clinicians recognize that people with ID may have other neurodevelopmental comorbidities, such as autism and attention deficit hyperactivity disorder (ADHD), the extent of these comorbidities is still not well established. In recent years, several large record linkage cohorts have helped understand the epidemiology of autism, and some have the ability to identify the presence of ID (57). A recent study based on the 2007 adult psychiatric morbidity survey in England highlighted that the rates of autism in people with moderate to profound ID disability were much greater than the general population (58). Both how to most effectively manage such comorbidities and how they influence outcomes are questions that still need to be addressed.

Studies suggest that the prevalence of ADHD in children with ID is higher than that in the general population (59) and increases with increasing severity of the ID (60). This is likely partially due to a number of chromosomal and genetic syndromes associated with increased rates of ADHD, such as fragile X, Smith-Magenis, Angelman, Prader-Willi, Turner, Williams, and Cornelia de Lange (61, 62). Furthermore, ID and ADHD may share similar risk factors, such as prematurity, or a low birth weight (60). Furthermore, while in the general population the prevalence of ADHD declines with age, research indicates the possibility of a longer and more persistent course of the disorder in those with ID. In adults with borderline or mild levels of ID, a more severe presentation and a less favourable pattern of improvement across the lifespan has been reported (63).

Nonetheless, some small-scale studies have highlighted positive responses to routine ADHD medication treatment among people with ID (64). As such, the identification of ADHD in people with ID is important in order to maximize outcomes. Yet at present, few diagnostic tools have been evaluated in relation to their clinical utility with this population. Malfa, Lassi, Bertelli, Pallanti, and Albertini evaluated the Conners' Adult ADHD Rating Scales (CAARS), a checklist of symptoms and behaviours designed to help assess, diagnose, and monitor treatment of ADHD in adults, with some success, yet the authors highlighted the need for future research in this area (65).

2. Both pharmacological and non-pharmacological.

Dementia, aging, and end of life care

Despite the disproportionate rates of early mortality, many people with ID are now living longer, and this has prompted more focus on aging and conditions occurring in later life, such as dementia (66). Making a diagnosis of dementia in persons with ID poses a clinical challenge, as it requires the recognition of a change in the individual's functioning from their specific baseline, rather than from a 'normal level', as would be typically the case in assessing an individual without ID (67, 68). A recent study concluded that a clinician with experience in Down syndrome was more accurate in identifying cases of dementia than through the use of ICD-10 or DSM-IV criteria, and may be able to pick up cases at an earlier stage (69). Indeed, the NICE guidelines on mental health problems in people with learning disabilities recommend referring individuals with ID and suspected dementia to a psychiatrist with specialist expertise in persons with ID (70). Further scrutiny of the diagnostic criteria and the development of methods of timely identification will therefore be important in future research.

Furthermore, much of the literature on this issue is focused on dementia in people with Down syndrome, and research gaps about the understanding and management of dementia for the wider population of people with ID will need to be addressed. Even for Down syndrome, a recent Cochrane review on the topic of pharmacological intervention identified a need for further trials on the topic, as the overall quality of the evidence was low (71). A recent feasibility study for an RCT comparing simvastatin to placebo for the prevention of Alzheimer's dementia in people with Down syndrome reported that a large scale RCT would be feasible but highlighted the potential challenges of recruiting a sufficiently large sample size required (72).

With regard to anti-dementia medications in persons with ID, while there is a lack of conclusive evidence to support the notion that they slow down cognitive decline, the limited evidence available appears to suggest that they can improve quality of life for both the afflicted individual and their carers (68).

The aging population and the challenges of dementia have also highlighted a need to address care of the dying patient. End of life issues and needs for people with ID have not been the focus of research until relatively recently. Communication and involvement in decision-making may be particular obstacles when compared to the non-ID population, and therefore joined-up working between palliative care/hospice and ID teams will be essential. A recent paper sought to establish consensus on research priorities in this area (73), finding that decision-making emerged as a top priority, including establishing pathways/framework and what factors may influence decision-making. This was closely followed by the need to compare palliative care with that of the general population (including societal attitudes, transitions, and cancer services). Thirdly, quality of palliative care provision was identified as an area for further work (including defining 'best practice', patient involvement, and service user perspective and experience). An important next step would be to clarify and help further develop these priorities with people with ID, their families, and other stakeholders.

Pharmacological and psychological interventions

At present, there is a relative paucity of high quality research evidence evaluating the efficacy of commonly used pharmacological and psychological interventions, which has presented long term challenges to the field of ID psychiatry. As such, much of the evidence is extrapolated from research carried out on the general population. Here, we highlight some of the recent successes, challenges, and opportunities in the areas most important for day to day clinical practice, that of evaluation of interventions.

Psychotropic medications

The prescribing of psychotropic medications, in particular antipsychotic medications, is common in people with ID (74). However, it is important that such prescription is judicious and appropriate, and indeed the NICE guidelines recommend that only individuals with specialist expertise in treating mental health problems in persons with ID should initiate psychotropic medications in those with more severe ID and/or children and adolescents with ID (70). Additionally, though prescribing guidelines specific to mental disorder in persons with ID have been developed (75), the ID-specific evidence base is often limited for many conditions, and in such instances, one should refer to the clinical evidence from studies conducted in non-ID patient groups (70).

A recent report using a large primary care database in the UK highlighted that people with ID are commonly prescribed antipsychotics without a clear psychiatric indication (74). Polypharmacy is also common, increasing the risks in respect of adverse outcomes related to drug interactions and drug-disease interactions. One of the concerns this has raised is of iatrogenic harm, such as anticholinergic burden (76) and adverse metabolic consequences (77), which may contribute to the increased mortality rates in persons with ID. Despite some evidence of short-term benefit in children with ID and behaviours that challenge (78), only a handful of RCTs have been conducted to investigate the efficacy of antipsychotic use in behaviours that challenge in adults, with no good quality evidence to support their continued use in this context (79–81). However, carrying out trials of medication use in this area has proven to be complex, with recruitment presenting a major challenge. Therefore, further work to understand the barriers and enhance feasibility of such trials is necessary. Furthermore, in the absence of RCTs there have been proposals for national audits of clinical practice (82), and opportunities to use observational cohort designs to assess outcomes. While there is broad consensus amongst clinicians working with people with ID about the need to reduce inappropriate prescribing of antipsychotic medication, it remains hotly disputed whether antipsychotics should be used in behaviours that challenge. The NICE guidance recommends their use in this context only in specific circumstances, including the absence of adequate change being produced by non-pharmacological interventions, treatment for co-existing problems having not reduced the behaviour and where this risk to the individual or others is severe (55).

A further priority for research, as recommended in the NICE guidance for mental health problems in people with learning disabilities, was for pharmacological treatment for anxiety in people with ID and autism spectrum disorders (70). Anxiety disorders are particularly prevalent in this patient group, who additionally often have concurrent issues pertaining to communication which further complicate management. Again, the recommended approach would be an RCT wherever possible, and this may require collaboration of several centres in order to obtain a sufficiently large sample size.

Conducting large-scale RCT's pertaining to psychopharmacological interventions in people with ID has proven problematic for many reasons, including capacity to consent, obtaining funding, obtaining ethical approval, and obtaining sufficient sample sizes to potentially attain clinically meaningful results (83). However, the lack of evidence is to the likely detriment of patients, carers, and professionals alike, as all would stand to benefit from further high-quality research into the effectiveness of psychopharmacological interventions in persons with ID.

Psychological and non-pharmacological interventions

Although it was initially believed that psychological therapies may have a limited role in people with ID, it is now clear that a range of such therapies could be usefully adapted and successfully used in this patient group. Adapting and developing psychological therapies for people with ID is a field that has shown promise, with a range of recently completed trials. A systematic review identified 22 trials evaluating the efficacy of psychological therapies for people with ID, and including 14 in a meta-analysis (84). The quality of reporting of methodology within the included studies was poor, with many failing to include adequate detail about their participants, particularly the level of ID, information about masked assessment, and therapy fidelity. However, thematic analysis yielded an overall moderate between-group effect size of all the therapies evaluated, while group-based interventions had a moderate but smaller treatment effect than individual-based interventions. Cognitive-behaviour therapy (CBT) was effective for both anger and depression, while interventions aimed at improving interpersonal functioning were not effectual. When CBT was excluded, there was insufficient evidence regarding the efficacy of other psychological therapies, or psychological therapies intended to treat mental health problems in children and young people with ID. Adults with ID and concurrent mental health problems appear to benefit from psychological therapies. However, clinical trials need to make use of improved reporting standards and larger samples. Further studies have subsequently been published, including RCTs for anger control (85) and a group intervention for depression (86, 87). However, much of the evidence relates to patients with mild rather than more severe levels of ID, and to adults rather than children and young people, and the overall literature is sparse. More research is needed on the actual delivery of modified interventions within community services, including mainstream services.

Research into non-pharmacological approaches to managing behaviours that challenge in people with ID continues to be a developing area. For example, positive behaviour support (PBS) is an intervention which is aimed at addressing behaviours that challenge through the use of functional behavioural analysis, though a recently published multicentre cluster randomized controlled trial found that it was no more effective than treatment as usual in terms of reducing behaviours that challenge over a 12-month period (88).

Non-pharmacological interventions that promote healthier lifestyles, including opportunities to increase physical activity or manage weight, will be another research focus, and may be particularly relevant to those individuals for whom antipsychotic medications are part of a long-term treatment plan. For example, one planned trial aims to test an intervention to embed sustainable physical activity in the day-to-day routines of adults with ID (89). However, a cluster randomized trial of a walking intervention reported that this was not effective in increasing levels of physical activity, and recommended that more intensive programmes may be required (90).

Service models and health services research

Although few would argue that service design should not be evidence-based in nature, there has been little research in this area to address this, and provision of specialist services for people with ID varies widely across the UK. The recent UK NICE guidelines recommended further research on evaluating different models of service delivery for effectiveness (clinical outcome) but also highlighted the importance of understanding patient experience within such services (70). This is a topical area, considering England is currently implementing the transforming care programme following the Winterbourne View scandal, which aims to enable system-wide changes in order to reduce the number of in-patient admissions for people with ID, and increase the local provision of care so that the need for out-of-area care is minimized. The widespread policy changes also offer research opportunities to study the organization of services, the needs of people placed in out-of-area care, and the evaluation of alternative local provisions. Understanding the specifications and key elements for 'gold standard' residential care for people with behaviours that challenge has been recommended as a research priority by NICE (55).

A current research stream is investigating the efficacy of secure, or forensic services for people with ID. Such services were established for patients whose presentation rendered their management unsafe in the community (91). Previous research in this area has relied on single service outcome studies, and have varied in terms of the outcome measures used, including domains such as length of stay, which are affected by variables other than the effectiveness of treatment (92). More recently, a systematic review and evidence synthesis aimed to evaluate the outcome domains of relevance when assessing treatment efficacy at the whole service level (93, 94). The study highlighted a broad range of domains and incorporated these into an outcomes framework, within overarching themes of patient safety, effectiveness, and patient and carer experience. The authors recommended that any future prospective outcome studies should utilize the outcomes framework, in order to assess patient progress on a holistic array of variables.

Another related area of health service research is in provision of effective care for people with ID within mainstream settings. There has been little research on the benefits of 'mainstreaming care', or whether specialists and specialist teams provide superior care for people with ID. Considering that service models in the UK are currently diverse and varied, there may be opportunities to carry out naturalistic evaluations or pragmatic trials of these different approaches to service provision.

People with ID often have comorbid physical health conditions such as epilepsy, endocrine dysfunction, and mobility problems. Community teams for people with ID provide support for a range of these conditions. For example, epilepsy care is often provided by community nurses and psychiatrists, although little research has been carried out with regard to its clinical efficacy and cost effectiveness. A cluster RCT is currently being conducted to investigate nurse-led epilepsy management compared to treatment as usual (53). Understanding effective care pathways between ID services and acute medical or surgical services, and residential and support services may help identify best practice and address disparity in outcomes such as mortality. For example, an audit into the quality of in-patient care within both acute general hospital and mental health settings highlighted the potential benefits of ID liaison nursing, as well as suggesting the need for further research, including effective provision of accessible information and expert advice relating to the Mental Capacity Act (95).

Building capacity and addressing arriers to research

Research into training of doctors and healthcare professionals

One important but often overlooked area of research in relation to ID is on providing high quality training opportunities and attracting the most talented professionals to the field. Some research has been carried out with regards to medical undergraduate training, including developing competence and confidence in communication (96) and attitudes (97, 98), as well as recommendations on what medical students should learn in relation to ID (99). Work on improving attitudes can be seen as a way to address the broader issue of stigma, which is likely to improve access to good quality healthcare (100). The subject of training needs for mainstream healthcare services has recently been systematically reviewed, which set out key areas of interest for future research, including a focus on training for GPs and primary care, assessing the training needs of psychological therapists within mainstream mental health services, and assessing the delivery of training for healthcare professionals (101).

Research in low and middle income countries and migrant communities

Outside of high income countries, research in relation ID is very limited. There are likely to be major limitations in translating research findings from higher income countries to aid service delivery, clinical practice, or policy related to ID in lower and middle income countries (LMIC). Recent reports have highlighted the key questions and themes which emerge as top global priorities, include early identification of ID, early intervention and rehabilitation, health needs, and empowerment of families and carers (102). It is notable that many of these issues are still important subjects of ongoing research in higher-income countries. Although much of the focus of the recommendations appears to be on early life, adult and later life issues are increasingly important areas of research internationally.

Stigma is a major issue in individuals with ID, as well as their families and carers (103). Issues related to stigma continue to exist in the developed world, though are likely to be an even bigger problem in the developing world; as such, the prioritization of research and policy in addressing this on a global scale has been suggested (104). The under-representation in terms of government policy and the need for both strong parental/carer advocacy and developing self-advocacy are particular issues worthy of further study.

Even within developed countries, there are big cross-cultural differences in the perceptions of ID and other neurodevelopmental problems such as autism (105, 106). There is also a need to understand the perceptions and needs of migrant and minority ethnic communities, and how clinicians and services could provide culturally sensitive care to reduce health inequalities and improve engagement.

Overcoming barriers to research

It is well known that carrying out high quality research with people with ID can be challenging, and that they are often actively excluded from research (107). The number of researchers in the field is also limited, and the lack of funding opportunities compared to other areas is a practical challenge (83).

One important barrier to inclusion has been the reluctance of professionals as well as carers and families in involving people with ID in research (108). Issues over mental capacity and consent can be contentious, although it is known that given enough information in an accessible way, people with ID may be able to provide fully informed consent. In contrast, an assumption of a lack of capacity can therefore be a barrier to involving people with ID in research (109). The safeguards in place around research involving subjects with ID may be a double-edged sword, as they provide a level of protection from potential abuse whilst likely having a negative effect on inclusion into studies (110). While there is an understandable widely held wish to protect persons with ID from potential harm, this can be a double-edged sword when it prevents them from contributing to research that could increase understanding of how to provide them with improved clinical care; such benefits should be proportionately weighed against potential risks (111).

There are difficulties in recruiting and retaining people with ID into research studies (107, 112), and this may be a particular challenge in experimental designs involving medications. Carrying out research with people with ID usually entails greater investments in relation to researcher time, adaptation, or adjustment of methods or measures, as well as costs, which may prove to be hindrances to research (112). A qualitative study looking into views of people with ID and their carers identified the 'need for policies and practices that promote respect and safety' (113).

A recent study from Australia looked into the factors which may have a negative effect on recruitment into research in the ID population, particularly randomized controlled trials (114). It reported barriers resulting from the organization of the ID sector as well as those arising due to research process. In terms of 'sectoral' factors, the authors concluded that recruitment may be best achieved with use of an 'insider' and via staff/service providers with whom patients are already involved. They also highlighted that regional registries may help overcome difficulty in identifying members of the population to be included, particularly those with milder ID, who may be living independently. Barriers which arose from the research process itself included preconceived ideas or a lack of clear understanding about the intervention (advocacy), and ethical constraints which prevented a direct approach to potential participants (114). Another recent qualitative study aiming to look at stakeholder views (108), identified that improving knowledge on the principles of RCTs amongst service users and carers may overcome some barriers, as generally the results suggested that stakeholders were supportive of the aims of RCTs, particularly where they could appreciate a potential improvement in practice or service delivery.

These studies would suggest that time and resources spent in engaging and fully informing stakeholders about research will be a good investment in terms of improving recruitment to trials. Therefore, further research identifying effective ways of informing and engaging participants with ID throughout the whole process of research, as well as involving them as partners in the process may help recruitment and retention (115–117). Finally, collaborative working between researchers and ID representative groups may enhance opportunities in both implementation of research and development of ethical and acceptable study designs (118).

In conclusion, though there have been many exciting recent developments in ID research, there is much work still to be done. Table 26.2 provides an overview of current research priorities in persons with ID. Recent successes have demonstrated that it is possible to conduct complex studies, including high quality RCTs with this patient group. However, as well as studies involving solely ID-specific patient groups, collaboration with non-ID specialists is required to bring about a culture change whereby persons with ID are not routinely excluded from general psychiatry research.

We hope that this chapter has encouraged readers to consider questions that resonate with them, and pursue their own research projects, contributing to addressing the knowledge gaps in our

Table 26.2 Current research priorities for mental disorder and/or behaviours that challenge in persons with ID.

Category	Subcategory	Research Priorities
Prevention		• Preventing behaviours that challenge from developing in children aged under 5 years with ID (55)
Diagnosis		• Development of case identification tools for common mental health problems (70)
Interventions	General	• Interventions to reduce the frequency and extent of moderate to severe behaviours that challenge within community settings(55)
	Psychological	• Children and young people with internalizing disorders (70) • Depression and anxiety in adults with mild to moderate ID (70) • Psychological strategies in dementia (e.g. cognitive stimulation) (68)
	Pharmacological	• Anxiety disorders in people with ID and autism (70) • Preventative treatment for dementia in persons with Down syndrome (68)
	Other	• Psychosocial interventions for people with more severe ID (70) • Environmental strategies in dementia (68)
Care Provision		• Understanding the experiences of people with ID and mental disorders within services (70) • Locally accessible care (55) • Factors associated with sustained, high quality residential care (55)

understanding of how best to understand and address the challenges facing individuals with ID.

MULTIPLE CHOICE QUESTIONS

Questions

Please select the single most appropriate answer.

1. There is some evidence to support the effect of anti-dementia medications in people with intellectual disability in which of the following?

A. Slowing cognitive decline
B. Maintaining their level of global functioning for greater time when compared with placebo
C. Improving quality of life for the afflicted individual and their carers*

2. Which of the following psychological treatments is supported by evidence both in management of depression and anger in people with intellectual disability?

A. Interpersonal therapy
B. Cognitive analytic therapy
C. Cognitive behavioural therapy*
D. Positive behaviour support
E. Psychodynamic psychotherapy

3. Which of the following would suggest that a project you are planning would be defined as research, rather than audit, or service evaluation?

A. Analysis of existing data
B. Randomization*
C. Measurement against a set standard
D. Administration of a questionnaire
E. Measurement of current care

4. Which of the following is true regarding large scale randomized controlled trials in people with intellectual disability?

A. There are many published studies
B. There is adequate funding available
C. Obtaining large enough sample sizes is a challenge*
D. Results available from studies in the general population mean they are not necessary

5. Which of the following studies is most useful in assessing the environmental factors associated with intellectual disability?

A. Qualitative research
B. Large population-based studies*
C. Randomized controlled trial
D. Case series
E. Systematic review

Answers

1. C. In the ID population, there is evidence of improvement of quality of life for the afflicted individual and their carers.
2. C. CBT is supported by evidence for the management of depression, and in control of anger in people with ID.
3. B. Randomization is only used in research whereas other approaches could be used in audit or service evaluation.
4. C. Recruiting enough participants to provide a sufficient sample size is a challenge when conducting RCTs in people with intellectual disability.
5. B. Large population-based studies enable researchers to identify environmental factors which may be associated with intellectual disability.

REFERENCES

1. UK Policy Framework for Health and Social Care Research. London: NHS Health Research Authority; 2018. https://www.hra.nhs.uk/planning-and-improving-research/policies-standards-legislation/uk-policy-framework-health-social-care-research/.
2. Research, Audit and Service Evaluation: A practical guide for Clinician Researchers. London: Royal College of Psychiatrists; 2015. http://www.rcpsych.ac.uk/workinpsychiatry/faculties/intellectualdisability/professional/research/researchauditand evaluation.aspx.
3. Emerson E, Hatton C, Robertson J. Prevention and social care for adults with learning disabilities. NIHR School for Social Care Research, 2011.
4. Knox WE. An evaluation of the treatment of phenylketonuria with diets low in phenylalanine. *Pediatrics.* 1960; 26: 1–11.
5. AlSagob M, Colak D, Kaya N. Genetics of autism spectrum disorder: An update on copy number variations leading to autism in the next generation sequencing era. *Discov Med.* 2015; 19(106): 367–379.
6. Torres F, Barbosa M, Maciel P. Recurrent copy number variations as risk factors for neurodevelopmental disorders: Critical overview and analysis of clinical implications. *J Med Genet.* 2016; 53(2): 73–90.
7. Mullen SA, Carvill GL, Bellows S, Bayly MA, Trucks H, Lal D et al. Copy number variants are frequent in genetic generalized epilepsy with intellectual disability. *Neurology.* 2013; 81(17): 1507–1514.
8. Wolfe K, Strydom A, Morrogh D, Carter J, Cutajar P, Eyeoyibo M et al. Chromosomal microarray testing in adults with intellectual disability presenting with comorbid psychiatric disorders. *Eur J Hum Genet.* 2016.
9. Gilissen C, Hehir-Kwa JY, Thung DT, van de Vorst M, van Bon BW, Willemsen MH et al. Genome sequencing identifies major causes of severe intellectual disability. *Nature.* 2014; 511(7509): 344–347.
10. Carvill GL, Mefford HC. Next-generation sequencing in intellectual disability. *J Pediatr Genet.* 2015; 4(3): 128–135.
11. Brian J, Doyle-Thomas K, Baribeau D, Anagnostou E. Novel mechanisms and treatment approaches in autism spectrum disorder. *Discov Med.* 2016; 22(119): 47–54.
12. Comi A. Current therapeutic options in Sturge-Weber syndrome. *Semin Pediatr Neurol.* 2015; 22(4): 295–301.
13. French JA, Lawson JA, Yapici Z, Ikeda H, Polster T, Nabbout R et al. Adjunctive everolimus therapy for treatment-resistant focal-onset seizures associated with tuberous sclerosis (EXIST-3): A phase 3, randomised, double-blind, placebo-controlled study. *Lancet.* 2016; 388(10056): 2153–2163.
14. Jeong A. Tuberous sclerosis complex: A roadmap for future research. *Pediatr Neurol Briefs.* 2016; 30(7): 32.
15. Huang J, Zhu T, Qu Y, Mu D. Prenatal, perinatal and neonatal risk factors for intellectual disability: A systemic review and meta-analysis. *PLoS One.* 2016; 11(4): e0153655.

16. Mackay DF, Smith GC, Dobbie R, Cooper SA, Pell JP. Obstetric factors and different causes of special educational need: Retrospective cohort study of 407,503 schoolchildren. *BJOG*. 2013; 120(3): 297–307; discussion 8.
17. Mackay DF, Smith GC, Cooper SA, Wood R, King A, Clark DN et al. Month of conception and learning disabilities: A record-linkage study of 801,592 children. *Am J Epidemiol*. 2016; 184(7): 485–493.
18. Schendel DE, Bresnahan M, Carter KW, Francis RW, Gissler M, Gronborg TK et al. The International Collaboration for Autism Registry Epidemiology (iCARE): Multinational registry-based investigations of autism risk factors and trends. *J Autism Dev Disord*. 2013; 43(11): 2650–2663.
19. Idring S, Magnusson C, Lundberg M, Ek M, Rai D, Svensson AC et al. Parental age and the risk of autism spectrum disorders: Findings from a Swedish population-based cohort. *Int J Epidemiol*. 2014; 43(1): 107–115.
20. Abel KM, Dalman C, Svensson AC, Susser E, Dal H, Idring S et al. Deviance in fetal growth and risk of autism spectrum disorder. *Am J Psychiatry*. 2013; 170(4): 391–398.
21. Magnusson C, Rai D, Goodman A, Lundberg M, Idring S, Svensson A et al. Migration and autism spectrum disorder: Population-based study. *Br J Psychiatry*. 2012; 201: 109–115.
22. Magnusson C, Lundberg M, Lee BK, Rai D, Karlsson H, Gardner R et al. Maternal vitamin D deficiency and the risk of autism spectrum disorders: Population-based study. *BJPsych Open*. 2016; 2(2): 170–172.
23. Lee BK, Magnusson C, Gardner RM, Blomstrom A, Newschaffer CJ, Burstyn I et al. Maternal hospitalization with infection during pregnancy and risk of autism spectrum disorders. *Brain Behav Immun*. 2015; 44: 100–105.
24. Heuvelman H, Abel K, Wicks S, Gardner R, Johnstone E, Lee B et al. Gestational age at birth and risk of intellectual disability without a common genetic cause. *Eur J Epidemiol*. 2018;33(7): 667–678.
25. Krahn GL, Fox MH. Health disparities of adults with intellectual disabilities: What do we know? What do we do? *J Appl Res Intellect Disabil*. 2014; 27(5): 431–446.
26. Emerson E, Baines S, Allerton L, Welch V. *Health Inequalities and People with Learning Disabilities in the UK: 2012*. Improving Health and Lives: Learning Disabilities Observatory, 2012.
27. Emerson E. Underweight, obesity and exercise among adults with intellectual disabilities in supported accommodation in Northern England. *J Intellect Disabil Res*. 2005; 49(Pt 2):134–143.
28. Perry BI, Cooray SE, Mendis J, Purandare K, Wijeratne A, Manjubhashini S et al. Problem behaviours and psychotropic medication use in intellectual disability: A multinational cross-sectional survey. *J Intellect Disabil Res*. 2018; 62(2): 140–149.
29. Balogh R, Brownell M, Ouellette-Kuntz H, Colantonio A. Hospitalisation rates for ambulatory care sensitive conditions for persons with and without an intellectual disability—a population perspective. *J Intellect Disabil Res*. 2010; 54(9): 820–832.
30. Balogh RS, Lake JK, Lin E, Wilton A, Lunsky Y. Disparities in diabetes prevalence and preventable hospitalizations in people with intellectual and developmental disability: A population-based study. *Diabet Med*. 2015; 32(2): 235–242.
31. Heslop P, Blair PS, Fleming P, Hoghton M, Marriott A, Russ L. The confidential inquiry into premature deaths of people with intellectual disabilities in the UK: A population-based study. *Lancet*. 2014; 383(9920): 889–895.
32. Glover G, Williams R, Heslop P, Oyinlola J, Grey J. Mortality in people with intellectual disabilities in England. *J Intellect Disabil Res*. 2017;61(1): 62–74.
33. Heslop P, Glover G. Mortality of people with intellectual disabilities in England: A comparison of data from existing sources. *J Appl Res Intellect Disabil*. 2015; 28(5): 414–422.
34. Hosking FJ, Carey IM, Shah SM, Harris T, DeWilde S, Beighton C, et al. Mortality among adults with intellectual disability in England: Comparisons with the general population. *Am J Public Health*. 2016; 106(8): 1483–1490.
35. Burtner AP, Wakham MD, McNeal DR, Garvey TP. Tobacco and the institutionalized mentally retarded: Usage choices and ethical considerations. *Spec Care Dentist*. 1995; 15(2): 56–60.
36. MENCAP. Treat me right! Better healthcare for people with a learning disability. MENCAP, 2004.
37. Beacroft M, Dodd K. 'I Feel Pain'—audit of communication skills and understanding of pain and health needs with people with learning disabilities. *British Journal of Learning Disabilities*. 2011; 39(2): 139–147.
38. Chester V, Green F, Alexander R. An audit of a smoking cessation programme for people with an intellectual disability resident in a forensic unit. *Advances in Mental Health and Intellectual Disabilities*. 2011; 5(1): 33–41.
39. Plant A, McDermott E, Chester V, Alexander RT. Substance misuse among offenders in a forensic intellectual disability service. *Journal of Learning Disabilities and Offending Behaviour*. 2011; 2(3): 127–135.
40. Kalyva E. Prevalence and influences on self-reported smoking among adolescents with mild learning disabilities, attention deficit hyperactivity disorder, and their typically developing peers. *J Intellect Disabil*. 2007; 11(3): 267–279.
41. Buszewicz M, Welch C, Horsfall L, Nazareth I, Osborn D, Hassiotis A et al. Assessment of an incentivised scheme to provide annual health checks in primary care for adults with intellectual disability: A longitudinal cohort study. *Lancet Psychiatry*. 2014; 1(7): 522–530.
42. Cooper SA, Morrison J, Allan LM, McConnachie A, Greenlaw N, Melville CA et al. Practice nurse health checks for adults with intellectual disabilities: A cluster-design, randomised controlled trial. *Lancet Psychiatry*. 2014; 1(7): 511–521.
43. Cooper SA, Smiley E, Morrison J, Williamson A, Allan L. Mental ill-health in adults with intellectual disabilities: Prevalence and associated factors. *Br J Psychiatry*. 2007; 190: 27–35.
44. Deb S, Thomas M, Bright C. Mental disorder in adults with intellectual disability. 1: Prevalence of functional psychiatric illness among a community-based population aged between 16 and 64 years. *J Intellect Disabil Res*. 2001; 45(Pt 6): 495–505.
45. Buckles J, Luckasson R, Keefe E. A Systematic Review of the Prevalence of Psychiatric Disorders in Adults With Intellectual Disability, 2003–2010. In: *Journal of Mental Health Research in Intellectual Disabilities*: 181–207. Routledge, 2013.
46. Marston GM, Perry DW, Roy A. Manifestations of depression in people with intellectual disability. *J Intellect Disabil Res*. 1997; 41 (Pt 6): 476–480.
47. Bouras N, Martin G, Leese M, Vanstraelen M, Holt G, Thomas C et al. Schizophrenia-spectrum psychoses in people with and without intellectual disability. *J Intellect Disabil Res*. 2004; 48(Pt 6): 548–555.
48. Cooper SA, Melville CA, Einfeld SL. Psychiatric diagnosis, intellectual disabilities and Diagnostic Criteria for Psychiatric Disorders for Use with Adults with Learning Disabilities/Mental

Retardation (DC-LD). *J Intellect Disabil Res.* 2003; 47 Suppl 1: 3–15.
49. Smiley E, Cooper SA. Intellectual disabilities, depressive episode, diagnostic criteria and Diagnostic Criteria for Psychiatric Disorders for Use with Adults with Learning Disabilities/Mental Retardation (DC-LD). *J Intellect Disabil Res.* 2003; 47 Suppl 1: 62–71.
50. Fletcher RJ, Havercamp SM, Ruedrich SL, Benson BA, Barnhill LJ, Cooper SA et al. Clinical usefulness of the diagnostic manual-intellectual disability for mental disorders in persons with intellectual disability: Results from a brief field survey. *J Clin Psychiatry.* 2009; 70(7): 967–974.
51. Koslowski N, Klein K, Arnold K, Kosters M, Schutzwohl M, Salize HJ et al. Effectiveness of interventions for adults with mild to moderate intellectual disabilities and mental health problems: Systematic review and meta-analysis. *Br J Psychiatry.* 2016; 209(6): 469–474.
52. Waite J, Heald M, Wilde L, Woodcock K, Welham A, Adams D et al. The importance of understanding the behavioural phenotypes of genetic syndromes associated with intellectual disability. In: *Paediatrics and Child Health*: 468–472. Elsevier.
53. Royston R, Howlin P, Waite J, Oliver C. Anxiety disorders in Williams syndrome contrasted with intellectual disability and the general population: A systematic review and meta-analysis. *J Autism Dev Disord.* 2017;47(12): 3765–3777.
54. O'Brien G. Behavioural phenotypes: Causes and clinical implications. *Advances in Psychiatric Treatment.* 2006; 12(5): 338–348.
55. NICE guideline [NG11]. Challenging behaviour and learning disabilities: Prevention and interventions for people with learning disabilities whose behaviour challenges. *National Institute for Health and Care Excellence*, 2015.
56. Aman MG, Singh NN, Stewart AW, Field CJ. The aberrant behavior checklist: a behavior rating scale for the assessment of treatment effects. *Am J Ment Defic.* 1985; 89(5): 485–491.
57. Idring S, Rai D, Dal H, Dalman C, Sturm H, Zander E, et al. Autism spectrum disorders in the Stockholm Youth Cohort: Design, prevalence and validity. *PLoS One.* 2012; 7(7): e41280.
58. Brugha TS, Spiers N, Bankart J, Cooper SA, McManus S, Scott FJ et al. Epidemiology of autism in adults across age groups and ability levels. *Br J Psychiatry.* 2016; 209(6): 498–503.
59. Hastings RP, Beck A, Daley D, Hill C. Symptoms of ADHD and their correlates in children with intellectual disabilities. *Res Dev Disabil.* 2005; 26(5): 456–468.
60. Bretherton K. ADHD and learning disability. *Cutting edge Psychiatry in Practice.* 2012; (2): 113–117.
61. Seager MC, O'Brien G. Attention deficit hyperactivity disorder: Review of ADHD in learning disability: the Diagnostic Criteria for Psychiatric Disorders for Use with Adults with Learning Disabilities/Mental Retardation[DC-LD] criteria for diagnosis. *J Intellect Disabil Res.* 2003; 47 Suppl 1: 26–31.
62. Reilly C, Holland N. Symptoms of attention deficit hyperactivity disorder in children and adults with intellectual disability: A review. *Journal of Applied Research in Intellectual Disabilities.* 2011; 24(4): 291–309.
63. Xenitidis K, Paliokosta E, Rose E, Maltezos S, Bramham J. ADHD symptom presentation and trajectory in adults with borderline and mild intellectual disability. *J Intellect Disabil Res.* 2010; 54(7): 668–677.
64. Jou R, Handen B, Hardan A. Psychostimulant treatment of adults with mental retardation and attention-deficit hyperactivity disorder. *Australas Psychiatry.* 2004; 12(4): 376–379.
65. La Malfa G, Lassi S, Bertelli M, Pallanti S, Albertini G. Detecting attention-deficit/hyperactivity disorder (ADHD) in adults with intellectual disability: The use of Conners' Adult ADHD Rating Scales (CAARS). *Res Dev Disabil.* 2008; 29(2): 158–164.
66. Dieckmann F, Giovis C, Offergeld J. The life expectancy of people with intellectual disabilities in Germany. *J Appl Res Intellect Disabil.* 2015; 28(5): 373–382.
67. Aylward EH, Burt DB, Thorpe LU, Lai F, Dalton A. Diagnosis of dementia in individuals with intellectual disability. *J Intellect Disabil Res.* 1997; 41 (Pt 2): 152–164.
68. Dementia and People with Intellectual Disabilities. Guidance on the assessment, diagnosis, interventions and support of people with intellectual disabilities who develop dementia. British Psychological Society, Division of Clinical Psychology and Royal College of Psychiatrists 2015.
69. Sheehan R, Sinai A, Bass N, Blatchford P, Bohnen I, Bonell S et al. Dementia diagnostic criteria in Down syndrome. *Int J Geriatr Psychiatry.* 2015; 30(8): 857–863.
70. NICE guideline [NG54]. Mental health problems in people with learning disabilities: Prevention, assessment and management. National Institute for Health and Care Excellence, 2016.
71. Livingstone N, Hanratty J, McShane R, Macdonald G. Pharmacological interventions for cognitive decline in people with Down syndrome. *Cochrane Database Syst Rev.* 2015; (10): CD011546.
72. Cooper SA, Ademola T, Caslake M, Douglas E, Evans J, Greenlaw N et al. Towards onset prevention of cognition decline in adults with Down syndrome (The TOP-COG study): A pilot randomised controlled trial. *Trials.* 2016; 17: 370.
73. Tuffrey-Wijne I, Wicki M, Heslop P, McCarron M, Todd S, Oliver D et al. Developing research priorities for palliative care of people with intellectual disabilities in Europe: A consultation process using nominal group technique. *BMC Palliat Care.* 2016; 15: 36.
74. Sheehan R, Hassiotis A, Walters K, Osborn D, Strydom A, Horsfall L. Mental illness, challenging behaviour, and psychotropic drug prescribing in people with intellectual disability: UK population based cohort study. *BMJ.* 2015; 351: h4326.
75. Bhaumik S, Branford D, Barrett M, Gangadharan SK. The Frith prescribing guidelines for people with intellectual disability. John Wiley & Sons Inc., 2015.
76. O'Dwyer M, Maidment ID, Bennett K, Peklar J, Mulryan N, McCallion P et al. Association of anticholinergic burden with adverse effects in older people with intellectual disabilities: An observational cross-sectional study. *Br J Psychiatry.* 2016; 209(6): 504–510.
77. Vigod SN, Lunsky Y, Cobigo V, Wilton AS, Somerton S, Seitz DP. Morbidity and mortality of women and men with intellectual and developmental disabilities: Newly initiating antipsychotic drugs. *BJPsych Open.* 2016; 2(2): 188–194.
78. McQuire C, Hassiotis A, Harrison B, Pilling S. Pharmacological interventions for challenging behaviour in children with intellectual disabilities: A systematic review and meta-analysis. *BMC Psychiatry.* 2015; 15: 303.
79. Gagiano C, Read S, Thorpe L, Eerdekens M, Van H, I. Short- and long-term efficacy and safety of risperidone in adults with disruptive behavior disorders. *Psychopharmacology (Berl).* 2005; 179(3): 629–636.

80. McDougle CJ, Holmes JP, Carlson DC, Pelton GH, Cohen DJ, Price LH. A double-blind, placebo-controlled study of risperidone in adults with autistic disorder and other pervasive developmental disorders. *Arch Gen Psychiatry*. 1998; 55(7): 633–641.
81. Tyrer P, Oliver-Africano PC, Ahmed Z, Bouras N, Cooray S, Deb S et al. Risperidone, haloperidol, and placebo in the treatment of aggressive challenging behaviour in patients with intellectual disability: A randomised controlled trial. *Lancet*. 2008; 371(9606): 57–63.
82. Glover G, Bernard S, Branford D, Holland A, Strydom A. Use of medication for challenging behaviour in people with intellectual disability. *Br J Psychiatry*. 2014; 205(1): 6–7.
83. Dalton AJ, McVilly KR. Ethics Guidelines for International, Multicenter Research Involving People with Intellectual Disabilities 1, 2, 3, 4. *Journal of Policy and Practice in Intellectual Disabilities*. 2004; 1(2): 57–70.
84. Vereenooghe L, Langdon PE. Psychological therapies for people with intellectual disabilities: A systematic review and meta-analysis. *Res Dev Disabil*. 2013; 34(11): 4085–4102.
85. Willner P, Rose J, Jahoda A, Kroese BS, Felce D, Cohen D et al. Group-based cognitive-behavioural anger management for people with mild to moderate intellectual disabilities: Cluster randomised controlled trial. *Br J Psychiatry*. 2013; 203(3): 288–296.
86. Jahoda A, Melville C, Cooper SA, Hastings R, Briggs A, Dagnan D et al. BEAT-IT. Comparing a behavioural activation treatment for depression in adults with intellectual disabilities with an attention control: Study protocol for a randomised controlled trial. *Trials*. 2015; 16: 595.
87. Jahoda A, Melville CA, Pert C, Cooper SA, Lynn H, Williams C et al. A feasibility study of behavioural activation for depressive symptoms in adults with intellectual disabilities. *J Intellect Disabil Res*. 2015; 59(11): 1010–1021.
88. Hassiotis A, Poppe M, Strydom A, Vickerstaff V, Hall IS, Crabtree J et al. Clinical outcomes of staff training in positive behaviour support to reduce challenging behaviour in adults with intellectual disability: Cluster randomised controlled trial. *Br J Psychiatry*. 2018; 212(3): 161–168.
89. Lante K, Stancliffe RJ, Bauman A, van der Ploeg HP, Jan S, Davis GM. Embedding sustainable physical activities into the everyday lives of adults with intellectual disabilities: A randomised controlled trial. BMC Public Health. 2014; 14: 1038.
90. Melville CA, Mitchell F, Stalker K, Matthews L, McConnachie A, Murray HM et al. Effectiveness of a walking programme to support adults with intellectual disabilities to increase physical activity: Walk well cluster-randomised controlled trial. *Int J Behav Nutr Phys Act*. 2015; 12: 125.
91. Alexander R, Hiremath A, Chester V, Green F, Gunaratna I, Hoare S. Evaluation of treatment outcomes from a medium secure unit for people with intellectual disability. *Advances in Mental Health and Intellectual Disabilities*. 2011; 5(1): 22–32.
92. Alexander RT, Crouch K, Halstead S, Piachaud J. Long-term outcome from a medium secure service for people with intellectual disability. *J Intellect Disabil Res*. 2006; 50(Pt 4): 305–315.
93. Morrissey C, Geach N, Alexander R, Chester V, Devapriam J, Duggan C et al. Researching outcomes from forensic services for people with intellectual or developmental disabilities: A systematic review, evidence synthesis and expert and patient/carer consultation. *Health Services and Delivery Research*. 2017; 5(3).
94. Morrissey C, Langdon PE, Geach N, Chester V, Ferriter M, Lindsay WR et al. A systematic review and synthesis of outcome domains for use within forensic services for people with intellectual disabilities. *BJPsych Open*. 2017; 3(1): 41–56.
95. Sheehan R, Gandesha A, Hassiotis A, Gallagher P, Burnell M, Jones G et al. An audit of the quality of inpatient care for adults with learning disability in the UK. *BMJ Open*. 2016; 6(4): e010480.
96. Thomas B, Courtenay K, Hassiotis A, Strydom A, Rantell K. Standardised patients with intellectual disabilities in training tomorrow's doctors. *Psychiatr Bull* (2014). 2014; 38(3): 132–136.
97. Ryan TA, Scior K. Medical students' attitudes towards people with intellectual disabilities: a literature review. *Res Dev Disabil*. 2014; 35(10): 2316–2328.
98. Tracy J, Iacono T. People with developmental disabilities teaching medical students—does it make a difference? *J Intellect Dev Disabil*. 2008; 33(4): 345–348.
99. Spackman R, Qureshi A, Rai D. A review of recommendations for medical undergraduate intellectual disability psychiatry teaching from UK reports. In: *Advances in Mental Health and Intellectual Disabilities*: 158–163. Emerald, 2016.
100. Lewis S, Stenfert-Kroese B. An investigation of nursing staff attitudes and emotional reactions towards patients with intellectual disability in a general hospital setting. *Journal of Applied Research in Intellectual Disabilities*. 2010; 23(4): 355–365.
101. Hemm C, Dagnan D, Meyer TD. Identifying training needs for mainstream healthcare professionals, to prepare them for working with individuals with intellectual disabilities: A systematic review. *J Appl Res Intellect Disabil*. 2015; 28(2): 98–110.
102. Tomlinson M, Yasamy MT, Emerson E, Officer A, Richler D, Saxena S. Setting global research priorities for developmental disabilities, including intellectual disabilities and autism. *J Intellect Disabil Res*. 2014; 58(12): 1121–1130.
103. Ali A, Hassiotis A, Strydom A, King M. Self stigma in people with intellectual disabilities and courtesy stigma in family carers: A systematic review. *Res Dev Disabil*. 2012; 33(6): 2122–2140.
104. Scior K, Hamid A, Hastings R, Werner S, Belton C, Laniyan A et al. Consigned to the margins: A call for global action to challenge intellectual disability stigma. *Lancet Glob Health*. 2016; 4(5): e294–e5.
105. Fox F, Aabe N, Turner K, Redwood S, Rai D. 'It was like walking without knowing where I was going': A qualitative study of autism in a UK Somali migrant community. *J Autism Dev Disord*. 2017; 47(2): 305–315.
106. Selman LE, Fox F, Aabe N, Turner K, Rai D, Redwood S. 'You are labelled by your children's disability'—A community-based, participatory study of stigma among Somali parents of children with autism living in the United Kingdom. *Ethn Health*. 2017: 1–16.
107. Lewis K. Participation of people with a learning disability in medical research. Scoping review. London: MenCap. 2014.
108. Robotham D, King M, Canagasabey A, Inchley-Mort S, Hassiotis A. Social validity of randomised controlled trials in health services research and intellectual disabilities: A qualitative exploration of stakeholder views. *Trials*. 2011; 12: 144.
109. Iacono T, Carling-Jenkins R. The human rights context for ethical requirements for involving people with intellectual disability in medical research. *J Intellect Disabil Res*. 2012; 56(11): 1122–1132.
110. Carlson L. Research ethics and intellectual disability: Broadening the debates. *Yale J Biol Med*. 2013; 86(3): 303–314.
111. Iacono T. Ethical challenges and complexities of including people with intellectual disability as participants in research. *J Intellect Dev Disabil*. 2006; 31(3): 173–179; discussion 80–91.
112. Feldman MA, Bosett J, Collet C, Burnham-Riosa P. Where are persons with intellectual disabilities in medical research?

A survey of published clinical trials. *J Intellect Disabil Res*. 2014; 58(9): 800–809.

113. McDonald KE, Schwartz NM, Gibbons CM, Olick RS. 'You can't be cold and scientific': Community views on ethical issues in intellectual disability research. *J Empir Res Hum Res Ethics*. 2015; 10(2): 196–208.
114. Lennox N, Taylor M, Rey-Conde T, Bain C, Purdie DM, Boyle F. Beating the barriers: Recruitment of people with intellectual disability to participate in research. *J Intellect Disabil Res*. 2005; 49(Pt 4): 296–305.
115. Nicholson L, Colyer M, Cooper SA. Recruitment to intellectual disability research: A qualitative study. *J Intellect Disabil Res*. 2013; 57(7): 647–656.
116. Oliver-Africano P, Dickens S, Ahmed Z, Bouras N, Cooray S, Deb S, et al. Overcoming the barriers experienced in conducting a medication trial in adults with aggressive challenging behaviour and intellectual disabilities. *J Intellect Disabil Res*. 2010; 54(1): 17–25.
117. Turk V, Leer G, Burchell S, Khattram S, Corney R, Rowlands G. Adults with intellectual disabilities and their carers as researchers and participants in a RCT. *J Appl Res Intellect Disabil*. 2012; 25(1): 1–10.
118. McDonald KE, Kidney CA. What Is Right? *Ethics in Intellectual Disabilities Research. Journal of Policy and Practice in Intellectual Disabilities*. 2012; 9(1): 27–39.

27

Models of Service Development and Delivery for People with Intellectual Disability

Sujeet Jaydeokar, John Devapriam, Jane McCarthy, Chaya Kapugama, and Sabyasachi Bhaumik[†]

Introduction

Intellectual disability (ID) is a condition characterized by significant impairments of both intellectual and adaptive functioning and an onset before 18 years of age (1). It affects about 1–2 per cent of the general population (2). The degree of ID can be mild, moderate, severe, or profound, with over 90 per cent of those affected falling within the mild range (3). People with ID have high rates of mental health (4) and physical health comorbidities (5).

Around the world, health services have found their own solutions depending on availability of resources and specialism. In some European countries, there are physicians specializing in ID, who have responsibility for both physical and mental health of people with ID; the same is also seen in children's services in the UK where community paediatricians are involved managing both physical and mental healthcare issues in children with ID. The international perspective is that some form of service specialization is required along with community outreach services and in-patient facilities with strong links between general mental health and ID services (6). However in countries which are still dependent on large institutions or where the families have been the main support, there has been limited access to more specialist services (7). In many countries, there are no specialist ID community teams and people with ID utilize mainstream health services in which there may or may not be ID specialists. Where there are no specialists available, or where specialism is not routinely available, health services have developed innovative solutions like the 'Hub and Spoke' model, where a specialist centre provides consultation along with teaching and training to the frontline staff with a view to develop their skills in some of the multi-disciplinary interventions, and thus provide therapeutic input to resource deficient areas. The type of service model required will therefore differ from country to country, and even within each individual country, due to the different needs of local populations and the model of health care for the wider community.

In some low and middle income countries ID is recognized as a social disorder. Hence health service provision, and more specifically mental health service provision is not well organized and sometimes rudimentary. A lack of prevalence data due to a lack of systematic research is a significant drawback in many countries. Therefore, many individuals with ID are not under the radar of health surveillance. In addition, the majority of these countries have extremely limited resources for health provision, and a service model for a group of marginalized individuals (i.e. people with ID) is not seen as a priority in the health sector. There have been some examples of developing and creating service models that may be appropriate for a low or medium resource country. However, the best examples as described in detail below have mostly arisen from high income countries like UK, Australia, New Zealand, and parts of China such as Hong Kong.

Models of service provision—a United Kingdom perspective

In the United Kingdom (UK), policies for people with ID began with a focus on illness and disability, leading to services aligned with care, custody, and education. They have also largely been influenced by the evolution of mental health and mental capacity legislation. Policies have tended to focus on access pathways between hospitals, the community and diversion from criminal justice systems, and influenced by public opinion, political will, and legislation.

Historically, most people with ID were cared for in long stay institutions—from workhouses and prisons during the industrial revolution to Local Authority built special asylums in the late nineteenth century. Édouard Séguin in France, with the influence of Jean Mark Gaspard Itard, worked on methods of training people with ID and opened the first private school in Paris dedicated for this purpose (8). This led to an interest in people with ID as a separate entity. Later on Séguin continued the same work in the United States, and founded in 1876 what is known today as the American Association on Intellectual and Developmental Disabilities which is the oldest professional association concerned with intellectual and developmental disabilities.

In the early twentieth century, the shift was towards life-long segregation. Legislation in England led to care of people with ID being

[†] It is with great regret that we report the death of Sabyasachi Bhaumik during the production of this textbook.

in special asylums, with the majority being built between 1880 and 1910. They focused on training and rehabilitation and later on lifelong containment and isolation from society. In the 1920s and 1930s medical interest in the research into the biological basis of 'mental deficiency' and involvement of prominent people of the medical profession such as Professor Lionel Penrose led to these asylums becoming designated as hospitals when the National Health Service was introduced in 1948.

With the Mental Health Act 1959, compulsory admission to hospital was possible on the basis of mental sub-normality and care became polarized between hospitals and the community, with numbers in hospital increasing till the 1970s. When people with ID were cared for in hospitals it was assumed that all the healthcare needs could be met in that setting. However the segregated nature of the hospitals made access to mainstream health services difficult and inequitable. Two large-scale hospital inquiries by the Department of Health and Social Security (Ely hospital in 1969 and Farleigh hospital in 1971) revealed overcrowding, understaffing, and serious ill-treatment. Influential publications by Goffman (9) and Morris (10) describing the dehumanizing effects of institutions coupled with changing attitudes throughout the Western world led to closure of large-scale asylums and shift of care to the community.

Following the deinstitutionalization movement of the 1980s, these hospitals were closed and patients moved into the community. By the 1990s there was greater acknowledgement of both the basic and special health care needs of people with ID and that people with ID have the same rights of access to NHS services as everyone else, but that they may require assistance to use such services. This was accompanied by an increasing focus on community ID teams providing a range of services, including those for mental health and behavioural difficulties (11). These teams were multidisciplinary, offering advice and support to families and carers as well as direct work with individuals with an ID. They varied in composition but usually included social workers, nurses, speech and language therapists, occupational therapists, physiotherapists, clinical psychologists, psychiatrists, and other therapists.

More recently, following institutional abuse uncovered in Sutton and Merton Trust, Cornwall ID services, and Winterbourne View hospital, there has been increasing scrutiny. Specialist in-patient units for people with ID and mental health or behavioural problems (described as assessment and treatment units) have attracted particular attention following the broadcast of the BBC Panorama programme 'Undercover Care: the Abuse Exposed'. Following this scandal a serious case review was published by the South Gloucestershire Adult Safeguarding Board followed by the interim (12) and final (13) reports from the Department of Health in 2012. These reports described hospital-based assessment and treatment units as a new form of institutional care which had no place in the twenty-first century, and concluded that there were too many people staying for too long within these units. A general theme that has emerged from abuse scandals and inquiries is that there is a widespread failure to design, commission, and provide services locally and a failure to assess the quality and outcomes being delivered in ID hospitals.

The current service model in the UK is a combination of generic and specialist services spanning across hospital-based and community services. In England, the vast majority of people with ID live fairly independent lives in the community. Of the 900,000 adults with the condition, 191,000 (21%) have contact with specialist ID services and 3,035 (0.3%) receive treatment in psychiatric in-patient settings, including specialist ID hospitals (14). The latter number is subject to fluctuations and is expected to reduce further.

Models of service provision—an international perspective

Data on prevalence of ID and studies on services is generally scarce in many Middle Eastern countries. There are limited specialist services specifically designed for people with ID, and those that are available are mainly through institutional care. People with ID are expected to access generic services like the rest of the population. Despite these less than optimal conditions, in Israel, there have been some attempts in developing community-based services for young persons with disabilities (including ID) since the 1990s. Methods such as vocational rehabilitation, independent living education, recreational activities, social skills training, and sexuality education have been utilized in these services (15). The willingness of clinicians to treat psychiatric problems arising in this population is low and almost exclusively biologically driven. Some residential care settings and special schools may have psychiatrists and psychologists visiting them. Families of people with ID are noted to seek psychiatric care in the private sector in search of better care (16).

In Asia, similarly, the biggest challenge in ascertaining the epidemiology, policies, and services for people with ID is the lack of literature and statistics. The available studies are sporadic and the different terminology (e.g. mental retardation, mental handicap, learning disabilities, mental deficiency, mental sub normality) used to describe this group has led to a degree of unreliability in epidemiological surveys. In addition, most of these study designs did not serve the purpose of getting good quality and reliable prevalence data from the population at large. All Asian countries have at least one law or policy that promotes the wellbeing of this population group. Japan leads in this aspect by being the only Asian country with a law enacted specifically for people with ID. Most policies in this regard are related to the states' participation in international programmes and conventions, for example the UN Convention on the Rights of Persons with Disabilities. Most countries have special employment and pension schemes for this population (17).

There have been various attempts in Asian countries to bridge the large gap in treatment of developmental disorders through using innovative methods. For example, in rural Pakistan, a system was tried out successfully where volunteers from families with developmental disorders (including ID) were trained in evidence-based interventions, who worked under the supervision of specialists to provide care and work with 'family networks' (18). In Kerala, India, a child development centre has been successfully established using a lifecycle approach, which is easily replicable all over the country (19). Additionally in Northern India, a study was carried out to assess the satisfaction level of parents/attendees at a child development clinic. This showed that despite a reportedly good level of satisfaction, the attendees travel long distances, face hardships in carrying their children to clinics, and lose earnings in doing so (20). This is a result of centralized service structures that prevail in many Asian countries. In Sri Lanka, there are no specialized services for people with ID; people with ID utilize mainstream healthcare services, including psychiatric services. The healthcare staff do not usually have special training in care provision for people with ID.

In the People's Republic of China, there have been encouraging developments in services for people with ID in recent years. Two nationwide disability surveys have been conducted in 1987 and 2006. Several laws and policies for the protection of the rights of this vulnerable group have been formulated and the country has seen the beginnings of a variety of services, including early intervention, education, training, employment, and rehabilitation. However, there is still room for improvement in continuity of care and transitioning smoothly from different services. The geographical distribution of services is uneven in that most services are congregated in urban areas. The mental health services for this population is still rudimentary, and there are no specialized psychiatric services dedicated to the diagnosis and treatment of psychiatric disorders and the management of challenging behaviours (21).

In Hong Kong, Kwai Chung Hospital (KCH) is one of the first in Asia to set up a service for patients with ID. Originally opened as a general psychiatry hospital in 1981, it has been keeping up with the global de-institutionalization movement by gradually reducing numbers of in-patient beds. Recognizing the need for specialist ID services to meet the complex demands of this population, KCH set up a specialist unit dubbing it 'Psychiatric Unit for Learning Disabilities (PULD)' in 1995. This comprised of two in-patient wards with 90 beds in total, an outpatient clinic, outreach service, and respite service. PULD aims to meet the mental health needs of people with ID by providing a high quality, comprehensive psychiatric service that incorporates principles of normalization and integration. Over the years there has been an increase in the facilities provided, with a growth in manpower, service elements, and an inclination towards training and research. The staff have gained tremendous experience in dealing with this patient group (22).

The healthcare system in Australia is funded by Commonwealth and State Governments. The mainstream public mental health services bear the bulk of the responsibility in meeting the mental health needs of people with ID. Only a handful of services and clinicians are available in the public sector for providing specialist ID mental healthcare. Admissions occur to general mental health facilities since no special in-patient facilities for ID are available, and staff have limited experience in working with this patient group. As a way of rising to the above challenges, in 2007 New South Wales (NSW) Department of Health and NSW Department of Ageing, Disability, and Home Care together with NSW Council for ID developed the NSW Health Service Framework to Improve Health Care of People with ID, which promoted a five-tiered structure to address the health needs of people with ID. The costs of implementation have hindered its full realization. However, several smaller projects have arisen out of this framework. Other states have also taken initiative in developing specialized services for this group. For example, a tertiary dual disability service for those with ID and mental illness has been developed in Victoria. Queensland has established a Forensic Disability Service. Australia has also realized the increased need to train professionals in ID in medical schools, particularly general practitioners and psychiatrists (23).

In New Zealand, there seems to have been interest into carers' satisfaction with ID services, as well as the prevalence, health, and educational needs of various subgroups with ID for a few decades (23, 24, 25). More recent research into the current service and delivery structures seem to be scarce.

A framework to understand specialist ID service delivery

Specialist ID care provision can be best described by a tiered model of care, where tiers 1 to 3 constitute the community element of care provision and tier 4 constitutes hospital-based element of care provision (26) (Box 27.1). The tiered care model and care pathway strives to enable the right care to be delivered by the right people and at the right time and place. This model will be helpful only if changing needs, crises, and circumstances allow for timely and appropriate moving 'up' or 'down' the tiers. Such a model recognizes a range of levels of need—including people with less severe needs, who are able to manage and thrive with the support of their family and friends, primary care, and community services, through to people whose difficulties require intensive specialist support or in-patient care. Tier 4 is further categorized into six types of in-patient beds, ranging from secure beds and high medium and low secure units, acute admission beds in specialist and mainstream mental-health settings, and forensic and complex care rehabilitation beds (Box 27.1) (27).

Countries such as the UK have high numbers of specialist mental health professionals including psychiatrists, nurses, and psychologists trained to work with people with ID (28). This approach also ensures training is available to support care staff and family carers as well as the professionals. This rich availability of specialists has supported a model of designated ID teams at a secondary care level providing specialist mental health assessments and interventions delivered in the community alongside a clinic-based service. These teams also provide other secondary healthcare interventions such as communication assessments, functional assessments, and social care. Other centres have provided more specialist mental health ID

Box 27.1 Tiered model of care for ID services

Tier 1 encompasses primary care and other mainstream services. It is the tier of service provision that serves the general health, social care, and educational needs of people with ID and their families. The community ID team and the psychiatrist have limited direct clinical contact in this tier. Nevertheless, they are involved in activities which may influence patients' care, and interacting with this tier is essential to the training of ID psychiatrists.

Tier 2 is general community ID services. At this level the person with ID starts to use specialist ID services. Most specialist services are provided jointly between health and social services or are moving towards such a model.

Tier 3 is a highly specialized element of community ID service. This includes areas of specialized needs such as epilepsy, dementia, challenging behaviour, pervasive developmental disorders, and outpatient forensic services.

Tier 4 is specialist in-patient services. It includes all specialist in-patient services for people with ID, ranging from local assessment and treatment services to high secure forensic services (see Box 27.2).

Box 27.2 Categories of in-patient beds within Tier 4 for people with ID and mental health and/or severe behavioural problems

Category 1: High, medium, and low secure forensic beds.
Category 2: Acute admission beds within specialized ID units.
Category 3: Acute admission beds within generic mental health settings.
Category 4: Forensic rehabilitation beds.
Category 5: Complex continuing care and rehabilitation beds.
Category 6: Other beds, including those for specialist neuropsychiatric conditions and short breaks.

teams alongside these community ID teams (29, 30, 31) although their availability is limited to specific geographical areas such as London, England. The access to primary health care in the UK is through general practitioners.

Developing services for people with ID

The essentials of any service model should aim to meet the needs of people with ID through the effective use of available resources—ensuring quality and sustainability of services. This is usually achieved by using the commissioning cycle framework and the five-stage model of care pathway development. The commissioning cycle consists of the following stages:

1. Assessing the needs of the local population, engaging stakeholders (including patients and their families) and clinical leaders/champions,
2. Reviewing services and undertaking a gap in service analysis,
3. Understanding key health and care risks and develop a strategy to mitigate risk,
4. Deciding on commissioning priorities by using evidence-based and cost-effectiveness analysis,
5. Strategic planning using local and national drivers,
6. Contract implementation with providers of services with clear objectives and outcomes,
7. Provider development through identifying workforce and resource needs to deliver services,
8. Managing provider performance from a quality and financial perspective.

A care pathway-based approach to service development addresses variation in practice and ensures standardization and personalization (through use of personalized care plans) of services. Care pathways can be both operational and clinical in nature and developed usually in five stages:

- Stage 1: Mapping patient's journey through the care system.
- Stage 2: Embedding standards across mental health and physical health. The standards could include regulatory, contractual, clinical, continuous learning from incidents and values-based standards.
- Stage 3: Develop the service structure around the patient's journey.
- Stage 4: Develop the workforce—identify tasks and level of skills required to undertake the tasks (e.g. functional mapping by Skills for Health).
- Stage 5: Operationalize, evaluate, improvise.

There are no one size fits all models, so a strategic approach is required in developing services at a local level which are person-centred and outcome-focused, with evidence of improved quality of life for people with mental health needs and/or challenging behaviours. A recent review of the literature (32) of the diverse models in place for community-based services found that those services which provided the most effective care were: person-centred, multi-agency, and providing therapeutic approaches based on behaviour support plans.

A strategic approach therefore needs to include a person-centred approach within a tiered model of service delivery. A proactive and preventative approach at Tiers 1 and 2 should lead to less pressure on specialist Tier 3 and Tier 4 services. At the same time, any significant gaps at any level would result in services dealing with more crisis and emergency situations and risks of prolonged hospital care. A strategic approach must also identify the workforce required to develop the service model in terms of professional skills of the specialist but also in the training of non-specialist carers (33). The development of services must be based on an assessment of local needs of the population. This will also need to be set in the context of how the current service model is working and the availability of professionals who are specialists in the field of ID.

Co-production, involving partnership working with service users and carers, is an essential element of any service developments and innovations, as it allows focusing the service delivery on outcomes that were relevant and important to patients, service users, and their carers. Such an approach would give any service development initiative a better understanding of what was needed to deliver those outcomes and the gaps in the current service provision. It also facilitates innovation, as it becomes clear as to what input was needed to achieve certain outcomes. Additionally, it makes it easy to identify elements of skills, competencies, specialism, and agencies needed that could deliver outcomes.

Considering wide variations in the availability of resources, both in terms of workforce competencies and capabilities and social care, any service delivery model should ensure that the available resources were used to meet the person-centred needs of most in a most efficient way. With changing needs of the population and changing resources, service delivery models should be able to adapt and innovate to meet changing demands. Thus, while underpinning the principles of a person-centred and rights-based approach to service delivery, service models should also focus on advocacy on behalf of people with ID, performance management, and sustainability through development of competencies and capabilities. Health services where possible should advocate development of specialism in ID, as they deliver better outcomes for people with ID, while keeping in mind that those with mild to borderline ID and severe mental illness seem to have better outcomes with intensive support within the context of generic mental health services (34).

Conclusion

Ensuring the availability of high quality healthcare for people with ID should be a priority of any healthcare service (35). However, services have developed differently in different parts of the world based on availability of resources in terms of organization of health services, availability of specialists in the field, training availability, prevailing social attitudes towards disability, and legal frameworks. This has also resulted in large variations in approaches to service delivery including generic services, specialist ID services, development of specialists like ID physicians, private/public partnerships, and reliance on voluntary sectors/Non-Governmental Organizations (NGOs). High income countries have access to greater provision compared to low income countries; the availability of specialist services is distinctly less for adults living in South East Asia, Africa, and the Western Pacific. It would not be appropriate to advocate one service delivery model as a preferred one as all these models would have their advantages and disadvantages and have evolved in response to local circumstances. However, it is important to agree on some principles that should underpin all the service delivery models, developments, and innovations. This discrepancy also highlights the need for reasonable adjustments from generic services to ensure access to the services for people with ID.

Any service development or delivery model should take an approach that is person-centred and outcome-focused. It is important that when we consider person centredness and outcomes for service delivery, it takes into account the 'rights' of people with ID. At the same time services are needed to be delivered within the available legal framework and available resources. Advocacy and sustainability are two important components of service delivery, and as professionals involved in the development of and delivery of services for people with ID, we have to ensure that we advocate and challenge attitudes and inadequate legal frameworks as well as invest in the development of competency and capability developments.

Finally, even though there is a wide variation in service provision in high income countries compare to low- and middle-income countries, there are numerous examples of innovation and good practices globally. It is important that we learn from these and incorporate them in our practices where appropriate.

MULTIPLE CHOICE QUESTIONS

Questions

Answer True or False for each of the statements

1. 'Hub and Spoke' model used in some countries:

A. Provides interventions through specialist community multidisciplinary ID teams
B. Consists of specialist centre providing consultation along with teaching and training to frontline staff
C. Focuses on providing tiered approach to the care delivery
D. Provides therapeutic input to resource deficient areas
E. Train frontline staff to provide some of the multidisciplinary interventions

2. Tiered model of specialist ID care provision:

A. Mainly focuses on various types of inpatient services for people with ID
B. Recognizes range of levels of needs of people with ID
C. Strives to enable the right care to be delivered by the right people at the right time and place
D. Could be used anywhere in the world
E. Does not need any specialist ID healthcare provision

3. When developing services for people with ID:

A. A service model should aim at meeting the needs of people with ID through effective use of available resources
B. Service provision should revolve around specialist in-patient services
B. It is important to engage local stakeholders
D. Any form of service specialism is not essential
E. There should be a review of available services and a gap analysis

4. Following principles are important when developing services at a local level:

A. Person centred approach
B. Outcome focus
C. Focus on quality of life of people with ID
D. Multi-agency service provision
E. One size fits all

5. Co-production:

A. Meant developing care pathways with social services
B. Is about partnership working with service users and carers
C. Allows service delivery to focus on outcomes relevant and important to patients and carers
D. Facilitates innovation
E. Doesn't identify gaps in service provision

Answers

1.

A. False—model is used where there are limited specialist resources by skilling up frontline staff
B. True
C. False—tiered approach is used where there are multidisciplinary resources available at various levels
D. True
E. True

2.

A. False—tiered model focused on various levels of specialist service provision including community service provisions
B. True
C. True
D. False—tiered model will not be suitable for resource deficient countries
E. False—services revolve around specialist provisions

3.

A. True
B. False—focus of service provision should be on providing care in the community
C. True
D. False—there should be some form of service specializations along with community outreach services and in-patient facilities
E. True

4.

A. True
B. True
C. True
D. True
E. False—services should reflect on local needs and available resources; one size fits all model are not appropriate

5.

A. False—co-production is about partnership with patients and carers. Other agencies are involved as important stakeholders
B. True
C. True
D. True
E. False—co-production does help identify gaps in service provision by involving patients and carers right from the beginning of service development and commissioning cycle

REFERENCES

1. World Health Organization (2008) ICD-10. International statistical classification of diseases and related health problems (10th Rev. ed.). New York, NY: Author.
2. Learning Disability Observatory (2012). Health Inequalities and People with Learning Disabilities in the UK. Available from: http://www.improvinghealthandlives.org.uk/uploads/doc/vid_7479_IHaL2010-3HealthInequality2010.pdf.
3. Department of Health (2001). Valuing people: A new strategy for learning disability for the 21st century—a White Paper. London: Author.
4. Cooper S-A, Smiley E, Morrison J, Williamson A, Allan L. Mental ill-health in adults with ID: Prevalence and associated factors. *Br J Psychiatry* 2007; 190: 27–35.
5. Hughes-McCormack LA, Rydzewska E, Henderson A, MacIntyre C, Rintoul J, Cooper S. Prevalence of mental health conditions and relationship with general health in a whole-country population of people with ID compared with the general population. *BJPsych Open* 2017; 3: 243–248
6. Cain N, Davidson P, Dosen A, Garcia-Ibanez J, Giesow V, Hillery J, Kwok, H et al. (2010). In: *Mental Health Services for Adults with Intellectual Disability: Strategies and Solutions*. Eds: N Bouras, G Holt. Psychology Press, East Sussex, UK.
7. Bhaumik S et al. (2016). Intellectual disability and mental health: An overview. *International Journal of Culture and Mental Health*, 9, 417–444.
8. Maulik P, Harbour CK, McCarthy J (2014). Epidemiology. In: *Handbook of Psychopathology in Adults with Developmental and Intellectual Disability: Research, Policy and Practice*. Editors: E Tsakanikos and J McCarthy. New York, NY: Springer Science.
9. Goffman E. Asylums: Essays on the Social Situation of Mental Patients and Other Inmates. Doubleday Anchor, New York, 1961.
10. Morris P (1969). Put Away: A Sociological Study of Institutions for the Mentally Retarded. London: Routledge and Kegan Paul.
11. Lindsey M (2000) Services for people with learning disability and mental health problems. *Mental Health Review*, 5, 5–18.
12. Department of Health (2012a). *Department of Health Review: Winterbourne View Hospital: Interim Report*, Department of Health.
13. Department of Health (2012b). *Transforming care: A national response to Winterbourne View Hospital: Department of Health Review Final Report*, London.
14. Devapriam J, Rosenbach A, Alexander R (2015). In-patient services for people with intellectual disability and mental health or behavioural difficulties. *BJPsych Advances*, 21(2) 116–123.
15. Hardoff D, Chigier E (1991). Developing community-based services for youth with disabilities. *Paediatrician*, 18, 157–162.
16. Stawski M, Merrick J (2006). Mental health services for people with intellectual disability in Israel—a review of options. *Isr J Psychiatry Relat Sci*, 43, 237–240.
17. Jeevanandam L (2009). Perspectives of intellectual disability in Asia: Epidemiology, policy, and services for children and adults. *Curr Opin Psychiatry*, 22, 462–468.
18. Hamdani SU, Minhas FA, Iqbal Z, Rahman A (2015). Model for service delivery for developmental disorders in low-income countries. *Paediatrics*, 136, 1166–1172.
19. Nair M K, George B, Nair GS, Bhaskaran D, Leena ML, Russell PS (2014). CDC Kerala 1: Organization of clinical child development services (1987–2013). *Indian J Pediatr*, 81 Suppl 2, S66–72.
20. Juneja M, Jain R, Singhal S, Mishra D (2012). Availing services for developmental disabilities: Parental experiences from a referral center in developing country. *Indian J Pediatr*, 79, 1213–1217.
21. Kwok HW, Cui Y, Li J (2011). Perspectives of intellectual disability in the People's Republic of China: Epidemiology, policy, services for children and adults. *Curr Opin Psychiatry*, 24, 408–412.
22. Kwok H (2006). A 10-year review of a Hong Kong model for mental health care of people with intellectual disability. *Isr J Psychiatry Relat Sci*, 43, 252–257.
23. Evans E, Howlett S, Kresmer T, Simpson J, Kayess R, Trollor J (2012). Service development for intellectual disability mental health: A human rights approach. *J Intellect Disabil Res*, 56, 1098–1109.
24. Pulman RM (1980). Medical services for parents of the mentally retarded as perceived by New Zealand parents. *Australian Journal of Developmental Disabilities*, 6, 39–42.
25. Hand JE, Reid PM (1996). Older adults with lifelong intellectual handicap in New Zealand: Prevalence, disabilities and implications for regional health authorities. *NZ Med J*, 109, 118–121.
26. Royal College of Psychiatrists (2011). Future role of psychiatrists working with people with learning disabilities. Faculty of psychiatry of learning disability, Faculty report FR/LD/1.
27. Royal College of Psychiatrists (2013). People with learning disability, mental health and behavioural or forensic problems—the role of inpatient services, Faculty report (FR/ID/03) Royal College of Psychiatrists.
28. Costello H, Hardy S, Tsakanikos E, McCarthy J. (2010). Training professionals, family carers and support staff to work effectively with people with intellectual disability and mental health problems. In: *Mental Health Services for Adults with Intellectual Disability: Strategies and Solutions*. Eds: N Bouras, G Holt. Psychology Press, East Sussex, UK.
29. O'Hara J, Chaplin E, Lockett J, Bouras N (2014). Community Mental Health Services. In: *Handbook of Psychopathology in Adults with Developmental and Intellectual Disability: Research, Policy and Practice*. Editors: E Tsakanikos, J McCarthy. New York, NY: Springer Science.

30. Hemmings CP et al. (2009). Comparison of adults with intellectual disabilities and mental health problems admitted to specialist and generic inpatient units. *British Journal of Learning Disabilities*, 37, 123–128.
31. Sheehan R, Paschos D (2013). A comparison of different models to meet the mental health needs of adults with intellectual disabilities. *Advances in Mental Health and Intellectual Disabilities*, 7, 161–168.
32. Royal College of Psychiatrists (2014). Community-based services for people with intellectual disability and mental health problems. Faculty Report 06. April 2014. www.rcpsych.ac.uk.
33. Costello H, Hardy S, Tsakanikos E, McCarthy J. (2010). Training professionals, family carers and support staff to work effectively with people with intellectual disability and mental health problems. In: *Mental Health Services for Adults with Intellectual Disability: Strategies and Solutions*. Eds: N Bouras, G Holt. Psychology Press, East Sussex, UK.
34. Hassiotis A (2001). Intellectual Functioning: Report from the UK 700 Case Management Trial. *British Journal of Psychiatry*, 178, 166–171.
35. McCarthy J, Bouras N (2011). Intellectual Disability: Lifetime Course and Strategy for Intervention. In: *The Sage Handbook of Developmental Disorders*. (Eds: PA Howlin, T Charman, M Ghaziuddin. Sage Publications Ltd, London.

28

Safeguarding and Ethical Practice for People with Intellectual Disability

Meera Roy, Ashok Roy, Priyanka Tharian, and Ameeta Retzer

Legal principles of safeguarding and ethical practice

Safeguarding principles and ethical practice when working with people with intellectual disability (ID) have their foundations in human rights law. Human rights have a long history and were first enshrined in the Universal Declaration of Human Rights (UDHR). It came into being following the atrocities of the Second World War and was drafted by representatives from a variety of legal and cultural backgrounds from all over the world. It was proclaimed by the United Nations General Assembly in 1948 to be a common standard of fundamental human rights that were to be universally protected (http://www.un.org/en/universal-declaration-human-rights/). The understanding and interpretation of human rights is an ongoing and constantly evolving field, different countries and regions interpret them in different ways and the subsequent legal frameworks vary from place to place. The UDHR is the founding document for human rights and there have since been additional conventions introduced into the canon, including the Convention on the Rights of Persons with Disabilities. These serve as a resource but the laws that each country choose to enact, or fail to enact, for their fulfilment determine how these rights can be upheld and called upon by a country's citizens.

A human right constitutes a right that is owed to a person on the basis of their being a human being, for example the right to life, liberty, and security of person (Article 3 UDHR). A human right is legally upheld when it is a recognized claim that is delimited by law for the purpose of securing that right. If a government ratifies a human rights law, it must observe its tenets and respect its subsequent duties. These duties fall to all public institutions such as governmental departments, councils, or the police. The UK, as part of Europe, is subject to its regional interpretation of human rights as detailed in the European Convention on Human Rights (1950). UK legislation in the form of the Human Rights Act (1998) integrated the European Convention on Human Rights into domestic law. The Human Rights Act states that all UK law should be compatible with the rights detailed in the European Convention and cases where law does not fit would be subject to a decision by Parliament.

Many of the rights outlined in the Human Rights Act can be subject to limitation. This is so they do not infringe unnecessarily on the rights of other people. Upholding human rights requires carefully balancing the rights of everyone involved to ensure that everyone is treated fairly. As such, this human rights legislation makes it illegal for public bodies to overlook the rights of people unless there are legal factors prohibiting them from doing so. The Human Rights Act includes rights relating to life, death and freedom but also rights that impact on everyday life, and covers all people equally including those with ID (6, 7).

The Mental Capacity Act

The ongoing interpretation of the rights of those with ID continually unearths new areas where protections are required. One such area relates to capacity. A person's capacity dictates their authority under law to engage in particular activity, for example to get married or accept a form of medical treatment. Capacity relates to specific decisions and a person may have capacity in one area but not have capacity in another. This means that where capacity is in question, the person must be considered within their own specific context and in relation to a particular decision. As such, capacity is determined in a two-stage test. The first stage poses the question of whether there an impairment of or disturbance in the functioning of a person's mind or brain? If impairment or disturbance is identified, such as when a person has ID, the second stage requires the practitioner to determine whether the impairment or disturbance is such that the person lacks capacity to make a particular decision. If a person is unable to do one or more of the following four actions, they are found not to have capacity to make the decision in question:

1. Understanding the information relevant to the decision,
2. Retaining the necessary information,
3. Weighing up that information and can decide for themselves,
4. Communicating their decision.

Finally, it must be established whether the person can do any of the above actions alone or with support.

In England and Wales, the Mental Capacity Act 2005 (MCA) provides the legal framework for acting and making decisions for people who lack mental capacity to make particular decisions for themselves. The guiding principles of MCA enshrine the person's right to autonomy from the Human Rights Act, in particular the Right to Freedom from Inhumane and Degrading Treatment (Article 3), Right to Liberty and Security (Article 5), and Respect for Private and Family Life (Article 8). The statutory principles are:

1. A person must be assumed to have capacity unless it is established that they lack capacity.
2. A person is not to be treated as unable to make a decision unless all practicable steps have been taken to help to do so without success.
3. A person is not to be treated as unable to make a decision merely because they make an unwise decision.
4. A decision or act made on behalf of the person without capacity must be in their best interests.
5. The act or the decision made must be the least restrictive of the person's rights and freedom.

The Act covers a wide range of decisions made or actions taken on behalf of people without capacity, ranging from day to day matters such as what to wear or what to buy when shopping to major life-changing events such as whether the person should go into a care home or undergo a major surgery. However, there are certain decisions which cannot be taken under MCA either because they are very personal, such as consenting to marriage, divorce, or matters relating to children or because they are governed by other legislation, such as the Mental Health Act (MHA).

The MCA allows a person to give another person (the attorney or donee) the authority to act on their behalf on financial and welfare matters under Lasting Power of Attorney, registered with the Public Guardian, should they lose capacity in future. The Independent Mental Capacity Advocate (IMCA) is a service created under the Act to help vulnerable people who lack capacity make important decisions about serious medical treatment or changes of accommodation when they have no family or friends who it would be appropriate to consult. They will support and represent their views to those who are looking at their best interests.

The MCA protects the person without capacity and their carers. The way MCA impinges on the everyday life of a person with ID is through Deprivation of Liberty Safeguards (DoLS). This is the process by which a care plan which potentially breaches Article 3 and Article 5 rights under the Human Rights Act may be delivered to a person lacking capacity to consent to it (8, 9, 10).

Case study 1

Neal is a 30-year-old man with severe ID and autism. He needs one to one support to meet all aspects of personal care and daily living. He is not safe in the kitchen and has to be supervised when he goes in to get a drink as he will drink anything he can get hold of. He has no idea of road safety and will run across the road. He is usually accompanied by two carers when he goes out. The front door is operated with a numbered keypad. Neal has no number skills and cannot open the door. In the above scenario, Neal is clearly being deprived of his liberty. The managing authority which is responsible for the care home, made an urgent authorization for seven days and made an application to the supervisory body—the City Council for a standard authorisation which needed to be completed within 28 days. During this period, six assessments were carried out. A psychiatrist undertook the Mental Health Assessment to establish that Neal had a mental disorder, that is, severe ID and autism. Eligibility Assessment established that he was not under any part of the MHA at the time or indeed eligible to be under MHA and was not presenting risks to himself or others to a degree so that care was best provided under MCA and not under MHA. The Best Interests Assessor undertook Age Assessment to ensure that he was over the age of 18, No Refusals Assessment that the deprivation would not conflict with any other existing authority, Mental Capacity Assessment that he did not have capacity to consent to be accommodated to receive care he needed, and Best Interests Assessment that it was in his best interests and the least restrictive option for him to be accommodated at the home. The care home was given a standard authorisation for their care plans for a year, a further authorization to be applied for if necessary before the current one expires.

The new Court of Protection set up by MCA to establish precedent and build up expertise in all issues related to lack of capacity is a superior court of record with powers, rights, privileges, and authority as the High Court and is:

1. Able to decide whether a person has capacity to make a particular decision for themselves.
2. Make declarations on financial and welfare matters of people lacking capacity.
3. Appoint deputies to make decisions for those who lack capacity.
4. Decide whether a last Power of Attorney is valid and
5. Remove deputies or attorneys who fail to carry out their duties.

Interface between MHA and MCA

The MHA has jurisdiction over non-compliant patients with mental disorder who pose risk to themselves or others and have to be admitted, detained, and treated in hospital against their wishes. In a psychiatric hospital setting, if a person lacking capacity refuses care and treatment, particularly medication for a psychiatric disorder which then has to be given covertly, then MHA may be the more suitable legal frame-work (11). By the same token, a compliant person lacking capacity may also be cared for under DoLS in a psychiatric hospital.

Origins of safeguarding principles relating to people with ID

Historically, the rights of people with ID in the UK have been overlooked. The eugenics movement, founded in the nineteenth century by Sir Francis Galton, promoted the 'science for the biological improvement of the human race' (1). This was based upon the belief that physical, mental, and moral traits were inherited and that human progress depended upon ensuring that 'positive' characteristics were passed on to subsequent generations. This could be accomplished either by using positive eugenics, whereby those with desirable characteristics are encouraged to reproduce, or negative eugenics, whereby those with 'undesirable' traits are discouraged from reproducing. As a result of these views, it was considered that people with ID should be separated from society and prevented from reproducing (2). This was accomplished through policies of sterilization, institutionalization, and segregation; and protection and prevention of harm to people with ID.

The 1950s and 1960s marked a point of significant evolution in how ID was understood and as a result, services for people with ID were transformed. The shift towards greater use of a 'care in the community' model rather than institutional care was driven by research unearthing the extent to which people with ID could learn, challenging traditional assumptions about the capacity of people with ID to acquire new skills (2). At the same time, the 'normalization' principles emerged as a practical alternative to institutional care, encouraging people with ID to experience 'normal' patterns of life (3, 4, 12). This, paired with concerns arising during the 1970s regarding the treatment of people in institutional hospitals, lead to dramatic changes in policy relating to people with ID (5). In the wider context of civil and human rights movements, significant improvements in integration, participation, inclusion, and choice for people with ID have taken place. This history continues to serve as a significant source of concern and drives development and activism in this area to ensure ethical, moral, and legal practice takes place. Policy relating to people with ID is continually evolving and practitioners and individuals working in the field continue to draw from the lessons to be learned from the past.

Current safeguarding practice

Progress in how ID is understood in the UK has led to the foundation of basic standards for care. These standards are informed by key principles that should articulate and inform good practice in relation to safeguarding vulnerable adults (13).

Principle 1—Empowerment

Adults should be in charge of their care and of any decisions that affect their lives. Safeguarding must involve promoting the independence and quality of life of adults and must maximize their ability to control their own lives. Where adults cannot make decisions, as a result for example of a lack of capacity to make the specified decision due to severe ID, they should still be involved in the decision as far as possible.

Principle 2—Protection

Patients should be offered the support necessary for them to protect themselves. Where adults are less able to protect or promote their own interests, psychiatrists should take reasonable and appropriate measures to ensure their protection. This also involves assessing whether more proactive measures are required to protect a person, where for example, an adult lacks the capacity to make a specified decision due to the presence of an ID.

Principle 3—Prevention

Prevention of harm or abuse is the primary goal. Prevention involves working with individuals to reduce risks of harm or abuse that they find unacceptable. Prevention involves delivering high quality person-centred services in safe environments. All adults have a right to holistic care that is focused on their individual needs and to be kept safe.

Principle 4—Proportionality

Safeguarding responses should be proportional to the nature and seriousness of the concern. Options should be presented that are the least restrictive of individual rights and choices.

Principle 5—Partnership

Safeguarding adults is most effective where individuals, professionals, and communities work together to prevent, detect and respond to harm and abuse.

Principle 6—Transparency and accountability

As with all other areas of health care, responsibilities for safeguarding should form part of ongoing assessment and clinical audit in order to identify areas of concern and to improve delivery. Good safeguarding requires collaboration and transparency with partner agencies.

In addition to these principles, care providers must avoid discriminating unfairly between groups of patients. Care and treatment decisions must be made on the basis of a fair and objective assessment of individual needs and not on assumptions about ID. The current process of safeguarding the liberty of those without capacity has been considered cumbersome. In England & Wales, the Mental Capacity (Amendment) Act 2019 will introduce Liberty Protection Safeguards which is said to run alongside the present arrangements for a year in from Spring 2020. The advantages are that the individual will not need repeated assessments when they move from one setting to the next, e.g. from care home to hospital, but carry the safe guard with them and will not need repeated medical assessments as they do now; once a mental disorder has been diagnosed, there isn't a need for repeated assessment, making the process more stream lined.

Case study 2

A 25-year-old woman with a moderate ID and an autism spectrum disorder accused a member of staff of entering her shower cubicle and touching her. A safeguarding referral was made and the member of staff in question was suspended. Initially it was assumed that the patient was not capable of providing a reliable history and her account would not be accepted by the police and the courts. However, she was supported by the communication therapist and her evidence was deemed admissible in court and the outcome was a successful prosecution.

Case study 3

A 33-year-old man with severe ID, epilepsy, and dysphagia living in his family home was referred for severe weight loss. Professionals stated that the family were not spending enough time with him and encouraging him to eat to the best of his ability. They also said that the family carers were not skilled enough to administer his medication and this had led to him being taken twice in the last two months to casualty with status epilepticus. A safeguarding referral was made. On further investigation, it was apparent that the family were not cooperating with professionals as they were worried that they would be seen as providing poor care and their loved one would be taken away and put into a hospital. An advocate was appointed and this led to clearer communication between the family and professionals with his family carers improving their skills and working with the dysphagia team and the epilepsy nurse to effect an improvement in his weight and seizure control. The safeguarding referral was not acted on any further.

Key points

- Human rights were first enshrined in the Universal Declaration of Human Rights in 1948.
- A human right is a right owed to a person on the basis of their being a human being, including the right to life, liberty, and security of a person.
- In England & Wales, the principles of the Mental Capacity Act enshrine the person's right to autonomy from the Human Rights Act. The Mental Capacity (Amendment) Act 2019 will introduce Liberty Protection Safeguards which is said to run alongside the present arrangements for a year in from Spring 2020.
- Deprivation of liberty safeguards relates to how the Mental Capacity Act impacts on the everyday life of a person with intellectual disability.
- When a person lacking capacity refuses treatment, especially medication for a psychiatric disorder, which then has to be given covertly, the Mental Health Act is the more suitable legal framework.
- Current safeguarding practice is governed by basic standards/principles: empowering the client, protecting and promoting their interests, preventing abuse/harm, enacting proportional responses to safeguarding concerns, working in partnership with other teams, and providing a transparent service where all parties take responsibility for safeguarding.

MULTIPLE CHOICE QUESTIONS

Questions

Please select the single most appropriate answer.

1. The Humans Rights Act covers all people:

A. Differently depending on their level of intellectual functioning.
B. Differently, with greater consideration needed for minority groups.
C. Equally and includes those with intellectual disability.
D. Except for sentenced prisoners.
E. With absolute rights regardless of public concerns.

2. When assessing a person's capacity to make a particular decision after identifying impairment or disorder in the functioning of their mind or brain, they must be able to do all of the following except:

A. Understand information relevant to the decision.
B. Retain the necessary information.
C. Make a decision in line with medical advice.
D. Weigh up the information and decide for themselves.
E. Communicate that decision.

3. The statutory principles of the Mental Capacity Act include all except:

A. The decision made must be the least restrictive option.
B. Patient must have insight into their illness.
C. The decision made for a patient lacking capacity must be in their best interests.
D. Assume the patient has capacity unless proven otherwise.
E. All practicable steps must be taken to enable the patient to make their own decision.

4. The eugenics movement was based on the belief/s that:

A. Challenged traditional assumptions about the capacity of people with ID to acquire new skills.
B. Raised concerns about the treatment of people in institutional hospitals leading to changes in policy.
C. All traits were inherited and human progress relied on passing these on to the next generation.
D. Enshrined normalization principles as a practical alternative to institutional care.
E. Measures like forced sterilization and marriage prohibitions violated people's human rights.

5. Which of these is not a principle in current safeguarding practice:

A. Prevention of abuse.
B. Protection with proactive measures.
C. Families can make decisions on behalf of clients lacking capacity.
D. Proportional response.
E. Transparency and collaboration.

Answers

1. C. See paragraph 3 of *Legal principles of safeguarding and ethical practice*. The Human Rights Act includes rights relating to life, death, and freedom but also rights that impact on everyday life, and covers all people equally including those with ID.
2. C. A patient does not have to make a decision in line with medical advice to be deemed capacitous. If they are able to show evidence of weighing up the risks and benefits linked with their decision, along with the other components then they are entitled to make what clinicians may deem as 'an unwise decision."'. This would then be seen as a capacitous decision which goes against medical advice.
3. B. A patient does not need to have insight into their illness in order to make a capacitous decision. Capacity is decision-specific and a mental illness does not preclude them from making all decisions so their capacity must be assessed for the relevant decision using a formal capacity assessment. This will usually be done by the treating team who are able to inform the patient about the intended benefits and relevant risks, for example, in the case of a decision about an operation, the surgeons should assess a mentally unwell patient's capacity rather than their psychiatry team.

4. C. See first paragraph in *Origins of safeguarding principles relating to people with ID.* Eugenics was based upon the belief that physical, mental, and moral traits were inherited and that human progress depended upon ensuring that 'positive' characteristics were passed on to subsequent generations. As a result of these views, it was considered that people with ID should be separated from society and prevented from reproducing.

   During WW2 nazi eugenics were racially-based social policies that placed the biological improvement of the Aryan race as the centre of Nazi ideology, and included a legalized forced sterilization programme for people with intellectual disability. Other Nazi institutions included the Hadamar Clinic, which was a mental hospital, used as a site for their euthanasia programme ("Action T4").

   In the 1950s/60s these views were replaced with '"normalization' principles which emerged as a practical alternative to institutional care, encouraging people with ID to experience 'normal' patterns of life and have access to community-based care.
5. C. Families cannot make decisions on behalf of clients lacking capacity. In these situations, the treating team usually hold a best-interests meeting with professionals involved in the client's care. The family members' viewpoints should be taken into account in the decision-making process by the MDT. Where there are safeguarding concerns regarding the family, an advocate can facilitate constructive communication between the family and treating team and work towards empowering solutions for both the patient and their families.

REFERENCES

1. Garver KL Garver B (1991). Eugenics: Past, present, and the future. *American Journal of Human Genetics*, **49**, 1109–1118.
2. Hall J (2008). Mental Deficiency—changing the outlook. *The Psychologist*, **21**(11), 1006–1007.
3. Alaszewski A, Roughton H (1990). The development of residential care for children with a mental handicap. In: Alaszewski A, Ong BN (eds). *Normalisation in Practice: Residential care for children with a profound mental handicap*. London: Routledge.
4. Nirje B (1980). *The Normalization Principle in Normalization, Social Integration and Community Service* (pp. 117–129). Baltimore, MD: Paul Brookes; 1980.
5. Chappell AL (1992). Towards a sociological critique of the normalisation principle. *Disability, Handicap and Society*, **7**(1), 35–51.
6. Council of Europe (1988). *Protocol to the Convention for the Protection of Human Rights and Fundamental Freedoms* (European Convention on Human Rights) as amended by Protocol No. 11. [Online]. Available from: http://www.echr.coe.int/Documents/Convention_ENG.pdf [Accessed 26 October 2016).
7. HM Government (1998). *Human Rights Act* [Online]. Available from http://www.legislation.gov.uk/ukpga/1998/42/contents [Accessed 26 October 2016].
8. HM Government (2005). *Mental Capacity Act* [Online]. Available from: http://www.legislation.gov.uk/ukpga/2005/9/contents [Accessed 26 October 2016].
9. *Mental Capacity Act 2005. Code of Practice.*
10. *Mental Capacity Act 2005. Deprivation of liberty, safeguards, Code of Practice, supplement, the main Mental Capacity Act 2005, Code of Practice.*
11. HM Government (2007). *Mental Health Act* [Online]. Available from: http://www.legislation.gov.uk/ukpga/2007/12/contents [Accessed 26 October 2016].
12. Nirje B (1980). *The Normalization Principle in Normalization, Social Integration and Community Service* (pp. 117–129). Baltimore MD: Paul Brookes; 1980.
13. *Safeguarding Vulnerable Adults*. British Medical Association.
14. UN General Assembly. (1948) *Universal declaration of human rights*. [Online]. Available from: http://www.un.org/en/universal-declaration-human-rights/ [Accessed 26 October 2016].

Name Index

Note: Tables and boxes are indicated by an italic *t* and *b* following the page number.

For the benefit of digital users, indexed terms that span two pages (e.g., 52–53) may, on occasion, appear on only one of those pages.

Subject Index

Note: Tables, figures, and boxes are indicated by an italic *t*, *f*, and *b* following the page number.

For the benefit of digital users, indexed terms that span two pages (e.g., 52–53) may, on occasion, appear on only one of those pages.

www.ingramcontent.com/pod-product-compliance
Lightning Source LLC
Chambersburg PA
CBHW082033280826
50591CB00005B/197
* 9 7 8 0 1 9 8 7 9 4 5 8 5 *